POLIT & BECK'S

ESSENTIALS OF
Nursing Research

APPRAISING EVIDENCE FOR NURSING PRACTICE

Eleventh Edition

POLIT & BECK'S

ESSENTIALS OF
Nursing Research

APPRAISING EVIDENCE FOR NURSING PRACTICE

Eleventh Edition

Jane Flanagan, PhD, RN, ANP-BC, AHN-B, FNI, FNAP, FAAN

Associate Professor
William F. Connell School of Nursing
Chestnut Hill, Massachusetts

Cheryl Tatano Beck, DNSc, CNM, FAAN

Distinguished Professor, School of Nursing
University of Connecticut
Storrs, Connecticut

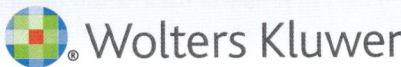

Philadelphia • Baltimore • New York • London
Buenos Aires • Hong Kong • Sydney • Tokyo

Not authorised for sale in United States, Canada, Australia, New Zealand, Puerto Rico, and U.S. Virgin Islands.

Vice President, Nursing Segment: Julie K. Stegman
Director, Content Management: Jamie Blum
Acquisitions Editor: Joyce Berendes
Senior Development Editor: Rachel Lucke
Editorial Coordinator: Janet Jayne
Marketing Manager: Wendy Mears
Editorial Assistant: Sara Thul
Production Project Manager: Jennifer L. Harper
Manager, Graphic Arts & Design: Steve Druding
Art Director: Jennifer Clements
Manufacturing Coordinator: Margie Orech-Zeranko
Prepress Vendor: S4Carlisle Publishing Services

Eleventh edition

Copyright © 2027 Wolters Kluwer.

Copyright © 2022 Wolters Kluwer. Copyright © 2018 Wolters Kluwer. Copyright © 2014, 2010 by Wolters Kluwer Health | Lippincott Williams & Wilkins. Copyright © 2006, 2001 by Lippincott Williams & Wilkins. Copyright © 1997 Lippincott-Raven Publishers. Copyright © 1993, 1989, 1985 J. B. Lippincott Company. All rights reserved. This book is protected by copyright. No part of this book may be reproduced or transmitted in any form or by any means, including as photocopies or scanned-in or other electronic copies, or utilized by any information storage and retrieval system without written permission from the copyright owner, except for brief quotations embodied in critical articles and reviews. Materials appearing in this book prepared by individuals as part of their official duties as U.S. government employees are not covered by the above-mentioned copyright. To request permission, please contact Wolters Kluwer at Two Commerce Square, 2001 Market Street, Philadelphia, PA 19103, via email at permissions@lww.com, or via our website at shop.lww.com (products and services).

9 8 7 6 5 4 3 2 1

Printed in Mexico

Library of Congress Cataloging-in-Publication Data

North American ISBN-13: 978-1-975262-90-7
International ISBN-13: 978-1-9752-6291-4

Cataloging in Publication data available on request from publisher.

This work is provided "as is," and the publisher disclaims any and all warranties, express or implied, including any warranties as to accuracy, comprehensiveness, or currency of the content of this work.

This work is no substitute for individual patient assessment based upon healthcare professionals' examination of each patient and consideration of, among other things, age, weight, gender, current or prior medical conditions, medication history, laboratory data and other factors unique to the patient. The publisher does not provide medical advice or guidance and this work is merely a reference tool. Healthcare professionals, and not the publisher, are solely responsible for the use of this work including all medical judgments and for any resulting diagnosis and treatments.

Given continuous, rapid advances in medical science and health information, independent professional verification of medical diagnoses, indications, appropriate pharmaceutical selections and dosages, and treatment options should be made and healthcare professionals should consult a variety of sources. When prescribing medication, healthcare professionals are advised to consult the product information sheet (the manufacturer's package insert) accompanying each drug to verify, among other things, conditions of use, warnings and side effects and identify any changes in dosage schedule or contraindications, particularly if the medication to be administered is new, infrequently used or has a narrow therapeutic range. To the maximum extent permitted under applicable law, no responsibility is assumed by the publisher for any injury and/or damage to persons or property, as a matter of products liability, negligence law or otherwise, or from any reference to or use by any person of this work.

shop.lww.com

TO

The memory of Denise F. Polit

1946–2021

From Denise's son:

Denise Polit was, above all, a force of nature. She was brilliant and kind, giving and strong, and passionate to the point of danger. She tasked herself with constant improvement so that she could lift up others. She would agonize for hours over a sentence, trying to find the perfect way to help others understand a difficult concept. As you read these pages, I hope that you can catch a glimpse of the passion she had for this material, for the desire she had to make a difference to those who dedicated themselves to trying to learn a difficult subject. She cared, deeply, about the book you're about to read, and I hope that, like myself and so many others, you will find her passion and dedication help guide you and make you a better version of yourself.

Denise is survived by her stepdaughters Norah, Lauren, and Alaine and their wonderful families, as well as by her son Alex, who still hopes that, one day, he will be worthy of all that she did for him.

Respectfully,

N. Alexander O'Hara

ABOUT THE AUTHORS

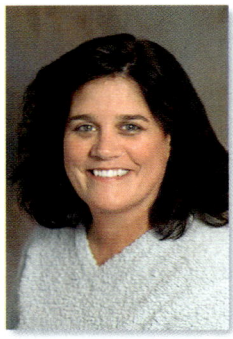

Jane Flanagan, PhD, RN, AHN-BC, ANP-BC, FNI, FNAP, FAAN

Jane Flanagan, PhD, RN, AHN-BC, ANP-BC, FNI, FNAP, FAAN, is an associate professor and department chairperson at the Connell School of Nursing and a nurse scientist at the Massachusetts General Hospital (MGH) Yvonne Munn Center for Nursing Research. She holds appointments as a member of the Board of Directors at the Sherrill House in Boston; volunteer faculty in the School of Nursing at the Health Science Center at the University of Tennessee Memphis; an associate clinical scientist at the Phyllis Cantor Center at the Dana Farber Cancer Institute.

Jane is the editor of the *International Journal of Nursing Knowledge* and serves on the editorial board of the *International Journal for Human Caring*. She is an appointed fellow in NANDA-I, the National Academy of Practice, and the American Academy of Nursing. Dr. Flanagan's work is focused on lifestyle interventions to improve the health of those caring for people with chronic health conditions with a focus on older adults.

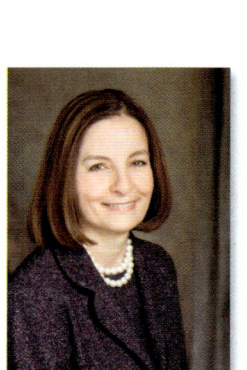

Cheryl Tatano Beck, DNSc, CNM, FAAN

Cheryl Tatano Beck, DNSc, CNM, FAAN, is a distinguished professor at the University of Connecticut, School of Nursing, with a joint appointment in the Department of Obstetrics and Gynecology at the School of Medicine. She received her master's degree in maternal–newborn nursing from Yale University and her doctor of nursing science degree from Boston University. She has received numerous awards such as the Association of Women's Health, Obstetric and Neonatal Nurses' Distinguished Professional Service Award; Eastern Nursing Research Society's Distinguished Researcher Award; the Distinguished Alumna Award from Yale University School of Nursing; and the Marcé Medal from the International Marcé Society for Perinatal Mental Health in recognition of her program of research. She was inducted into the American Academy of Nursing, the Sigma Theta Tau International Nurse Researcher Hall of Fame, and Sigma Xi: The Scientific Research Honor Society.

Over the past 35 years, Cheryl has focused her research efforts on developing a research program on postpartum mood and anxiety disorders. Based on the findings from her series of qualitative studies, Cheryl developed the Postpartum Depression Screening Scale (PDSS). She is a prolific writer who has published over 200 journal articles. In addition to coauthoring award-winning research methods books with Denise Polit, Cheryl coauthored with Dr. Jeanne Driscoll *Postpartum Mood and Anxiety Disorders: A Clinician's Guide*, which received the 2006 *American Journal of Nursing* Book of the Year Award. In addition, Cheryl has published six other books: *Traumatic Childbirth*, *Routledge International Handbook of Qualitative Nursing Research*, *Developing a Program of Research in Nursing*, *Secondary Qualitative Analysis in the Health and Social Sciences*, *Introduction to Phenomenology: Focus on Methodology*, and *Using Grounded Theory Research Methods: A Guide for the Health and Social Sciences*.

PREFACE

Polit and Beck's Essentials of Nursing Research, 11th edition, helps students learn how to read and critically appraise research reports and to develop an appreciation of research as a path to enhancing nursing practice.

We continue to enjoy updating this book with important innovations in research methods and with examples of nurse researchers' use of emerging research strategies. Feedback from our loyal adopters has inspired several important changes to the content and organization of this book. We are convinced that these revisions introduce important improvements—while at the same time retaining many features that have made this book a classic best-selling textbook throughout the world. The 11th edition of this book and its online resources will make it easier and more satisfying for nurses to pursue a professional pathway that incorporates thoughtful appraisals of evidence.

LEGACY OF *ESSENTIALS OF NURSING RESEARCH*

This edition, like its predecessors, is focused on the art—and science—of critically appraising studies conducted by nurses and other health care professionals. The textbook offers guidance to students who are learning to assess research reports and to use research findings in practice.

Among the basic principles that helped to shape this and earlier editions of this book are the following:

1. Confidence in the idea that competence in doing and appraising research is critical to the nursing profession
2. A conviction that research inquiry is intellectually and professionally rewarding to nurses
3. An unswerving belief that learning about research methods need be neither intimidating nor dull

Consistent with these principles, we have tried to present research fundamentals in a way that both facilitates understanding and arouses curiosity and interest. We hope that, for some, it will arouse passion for the pursuit of research-based knowledge to guide practice.

NEW TO THIS EDITION

New Organization

A lot has happened in the world of research since the tenth edition. A particularly salient issue is patient (and other stakeholder) involvement in identifying important questions and translating research evidence into local settings. Relatedly, standard methods of appraising evidence for the **rigor** of study methods (which has been a focus of evidence-based practice, or EBP, initiatives) are being supplemented by a new emphasis on the **relevance** and **applicability** of research evidence for individual patients or small groups of patients (as espoused by the movement for **practice-based evidence** and **patient-centered research**).

Enhanced Accessibility

To make this edition even more user-friendly than in the past, we have made a concerted effort to simplify the presentation of complex topics. For example, we reduced and simplified the coverage of statistical information. In addition, throughout the book we have used more straightforward, concise language.

New Content

Throughout this 11th edition, we have included up-to-date information on methodologic innovations that have arisen in nursing, medicine, and the social sciences since the previous edition was published. These changes reflect the 2022–2026 National Institute of Nursing Research (NINR) Strategic Plan and the American Association of Colleges of Nursing (AACN) Essentials. In addition to updating the book with new information on conventional research methods, all new recent examples of nursing studies are included. The many additions and changes are too numerous to describe here, so here are just some examples.

In Chapter 1, we highlight the research priorities articulated by the NINR and Sigma Theta Tau International, and other nursing organizations. We describe the nature of the 2022–2026 NINR strategic plan as a living document that provides a research lens for research concerned with health-related questions of concern to nurses. In Chapter 2, we include a schedule for a qualitative study to help students understand the amount of time needed to plan such a study. Chapter 4 discusses the updated American Nurses Association (2025) *Code of Ethics for Nurses* and its relevance to nursing research. Chapter 6, which focuses on retrieving and reviewing the research literature, now includes a section on artificial intelligence and its use in literature reviews. Also discussed in this chapter is the issue around predatory journals and guidance on avoiding them. Chapter 7 introduces the website Nursology.net and the purpose it serves in keeping nurses abreast on the development and use of nursing theory in research.

In Chapter 10, we include information on additional types of ethnography such as institutional ethnography, autoethnography, and netnography. Also described is situational analysis, which is a type of grounded theory. In Chapter 11, we added discussions of the think-aloud method, joint interviews, and differing perspectives on data saturation. We have added information about collecting data via the Internet such as data that are available directly on the Internet (e.g., blogs). Chapter 12 provides updated information and examples of mixed methods research. In Chapter 15, we include a discussion of artificial intelligence for qualitative data analysis and updated information on computer-assisted qualitative data analysis software. Qualitative content analysis is expanded to include a description of Krippendorff and Kyngäs et al.'s methods of both inductive and deductive content analysis. Also in Chapter 15, secondary qualitative data analysis and its different types are explained. In Chapter 16, positionality and the writing of positionality statements to help with qualitative researchers' reflexivity are addressed.

A Note About the Language Used in This Book

Wolters Kluwer recognizes that people have a diverse range of identities, and we are committed to using inclusive and nonbiased language in our content. In line with the principles of nursing, we strive not to define people by their diagnoses, but to recognize their personhood first and foremost, using as much as possible the language diverse groups use to define themselves, and including only information that is relevant to nursing care.

We strive to better address the unique perspectives, complex challenges, and lived experiences of diverse populations traditionally underrepresented in health literature. When describing or referencing populations discussed in research studies, we will adhere to the identities presented in those studies to maintain fidelity to the evidence presented by the study investigators. We follow best practices of language set forth by *the Publication Manual of the American Psychological Association, 7th edition*, but acknowledge that language evolves rapidly, and we will update the language used in future editions of this book as necessary.

THE TEXT

The content of this edition is as follows:

- **Part 1, Overview of Nursing Research and Its Role in Evidence-Based Practice**, introduces fundamental concepts in nursing research. Chapter 1 summarizes the background of nursing research, discusses the philosophical underpinnings of qualitative research versus quantitative research, describes major purposes of nursing research, and introduces key concepts relating to EBP. Chapter 2 introduces readers to key research terms and presents an overview of steps in the research process for both quantitative and qualitative studies. Chapter 3 focuses on research journal articles, explaining what they are and how to read them. Chapter 4 discusses ethics in nursing studies.

- **Part 2, Preliminary Steps in Quantitative and Qualitative Research**, further sets the stage for learning about the research process by considering aspects of a study's conceptualization. Chapter 5 focuses on the development of research questions and the formulation of research hypotheses. Chapter 6 discusses how to retrieve research evidence (especially in electronic bibliographic databases) and the role of research literature reviews. Chapter 7 presents information about theoretical and conceptual frameworks for nursing studies.

- **Part 3, Designs and Methods for Quantitative and Qualitative Nursing Research**, presents material on the design and conduct of all types of nursing studies. Chapter 8 describes fundamental design principles and discusses many specific aspects of quantitative research design, including efforts to enhance rigor. Chapter 9 introduces the topics of sampling and data collection in quantitative studies. Concepts relating to quality in measurements—reliability and validity—are introduced in this chapter. Chapter 10 describes the various qualitative research traditions that have contributed to the growth of constructivist inquiry and presents the basics of qualitative design. Chapter 11 covers sampling and data collection methods used in qualitative research, describing how these differ from approaches used in quantitative studies. Chapter 12 provides an overview of several distinctive types of research, with a special emphasis on mixed methods research. This chapter also discusses other special types of research such as surveys, comparative effectiveness studies, evaluation research, and outcomes research. Methods of undertaking quality improvement projects are also described.

- **Part 4, Analysis, Interpretation, and Application of Nursing Research**, presents tools for making sense of—and using—research data. Chapter 13 reviews methods of statistical analysis. The chapter assumes no prior instruction in statistics and focuses primarily on helping readers to understand why statistics are useful, what test might be appropriate in a given situation, and what statistical information in a research article means. Chapter 14 discusses approaches to interpreting statistical results, including interpretations linked to assessments of clinical significance. Chapter 15 discusses qualitative analysis, with an emphasis on ethnographic, phenomenologic, and grounded theory studies. In this edition, we offer an expanded discussion of the coding of qualitative data. Chapter 16 elaborates on criteria for appraising trustworthiness and integrity in qualitative studies. Chapter 17 describes systematic reviews, including how to understand and appraise meta-analyses and meta-syntheses—and how the GRADE system works in the context of systematic reviews. Finally, Chapter 18 describes key steps in EBP and also explains emerging ideas about how to improve EBP by striving for evidence that is more practice-based and patient-centered—that is, how to enhance the applicability of evidence to individual patients or well-defined subgroups of patients.

- **In the appendices, we offer two full-length research articles**—one quantitative and one qualitative—that students can read, analyze, and appraise. Some of the Critical Thinking Exercises in each chapter focus on these two studies. A **glossary** at the end of the book provides additional support for those needing to look up the meaning of a methodologic term.

FEATURES OF THE TEXT

We have retained many of the classic features that were successfully used in previous editions to assist those learning to read and apply evidence from nursing research:

- **Clear, User-Friendly Style.** Our writing style is easily digestible and nonintimidating—and we have worked even harder in this edition to write clearly and simply. Concepts are introduced carefully, difficult ideas are presented thoughtfully, and readers are assumed to have no prior knowledge of technical terms.
- **Critical Appraisal Guidelines.** Each chapter includes guidelines for conducting a critical appraisal of various aspects of a research report. The guidelines sections provide a list of questions that walk students through a study, drawing attention to aspects of the study that are amenable to evaluation by research consumers.
- **Research Examples and Critical Thinking Exercises.** Each chapter concludes with summaries of one or two research examples designed to highlight important points made in the chapter and to sharpen the reader's critical thinking skills. In addition, many research examples are used to illustrate key points in the text and to stimulate students' thinking about areas of research inquiry. We have chosen many international examples to communicate to students that nursing research is growing in importance worldwide. Some of the Critical Thinking Exercises focus on the full-length articles in the two appendices.
- **Tips for Students.** The textbook is filled with practical guidance and tips on how to translate the abstract notions of research methods into more concrete applications. In these tips, we have paid special attention to helping students *read* research reports, which are often daunting to those without specialized research training.
- **Graphics.** Colorful graphics—in the form of supportive tables, figures, and examples—reinforce the text and offer visual stimulation.
- **Chapter Objectives.** Learning objectives are identified in the chapter opener to focus students' attention on critical content.
- **Key Terms.** Each chapter opener includes a list of new research terms. In the text, new terms are defined in context (and bolded) when used for the first time; terms of lesser importance are italicized. Key terms are also defined in our glossary.
- **Bulleted Summary Points.** A succinct list of summary points that focus on salient chapter content is provided at the end of each chapter.

A COMPREHENSIVE PACKAGE FOR TEACHING AND LEARNING

To further facilitate teaching and learning, a carefully designed ancillary package has been developed to assist faculty and students.

Resources for Instructors

Tools to assist with teaching this text are available at http://thePoint.lww.com/PolitEssentials11e.

- NEW! **Test Generator Questions** include hundreds of multiple-choice questions that aid instructors in assessing their students' understanding of the chapter content.
- An **Image Bank** includes figures from the text.
- A **Sample Syllabus** is provided for a 14-week course.
- **Answers to Critical Thinking Exercises** are provided for selected questions related to the studies in the appendices of the textbook and others summarized throughout the chapters.
- **PowerPoint Slides** offer summaries of key points in each chapter for use in class presentations. At the end of each slide deck, five multiple-choice **Self-Test** questions relating to key concepts in the chapter are followed by answers to the questions. (A few chapters have two sets of **Self-Test** slides.) The aim of these slides is not to evaluate student performance. We recommend these slides be given to students for self-testing, or they can be used in the classroom with iClicker to assess students' grasp of important concepts. To enhance the likelihood that students will see the relevance of the concepts to clinical practice, all the questions are application-type questions. We hope instructors will use the slides to clarify any misunderstandings and, just as importantly, to reward students with immediate positive feedback about newly acquired skills.
- **AACN Essentials Map** shows how the book content integrates AACN Essentials of Baccalaureate Education for Professional Nursing Practice competencies.

A COMPREHENSIVE, DIGITAL, INTEGRATED COURSE SOLUTION: LIPPINCOTT® COURSEPOINT

The same trusted solution, innovation, and unmatched support that you have come to expect from *Lippincott CoursePoint* is now enhanced with more engaging learning tools and deeper analytics to help prepare students for practice. This powerfully integrated, digital learning solution combines learning tools, case studies, real-time data, and the most trusted nursing education content on the market to make curriculum-wide learning more efficient and to meet students where they're at in their learning. The solution connects learning to real-life application by integrating content from *Polit and Beck's Essentials of Nursing Research* with video cases, interactive modules, and research journal articles. Ideal for active, case-based learning, this powerful solution helps students develop higher level cognitive skills and asks them to make decisions related to simple-to-complex scenarios. And now, it's easier than ever for instructors and students to use, giving them everything they need for course and curriculum success! To learn more about this solution, contact your local Wolters Kluwer representative.

Lippincott CoursePoint for Polit and Beck's: Essentials of Nursing Research, 11th edition includes the following:

- Leading Content in Context, with digital content from *Polit and Beck's Essentials of Nursing Research*, 11th edition, is embedded in our powerful tools, engaging students and encouraging interaction and learning on a deeper level.
  - The complete interactive e-book provides students with anytime, anywhere access on multiple devices.
  - Full online access to *Stedman's Medical Dictionary for the Health Professions and Nursing* ensures students work with the best medical dictionary available.
- Engaging course content provides a variety of learning tools to engage students of all learning styles.
- A more personalized learning approach gives students the content and tools they need at the moment they need it, giving them data for more focused remediation and helping to boost their confidence and competence.
- Powerful tools help students learn the critical thinking and clinical judgment skills to help them become practice-ready nurses, including the following:
  - Video Cases show how nursing research and EBP relate to real-life nursing practice. By watching the videos and completing related activities, students will flex their nursing research skills and build a spirit of inquiry.

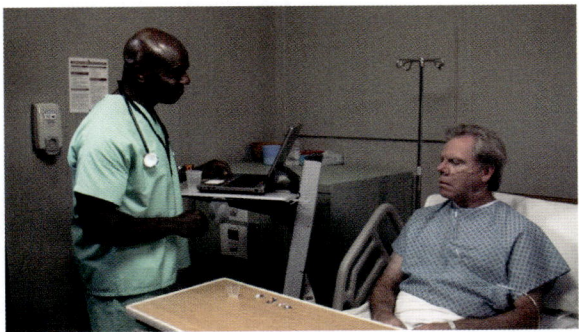

  - Interactive Modules help students quickly identify what they do and do not understand, so they can study smartly. With exceptional instructional design that prompts students to discover, reflect, synthesize, and apply, students actively learn. Remediation links to the digital textbook are integrated throughout.
- Unparalleled reporting provides in-depth dashboards with several data points to track student progress and help identify strengths and weaknesses.
- Unmatched support includes training coaches, product trainers, and nursing education consultants to help educators and students implement CoursePoint with ease.

CLOSING NOTE

It is our hope and expectation that the content, style, and organization of this 11th edition of *Polit and Beck's Essentials of Nursing Research* will be helpful to those students who want to become skillful, thoughtful readers of nursing studies and to those wishing to enhance their clinical performance based on research findings. We also hope that this textbook will help to develop an enthusiasm for the kinds of discoveries and knowledge that research can produce.

Jane Flanagan, PhD, RN, AHN-BC, ANP-BC, FNI, FNAP, FAAN
Cheryl Tatano Beck, DNSc, CNM, FAAN

USER'S GUIDE

Learning Objectives focus students' attention on critical content

10 Appraising Qualitative Designs and Approaches

Learning Objectives

On completing this chapter, you will be able to:

- Discuss the rationale for an emergent design in qualitative research and describe qualitative design features
- Identify the major research traditions for qualitative research and describe the domain of inquiry of each
- Describe the main features and methods associated with ethnographic, phenomenologic, and grounded theory studies
- Describe key features of case studies, narrative analyses, and descriptive qualitative studies
- Discuss the goals and features of research with ideologic perspectives
- Define new terms in the chapter

Key Terms

- Autoethnography
- Basic social process (BSP)
- Bracketing
- Case study
- Constant comparison
- Constructivist grounded theory
- Core variable
- Critical ethnography
- Critical theory
- Descriptive phenomenology
- Descriptive qualitative study
- Emergent design
- Ethnonursing research
- Feminist research
- Grounded theory
- Hermeneutics
- Historical research
- Institutional ethnography
- Interpretive phenomenology
- Narrative analysis
- Netnography
- Participant observation
- Participatory action research (PAR)
- Reflexive journal
- Situational analysis

Key Terms alert students to important terminology

Examples help students apply content to real-life research

Example of an ethnonursing study
Strange and colleagues (2024) conducted an ethnonursing study to discover the influences of faith on rural Appalachian older adult health. Interviews were conducted with 12 key and 20 general informants.

Tip boxes describe what is found in actual research articles

TIP Systematic reviews of qualitative studies on a specific topic can lead to substantive theory development. In metasyntheses, qualitative studies are combined to identify their essential elements used for theory building.

How-to-Tell Tip boxes explain confusing issues in actual research articles

HOW-TO-TELL TIP How can you tell a variable's measurement level? A variable is *nominal* if the values could be interchanged (e.g., 1 = male, 2 = female OR 1 = female, 2 = male). A variable is usually *ordinal* if there is a quantitative ordering of values AND if there are a small number of values (e.g., excellent, good, fair, poor). A variable is usually considered *interval* if it is measured with a composite scale or test. A variable is *ratio* level if it makes sense to say that one value is twice as much as another (e.g., 100 mg is twice as much as 50 mg).

User's Guide   **xv**

Critiquing Guidelines boxes lead students through key issues in a research article

Box 7.1 Guidelines for Critically Appraising Theoretical/Conceptual Frameworks in a Research Report

a. Did the report describe an explicit theoretical or conceptual framework for the study? If not, does the absence of a framework detract from the study's conceptual integration?
b. Did the report adequately describe the major features of the theory or model so that readers could understand the conceptual basis of the study?
c. Is the theory or model appropriate for the research problem? Does the purported link between the problem and the framework seem contrived?
d. Was the theory or model used for generating hypotheses, or is it used as an organizational or interpretive framework? Do the hypotheses (if any) naturally flow from the framework?
e. Were concepts defined in a way that is consistent with the theory? If there was an intervention, were intervention components consistent with the theory?
f. Did the framework guide the study methods? For example, was the appropriate research tradition used if the study was qualitative? If quantitative, do the operational definitions correspond to the conceptual definitions?
g. Did the researcher tie the study findings back to the framework at the end of the report? Were the findings interpreted within the context of the framework?

Research Examples highlight critical points made in the chapter and sharpen critical thinking skills

RESEARCH EXAMPLES WITH CRITICAL THINKING EXERCISES

Abstracts for a quantitative and a qualitative nursing study are presented in the following sections. Read the abstracts for Examples 1 and 2, and then answer the critical thinking questions that follow. The critical thinking questions for Examples 3 and 4 are based on the studies that appear in their entirety in Appendices A and B of this book.

EXAMPLE 1: QUANTITATIVE RESEARCH

Study: "Effects of a web-based pediatric oncology legacy intervention on the coping of children with cancer" (Cho et al., 2023)

Objective: The objective of this study was to examine the effects of a legacy intervention using digital storytelling on the coping strategies of children with recurrent or refractory cancer.

Background: Legacy interventions are evidence-based, family-centered palliative care strategies that help children with serious illness to cope. However, the impact of legacy interventions on coping in children with recurrent or refractory cancer is poorly understood.

Methods: This study used a two-arm randomized waitlist control clinical trial. Children with recurrent or refractory cancer and their parents were recruited via Facebook. They were randomly assigned to the intervention or control group through the use of a computer-generated permuted-block randomization sequence. The primary end point was the response to stress questionnaire (RSQ).

Results: The sample included 92 parent–child dyads (35—intervention group, 57—control group). Results indicate that the legacy intervention resulted in small and statistically nonsignificant effects on coping among children with recurrent or refractory cancer.

Conclusions: Although the findings indicated a small and statistically nonsignificant change in coping, this is the first RCT to test a legacy intervention in this population. More work is needed to understand if expanding the options for legacy interventions may yield better outcomes.

Critical Thinking Exercises

Critical Thinking Exercises provide opportunities to practice critiquing actual research articles

1. What were the independent and dependent variables in this study?
2. What are the PICO components?
3. Is this study experimental or nonexperimental?
4. How, if at all, was *randomness* used in this study?
5. How, if at all, was *blinding* used in this study?
6. Did the researchers use any statistical tests? If yes, were any of the results statistically significant?
7. If the results of this study are valid and generalizable, what might be some of the ways the findings could be used in clinical practice?

EXAMPLE 2: QUALITATIVE RESEARCH

Study: "Parents' shared experiences of separation from their newborns after birth in Denmark" (Brodsgaard et al., 2024).

Summary Points
review chapter content to ensure success

Summary Points

- High-quality research requires *conceptual integration*, one aspect of which is having a defensible theoretical rationale for the study.

- As classically defined, a **theory** consists of two or more concepts and propositions that form a logically interrelated system, providing a mechanism for deducing hypotheses. **Descriptive theory** thoroughly describes a phenomenon.

- *Grand theories* (or *macrotheories*) attempt to describe or explain large segments of the human experience. **Middle-range theories** are specific to certain phenomena; examples include Pender's HPM and Mishel's Uncertainty in Illness Theory.

- Concepts are also the basic elements in **conceptual models**, but concepts are not linked in a logically ordered, deductive system.

- In research, the goals of theories and models are to make findings meaningful, to integrate knowledge into coherent systems, to stimulate new research, and to explain phenomena and relationships among them.

- **Schematic models** (or **conceptual maps**) are graphic representations of phenomena and their interrelationships using symbols or diagrams and a minimal use of words.

- A **framework** is the conceptual underpinning of a study, including an overall rationale and conceptual definitions of key concepts. In qualitative studies, the framework often springs from distinct research traditions.

- Several conceptual models of nursing have been used in nursing research. The concepts central to models of nursing are *human beings, environment, health,* and *nursing*. An example of a model of nursing used by nurse researchers is RAM. Nonnursing models are also used by nurse researchers (e.g., Bandura's Social Cognitive Theory).

- In some qualitative research traditions (e.g., phenomenology), the researcher strives to suspend previously held *substantive theories* of the specific phenomena under study, but each tradition has rich theoretical underpinnings.

- Some qualitative researchers seek to develop *grounded theories*, data-driven explanations to account for phenomena under study through inductive processes.

- In the classical use of theory, researchers test hypotheses deduced from an existing theory. An emerging trend is the testing of theory-based interventions.

- In both qualitative and quantitative studies, researchers sometimes use a theory or model as an organizing framework or as an interpretive tool.

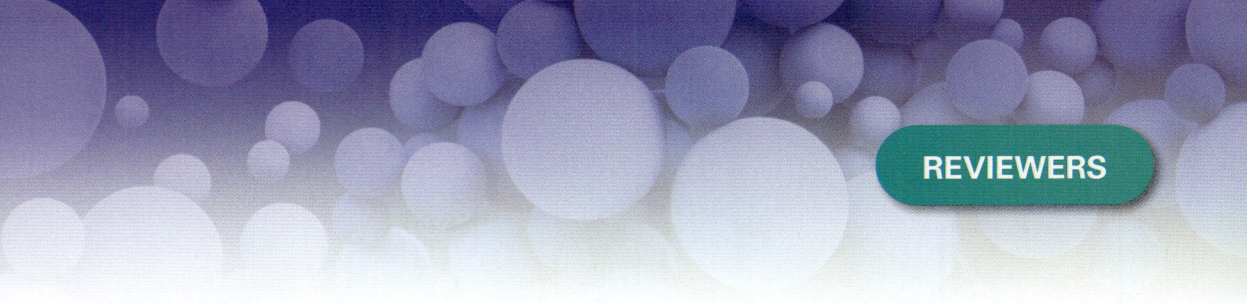

REVIEWERS

Linda Eanes, EdD, MSN, PMHNP
The University of Texas Rio Grande Valley
Edinburg, Texas

April Folgert, PhD, MSN, BSN, RN
Carroll University
Waukesha, Wisconsin

Carlene Galanopulo, MSN, RN, PhD Candidate
Xavier University
Cincinnati, Ohio

Jamie Hansen, PhD, RN, CNE
Carroll University
Waukesha, Wisconsin

Gaynelle Kahigian, EdD, MSN, RN
Delaware State University
Dover, Delaware

Kristen McCook, MSN, FNP-BC (Pending DNP Completion)
Harding University
Searcy, Arkansas

Stacy Mikel, DNP, MSN, RN
Jacksonville State University
Jacksonville, Alabama

Patricia Munno, DNP, CNE, RN
Felician University
Rutherford, New Jersey

Dania Ochoa, MSN, BSN, RN
The University of Texas Rio Grande Valley
Edinburg, Texas

Mae Ann Pasquale, PhD, MSN, RN
Cedar Crest College
Allentown, Pennsylvania

Debra Penrod, MSN
William Jewell College
Liberty, Missouri

Shelly Randall, PhD, RN
Arkansas Tech University
Russellville, Arkansas

Debra Renna, PhD, RN, CNE
Broward College
Davie, Florida

Kathyann Sager, DNP, MSN-Ed, RN
Alfred State, SUNY College of Technology
Alfred, New York

Melissa Vander Stucken, AAS, BSN, MSN
University of Houston-Victoria
Victoria, Texas

Lisa Walsh, PhD, RN
Emmanuel College
Boston, Massachusetts

ACKNOWLEDGMENTS

We must start this 11th edition of the book by acknowledging the tremendous loss of Dr. Denise Polit not only for her family but also for the discipline of nursing. Dr. Polit was not a nurse, but how extremely fortunate our discipline has been to have had her devote her career to supporting the learning, knowledge, and professional development of nurses, specifically in the field of nursing research. Since Denise wrote the first edition of this book in 1985, there has been no other individual who we believe has had more of an impact on the development of generations of nurses in regard to nursing research than Dr. Denise Polit. Denise would often call this book "her baby," which she tenderly cared for throughout each of the first 10 editions. She will be deeply missed!

This 11th edition, like the previous editions, depended on the contributions of dozens of people. Many faculty and students who have used the text have made invaluable suggestions for its improvement, and to all of you we are very grateful. In addition to all those who assisted us over the past 40 plus years with the earlier editions, the following individuals deserve special mention.

We would like to acknowledge the comments of reviewers of the previous edition of this book, anonymous to us initially, whose feedback influenced our revisions. We would like to thank Dr. Carrie Morgan Eaton at the University of Connecticut who provided regular feedback and updates to computer-assisted qualitative data analysis software.

We also extend our thanks to those who helped to turn the manuscript into a finished product. The staff at Wolters Kluwer has been of great assistance to us over the years. We are indebted to Joyce Berendes, Rachel Lucke, Janet Jayne, and all the others behind the scenes for their fine contributions.

Finally, we thank our family and friends. Our husbands, Richard Naegle and Chuck Beck, and Cheryl's children, Lisa and Curt, have become accustomed to our demanding schedules, but we recognize that their support involves a lot of patience and many sacrifices.

CONTENTS

Part 1 — Overview of Nursing Research and Its Role in Evidence-Based Practice

1. Introducing Nursing Research for Evidence-Based Practice 1
2. Understanding Key Concepts and Steps in Quantitative and Qualitative Research 23
3. Reading and Critically Appraising Research Articles 42
4. Attending to Ethics in Research 59

Part 2 — Preliminary Steps in Quantitative and Qualitative Research

5. Identifying Research Problems, Research Questions, and Hypotheses 73
6. Finding and Reviewing Research Evidence in the Literature 89
7. Understanding Theoretical and Conceptual Frameworks 105

Part 3 — Designs and Methods for Quantitative and Qualitative Nursing Research

8. Appraising Quantitative Research Design 117
9. Appraising Sampling and Data Collection in Quantitative Studies 141
10. Appraising Qualitative Designs and Approaches 162
11. Appraising Sampling and Data Collection in Qualitative Studies 177
12. Understanding Mixed Methods Research, Quality Improvement, and Other Special Types of Research 192

Part 4 — Analysis, Interpretation, and Application of Nursing Research

13. Understanding Statistical Analysis of Quantitative Data 209
14. Interpreting Quantitative Findings and Evaluating Clinical Significance 241
15. Understanding the Analysis of Qualitative Data 257
16. Appraising Trustworthiness and Integrity in Qualitative Research 274
17. Learning From Systematic Reviews 289
18. Putting Research Evidence Into Practice: Evidence-Based Practice and Practice-Based Evidence 310

Appendix A Advance Care Planning Affects End-of-Life Treatment Preferences Among Patients With Heart Failure   331

Appendix B Lived Experiences of Fatherhood After Infertility   339

Glossary   349
Index   379

Part 1: Overview of Nursing Research and Its Role in Evidence-Based Practice

1 Introducing Nursing Research for Evidence-Based Practice

Learning Objectives

On completing this chapter, you will be able to:

- Describe why research is important in nursing and discuss the importance of evidence-based practice
- Describe broad historical trends and future directions in nursing research
- Describe alternative sources of evidence for nursing practice
- Describe major characteristics of the positivist and constructivist paradigm and discuss similarities and differences between the traditional scientific method (quantitative research) and constructivist methods (qualitative research)
- Identify several purposes of qualitative and quantitative nursing research
- Understand sources of information for evidence-based practice
- Describe evidence hierarchies and level of evidence scales
- Identify a well-worded clinical question for evidence-based practice
- Define new terms in the chapter

Key Terms

- Applicability
- Assumption
- Cause-probing research
- Clinical nursing research
- Clinical significance
- Constructivist paradigm
- Empirical evidence
- Evidence-based practice (EBP)
- Evidence hierarchy
- Generalizability
- Journal club
- Level of evidence (LOE)
- Meta-aggregation
- Meta-analysis
- Metasynthesis
- Mixed methods research
- Mixed studies review
- Nursing research
- Paradigm
- Patient centeredness
- PICO format
- Positivist paradigm
- Primary studies
- Qualitative research
- Quantitative research
- Research
- Research methods
- Scientific method
- Systematic review

NURSING RESEARCH IN PERSPECTIVE

We know that most readers are not reading this book because they plan to become nurse researchers. Yet, we are confident that many of you *will* participate in research-related activities during your careers, and virtually all of you will be expected to be research-savvy at a basic level. We hope that you will come to see the value of nursing research and will be inspired by the efforts of the thousands of nurse researchers now working worldwide to improve patient care. You are embarking on a lifelong voyage in which research will play a role. We hope to help you enjoy the journey.

What Is Nursing Research?

Research is systematic inquiry that relies on disciplined methods to answer questions and solve problems. The ultimate goal of research is to gain knowledge that can benefit many people. **Nursing research** is systematic inquiry designed to develop evidence about issues of importance to nurses and their patients. Nurses undertake research to address problems relating to nursing education and nursing administration, but in this book, we emphasize **clinical nursing research**—that is, research designed to guide nursing practice and to improve the health and quality of life of nurses' patients. Clinical nursing research typically begins with questions stemming from practice problems—problems you may have already encountered.

> **Examples of nursing research questions**
> - What are the trajectories of spiritual distress and religious involvement among patients suffering from cancer during chemotherapy? (Martins et al., 2024)
> - What factors are associated with the intention to obtain the HPV vaccine among those who have never been vaccinated? (Allen et al., 2024)

 TIP You may think that research is too abstract to have a bearing on patient care. But nursing research focuses on *real* people with *real* problems, and studying those problems offers opportunities to address them through improvements to nursing care.

The Importance of Research to Evidence-Based Nursing

Nursing has experienced profound changes in the past few decades. Nurses are increasingly expected to understand research and to base their practice on evidence from research—that is, to adopt an **evidence-based practice (EBP)**. EBP involves using the best evidence in making patient care decisions, and such evidence typically comes from research conducted by nurses and other health care professionals. Nurse leaders recognize the need to base specific nursing decisions on evidence indicating that the decisions are clinically appropriate, resulting in positive patient outcomes, as well as cost-effective. We will discuss EBP in greater detail later in this chapter.

In some countries, research plays a role in nursing credentialing and status. For example, the American Nurses Credentialing Center—an arm of the American Nurses Association—has developed a Magnet Recognition Program to recognize health care organizations that provide high-quality nursing care. To achieve Magnet status, practice environments must demonstrate a sustained commitment to EBP; the 2023 Magnet application manual continues to strengthen evidence-based requirements. Changes to nursing practice are happening every day because of EBP efforts.

Example of evidence-based practice •
Many clinical practice changes reflect the impact of research. For example, "kangaroo care," the holding of diaper-clad preterm infants skin to skin, chest to chest by parents, is now widely practiced in neonatal intensive care units (NICUs), but before 2000, only a minority of NICUs offered kangaroo care options. Expanded adoption of this practice resulted from mounting evidence that early skin-to-skin contact has clinical benefits without negative side effects. Research on kangaroo care continues to reinforce the benefits of this care for infants under a variety of circumstances (Çaka et al., 2023; Pathak et al., 2023; Zengin et al., 2023; Zhao et al., 2022).

Roles of Nurses in Research

Nurses are likely to engage in one or more activities along a continuum of research participation. At one end of the continuum are *consumers of nursing research*—nurses who read research reports to keep up-to-date on findings that may affect their practice. EBP depends on well-informed nursing research consumers.

At the other end of the continuum are the *producers of nursing research*—nurses who actively undertake studies. Research is increasingly being conducted by practicing nurses who want to find what works best for their patients.

Between these two end points on the continuum lie a variety of research activities in which nurses engage. Even if you never carry out a study, you may do one of the following:

1. Contribute an idea for a study.
2. Gather information from those taking part in a study.
3. Advise patients about participating in a study.
4. Search for research evidence to address a practice problem.
5. Discuss the implications of a study in a **journal club** in your practice setting, which involves meetings (in groups or online) to discuss research articles.

In all these possible research-related activities, nurses who have some research skills are better able than those without them to make a contribution to nursing and to EBP.

Nursing Research: Past and Present

Florence Nightingale is credited with being the first nurse to use research techniques. Based on her skillful analysis of factors affecting soldier mortality and morbidity during the Crimean War (1854 to 1856), she was successful in bringing about changes in nursing care and public health. After Nightingale's work, however, research disappeared from the nursing literature until the early 1900s, but most studies at that time concerned nurses' education.

In the 1950s, research by nurses began to accelerate. Increased numbers of nurses with advanced degrees, the growth in research funding, and the establishment of the journal *Nursing Research* helped to propel nursing research at the mid-20th century. During the 1960s, practice-oriented research began to emerge, and research-oriented journals started publication in several countries. During the 1970s, there was a change in research emphasis from areas such as teaching and nurses' characteristics to improvements in patient care. Nurses also began to pay attention to the utilization of research findings in nursing practice.

In 1986, the National Center for Nursing Research (NCNR) was established at the National Institutes of Health (NIH) in the United States. A key purpose of NCNR was to promote and financially support research relating to patient care. In 1993, nursing research was strengthened when NCNR was promoted to full institute status within the NIH: the *National Institute of Nursing Research* (NINR) was created. NINR helped put nursing research into the mainstream of activities enjoyed by other health disciplines. Funding opportunities for nursing research also expanded in other countries. The 1990s witnessed the birth of several more journals for nurse researchers, and the growth of journals focused on nursing research continues to expand. Additionally, as members of interdisciplinary research teams, more nurses are publishing in health science journals with colleagues from other fields.

Current and Future Directions for Nursing Research

Nursing research continues to develop at a rapid pace as research is increasingly embedded into the nurse's professional role. In 1986, NCNR had a budget of $16 million, whereas NINR's funding request for fiscal year 2024 was $197.7 million. Among the trends we foresee for the near future are the following:

- *Continued focus on EBP*. Nurses' use of research findings in their practice will continue to be encouraged. This means that improvements will be needed in nurses' skills in locating, understanding, critically appraising, and using relevant study results.
- *Ongoing growth of research syntheses*. Systematic reviews, which are a cornerstone of EBP, rigorously integrate research information on a topic so that conclusions about the state of evidence can be reached.
- *Increased emphasis on patient centeredness*. **Patient centeredness** has become a central concern in health care and in research. Efforts are increasing to ensure that research is relevant to patients and that patients play a role in setting research priorities.
- *Relatedly, greater interest in the* **applicability** *of research*. More attention is being paid to figuring out how study results can be applied to individual patients or subgroups of patients. A limitation of the current EBP model is that evidence typically is based on the *average effects* of health care interventions implemented under ideal circumstances.
- *Expanded local research and quality improvement efforts in health care settings*. Small studies designed to solve local problems are increasing. This trend will be reinforced as more hospitals apply for (and are recertified for) Magnet status in the United States and other countries. Mechanisms are being developed to ensure that evidence from local projects becomes available to others facing similar problems.
- *Increased focus on health disparities*. Health disparities continue to be a crucially important concern, and this in turn has raised consciousness about the cultural sensitivity of health interventions. Research (and health care more generally) must be sensitive to the beliefs, life experiences, barriers, and values of racially, culturally, and linguistically diverse populations.
- *Growing interest in defining and ascertaining* **clinical significance**. Research findings increasingly must meet the test of being clinically significant, and patients have taken center stage in efforts to define clinical significance.
- *Nurse researchers contributing to interdisciplinary team science*. Nurses have a unique focus on people's health experiences. As nurses become more adept at articulating the distinct perspective of the discipline and in the conduct of nursing research, they increasingly serve as valuable members of interdisciplinary research teams.

What are nurse researchers likely to be studying in the future? Although there is tremendous diversity in research interests, research priorities have been articulated by NINR, Sigma Theta Tau International, and other nursing organizations. For example, NINR's 2022 to 2026 strategic plan is a living document that provides a research lens for research concerned with health-related questions aimed at achieving NINR's mission (NINR, 2022). The research lens is as follows:

- Health equity
- Social determinants of health
- Population and community health

- Prevention and health promotion
- Systems and models of care

KNOWLEDGE SOURCES FOR NURSING PRACTICE

Nurses make clinical decisions based on a large repertoire of knowledge. As a nursing student, you are gaining skills in nursing practice from your instructors, textbooks, and clinical placements. When you become a registered nurse (RN), you will continue to learn from other nurses and health care professionals. Because evidence is constantly evolving, learning about best-practice nursing will be an ongoing quest throughout your career.

Some of what you have learned thus far is based on systematic research, but much of it is not. Where does knowledge for nursing practice come from? Until fairly recently, knowledge was based primarily on clinical experience, trial and error, tradition, and expert opinion. These alternative sources of knowledge are different from research-based information.

Tradition and "Experts"

Some nursing decisions are based on untested traditions and "unit culture" rather than on sound evidence. Another common source of knowledge is an authority, a person with specialized expertise. Reliance on experts (such as nursing faculty, mentors, or textbook authors) is unavoidable. Experts, however, are not infallible—particularly if their expertise is based primarily on personal experience or outdated information; yet, their knowledge is often unchallenged.

TIP The consequences of *not* using research-based evidence can be devastating. For example, from 1956 through the 1980s, Dr. Benjamin Spock published several editions of *Baby and Child Care*, a parental guide that sold over 19 million copies worldwide. Dr. Spock wrote the following advice: "I think it is preferable to accustom a baby to sleeping on his stomach from the beginning if he is willing" (Spock, 1979, p. 164). Research has demonstrated that this sleeping position is associated with a heightened risk of sudden unexplained infant death (SUID) (formerly known as sudden infant death syndrome [SIDS]). In their systematic review of the evidence, Gilbert and colleagues (2005) wrote, "Advice to put infants to sleep on the front for nearly half a century was contrary to evidence from 1970 that this was likely to be harmful" (p. 874). They estimated that if medical advice had been guided by research evidence, over 60,000 infant deaths might have been prevented. An updated systematic review continues to support the supine sleeping position for infants to reduce the risk of SUID (Priyadarshi et al., 2022).

Clinical Experience and Trial and Error

Clinical experience is a functional source of knowledge—indeed, it is a component of the EBP model. Yet, personal experience has limitations as a source of evidence for practice because each nurse's experience is too narrow to be generally useful, and personal experiences are often colored by biases. Trial and error—alternatives tried successively until a solution to a problem is found—can be practical, but the method tends to be haphazard and solutions may be idiosyncratic.

Disciplined Research

Disciplined research is considered the best method of acquiring reliable knowledge. Evidence-based health care compels nurses to base their clinical practice to the extent possible on rigorous research-based findings rather than on tradition, authority, or personal experience—although nursing will always remain a rich blend of art and science.

PARADIGMS AND METHODS FOR NURSING RESEARCH

The questions that nurse researchers ask, and the strategies they use to answer their questions, spring from a researcher's view of how the world "works." In research parlance, a **paradigm** is a worldview, a general perspective on the world's complexities.

Disciplined inquiry in nursing has been conducted mainly within two paradigms. The paradigm that dominated nursing research for decades is called the **positivist paradigm**. Positivism, rooted in 19th century thought, is a reflection of a broad cultural movement that emphasizes the rational and scientific. The **constructivist paradigm** (sometimes called the *naturalistic paradigm*) began as a countermovement to positivism and is a major alternative system for conducting research in nursing.

This section describes the two paradigms and outlines the research methods associated with them. **Research methods** are the techniques researchers use to structure a study and to gather and analyze relevant information. The two paradigms are associated with different methods of developing evidence.

The Positivist Paradigm

An **assumption** is a principle that is believed to be true without verification. Paradigms are associated with a set of assumptions that have implications for the kinds of research questions that researchers ask and the methods they use to answer them.

Worldview of the Positivist Paradigm

A fundamental assumption of positivists is that there is a reality *out there* that can be studied and known. Positivists assume that nature is ordered and regular, and that a reality exists independent of human observation. The assumption of *determinism* refers to the positivists' belief that phenomena are not haphazard but rather have antecedent causes. Within the positivist paradigm, research activity is often aimed at understanding the underlying causes of natural phenomena. Because they believe in a factual reality, positivists prize objectivity. Their approach involves the use of orderly, disciplined procedures with tight controls over the research situation to test hunches about the nature of the phenomena being studied and the relationships among them.

TIP What do we mean by *phenomena*? In a research context, *phenomena* are those things in which researchers are interested—such as a health event (e.g., a patient fall), a health outcome (e.g., pain), or a health experience (e.g., living with chronic pain).

Strict positivist thinking has been challenged. *Postpositivists* recognize the impossibility of total objectivity, but they view objectivity as a goal and strive to be as unbiased as possible. Postpositivists also appreciate the barriers to knowing reality with certainty and therefore seek *probabilistic* evidence—i.e., learning what the true state of a phenomenon *probably* is. This modified positivist position remains a dominant force in nursing research. For the sake of simplicity, we refer to it as positivism.

The Scientific Method and Quantitative Research

The traditional, positivist **scientific method** involves using orderly procedures to gather primarily quantitative information. Quantitative researchers typically move in a systematic fashion from the definition of a problem to a solution. By *systematic*, we mean that investigators progress through a series of steps, according to a prespecified plan. Quantitative researchers use methods designed to control the research situation with the goal of minimizing *bias* and maximizing validity.

Quantitative researchers gather **empirical evidence**—evidence that is rooted in objective reality and gathered through the senses rather than through personal beliefs. Evidence for a study using the traditional scientific method is gathered systematically, using instruments to collect needed information. Usually, the information is *quantitative*—numeric information that results from some type of formal measurement and that is analyzed statistically. Quantitative researchers strive to go beyond the specifics of a situation; the ability to generalize research findings to individuals who did not take part in the study (referred to as **generalizability**) is an important goal.

The traditional scientific method has been used productively by nurse researchers studying a wide range of questions. Yet, there are important limitations. For example, quantitative researchers must deal with problems of *measurement*. To study a phenomenon, scientists must measure it, that is, attach numeric values that express quantity. For example, if the phenomenon of interest were patient stress, researchers would want to assess if stress was high or low, or higher under certain conditions. Physiologic phenomena like blood pressure and temperature can be measured with accuracy and precision, but the same cannot be said of psychological phenomena, such as stress, resilience, or pain.

Nursing research focuses on human beings who are inherently complicated and diverse. Quantitative studies typically focus on only a few concepts (e.g., weight gain, depression). Complexities tend to be controlled and, if possible, eliminated rather than studied directly, and this narrowness of focus can sometimes obscure insights. **Quantitative research** within the positivist paradigm has been criticized for failing to capture the full breadth of human experience.

> **Example of a quantitative study** •••••••••••••••••••••••••••••••••••
> Tung et al. (2022) conducted a randomized clinical trial aimed at examining the effects of an exercise program on functional fitness and the ability to perform the activities of daily living (ADL) in 114 older adults with probable sarcopenia in 12 long-term care facilities. The findings suggested that functional fitness and ADL in the intervention group were significantly improved while the control group experienced a significant decline.

> **TIP** Students often find quantitative studies more intimidating than qualitative ones. Try not to worry too much about the jargon at first—remember that each study has a *story* to tell, and grasping the main point of the story is what is initially important.

The Constructivist Paradigm

This section describes the assumptions and research methods associated with the constructivist paradigm.

Worldview of the Constructivist Paradigm

For the naturalistic inquirer, reality is not a fixed entity but rather a construction of the people participating in the research; reality exists within a context, and many constructions are possible. Constructivists take the position of relativism: If there are multiple interpretations of reality that exist in people's minds, then there is no process by which the ultimate truth or falsity of the constructions can be determined.

The constructivist paradigm assumes that knowledge is maximized when the distance between the inquirer and participants in the study is minimized. The voices and interpretations of those under study are crucial to understanding the phenomenon of interest, and subjective interactions are the best way to access them. Findings from a constructivist inquiry are the product of the interaction between the inquirer and the participants.

Constructivist Methods and Qualitative Research

Researchers in the constructivist versus the positivist paradigm rely on different research methods (Table 1.1). Researchers in constructivist traditions emphasize the inherent complexity of humans, their ability to shape their own experiences, and the idea that truth is a composite of realities. Consequently, constructivist studies are focused on understanding the human experience as it is lived, through the careful collection and analysis of *qualitative* materials that are narrative and subjective.

Qualitative researchers believe that a major limitation of the traditional scientific method is that it is *reductionist*—that is, it reduces human experience to the few concepts under investigation, and those concepts are defined in advance rather than emerging from the experiences of those under study. Constructivist researchers tend to emphasize the dynamic, holistic, and individual aspects of human life and try to capture those aspects in their entirety, within the context of those who are experiencing them.

Flexible, evolving procedures are used to capitalize on findings that emerge during the study, which typically is undertaken in naturalistic settings. The collection and analysis of information usually progress concurrently. As researchers sift through information, insights are gained, new questions emerge, and further evidence is sought to confirm the insights. Through an inductive process (going from specifics to the general), researchers integrate information to develop a theory or description that illuminates the phenomena under observation.

Constructivist studies yield rich, in-depth information that can potentially clarify the dimensions of a complicated phenomenon. The findings are grounded in the real-life experiences of people with firsthand knowledge of a phenomenon. Nevertheless, the approach has several limitations. Human beings are used directly as the instrument through which information is gathered, and humans are highly intelligent—but fallible—tools.

Another issue involves the subjectivity of constructivist inquiry, which can raise concerns about the idiosyncratic nature of the judgments. Would two constructivist researchers studying the same phenomenon in similar settings arrive at comparable conclusions? The problem is exacerbated by the fact that most constructivist studies involve a small number of participants. Thus, the generalizability of findings from constructivist inquiries is a potential concern.

TABLE 1.1 Key Methodologic Differences in the Positivist and Constructivist Paradigms

Positivist Paradigm (Quantitative Research)	Constructivist Paradigm (Qualitative Research)
Deductive processes—hypothesis testing	Inductive processes—hypothesis generation
Emphasis on discrete, specific concepts	Emphasis on the entirety of a phenomenon; holistic
Focus on the objective and quantifiable	Focus on the subjective and nonquantifiable
Outsider knowledge—researcher is external, separate	Insider knowledge—researcher is part of the process
Fixed, prespecified research design	Flexible, emergent research design
Controls over context	Context bound
Large, representative samples	Small, information-rich samples
Measured (quantitative) information	Narrative (unstructured) information
Statistical analysis	Qualitative analysis
Seeks generalizations	Seeks in-depth understanding

> **Example of a qualitative study**
> Brooks and Savitch (2022) conducted qualitative interviews to explore the experience and motivations of six people living with dementia who were blogging about what this experience was like for them.

 TIP Researchers seldom discuss or even mention the underlying paradigm of their studies in their reports. The paradigm shapes the inquiry without being explicitly referenced.

Multiple Paradigms and Nursing Research

Paradigms are lenses that help to sharpen researchers' focus on phenomena of interest. The availability of alternative paradigms for studying nursing problems can maximize the breadth of new evidence for practice. Nursing is enriched by the use of diverse methods—methods that are often complementary in their strengths and limitations.

We have emphasized differences between the two paradigms and associated methods so that distinctions would be easy to understand. It is equally important, however, to note that the two paradigms have many features in common, some of which are mentioned here:

- *Ultimate goals*. The ultimate aim of disciplined research, regardless of paradigm, is to answer questions and solve problems. All researchers seek to capture the truth with regard to the phenomena in which they are interested.
- *External evidence*. The word *empiricism* is often associated with the scientific method, but qualitative researchers also gather and analyze evidence gathered empirically, that is, through their senses.
- *Reliance on human cooperation*. Human cooperation is essential in both qualitative and quantitative research. To understand people's characteristics and experiences, researchers must persuade them to participate in the study and to speak candidly.
- *Ethical constraints*. Regardless of paradigms or methods, research with human beings is guided by ethical principles that sometimes conflict with research goals.
- *Fallibility*. Virtually all studies have limitations. The fallibility of any single study makes it important to understand and critically appraise researchers' methods when evaluating evidence quality.

Thus, despite philosophic and methodologic differences, researchers using the traditional scientific or constructivist methods face many similar challenges. The selection of an appropriate method depends not only on researchers' worldview but also on the research question. If a researcher asks, "What are the effects of cryotherapy on oral mucositis in patients undergoing chemotherapy?" the researcher needs to examine effects through a careful quantitative assessment of patient outcomes. On the other hand, if a researcher asks, "What is the process by which parents learn to cope with the death of a child?" the researcher would be hard pressed to quantify the process. Personal worldviews of researchers help to shape the questions they ask.

In reading about the alternative paradigms, you likely were more attracted to one of the two paradigms—the one that corresponds to your view of the world. It is important, however, to learn about and value both approaches to disciplined inquiry and to recognize their respective strengths and limitations. This book will hopefully help you to become *methodologically bilingual*—a skill that is increasingly important because many nurse researchers are now undertaking **mixed methods research** that involves the collection and analysis of both qualitative and quantitative data in a single study, as we discuss in Chapter 12.

HOW-TO-TELL TIP How can you quickly tell if a study is qualitative or quantitative? As you progress through this book, you should be able to identify most studies as qualitative versus quantitative based on terms in the introductory summary or on the report title. At this point, though, it may be easiest to distinguish the two types of studies based on how many *numbers* appear in the article, especially in tables. Qualitative studies may have no tables with quantitative information, or only one numeric table describing participants' characteristics (e.g., the percentage who were male or female). Quantitative studies typically have several tables with numbers and statistical information. Qualitative studies often have "word tables" or diagrams and figures illustrating processes inferred from the narrative information gathered.

THE PURPOSES OF NURSING RESEARCH

Why do nurses do research? Several systems have been devised to classify research goals.

Research for Varying Levels of Explanation

One classification system concerns the extent to which studies provide explanatory information. The descriptive/explanatory continuum includes studies whose purposes are identification, description, exploration, prediction/control, and explanation of health-related phenomena. For each purpose, various types of question are addressed—some more amenable to qualitative than to quantitative inquiry, and vice versa. Here are some examples of questions researchers ask related to these purposes, with a designation of whether the inquiry would most likely be quantitative (Quan) or qualitative (Qual):

- *Identification*: What is this phenomenon? What is its name? (Qual)
- *Description*: How prevalent is the phenomenon? (Quan) What are the dimensions or characteristics of the phenomenon? (Qual)
- *Exploration*: What factors are related to the phenomenon? (Quan) What is the full nature of the phenomenon? (Qual)
- *Prediction/control*: If phenomenon X occurs, will phenomenon Y follow? Can the phenomenon be prevented? (Quan)
- *Explanation*: What is the underlying cause of the phenomenon? (Quan) What does the phenomenon mean? (Qual)

TIP Specific study goals can range along a descriptive/explanatory continuum, but a fundamental distinction is between studies whose primary intent is to *describe* phenomena and those that are cause-probing—i.e., designed to illuminate the underlying causes of phenomena. Questions in the prediction/control and explanation categories are used in **cause-probing research**.

Research Purposes Linked to Evidence-Based Practice

Another system for classifying studies has emerged in efforts to communicate EBP-related purposes (Melnyk & Fineout-Overholt, 2023). In this classification scheme, most purposes can best be addressed with quantitative research.

Therapy/Intervention

Therapy/intervention questions are addressed by health care researchers who want to learn the benefits of specific actions, treatments, products, or processes. Studies with a therapy purpose seek to identify effective treatments for ameliorating or preventing health problems. Such studies range from evaluations of highly specific treatments (e.g., comparing two types of cooling blankets for febrile patients) to complex multicomponent interventions designed to result in behavioral changes (e.g., testing a nurse-led smoking cessation intervention). Therapy questions are foundational for evidence-based decision-making; evidence for changes to nursing practice comes from studies that have tested the effects of intervening in a particular way.

> **Example of a study aimed at therapy**
> Does an evidence-based heart failure education program result in increased adherence to the treatment plan and decreased hospital readmissions in patients with heart failure after discharge posthospitalization (Rizzuto et al., 2022)?

Diagnosis and Assessment

Many nursing studies concern the rigorous development and testing of formal instruments to screen, diagnose, and assess patients and to measure clinical outcomes—that is, they address diagnosis/assessment questions. High-quality instruments with documented accuracy are essential for clinical practice and for research.

> **Example of a study aimed at diagnosis/assessment**
> Mendes and colleagues (2024) conducted a case-control study in 155 high-risk pregnant people to determine the clinical validity of the nursing diagnosis risk for disturbed maternal–fetal dyad in high-risk pregnancy.

Prognosis

Researchers who ask prognosis questions strive to understand the outcomes associated with a disease or a health problem (i.e., its consequences), to estimate the probability they will occur, and to predict the types of people for whom the outcomes are most likely. Such studies facilitate the development of long-term care plans for patients. They also provide valuable information for guiding patients to make beneficial lifestyle choices or to be vigilant for key symptoms.

> **Example of a study aimed at prognosis**
> Peng and colleagues (2023) examined whether enteral nutrition supplementation initiated in patients less than 24 hours after cardiac bypass surgery as compared to 24 to 48 hours and greater than 48 hours was associated with prognosis.

Etiology (Causation)/Prevention of Harm

It is difficult to prevent harm or treat health problems if we do not know what causes them—and this is the focus of etiology questions. For example, there would be no smoking cessation programs if research had not provided firm evidence that smoking cigarettes causes or contributes to many health problems. Thus, determining the factors and exposures that affect or cause illness, mortality, or morbidity is an important purpose of many studies.

> **Example of a study aimed at etiology/prevention of harm**
> Flanagan and colleagues (2023) examined the effects of occupational therapy, physical therapy, and a combination of the two on the change in physical function in patients with and without dementia admitted to skilled nursing facilities from acute care hospitals from the time of admission to quarterly assessment or discharge.

Description

Description questions are not in a category typically identified in EBP-related classification schemes, but so many nursing studies have a descriptive purpose that we include it here. Examples of phenomena that nurse researchers have described include patients' pain, physical function, confusion, and levels of depression. Quantitative description focuses on the prevalence, size, intensity, and measurable attributes of phenomena. Qualitative researchers, by contrast, describe the dimensions or the evolution of phenomena.

> **Example of a quantitative study aimed at description**
> Wang et al. (2024) described the sociodemographic characteristics of patients who missed their screening mammogram at a community health center in a 1-year period. They also sought to describe if and when the missed examinations were completed. Independent predictors of those who missed appointments included being non-Hispanic Black race, non-English speaking, and on Medicaid or other means-tested insurance. At 1-year follow-up, 40.6% of patients who missed appointments had not completed screening a *mammogram*.

> **Example of a qualitative study aimed at description**
> Hanan and colleagues (2024) used a qualitative descriptive design to describe health care professionals' perceptions of the barriers and facilitators to caring for long-term care residents with serious persistent mental illness.

Meaning and Processes

Many health care activities (e.g., motivating people to comply with treatments, designing appealing interventions) can benefit from gaining insight into the patients' perspectives, using **qualitative research** methods that address meaning/process questions. Research that offers evidence about what health and illness mean to patients, what barriers they face to positive health practices, and what processes they experience in a transition through a health care crisis are important to evidence-based nursing practice.

> **Example of a study aimed at meaning/process**
> Leone-Sheehan et al. (2024) used a qualitative descriptive design to explore intensive care unit nurses' experience of Watson's Theory of Human Caring Caritas Process III of developing spiritual self to meet the significant spiritual and existential needs of patients and their families.

 TIP Several EBP-related purposes involve *cause-probing* research. Therapy/intervention research focuses on whether an intervention *causes* improvements in key outcomes. Prognosis research examines whether a disease or health condition *causes* subsequent adverse consequences. Etiology research seeks explanations about the underlying *causes* of health problems.

Links Between Study Purposes and Evidence-Based Practice

Studies that address therapy/intervention questions provide the most direct evidence for EBP. If we want to know, for example, whether wedge-shaped foam cushions are more effective in preventing heel pressure ulcers than standard foam pillows, we would need to look for rigorous studies that have addressed this therapy question.

TABLE 1.2 Different Categories of Question Relating to Cigarette Smoking

Type of Question	Example of a Research Question on Cigarette Smoking
Therapy/intervention	Does a nurse-led smoking cessation program for young adults reduce smoking?
Diagnosis/assessment	Is our Smoking Susceptibility Index a valid and reliable measure of teenagers' propensity to initiate smoking?
Prognosis	Is a diagnosis of smoking-related lung cancer associated with increased risk of suicidal ideation?
Etiology (causation)/prevention of harm	Does smoking increase the risk of a fatality among people infected with the novel coronavirus?
Description	What percentage of high school students smoke ≥1 pack of cigarettes per week?
Meaning/process	What is it like for people who have smoked long term to attempt and fail at quitting?

Other questions also play a role in improving the quality of nursing care, although in different ways. Table 1.2 presents examples of different questions relating to cigarette smoking, using the EBP-related purpose categories. The findings from studies relating to only one of these questions is directly *actionable*—the therapy question. If there is good evidence that nurse-led smoking cessation programs are effective in reducing smoking among young adults, we might consider initiating such a program in our own community.

Strong evidence from studies addressing the other questions in Table 1.2 could also guide efforts to improve nursing practice—but not as directly. For example, evidence about suicide ideation from the prognosis question might prompt us to develop a program of emotional support for patients with lung cancer. Results from the etiology study might lead us to launch a smoking cessation initiative in communities hit hard by coronavirus infections. The stories from people who had been smoking long term and failed to quit despite efforts to do so (the meaning question) could lead us to involve them in the design of an intervention for people who smoke persistently.

Nurse researchers are making strides in addressing all types of questions about important health problems—but evidence regarding what "works" to improve nursing practice comes from studies addressing therapy questions. Evidence about the scope of a problem, factors affecting the problem, the consequences of the problem, and the meaning of the problem can, however, play a crucial role in efforts to design better interventions, to aim resources at those in greatest need, and to provide appropriate guidance to patients in everyday practice.

BASICS OF EVIDENCE-BASED NURSING PRACTICE

In this section, we describe some basic principles of EBP. We elaborate on EBP issues in Chapter 18.

Definition of Evidence-Based Practice

Dozens of definitions of EBP have been proposed. Most definitions describe EBP as a *decision-making* (or *problem-solving*) *process*. Most definitions also include the idea that EBP is built on a "three-legged stool," each "leg" of which is essential to the process: *best evidence*, *patient preferences and values*, and *clinical expertise*. Figure 1.1 depicts these concepts.

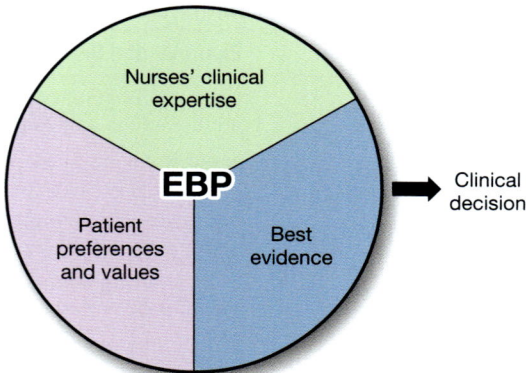

Figure 1.1 Model of evidence-based nursing practice.

Best Evidence

A basic feature of EBP as a clinical problem-solving strategy is that it de-emphasizes decisions based on tradition or expert opinion. The emphasis is on identifying and evaluating the best available research evidence as a tool for solving problems. There continues to be debate about what qualifies as "best" evidence. As we discuss in the next section, evidence is often evaluated in relation to *evidence hierarchies* that rank evidence sources according to the degree to which the evidence is unbiased. Evidence, however, whether "best" or not, is never by itself a sufficient basis for clinical decision-making.

Patient Preferences and Values

Patient input encompasses several concepts, including patient preferences for type of treatment, preferences for being involved in decision-making, social or cultural values, preferences about involving family members in health care decisions, priorities regarding quality-of-life issues, and spiritual or religious values. EBP decisions also require understanding patients' circumstances, such as the resources at their disposal. Nurses thus need the skills to elicit and understand patient preferences and their situations.

Nurses' Clinical Expertise

Decision-making in clinical practice also relies on clinicians' expertise, which is an amalgam of academic knowledge gained during training and continuing education, experiences with patient care, and interdisciplinary sharing of new knowledge. David Sackett, the pioneer of evidence-based medicine, strongly advocated for the importance of clinical expertise in making decisions because even very strong research evidence is seldom appropriate for all patients.

Sources of "Best" Research Evidence

Thousands of studies of relevance to nurses are published every month in professional journals. **Primary studies** must be critically appraised to determine if the evidence is sufficiently rigorous to warrant consideration in nursing practice. Finding evidence useful for practice is often facilitated by the availability of evidence that is preprocessed (synthesized) and sometimes pre-appraised. For example, several evidence-based journals publish synopses of original research (e.g., *Evidence-Based Nursing*, *The Online Journal of Knowledge Synthesis for Nursing*), and the synopses are occasionally accompanied by commentary about the clinical utility of the evidence.

Syntheses that integrate evidence from multiple studies on a given topic are an especially important resource for EBP. The most widely respected type of synthesis is the systematic review. A **systematic review** is not just a literature review—it is a methodical, scholarly inquiry that summarizes and evaluates current evidence on a research question. Systematic reviews are the basis for most clinical practice guidelines.

Systematic reviewers sometimes integrate findings from quantitative studies using statistical methods, in what is called a **meta-analysis**. Meta-analysts treat the findings from a study as one piece of information. The findings from multiple studies on the same topic are combined and analyzed statistically. Meta-analysis is an objective method of integrating a body of findings and of observing patterns that might otherwise have gone undetected (see Chapter 17).

Systematic reviews of qualitative studies often take the form of metasyntheses. A **meta-synthesis** is less about combining information and more about amplifying and interpreting it. For certain qualitative questions, an aggregative (rather than interpretive) approach to systematic synthesis called **meta-aggregation** may be appropriate. Strategies have also been developed for systematic **mixed studies review**, which are efforts to integrate and synthesize both quantitative and qualitative evidence on a topic.

Evidence Hierarchies and Level of Evidence Scales

Judgments about what evidence is "best" are often guided by evidence hierarchies. Evidence hierarchies rank evidence sources in terms of their risk of bias, focusing mainly on risk of bias in studies addressing therapy questions. Most evidence hierarchies are represented as pyramids, with the highest ranking sources—those presumed to have the least bias for making inferences about the effects of an intervention—at the top. The hierarchies form **level of evidence (LOE)** scales that rank order types of evidence. Level I evidence usually is considered the best (least biased) type of evidence.

Figure 1.2 shows our eight-level **evidence hierarchy** for therapy/intervention questions. In our scheme, the Level I evidence source is a systematic review of studies called *randomized controlled trials* (RCTs), which are the "gold standard" type of study for therapy questions. An individual RCT is a Level II evidence source. Going down the "rungs" of the evidence hierarchy for therapy questions results in evidence with a higher risk of bias in answering questions about "what works." (Technical terms in Figure 1.2, such as "quasi-experiment," are explained later in the book.)

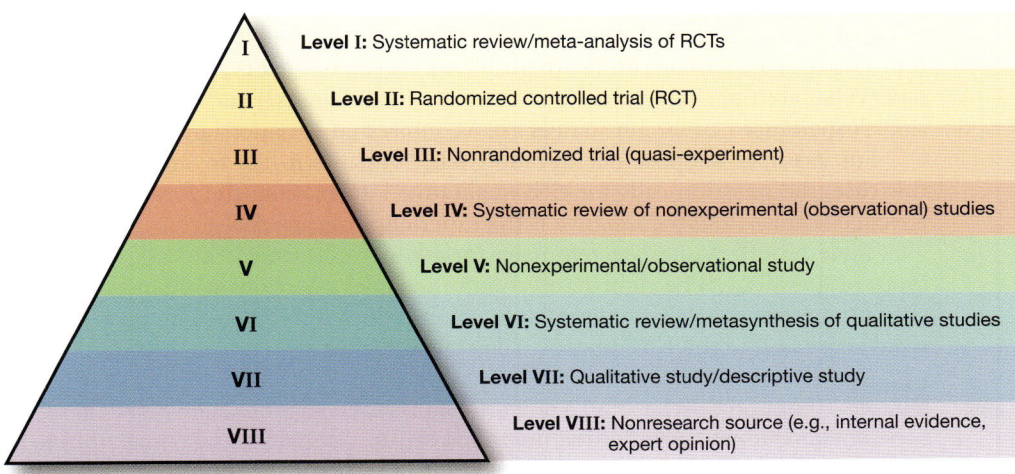

Figure 1.2 Polit–Beck evidence hierarchy/level of evidence scale for therapy questions.

TIP Sometimes, evidence hierarchies are used to "level" or grade evidence sources, with the implication that higher levels provide better quality evidence. As pointed out by Levin (2014), however, an evidence hierarchy "is not meant to provide a quality rating for evidence retrieved in the search for an answer" (p. 6). She noted that "leveling" a study is not a substitute for a critical appraisal of the evidence.

Asking Well-Worded Clinical Questions for Evidence-Based Practice

In Chapter 18, we describe a five-step process for putting research to use in clinical settings—the "5A" process: Ask, Acquire, Appraise, Apply, and Assess. Here, we focus on the first step.

The first activity in EBP involves asking well-worded clinical questions that can be answered with research evidence. For example, we may wonder, "Is a fish oil–enhanced nutritional supplement effective in stabilizing weight in cancer patients with cachexia?" The answer to such a therapy question may provide "best evidence" on how to address the needs of patients with cachexia.

Most guidance for EBP uses the acronyms PIO and PICO to help practitioners develop well-worded questions. In the PICO form, the clinical question is worded to identify four components:

P: the *Population* or *patients* (What are key characteristics of the patients or people?)
I: the *Intervention*, *influence*, or *exposure* (What is the intervention or therapy of interest? or, What is a potentially beneficial—or harmful—influence?)
C: an explicit *Comparison* to the "I" component (With what is the intervention or influence being compared?)
O: the *Outcome* (What is the outcome in which we are interested?)

Applying this scheme to our question about cachexia, our *population* (P) is cancer patients with cachexia; the *intervention* (I) is fish oil–enhanced nutritional supplements; and the *outcome* (O) is weight stabilization. In this question, the *comparison* is not formally stated, but the implied "C" is the *absence* of fish oil–enhanced supplements—the question is in a PIO format. However, when there is an explicit comparison of interest, the full **PICO format** is used. For example, we might be interested in learning whether fish oil–enhanced supplements (I) are better than melatonin (C) in stabilizing weight (O) in patients with cachexia (P).

For questions that can best be answered with qualitative information (e.g., about the meaning of an experience or health problem), two components are most relevant: the *population* (What are the characteristics of the patients or clients?) and the *situation* (What conditions, experiences, or circumstances are we interested in understanding?).

For example, suppose our question was, "What is it like to suffer from cachexia?" In this case, the question calls for rich qualitative information; the *population* is patients with advanced cancer, and the *situation* is the experience of cachexia.

Table 1.3 offers question templates for asking well-framed clinical questions for specific types of questions. The right-hand column includes questions with an explicit comparison (PICO questions), whereas the middle column does not (PIO). The questions are categorized according to the EBP purposes described earlier.

 TIP Although EBP has had a powerful and beneficial impact on health care practices, recent concerns have emerged regarding the applicability of evidence from systematic reviews for individual patients. In Chapter 18, we elaborate on new ideas for creating *practice-based evidence* that enhances *applicability* to individuals, small groups of people, and local contexts.

Chapter 1 Introducing Nursing Research for Evidence-Based Practice

TABLE 1.3 Question Templates for Clinical Questions: PIO and PICO

Type of Question	PIO Question Template (Questions Without an Explicit Comparison)	PICO Question Template (Questions With an Explicit Comparison)
Therapy/treatment/intervention	In _____ (Population), what is the effect of _____ (Intervention) on _____ (Outcome)?	In _____ (Population), what is the effect of _____ (Intervention), in comparison to _____ (Comparative/alternative intervention), on _____ (Outcome)?
Diagnosis/assessment	For _____ (Population), does _____ (Identifying tool/procedure) yield accurate and appropriate diagnostic/assessment information about _____ (Outcome)?	For _____ (Population), does _____ (Identifying tool/procedure) yield more accurate or more appropriate diagnostic/assessment information than _____ (Comparative tool/procedure) about _____ (Outcome)?
Prognosis	In _____ (Population), does _____ (Influence/exposure to disease or condition) increase the risk of _____ (Outcome)?	In _____ (Population), does _____ (Influence/exposure to disease or condition), relative to _____ (Comparative disease/condition OR absence of the disease/condition) increase the risk of _____ (Outcome)?
Etiology/harm	In _____ (Population), does _____ (Influence/exposure/characteristic) increase the risk of _____ (Outcome)?	In _____ (Population), does _____ (Influence/exposure/characteristic) compared to _____ (Comparative influence/exposure OR lack of influence or exposure) increase the risk of _____ (Outcome)?
Description (prevalence/incidence)	In _____ (Population), how prevalent is _____ (Outcome)?	Explicit comparisons are not typical, except to compare different populations.
Meaning or process	What is it like for _____ (Population) to experience _____ (condition, illness, circumstance)? OR What is the process by which _____ (Population) cope with, adapt to, or live with _____ (condition, illness, circumstance)?	Explicit comparisons are not typical in these types of questions.

ASSISTANCE FOR CONSUMERS OF NURSING RESEARCH

We hope that this book will help you develop skills that will allow you to read, appraise, use, and appreciate nursing studies. In each chapter, we present information about methods that nurse researchers use to conduct their studies and provide guidance in several ways. First, we offer tips that often explain what you can expect to find in actual research articles, identified by the icon 👉. There are also special "how-to-tell" tips (identified with the icon 👉) that help with some potentially confusing issues in research articles.

Second, we include guidelines for critically appraising various aspects of a study in every chapter. The guiding questions in Box 1.1 are designed to assist you in using the information in this chapter in a preliminary assessment of a research article.

> **Box 1.1 Questions for a Preliminary Overview of a Research Report**
>
> a. How relevant is the research problem to the practice of nursing?
> b. Was the study quantitative or qualitative?
> c. What was the underlying purpose (or purposes) of the study—therapy/intervention, diagnosis/Assessment, prognosis, etiology/harm, description, or meaning?
> d. What might be some clinical implications of this research? To what type of people and settings is the research most relevant? If the findings were accurate, how might *I* use the results of this study?

And third, we offer opportunities to apply your new skills. The Critical Thinking Exercises at the end of each chapter guide you through appraisals of examples of qualitative and quantitative studies. These activities also challenge you to think about how the findings from these studies could be used in nursing practice. Answers to some of these questions are in the Instructor Resources on website. Two journal articles for the Critical Thinking Exercises are found in the appendices to this book.

RESEARCH EXAMPLES WITH CRITICAL THINKING EXERCISES

This section presents examples of studies with different purposes. Read the research summaries for Examples 1 and 2, and then answer the critical thinking questions that follow. The critical thinking questions for Examples 3 and 4 are based on the studies that appear in their entirety in Appendices A and B of this book.

EXAMPLE 1: QUANTITATIVE RESEARCH

Study: "Using pet therapy to decrease patients' anxiety on two diverse inpatient units" (Mulvaney-Roth et al., 2023)

Purpose: The purpose of the study was to explore the impact of pet therapy on patients' anxiety levels on two diverse inpatient units: Behavioral Health (BHU) and Pediatrics (PEDS).

Methods: This quantitative study used a convenience sample of patients on each of the BHU and PEDS units. After patients consented to the study, they were assigned to either the experimental group (received pet therapy) or the control group (did not receive pet therapy). The researchers used the six-item State Anxiety Scale (SAS) to measure anxiety pre pet therapy and at 1 hour post pet therapy. The Pediatric Emoji Method was used to assist children with the SAS. The pet therapy session was 15 minutes.

Key Findings: The researchers found that patients on each inpatient unit who received the pet therapy session had lower levels of anxiety than patients who did not receive the therapy session.

Conclusions: The researchers concluded that a 15-minute pet therapy session was effective in reducing anxiety levels in patients on both the BHU and PEDS units.

Critical Thinking Exercises

1. Answer the questions from Box 1.1 regarding this study.
2. Why do you think the researchers used two groups to assess the effects of the pet therapy intervention?
3. Could this study have been undertaken as a qualitative study? Why or why not?

EXAMPLE 2: QUALITATIVE RESEARCH

Study: "Nursing staff perceptions of outcomes related to honoring residents' "risky" preferences" (Behrens et al., 2022)

Purpose: The purpose of this study was to describe staff's perspectives of the health and safety outcomes associated with honoring nursing home residents' risky preferences for everyday living and care activities.

Methods: This study used a qualitative descriptive approach and sequential focus groups of nursing staff to obtain in-depth description of the complex and sensitive phenomena of risk. The Preference-Based Person-Centered Risk Engagement Model (Behrens et al., 2020) guided the development of the interview guide and data analysis.

Key Findings: A total of 27 licensed and unlicensed nursing staff participated in 12 sequential focus groups. Each group had three to five participants. The age range of the participants was 18 to 60 years of age. Other characteristics of the sample include 85.2 % female, 59.3% White, 66.6% reporting that their highest level of education was high school, and 51.8% reporting over 11 years of experience working in nursing homes. Three themes were identified: potential harms to staff, potential harms to residents, and positive shared outcomes.

Conclusions: Findings from this study identified physical and psychosocial outcomes associated with delivering person-centered care that honors nursing home residents' risky preferences.

Critical Thinking Exercises

1. Answer the questions in Box 1.1 regarding this study.
2. Why do you think that the researchers audiotaped and transcribed their in-depth interviews with study participants?
3. Do you think it would have been appropriate for the researchers to conduct this study using quantitative research methods? Why or why not?

EXAMPLE 3: QUANTITATIVE RESEARCH IN APPENDIX A

Read the abstract and the introduction from Cheng and colleagues' (2024) study "Advance care planning affects end-of-life treatment preferences among patients with heart failure: A randomized controlled trial" in Appendix A of this book.

1. Answer the questions in Box 1.1 regarding this study.
2. Could this study have been undertaken as a qualitative study? Why or why not?
3. Was this study supported with funding? (This information appears on the first page of the report.)
4. What might a prognosis question for this study be?

EXAMPLE 4: QUALITATIVE RESEARCH IN APPENDIX B

Read the abstract and the introduction from Morrison et al.'s (2024) study "Lived experiences of fatherhood after infertility" in Appendix B of this book.

1. Answer the questions in Box 1.1 regarding this study.
2. Was Morrison et al.'s study conducted within the positivist paradigm or the constructivist paradigm? Provide a rationale for your choice.
3. What was the phenomenon that Morrison and colleagues were studying? How was it defined?

Summary Points

- **Nursing research** is systematic inquiry undertaken to develop evidence on problems of importance to nurses.
- Nurses in various settings are adopting an **evidence-based practice (EBP)** that incorporates research findings into their decisions and interactions with patients.
- Knowledge of nursing research enhances the professional practice of all nurses—including both *consumers of research* (who read and evaluate studies) and *producers of research* (who design and undertake studies).
- Nursing research began with Florence Nightingale but developed slowly until its rapid acceleration in the 1950s. Since the 1980s, a major focus has been on **clinical nursing research**—that is, on problems relating to clinical practice.
- The NINR, established at the U.S. National Institutes of Health in 1993, affirms the stature of nursing research in the United States.
- Contemporary issues in nursing research include the growth of EBP, expansion of local research and quality improvement efforts, research synthesis through systematic reviews, **patient centeredness**, interest in the **applicability** of research to individual patients or groups, and efforts to measure the **clinical significance** of research results.
- Disciplined research stands in contrast to other knowledge sources for nursing practice, such as tradition, authority, personal experience, and trial and error.
- Disciplined inquiry in nursing is conducted mainly within two **paradigms**—worldviews with underlying **assumptions** about reality: the positivist paradigm and the constructivist paradigm.
- In the **positivist paradigm**, it is assumed that there is an objective reality and that natural phenomena are regular and orderly. The assumption of *determinism* refers to the belief that phenomena result from prior causes and are not haphazard.
- **Quantitative research** (associated with positivism) involves the collection and analysis of numeric information. Quantitative research is typically conducted within the traditional **scientific method**, which is systematic and controlled. Quantitative researchers base their findings on **empirical evidence** (evidence collected by way of the human senses) and strive for **generalizability** beyond a single setting or situation.
- In the **constructivist paradigm**, it is assumed that reality is not a fixed entity but is rather a construction of human minds—and thus "truth" is a composite of multiple constructions of reality.
- Constructivist researchers emphasize understanding human experience as it is lived through the collection and analysis of subjective, narrative materials using flexible procedures; this paradigm is associated with **qualitative research**.
- A fundamental distinction that is especially relevant in quantitative research is between studies whose primary intent is to *describe* phenomena and those that are **cause-**

- **probing**—i.e., designed to illuminate underlying causes of phenomena. Specific purposes on a description/explanation continuum include identification, description, exploration, prediction/control, and explanation.

- Nursing studies can also be classified in terms of EBP-related aims: therapy/intervention, diagnosis/assessment, prognosis, etiology (causation)/prevention of harm, description, and meaning/processes. Therapy questions are foundational for evidence-based decision-making.

- EBP is the conscientious integration of current best evidence and other factors in making clinical decisions. The three "legs" of EBP are (1) best research evidence, (2) patient preferences and values, and (3) nurses' own clinical experience and knowledge.

- **Primary studies** of original research published in professional journals are one source of evidence for EBP, but preprocessed (synthesized) evidence is especially useful in addressing clinical queries. Systematic reviews, considered the cornerstone of EBP, are important sources of evidence.

- **Systematic reviews** are rigorous integrations of research evidence from multiple studies on a topic. Systematic reviews can involve either narrative approaches to integration (including **metasynthesis** and **meta-aggregation** of qualitative studies) or quantitative approaches (**meta-analysis**) that integrate findings statistically by using individual studies as the unit of analysis.

- There has been a proliferation of **evidence hierarchies** that provide a preliminary guide for finding "best" evidence—evidence with the lowest risk of bias. Evidence hierarchies reflect **level of evidence (LOE) scales** that rank order types of evidence source—primarily for therapy/intervention questions. In LOEs for therapy questions, systematic reviews of RCTs are considered Level I sources.

- EBP efforts typically start by asking a well-worded clinical question for which evidence is then sought. A widely used scheme for asking well-worded clinical questions involves four primary components, an acronym for which is **PICO**: population or patients (P), intervention or influence (I), comparison (C), and outcome (O).

REFERENCES

Allen, J. D., Abuelezam, N. N., Rose, R., Isakoff, K., Zimet, G., & Fontenot, H. B. (2024). HPV vaccine behaviors and intentions among a diverse sample of women aged 27–45 years: Implications for shared clinical decision-making. *BMC Public Health*, 24(1), 2154. https://doi.org/10.1186/s12889-024-18740-2

Behrens, L. L., Boltz, M., Kolanowski, A., Sciegaj, M., Madrigal, C., Abbott, K., & Van Haitsma, K. (2020). Pervasive risk avoidance: Nursing staff perceptions of risk in person-centered care delivery. *The Gerontologist*, 60(8), 1424–1435. https://doi.org/10.1093/geront/gnaa099

Behrens, L. L., Boltz, M., Sciegaj, M., Kolanowski, A., Jones, J. R., Paudel, A., & Van Haitsma, K. (2022). Nursing staff perceptions of outcomes related to honoring residents' "Risky" preferences. *Research in Gerontological Nursing*, 15(6), 271–281. https://doi.org/10.3928/19404921-20220930-01

Brooks, J., & Savitch, N. (2022). Blogging with dementia: Writing about lived experience of dementia in the public domain. *Dementia (London, England)*, 21(8), 2402–2417. https://doi.org/10.1177/14713012221112384

Çaka, S. Y., Topal, S., Yurttutan, S., Aytemiz, S., Çıkar, Y., & Sarı, M. (2023). Effects of kangaroo mother care on feeding intolerance in preterm infants. *Journal of Tropical Pediatrics*, 69(2), fmad015. https://doi.org/10.1093/tropej/fmad015

Cheng, H. C., Wu, S. V., Chen, Y. H., Tsan, Y. H., Sung, S. H., & Ke, L. S. (2024). Advance care planning affects end-of-life treatment preferences among patients with heart failure: A randomized controlled trial. *Journal of Hospice and Palliative Nursing*, 26(1), E13–E19. https://doi.org/10.1097/NJH.0000000000000988

Flanagan, J., Boltz, M. & Ji, M. Post-acute Rehabilitation in Persons with and without Dementia. *Annals of Long-term Care*. Published online September 12, 2023. https://www.hmpgloballearningnetwork.com/site/altc/practical-research/postacute-rehabilitation-patients-and-without-dementia

Gilbert, R., Salanti, G., Harden, M., & See, S. (2005). Infant sleeping position and the sudden infant death syndrome: Systematic review of observational studies and historical review of recommendations from 1940 to 2002. *International Journal of Epidemiology*, 34(4), 874–887. https://doi.org/10.1093/ije/dyi088

Hanan, D. M., Lyons, K. S., Mahoney, E. K., Irwin, K. E., & Flanagan, J. M. (2024). Barriers and facilitators to caring for individuals with serious persistent mental illness in long-term care. *Archives of Psychiatric Nursing*, 51, 25–29. https://doi.org/10.1016/j.apnu.2024.05.006

Leone-Sheehan, D., Flanagan, J., & Willis, D. (2024). Intensive care unit nurses' experience of Watson's Theory of Human Caring Caritas Process III: Developing spiritual self to provide spiritual nursing care. *ANS. Advances*

Levin, R. F. (2014). Levels, grades, and strength of evidence: "What's it all about, Alfie?" *Research and Theory for Nursing Practice*, *28*(1), 5–8. https://doi.org/10.1891/1541-6577.28.1.5

Martins, H., Domingues, T. D., & Caldeira, S. (2024). Spiritual distress and religious involvement among cancer patients receiving chemotherapy: A longitudinal study. *International Journal of Nursing Knowledge*, *35*(3), 272–280. https://doi.org/10.1111/2047-3095.12442

Melnyk, B. M., & Fineout-Overholt, E. (2023). *Evidence-based practice in nursing and healthcare: A guide to best practice* (5th ed.). Lippincott Williams & Wilkins.

Mendes, R. C. M. G., Morais, S. C. R. V., Pontes, C. M., Frazão, C. M. F. Q., França, M. S., Lopes, M. V. O., Silva, G. P., Mangueira, S. O., & Linhares, F. M. P. (2024). Clinical validation of the nursing diagnosis risk for disturbed maternal-fetal dyad in high-risk pregnancy: A case-control study. *International Journal of Nursing Knowledge*, *35*(3), 281–289. https://doi.org/10.1111/2047-3095.12444

Morrison, S., Bryanton, J., Murray, C., & Foley, V. (2024). Lived experiences of fatherhood after infertility. *Journal of Obstetric, Gynecologic, and Neonatal Nursing*, *53*(3), 245–254. https://doi.org/10.1016/j.jogn.2023.12.002

Mulvaney-Roth, P., Jackson, C., Bert, L., Eriksen, S., & Ryan, M. (2023). Using pet therapy to decrease patients' anxiety on two diverse inpatient units. *Journal of the American Psychiatric Nurses Association*, *29*(2), 112–121. https://doi.org/10.1177/10783903211999719

National Institute of Nursing Research. (2022). *National Institute of Nursing Research 2022–2026 strategic plan*. https://www.fninr.org/assets/NINR/NINR_One-Pager12_508c.pdf.

Pathak, B. G., Sinha, B., Sharma, N., Mazumder, S., & Bhandari, N. (2023). Effects of kangaroo mother care on maternal and paternal health: Systematic review and meta-analysis. *Bulletin of the World Health Organization*, *101*(6), 391–402G. https://doi.org/10.2471/BLT.22.288977

Peng, Y., Chen, M., Ni, H., Li, S., Chen, L., & Lin, Y. (2023). Effect of timing of enteral nutrition initiation on poor prognosis in patients after cardiopulmonary bypass: A prospective observational study. *Nutrition (Burbank, Los Angeles County, Calif.)*, *116*, 112197. https://doi.org/10.1016/j.nut.2023.112197

Priyadarshi, M., Balachander, B., & Sankar, M. J. (2022). Effect of sleep position in term healthy newborns on sudden infant death syndrome and other infant outcomes: A systematic review. *Journal of Global Health*, *12*, 12001. https://doi.org/10.7189/jogh.12.12001

Rizzuto, N., Charles, G., & Knobf, M. T. (2022). Decreasing 30-day readmission rates in patients with heart failure. *Critical Care Nurse*, *42*(4), 13–19. https://doi.org/10.4037/ccn2022417

Spock, B. (1979). *Baby and child care*. Dutton.

Tung, H. T., Chen, K. M., Huang, K. C., Hsu, H. F., Chou, C. P., & Kuo, C. F. (2022). Effects of Vitality Acupunch exercise on functional fitness and activities of daily living among probable sarcopenic older adults in residential facilities. *Journal of Nursing Scholarship*, *54*(2), 176–183. https://doi.org/10.1111/jnu.12723

Wang, G. X., Mercaldo, S. F., Cahill, J. E., Flanagan, J. M., Lehman, C. D., & Park, E. R. (2024). Missed screening mammography appointments: patient sociodemographic characteristics and mammography completion after 1 year. *Journal of the American College of Radiology: JACR*, *21*(10), 1645–1656. https://doi.org/10.1016/j.jacr.2024.03.017

Zengin, H., Suzan, O. K., Hur, G., Kolukısa, T., Eroglu, A., & Cinar, N. (2023). The effects of kangaroo mother care on physiological parameters of premature neonates in neonatal intensive care unit: A systematic review. *Journal of Pediatric Nursing*, *71*, e18–e27. https://doi.org/10.1016/j.pedn.2023.04.010

Zhao, Y., Dong, Y., & Cao, J. (2022). Kangaroo care for relieving neonatal pain caused by invasive procedures: A systematic review and meta-analysis. *Computational Intelligence and Neuroscience*, *2022*, 2577158. https://doi.org/10.1155/2022/2577158

2 Understanding Key Concepts and Steps in Quantitative and Qualitative Research

Learning Objectives

On completing this chapter, you will be able to:

- Define new terms presented in the chapter and distinguish terms associated with quantitative and qualitative research
- Distinguish experimental and nonexperimental research
- Identify three main disciplinary traditions for qualitative nursing research
- Describe the flow and sequence of activities in quantitative and qualitative research and discuss how and why they differ

Key Terms

- Associative relationship
- Cause-and-effect (causal) relationship
- Clinical trial
- Concept
- Conceptual definition
- Construct
- Data
- Dependent variable
- Emergent design
- Ethnography
- Experimental research
- Gaining entrée
- Grounded theory
- Hypothesis
- Independent variable
- Informant
- Intervention protocol
- Literature review
- Nonexperimental research
- Observational study
- Operational definition
- Outcome variable
- Phenomenology
- Population
- Qualitative data
- Qualitative descriptive research
- Quantitative data
- Relationship
- Research design
- Sample
- Saturation
- Statistical analysis
- Study participant
- Subject
- Theme
- Theory
- Variable

THE BUILDING BLOCKS OF RESEARCH

Research, like any discipline, has its own language—its own *jargon* that can sometimes be intimidating. We readily admit that the jargon is plentiful and can be confusing. Some research jargon used in nursing research has its roots in the social sciences, but sometimes, different terms are used in medical research. Also, some terms are used by both qualitative and quantitative researchers, but others are used mainly by one or the other group. Please bear with us as we cover key terms that you will likely encounter in the research literature.

23

The Faces and Places of Research

When researchers address a research question, they are doing a *study* (or an *investigation*). Studies with humans involve two sets of people: those who do the research and those who provide the information. In a quantitative study, the people being studied are called **subjects** or **study participants**, as shown in Table 2.1. In a qualitative study, the people cooperating in the study are called study participants or **informants**. The person who conducts the research is the *researcher* or *investigator*. Studies are often undertaken by a research team rather than by a single researcher.

 HOW-TO-TELL TIP How can you tell if an article appearing in a nursing journal is a *study*? In journals that specialize in research (e.g., the journal *Nursing Research*), most articles are original research reports, but in specialty journals, there is usually a mix of research and nonresearch articles. Sometimes you can tell by the title, but sometimes you cannot. You can tell, however, by looking at the major headings of an article. If there is no heading called "Method" or "Research Design" (the section that describes what a researcher *did*) and no heading called "Findings" or "Results" (the section that describes what a researcher *learned*), then it is probably not a study.

Research can be undertaken in a variety of *settings* (the types of place where information is gathered), such as clinics, homes, or other community settings. A *site* is the broad location for the research—it could be an entire community (e.g., a Haitian neighborhood in Miami) or an institution (e.g., a long-term care facility in Seattle). Researchers sometimes do *multisite studies* because the use of multiple sites yields a larger and often more diverse group of participants.

Concepts, Constructs, and Theories

Nursing research addresses real-world problems, but studies are conceptualized in abstract terms. For example, *pain*, *fatigue*, and *obesity* are abstractions of human attributes. These abstractions are called *phenomena* (especially in qualitative studies) or **concepts**.

Researchers sometimes use the term **construct**, which also refers to an abstraction, but often one that is deliberately invented (or constructed). For example, *self-care* in Orem's model of health maintenance is a construct. The terms *construct* and *concept* are sometimes used interchangeably, but a construct often refers to a more complex abstraction than a concept.

TABLE 2.1 Key Terms in Quantitative and Qualitative Research

Concept	Quantitative Term	Qualitative Term
Person contributing information	Subject Study participant —	— Study participant Informant, key informant
Person undertaking the study	Researcher Investigator	Researcher Investigator
That which is being investigated	— Concepts Constructs Variables	Phenomena Concepts — —
Information gathered	Data (numerical values)	Data (narrative descriptions)
Connections between concepts	Relationships (cause-and-effect, associative)	Patterns of association
Logical reasoning processes	Deductive reasoning	Inductive reasoning

A **theory** is an explanation of some aspect of reality. In a theory, concepts are knitted together into a coherent system to describe or explain some aspect of the world. Theories play a role in both qualitative and quantitative research. In a quantitative study, researchers sometimes start with a theory and, using deductive reasoning, make predictions about how phenomena would behave in the real world *if the theory were valid*. The specific predictions are then tested. In qualitative studies, theory often is the *product* of the research: The investigators use information from study participants inductively to develop a theory rooted in the participants' experiences.

TIP The reasoning process of *deduction* is associated with quantitative research, and *induction* is associated with qualitative research.

Variables

In quantitative studies, concepts are called **variables**. A variable, as the name implies, is something that varies, differs, or changes. Weight, anxiety, and nausea are all variables—they vary from one person to another and can also change over time within the same person. Most human characteristics are variables. If everyone weighed 150 lb, weight would not be a variable, it would be a *constant*. But it is precise because people and conditions *do* vary that most research is conducted. Quantitative researchers seek to understand how or why things vary and to learn how differences in one variable relate to differences in another. For example, in lung cancer research, lung cancer is a variable because not everybody has this disease. Researchers have studied factors that might be linked to lung cancer, such as cigarette smoking. Smoking is also a variable because not everyone smokes. A variable, then, is any quality of a person, group, or situation that varies or takes on different values. Variables are the central building blocks of quantitative studies.

TIP Every study focuses on one or more phenomena, concepts, or variables, but these terms per se are not necessarily used in research reports. For example, a report might say, "The purpose of this study is to examine the effect of nurses' workload on hand hygiene compliance." Although the researcher did not explicitly label anything as a variable, the variables under study are *workload* and *hand hygiene compliance*. Key concepts or variables are often indicated in the study title.

Characteristics of Variables

Variables are often inherent human traits, such as age or weight, but sometimes researchers create a variable. For example, if a researcher tests the effectiveness of patient-controlled analgesia compared to intramuscular analgesia in relieving pain after surgery, some patients would be given one type of analgesia and some would receive the other. In the context of this study, the method of pain management is a variable because different patients are given different methods.

Some variables take on a wide range of values that can be represented on a continuum (e.g., a person's age or weight). Other variables take on only a few values; sometimes such variables convey quantitative information (e.g., number of children), but others simply involve placing people into categories (e.g., blood type A, B, AB, or O).

Dependent and Independent Variables

As noted in Chapter 1, many studies seek to understand causes of phenomena. Does a nursing intervention *cause* improvements in patient outcomes? Does smoking *cause* lung cancer? The presumed cause is the **independent variable**, and the presumed effect is the **dependent**

variable or **outcome variable**. The dependent variable is the outcome that researchers want to understand, explain, or predict. In terms of the PICO scheme discussed in Chapter 1, the dependent variable corresponds to the "O" (outcome). The independent variable corresponds to the "I" (the intervention, influence, or exposure) and the "C" (the comparison).

TIP In searching for evidence, a nurse might want to learn about the effects of an intervention or influence (I), compared to *any* alternative, on an outcome (O) of interest. In a cause-probing study, however, researchers must always specify the comparator (the "C").

The terms *independent variable* and *dependent variable* also can be used to indicate *direction of influence* rather than cause and effect. For example, suppose we compared levels of depression among those diagnosed with pancreatic cancer and found those who identified as men to be more depressed than those who identified as women. We could not conclude that depression was *caused* by gender. Yet the direction of influence begins to link the person's gender identity to depression. In this situation, it is appropriate to consider depression as the dependent variable and gender as the independent variable.

TIP Few research reports explicitly label variables as dependent and independent. Moreover, variables (especially independent variables) are sometimes not fully spelled out. Take the following research question: What is the effect of exercise on heart rate? In this example, heart rate is the dependent variable. Exercise, however, is not in itself a variable. Rather, exercise versus something else (e.g., no exercise) is a variable; "something else" is implied rather than stated in the research question.

Most outcomes have multiple causes or influences. If we were studying factors that influence people's body mass index (BMI), the independent variables might be height, physical activity, and diet. And, two or more outcome variables often are of interest. For example, a researcher may compare the effects of alternative dietary interventions on participants' weight, lipid profile, and self-esteem. It is common to design studies with multiple independent and dependent variables.

Variables are not inherently dependent or independent. A dependent variable in one study could be an independent variable in another. For example, a study might examine the effect of an exercise intervention (the independent variable) on osteoporosis (the dependent variable) to answer a therapy question. Another study might investigate the effect of osteoporosis (the independent variable) on bone fracture incidence (the dependent variable) to address a prognosis question. In short, whether a variable is independent or dependent, it is a function of the role that it plays in a particular study.

Example of independent and dependent variables
Research question: Does magnesium supplementation effectively treat nocturnal leg cramps? (Kaufman et al., 2023)
Independent variable: Magnesium supplementation
Dependent variable: Leg cramps

Conceptual and Operational Definitions

The concepts of interest to researchers are abstractions, and researchers' worldviews shape how those concepts are defined. A **conceptual definition** is the theoretical meaning of a concept. Researchers need to conceptually define even seemingly straightforward terms. A classic example used by nurses, as well as many other health professionals, is the concept of self-care. Ferguson and colleagues (2024) conducted a review of papers describing self-care that were published between 2009 and 2021. In their review of 116 publications, they identified 91 definitions of self-care. Researchers undertaking studies concerning self-care need to clarify how they conceptualize it.

In qualitative studies, conceptual definitions of key phenomena may be a major end product, reflecting an intent to have concepts explained by those being studied. In quantitative studies, however, researchers must define concepts at the outset because they must decide how the variables will be measured. An **operational definition** specifies what the researchers must do to measure the concept and collect needed information.

Readers of research articles may not agree with how researchers conceptualized and operationalized variables. However, definitional precision is important in communicating what concepts mean within the context of the study.

> **Example of conceptual and operational definitions**
> Hou et al. (2022) examined the relationships among social capital, patient empowerment, and self-management in patients undergoing hemodialysis in China. Patient empowerment was conceptually defined as "the degree to which patients are able to act autonomously and think critically concerning their own treatment and care" (p. 2). The construct of patient empowerment was operationalized using the Chinese version of the Client Empowerment Scale.

Data

Research **data** (singular, datum) are the pieces of information gathered in a study. In quantitative studies, researchers identify and define their variables and then collect relevant data from participants. The actual *values* of the study variables constitute the data. Quantitative researchers collect primarily **quantitative data**—information in numeric form. For example, if we conducted a quantitative study in which a key variable was *depression*, we would need to measure how depressed participants were. We might ask, "Thinking about the past week, how depressed would you say you have been on a scale from 0 to 10, where 0 means 'not at all' and 10 means 'the most possible'?" Box 2.1 presents quantitative data for three fictitious people. Subjects provided a number on the 0 to 10 continuum corresponding to their degree of depression—9 for subject 1 (a high level of depression), 0 for subject 2 (no depression), and 4 for subject 3 (mild depression).

In qualitative studies, researchers collect primarily **qualitative data**, that is, narrative descriptions. Narrative data can be obtained by conversing with participants, by making notes about their behavior in naturalistic settings, or by obtaining narrative records, such as diaries. Suppose we were studying depression qualitatively. Box 2.2 presents qualitative data for three participants responding conversationally to the prompt, "Tell me about how

---

Box 2.1 Example of Quantitative Data

Question:	Thinking about the past week, how depressed would you say you have been on a scale from 0 to 10, where 0 means "not at all" and 10 means "the most possible"?	
Data:	9	(Subject 1)
	0	(Subject 2)
	4	(Subject 3)

> **Box 2.2 Example of Qualitative Data**
>
> **Question:** Tell me about how you have been feeling lately in terms of your mood.
> **Data:** "Well, actually, I've been pretty depressed lately, to tell you the truth. I wake up each morning and I can't seem to think of anything to look forward to. I mope around the house all day, kind of in despair. I just can't seem to shake the blues and I've begun to think I need to go see a shrink." (Participant 1)
>
> "I can't remember ever feeling better in my life. I just got promoted to a new job that makes me feel like I can really get ahead in my company. And I've just gotten engaged to a really great guy who is very special." (Participant 2)
>
> "I've had a few ups and downs the past week but basically things are on a pretty even keel. I don't have too many complaints." (Participant 3)

you have been feeling lately in terms of your mood." Here, the data consist of rich narrative descriptions of participants' emotional states. In reports on qualitative studies, researchers include excerpts from their narrative data to support their interpretations.

Relationships

Researchers usually study phenomena in relation to other phenomena—they examine relationships. A **relationship** is a connection between phenomena; for example, researchers repeatedly have found that there is a relationship between frequency of turning bedridden patients and the incidence of pressure injuries. Qualitative and quantitative researchers examine relationships in different ways.

In quantitative studies, relationships are often explicitly expressed in quantitative terms, such as *more than* or *less than*. For example, consider a person's weight as our outcome variable. What variables are related to (associated with) a person's weight? Some possibilities include height, caloric intake, and exercise. For each independent variable, we can make a prediction about its relationship to the outcome:

Height: Tall people will weigh more than short people.
Caloric intake: People with high caloric intake will be heavier than those with low caloric intake.
Exercise: The lower the amount of exercise, the greater will be the person's weight.

Each statement expresses a predicted relationship between weight (the outcome) and a measurable independent variable. Most quantitative research is conducted to assess whether relationships exist among variables and to measure how strong the relationship is.

 TIP Relationships are expressed in two basic forms. First, relationships can be expressed as "if more of Variable X, then more of (or less of) Variable Y." For example, there is a relationship between height and weight: With greater height, there tends to be greater weight, that is, tall people tend to weigh more than short people. The second form involves relationships expressed as group differences. For example, there is a relationship between sex and height: Males tend to be taller than females.

Variables can be related to one another in different ways, including **cause-and-effect (causal) relationships**. Within the positivist paradigm, natural phenomena are assumed to have antecedent causes that are discoverable. For example, we might speculate that there is a causal relationship between caloric intake and weight: All else being equal, eating more calories causes greater weight. As noted in Chapter 1, many quantitative studies are *cause-probing*—they seek to illuminate the causes of phenomena.

> **Example of a study of causal relationships**
> Yıldırım and Gerçeker (2023) studied whether the use of virtual reality and the application of a cold vibration device during intravenous insertion would improve the first-time attempt of intravenous insertion and procedure-related pain, fear, and anxiety in children.

Not all relationships can be interpreted as causal. There is a relationship, for example, between a person's pulmonary artery and tympanic temperatures: People with high readings on one tend to have high readings on the other. We cannot say, however, that pulmonary artery temperature *caused* tympanic temperature, or vice versa. This type of relationship is sometimes referred to as an **associative** (or *functional*) **relationship** rather than a causal one.

> **Example of a study of associative relationships**
> Van Wilder and colleagues (2023) examined psychosocial factors associated with health-related quality of life in 544 patients with chronic diseases. They found that the modifiable factors of illness perception and sense of coherence were associated with health-related quality of life.

Qualitative researchers are not concerned with quantifying relationships nor in testing and confirming causal relationships. However, qualitative researchers may seek patterns of association as a way of illuminating the underlying meaning and dimensionality of phenomena of interest. Patterns of interconnected concepts are identified as a means of understanding the whole.

> **Example of a qualitative study of patterns**
> Utilizing Newman's theory of health as expanding consciousness as the theoretical framework, Shipley and Falkenstern (2023) explored the life patterns of family caregivers of those with amyotrophic lateral sclerosis (ALS). They found nine patterns of the whole across all ALS family caregivers.

MAJOR CLASSES OF QUANTITATIVE AND QUALITATIVE RESEARCH

Researchers usually work within a paradigm that is consistent with their worldview and that gives rise to the types of questions that excite their curiosity. In this section, we briefly describe broad categories of quantitative and qualitative research.

Quantitative Research: Experimental and Nonexperimental Studies

A basic distinction in quantitative studies is between experimental and nonexperimental research. In **experimental research**, researchers actively introduce an intervention or treatment—usually to address therapy questions. In **nonexperimental research**, on the other hand, researchers are bystanders—they collect data without introducing treatments (most often, to address etiology, prognosis, diagnosis, or description questions). For example, if a researcher gave bran flakes to one group of subjects and prune juice to another to evaluate which method facilitated elimination more effectively, the study would be experimental because the researcher intervened. If, on the other hand, a researcher compared elimination patterns of two groups whose regular eating patterns differed, the study would be nonexperimental because there is no intervention. In medical and epidemiologic research, experimental studies usually are called **clinical trials**, and nonexperimental inquiries are called **observational studies**.

Experimental studies are explicitly designed to test causal relationships—to test whether an intervention causes changes in the outcome. Sometimes, nonexperimental studies also explore causal relationships, but causal inferences in nonexperimental research are tricky and less conclusive, for reasons we explain in a later chapter.

Example of experimental research
Leng et al. (2024) examined the impact of a yoga intervention on symptoms of depression and quality of life in the dyad of the care partner and care recipient. Findings suggest that there was a significant decrease in symptoms of depression and an improvement in quality of life with the yoga intervention.

Example of nonexperimental research
Gregory and colleagues (2024) examined data from the 2019 Behavioral Risk Factor Surveillance System (BRFSS). In the sample of 42,727 survey respondents who reported a previous diagnosis of cancer, the researchers explored the proportion of cancer survivors who met the health behavior guidelines recommended by the American Cancer Society (ACS). They found that 84.9% met guidelines for not smoking, 89.5% met guidelines for not drinking excessive alcohol, 66.8% met BMI guidelines, and 51.1% met recommended physical activity levels. However, only 15.1% met the guidelines for adequate fruit and vegetable intake. In this nonexperimental study to address a question about healthy lifestyle, the researchers did not intervene in any way. Their intent was to study the health behaviors in survivors of cancer.

Qualitative Research: Disciplinary Traditions

The majority of qualitative nursing studies can best be described as **qualitative descriptive research**. Many qualitative studies, however, are rooted in research traditions that originated in anthropology, sociology, and psychology. Three such traditions are briefly described here. Chapter 10 provides a fuller discussion of these and other traditions and the methods associated with them.

Grounded theory research seeks to describe and understand key social psychological processes. Grounded theory was developed in the 1960s by two sociologists, Glaser and Strauss (1967). The focus of most grounded theory studies is on a developing social experience—the social and psychological processes that characterize an event or situation. A major component of grounded theory is the discovery of a *core variable* that is central in explaining what is going on in that social scene. Grounded theory researchers strive to generate explanations of phenomena that are grounded in reality.

Example of a grounded theory study
Michaels and Meeker (2024) conducted a grounded theory study to help explain the process of family caregiving to older adults who lived at home in rural areas and

required daily assistance. Two interviews were conducted, each with 15 family caregivers. Results indicated that family caregivers engaged in the process of orchestrating care by growing into caregiving, integrating technology, and utilizing networks when providing and managing caregiving.

Phenomenology is concerned with the lived experiences of humans. Phenomenology is an approach to thinking about what people's life experiences are like and what they mean. Phenomenologic researchers ask questions such as, "What is the *essence* of this phenomenon as experienced by these people?" or "What is the meaning of the phenomenon to those who experience it?"

Example of a phenomenologic study
Bond and colleagues (2025) conducted a phenomenologic study to explore the experiences of racial microaggressions for eight Black individuals while seeking orthopedic-related care.

Ethnography, the primary research tradition in anthropology, provides a framework for studying the patterns and lifeways of a defined cultural group in a holistic fashion. Ethnographers typically engage in extensive *fieldwork*, often participating to the extent possible in the life of the culture under study. Ethnographers strive to learn from members of a cultural group, to understand their worldview, and to describe their customs and norms.

Example of an ethnographic study
Monari et al. (2025) conducted a focused ethnography in Canada to explore Black family members' experiences regarding access to culturally supportive resources for family members and their relatives who suffer from substance use disorders.

MAJOR STEPS IN A QUANTITATIVE STUDY

In quantitative studies, researchers move from the beginning point of a study (posing a question) to the end point (obtaining an answer) in a reasonably linear sequence of steps that is broadly similar across studies (Fig. 2.1). This section describes that flow, and the next section describes how qualitative studies differ.

Phase 1: The Conceptual Phase

The early steps in a quantitative study typically involve activities with a strong conceptual element. During this phase, researchers rely on creativity, deductive reasoning, and grounding in research evidence on the focal topic.

Step 1: Formulating and Delimiting the Problem

Quantitative researchers begin by identifying an interesting research problem and formulating *research questions*. The research questions identify what the study variables are. In developing questions, nurse researchers must attend to substantive issues (Is this problem important?), theoretical issues (Is there a conceptual framework for this problem?), clinical issues (Will findings be useful in clinical practice?), methodologic issues (How can this question be answered to yield high-quality evidence?), and ethical issues (Can this question be addressed in an ethical manner?).

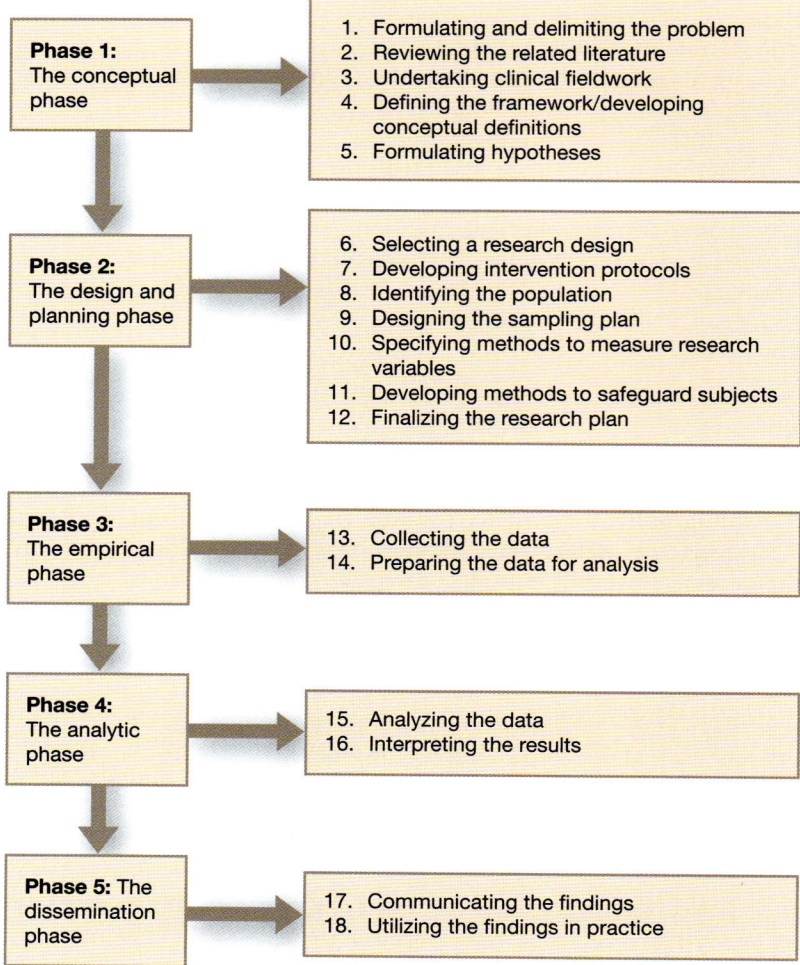

Figure 2.1 Flow of steps in a quantitative study.

Step 2: Reviewing the Related Literature

Quantitative research is conducted within the context of previous knowledge. Quantitative researchers typically strive to understand what is already known about a topic by undertaking a thorough **literature review** before any data are collected.

Step 3: Undertaking Clinical Fieldwork

Researchers embarking on a clinical study often benefit from spending time in relevant clinical settings (in the *field*), discussing the topic with clinicians, and observing current practices. Such clinical fieldwork can provide perspectives on clinicians' and patients' viewpoints.

Step 4: Defining the Framework and Developing Conceptual Definitions

When quantitative research is performed within the context of a theoretical framework, the findings may have broader significance and utility. Even when the research question is not embedded in a theory, researchers should have a conceptual rationale and a clear vision of the concepts under study.

Step 5: Formulating Hypotheses

A **hypothesis** states the researchers' expectations about relationships between study variables. Hypotheses are predictions of the relationships that researchers expect to observe in the study data. The research question identifies the concepts of interest and asks how the concepts might be related; a hypothesis is the predicted answer. Most quantitative studies are designed to test hypotheses through statistical analysis.

Phase 2: The Design and Planning Phase

In the second major phase of a quantitative study, researchers decide on the methods they will use to address the research question. Researchers make many methodologic decisions that have crucial implications for the quality of study evidence.

Step 6: Selecting a Research Design

The **research design** is the overall plan for obtaining answers to the research questions. Quantitative designs tend to be structured and controlled, with the goal of minimizing bias. Research designs also indicate how often data will be collected and what types of comparisons will be made. The research design is the architectural backbone of the study.

Step 7: Developing Protocols for the Intervention

In experimental research, researchers introduce an intervention. An **intervention protocol** for the study must be developed, specifying exactly what the intervention will entail (e.g., who will administer it, over how long a period will the treatment last, and so on) *and* what the comparative condition will be. In nonexperimental research, this latter step is not necessary.

Step 8: Identifying the Population

Quantitative researchers need to specify what characteristics study participants should possess—that is, they must identify the population to be studied. A **population** is *all* the individuals or objects with common, defining characteristics (the "P" component in PICO questions).

Step 9: Designing the Sampling Plan

Researchers collect data from a **sample**, which is a subset of the population. The researcher's *sampling plan* specifies how the sample will be selected and how many participants here will be. The goal is to have a sample that adequately reflects the population's traits.

Step 10: Specifying Methods to Measure Research Variables

Quantitative researchers must find methods to measure their research variables accurately. A variety of quantitative data collection approaches exist; the primary methods are *self-reports* (e.g., interviews and questionnaires), *observations* (e.g., watching and recording people's behavior), and *biophysiologic measures (biomarkers)*. The task of measuring research variables and developing a *data collection plan* is complex and challenging.

Step 11: Developing Methods to Safeguard Human/Animal Rights

Most nursing research involves humans, although some involves animals. In either case, procedures need to be developed to ensure that the study adheres to ethical principles.

Step 12: Reviewing and Finalizing the Research Plan

Before collecting data, researchers often undertake assessments to ensure that procedures will work smoothly. For example, they may evaluate the *readability* of written materials to see if participants with low reading skills can comprehend them. Researchers usually have their research plan critiqued by reviewers to obtain clinical or methodologic feedback. Researchers seeking financial support submit a *proposal* to a funding source.

Phase 3: The Empirical Phase

The third phase of quantitative research involves collecting the data. This phase is often the most time-consuming part of the study. Data collection often requires months or years of work.

Step 13: Collecting the Data

The actual collection of data in a quantitative study often proceeds according to a preestablished plan. The plan typically spells out procedures for training data collection staff, for implementing the sampling plan and collecting data (e.g., where and when the data will be gathered), and for recording information.

Step 14: Preparing the Data for Analysis

Data collected in a quantitative study must be prepared for analysis. For example, one preliminary step is *coding*, which involves translating verbal data into numeric form (e.g., coding sex information as "1" for females, "2" for males, and "3" for declined to answer).

Phase 4: The Analytic Phase

Quantitative data must be subjected to analysis and interpretation, which occur in the fourth major phase of a project.

Step 15: Analyzing the Data

To answer research questions and test hypotheses, researchers analyze their data in a systematic fashion. Quantitative data are analyzed through **statistical analyses**, which include some simple procedures (e.g., computing an average) as well as more complex methods.

Step 16: Interpreting the Results

Interpretation involves making sense of study results and examining their implications. Researchers attempt to explain the findings in light of prior evidence, theory, and clinical experience—and in light of the adequacy of the methods they used in the study. Interpretation also involves coming to conclusions about the *clinical significance* of the new evidence.

Phase 5: The Dissemination Phase

In the analytic phase, researchers come full circle: The questions posed at the outset are answered. The researchers' job is incomplete, however, until study results are disseminated.

Step 17: Communicating the Findings

A study cannot contribute evidence to nursing practice if the results are not communicated. Another—and often final—task of a research project is the preparation of a *research report* that can be shared with others. We discuss research reports in the next chapter.

Step 18: Putting the Evidence Into Practice

Ideally, the concluding step of a high-quality study is to plan for its use in practice settings. Although nurse researchers may not implement a plan for using research findings, they can contribute to the process by developing recommendations on how the evidence could be used in practice, by ensuring that adequate information has been provided for a meta-analysis, and by pursuing opportunities to disseminate the findings to practicing nurses.

ACTIVITIES IN A QUALITATIVE STUDY

Quantitative research involves a fairly linear progression of tasks—researchers plan what steps to take and then follow those steps. In qualitative studies, by contrast, the progression is closer to a circle than to a straight line. Qualitative researchers continually examine and interpret data and make decisions about how to proceed based on what has been discovered (Fig. 2.2).

As qualitative researchers have a flexible approach, we cannot show the flow of activities precisely—the flow varies from one study to another, and researchers themselves may not know in advance how the study will unfold. We provide a general sense of qualitative studies by describing major activities and indicating when they might be performed.

Conceptualizing and Planning a Qualitative Study

Identifying the Research Problem

Qualitative researchers usually begin with a general topic, often focusing on an aspect about which little is known. Qualitative researchers often proceed with a fairly broad initial question that allows the focus to be sharpened and delineated more clearly once the study is underway.

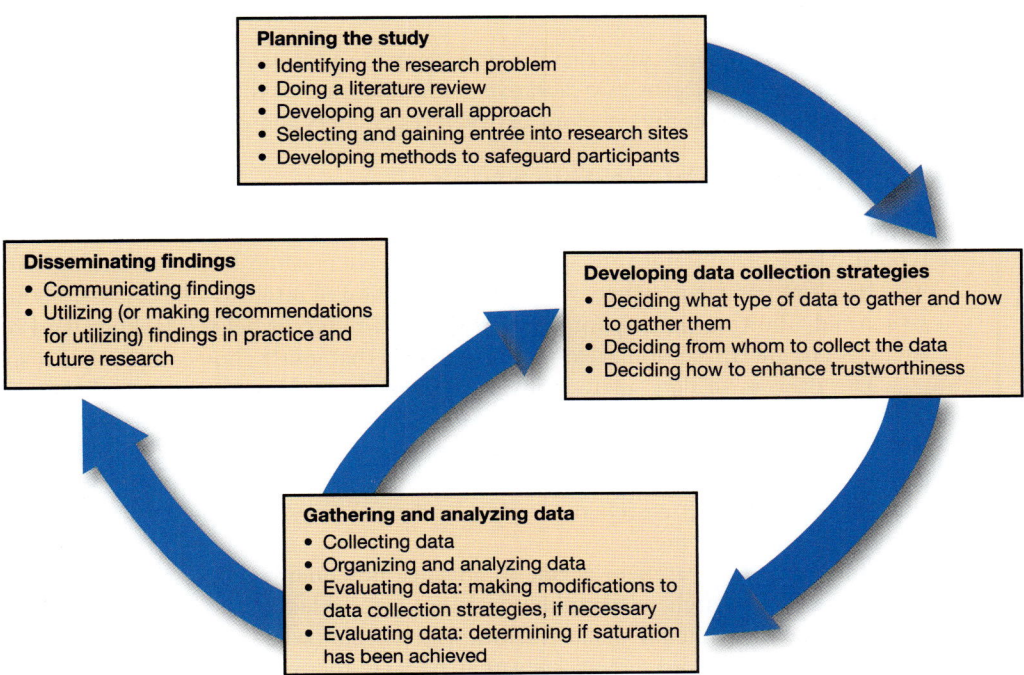

Figure 2.2 Flow of activities in a qualitative study.

Doing a Literature Review

Some qualitative researchers avoid consulting the literature before collecting data. They worry that prior studies might influence the conceptualization of the phenomenon under study, which they believe should be based on participants' viewpoints rather than on prior findings. Others believe that researchers should conduct at least a brief literature review at the outset. In any case, qualitative researchers typically find a relatively small body of relevant previous work because of the type of questions they ask.

Selecting and Gaining Entrée Into Research Sites

Before going into the field, qualitative researchers must identify an appropriate site. For example, if the topic is the health beliefs of people living in low-income urban areas, an inner-city neighborhood with a concentration of low-income residents must be identified. In some cases, researchers may have access to the selected site, but in others they need to gain entrée into it. **Gaining entrée** typically involves negotiations with *gatekeepers* who have the authority to permit entry into their world.

> **TIP** The process of gaining entrée is usually associated with doing fieldwork in qualitative studies, but quantitative researchers often need to gain entrée into sites for collecting data as well.

Developing an Overall Approach

Quantitative researchers do not collect data before finalizing their research design. Qualitative researchers, by contrast, use an **emergent design** that materializes during data collection. Certain design features are guided by the study's qualitative tradition, but qualitative studies rarely have rigid designs that prohibit changes while in the field.

Addressing Ethical Issues

Qualitative researchers must also develop plans for addressing ethical issues—and, indeed, there are special concerns in qualitative studies because of the more intimate nature of the relationship that typically develops between researchers and participants.

Conducting a Qualitative Study

In qualitative studies, the tasks of sampling, data collection, data analysis, and interpretation typically take place iteratively. Qualitative researchers often begin by talking with people who have firsthand experience with the phenomenon of interest. The discussions are loosely structured, allowing participants to express a full range of beliefs, feelings, and behaviors. Analysis and interpretation are ongoing activities that guide choices about "next steps."

The process of data analysis involves clustering related narrative information into a coherent scheme. Through inductive reasoning, researchers identify **themes** and categories, which are used to build a rich description or theory of the phenomenon. Data gathering becomes increasingly purposeful: As conceptualizations develop, researchers seek participants who can confirm and enrich theoretical understandings, as well as participants who can potentially challenge them.

Quantitative researchers decide in advance how many people to include in the study, but qualitative researchers' sampling decisions are guided by the data. Many qualitative researchers use the principle of **saturation**, which occurs when participants' accounts of their experiences become redundant, such that no new thematic development can occur from further data collection.

> **Box 2.3 Additional Questions for a Preliminary Review of a Study**
>
> a. What was the study all about? What were the main phenomena, concepts, or constructs under investigation?
> b. If the study was quantitative, what were the independent and dependent variables?
> c. Did the researcher examine relationships or patterns of association among variables or concepts? Did the report imply the possibility of a causal relationship?
> d. Were key concepts defined, both conceptually and operationally?
> e. What type of study does it appear to be, in terms of types described in this chapter—experimental or nonexperimental/observational? Grounded theory, phenomenologic, or ethnographic?
> f. Did the report provide information to suggest how long the study took to complete?

Quantitative researchers seek to collect high-quality data by measuring their variables with instruments that have been demonstrated to be accurate and valid. Qualitative researchers, by contrast, *are* the main data collection instrument and must take steps to demonstrate the trustworthiness of the data. The central feature of these efforts is to confirm that the findings accurately reflect the viewpoints of participants, rather than researchers' perceptions. One confirmatory activity, for example, involves going back to participants, sharing preliminary interpretations with them, and asking them to evaluate whether the researcher's thematic analysis is consistent with their experiences.

Qualitative nursing researchers also strive to share their findings at conferences and in journal articles. Qualitative studies help to shape nurses' perceptions of a problem, their conceptualizations of potential solutions, and their understanding of patients' concerns and experiences.

GENERAL QUESTIONS IN REVIEWING A STUDY

Box 2.3 presents some further suggestions for performing a preliminary overview of a research report, drawing on concepts explained in this chapter. These guidelines supplement those presented in Box 1.1, Chapter 1.

RESEARCH EXAMPLES WITH CRITICAL THINKING EXERCISES

In this section, we illustrate the progression of activities and discuss the time schedule of a study conducted by the second author of this book. Read the summary for Example 1, and then answer the critical thinking questions that follow. The critical thinking questions for Examples 2 and 3 are based on the studies that appear in their entirety in Appendices A and B of this book.

EXAMPLE 1: PROJECT SCHEDULE FOR A QUALITATIVE STUDY

Study: "Posttraumatic growth after postpartum psychosis" (Beck & Twomey, 2023)

Purpose: The purpose of the study was to explore positive changes in women's beliefs, emotions, and behaviors following their struggles with postpartum psychosis.

Methods: This study required 2 years and 6 months to complete. Key activities and methodologic decisions included the following:

- **Phase 1. Conceptualizing, designing, and planning phases (6 months):** Beck, one of the authors of this textbook, had conducted four other studies on posttraumatic growth and one study on postpartum psychosis. Twomey experienced postpartum psychosis and is an advocate for this serious mental health disorder after childbirth. Beck and Twomey were familiar with published research in these areas, so they did not need an extended period of time to review the literature. Beck and Twomey decided on a descriptive qualitative study with content analysis to analyze the data.
- **Phase 2. Empirical/analytic phases (11 months):** Beck and Twomey recruited through postings on three postpartum psychosis Facebook groups. Beck's university email address was posted, and individuals interested in learning more about the study and how to participate emailed her. After reading the information sheet, participants sent their narratives on attachment to the researchers which implied their informed consent. Thirteen mothers participated in the study. It took 8 months to recruit the sample and collect the data. Analysis of mothers' narratives of posttraumatic growth following postpartum psychosis took an additional 3 months.
- **Phase 3. Dissemination phase (13 months):** It took approximately 6 months to prepare the manuscript reporting this study. It took about 7 months to get the manuscript published. It was submitted to *MCN: The American Journal of Maternal Child Nursing* on March 29, 2023. This journal had an unusually rapid response, and 1 month later on April 28, 2023 Beck and Twomey received a revise and resubmit decision from the editor of the journal. Only minor revisions were needed, so on May 9, 2023 the authors submitted their revised manuscript. Only 1 day later on May 10, 2023 the authors received notification that their manuscript had been accepted for publication. The article was first published early online on July 23, 2023, and then published in the November/December issue of *MCN: The American Journal of Maternal Child Nursing*.

Critical Thinking Exercises

1. Answer the relevant questions from Box 2.3 regarding this study.
2. Do you think an appropriate amount of time was allocated to the various phases and steps in this study?
3. Would it have been appropriate for the researchers to address the research question using quantitative research methods? Why or why not?
4. If the results of this study are valid, what might be some of the ways the findings could be used in clinical practice?

EXAMPLE 2: QUANTITATIVE RESEARCH IN APPENDIX A

Read the abstract and the introduction in Cheng and colleagues' (2024) study "Advance care planning affects end-of-life treatment preferences among patients with heart failure: A randomized controlled trial" in Appendix A of this book.

Critical Thinking Exercises

1. Answer the relevant questions from Box 2.3 regarding this study.
2. Comment on the composition of the research team for this study.

3. Did this report present any actual data from the study participants?
4. Would it have been possible for the researchers to use an experimental design for this study?

EXAMPLE 3: QUALITATIVE RESEARCH IN APPENDIX B

Read the abstract and the introduction from Morrison and colleagues' 2024 study "Lived experiences of fatherhood after infertility" in Appendix B of this book.
1. Answer the relevant questions from Box 2.3 regarding this study.
2. Did this report present any actual data from the study participants? What is an example?
3. What information is provided in the article about the schedule for this project?

Summary Points

- The people who provide information to the researchers in a study are called **subjects** or **study participants** in quantitative research, and study participants or informants in qualitative research; collectively, they comprise the study **sample**.
- The *site* is the location for the research; researchers sometimes engage in *multisite studies*.
- Researchers investigate **concepts** and *phenomena* (or **constructs**), which are abstractions inferred from people's behavior or attributes.
- Concepts are the building blocks of theories. A **theory** is a systematic explanation of some aspect of the real world.
- In quantitative studies, concepts are called **variables**. A variable is a characteristic or quality that takes on different values (i.e., varies from one person or object to another).
- The **dependent (or outcome) variable** is the behavior, characteristic, or outcome the researcher is interested in explaining, predicting, or affecting (the "O" in the PICO format). The **independent variable** is the presumed cause of or influence on the dependent variable. The independent variable corresponds to the "I" and the "C" components in the PICO scheme.
- A **conceptual definition** describes the abstract meaning of a concept being studied. An **operational definition** specifies how a variable will be measured.
- **Data**—the information collected during the course of a study—may take the form of narrative information (**qualitative data**) or numeric values (**quantitative data**).
- A **relationship** is a connection or pattern of association between variables. Quantitative researchers study the relationship between independent variables and outcome variables.
- When the independent variable is a cause of the dependent variable, the relationship is a **cause-and-effect (causal) relationship**. In an **associative** (*functional*) **relationship**, variables are related in a noncausal manner.
- A key distinction in quantitative studies is between **experimental research**, in which researchers actively intervene to test an intervention or therapy, and **nonexperimental research** (**observational studies**), in which researchers collect data about phenomena without intervening.
- Qualitative research sometimes is rooted in research traditions that originate in other disciplines. Three such traditions are grounded theory, phenomenology, and ethnography.
- **Grounded theory** seeks to describe and understand key social psychological processes that occur in a social setting.

- **Phenomenology** focuses on the lived experiences of humans and is an approach to gaining insight into what the life experiences of people are like and what they mean.
- **Ethnography** provides a framework for studying the meanings, patterns, and lifeways of a culture in a holistic fashion.
- In a quantitative study, researchers usually progress in a series of linear steps, from asking research questions to answering them. The main phases in a quantitative study are the conceptual, planning, empirical, analytic, and dissemination phases.
- The *conceptual phase* involves (1) defining the problem to be studied, (2) doing a **literature review,** (3) engaging in *clinical fieldwork* for clinical studies, (4) developing a framework and conceptual definitions, and (5) formulating **hypotheses** to be tested.
- The *planning phase* entails (6) selecting a **research design,** (7) developing **intervention protocols** if the study is experimental, (8) specifying the **population** (the "P" in the PICO format), (9) developing a *sampling plan*, (10) specifying a *data collection plan* and methods to measure variables, (11) developing strategies to safeguard participants' rights, and (12) finalizing the research plan.
- The *empirical phase* involves (13) collecting data and (14) preparing data for analysis (e.g., *coding* data).
- The *analytic phase* involves (15) performing **statistical analyses** and (16) interpreting the results.
- The *dissemination phase* entails (17) communicating the findings and (18) promoting the use of the study evidence in nursing practice.
- The flow of activities in a qualitative study is flexible and less linear than in a quantitative study. Qualitative studies typically involve an **emergent design** that evolves during data collection.
- Qualitative researchers begin with a broad question regarding a phenomenon of interest, often focusing on a little-studied aspect. In the early phase of a qualitative study, researchers select a site and seek to **gain entrée** into it, which typically involves enlisting the cooperation of *gatekeepers* within the site.
- Once in the field, qualitative researchers select informants, collect data, and then analyze and interpret them in an iterative fashion; experiences during data collection help in an ongoing fashion to shape the design of the study.
- Early analysis in qualitative research leads to refinements in sampling and data collection, until **saturation** (redundancy of information) is achieved. Analysis typically involves a search for critical **themes** or categories in the data.
- Both qualitative and quantitative researchers disseminate their findings, most often by publishing their research reports in professional journals.

REFERENCES

Beck, C. T., & Twomey, T. (2023). Posttraumatic growth after postpartum psychosis. *MCN: The American Journal of Maternal Child Nursing*, 48(6), 303–311. https://doi.org/10.1097/NMC.0000000000000954

Bond, J., Julion, W. A., Shattell, M., Healey, W., & Reed, M. (2025). The lived experiences of racial microaggressions for Black individuals while seeking orthopedic-related care: A qualitative study. *Journal of Racial and Ethnic Health Disparities*, 12(4), 2424–2442. https://doi.org/10.1007/s40615-024-02063-4

Ferguson, L., Anderson, M. E., Satchi, K., Capron, A. M., Kaplan, C. D., Redfield, P., & Gruskin, S. (2024). The ubiquity of 'self-care' in health: Why specificity matters. *Global Public Health*, 19(1), 2296970. https://doi.org/10.1080/17441692.2023.2296970

Glaser, B. G., & Strauss, A. L. (1967). *The discovery of grounded theory: Strategies for qualitative research*. Aldine.

Gregory, K., Zhao, L., Felder, T. M., Clay-Gilmour, A., Eberth, J. M., Murphy, E. A., & Steck, S. E. (2024). Prevalence of health behaviors among cancer survivors in the United States. *Journal of Cancer Survivorship: Research and Practice*, 18(3), 1042–1050. https://doi.org/10.1007/s11764-023-01347-8

Hou, Y., Li, L., Zhou, Q., Wang, G., & Li, R. (2022). Relationships between social capital, patient empowerment, and self-management of patients undergoing hemodialysis: a cross-sectional study. *BMC Nephrology*, *23*(1), 71. https://doi.org/10.1186/s12882-022-02669-y

Kaufman, N., White, D., Bull, J., Radi, R., & DeSanto, K. (2023). Does magnesium supplementation treat nocturnal leg cramps? *American Family Physician*, *108*(6), 619–620. https://www.aafp.org/pubs/afp/issues/2023/1200/fpin-ci-magnesium-nocturnal-leg-cramps.html

Leng, Q. L., Lyons, K. S., Winters-Stone, K. M., Medysky, M. E., Dieckmann, N. F., Denfeld, Q. E., & Sullivan, D. R. (2024). Preliminary effects of a yoga intervention for lung cancer dyads: benefits for care partners. *Supportive Care in Cancer*, *32*(7), 447. https://doi.org/10.1007/s00520-024-08638-5

Michaels, J. A., & Meeker, M. A. (2024). Orchestrating care: A grounded theory study of family caregiving for older adults in rural areas. *Qualitative Health Research*, *34*(12), 1231–1242. https://doi.org/10.1177/10497323241236308

Monari, E. N., Booth, R., Forchuk, C., & Csiernik, R. (2025). Black family members' experiences and interpretations of supportive resources for them and their relatives with substance use disorders: A focused ethnography. *Qualitative Health Research*, *35*(3), 379–392. https://doi.org/10.1177/10497323241263261

Shipley, P. Z., & Falkenstern, S. K. (2023). Life patterns of family caregivers of patients with amyotrophic lateral sclerosis. *Nursing Science Quarterly*, *36*(4), 356–368. https://doi.org/10.1177/08943184231187903

Van Wilder, L., Vandepitte, S., Clays, E., Devleesschauwer, B., Pype, P., Boeckxstaens, P., Schrans, D., & De Smedt, D. (2023). Psychosocial factors associated with health-related quality of life in patients with chronic disease: Results of a cross-sectional survey. *Chronic Illness*, *19*(4), 743–757. https://doi.org/10.1177/17423953221124313

Yıldırım, B. G., & Gerçeker, G. Ö. (2023). The effect of virtual reality and buzzy on first insertion success, procedure-related fear, anxiety, and pain in children during Intravenous Insertion in the pediatric emergency unit: A randomized controlled trial. *Journal of Emergency Nursing*, *49*(1), 62–74. https://doi.org/10.1016/j.jen.2022.09.018

3 Reading and Critically Appraising Research Articles

Learning Objectives

On completing this chapter, you will be able to:

- Identify and describe the major sections of a research journal article
- Characterize the style used in quantitative and qualitative research reports
- Read a research article and broadly grasp its "story"
- Describe aspects of a critical appraisal of a study
- Understand the many challenges researchers face and identify some tools they use to address methodologic challenges
- Define new terms in the chapter

Key Terms

- Abstract
- Bias
- Blinding
- Confounding variable
- Credibility
- Critical appraisal
- Findings
- IMRAD format
- Inference
- Journal article
- Level of significance
- p
- Placebo
- Positionality statement
- Randomness
- Reflexivity
- Reliability
- Research control
- Scientific merit
- Statistical significance
- Statistical test
- Transferability
- Triangulation
- Trustworthiness
- Validity

Evidence from nursing studies is communicated through research reports that describe what was studied, how it was studied, and what was found. Research reports are often daunting to readers without research training. This chapter aims to make research reports more accessible and provides some guidance regarding critical appraisals of research reports.

TYPES OF RESEARCH REPORTS

Nurses are most likely to find research evidence in journals or at nursing conferences. Research **journal articles** are descriptions of studies published in professional journals. Competition for journal space is keen, so research articles are brief—generally only 10 to 20 double-spaced pages. This means that researchers must condense a lot of information about the study into a short report.

Usually, manuscripts are reviewed by two or more *peer reviewers* (other researchers) who make recommendations to the journal editor about accepting or requesting revisions to the manuscript. Reviews are usually *blind*—reviewers are not told researchers' names, and authors are not told reviewers' names. Consumers thus have some assurance that journals articles have been vetted by impartial nurse researchers. Nevertheless, publication does not mean that the findings can be uncritically accepted. Research methods courses help nurses evaluate the quality of evidence reported in journal articles.

At conferences, research findings are presented as oral presentations or poster sessions. In an *oral presentation*, researchers are typically allotted 10 to 20 minutes to describe key features of their study to an audience. In *poster sessions*, many researchers simultaneously present visual displays summarizing their studies, and conference attendees walk around the room looking at the displays. Conferences offer an opportunity for dialogue: Attendees can ask questions to help them better understand what the findings mean; moreover, they can offer and receive suggestions relating to clinical implications of the study. Thus, professional conferences are a valuable forum for clinical audiences.

THE CONTENT OF RESEARCH JOURNAL ARTICLES

Many research articles are structured using the **IMRAD format**. This format organizes content into four main sections—**I**ntroduction, **M**ethod, **R**esults, **a**nd **D**iscussion. The paper starts with a title and an abstract and concludes with references.

The Title and Abstract

Research reports have titles that succinctly convey key information. In qualitative studies, the title normally includes the central phenomenon and group under investigation. In quantitative studies, the title communicates key variables and the population (in other words, PICO components).

The **abstract** is a brief description of the study placed at the beginning of the article. The abstract answers questions like the following: What were the research questions? What methods were used to address those questions? What were the findings? and What are the implications for nursing practice? Readers can review an abstract to judge whether to read the full report.

The Introduction

The introduction to a research article acquaints readers with the research problem and its context. This section usually describes the following:

- The central phenomena, concepts, or variables under study
- The study purpose and research questions or hypotheses
- A brief review of related literature
- The theoretical or conceptual framework
- The significance of and need for the study

Thus, the introduction lets readers understand the problem the researcher sought to address.

> **Example of introductory material (modified)**
> "Most self-care studies … are focused on self-care maintenance and/or monitoring but not self-care management … [T]here is significant room for improvement in our ability to intervene with self-care interventions … and … close a key knowledge gap related to self-care management behaviors in cardiovascular disease" (Lee et al., 2024, p. 2; references removed).

In this paragraph, the researchers described the population of interest (people experiencing chronic cardiovascular disease), the central concept of the study (self-care management behaviors such as engaging in regular exercise and monitoring of signs and symptoms of change), and the gap in current knowledge.

 TIP The introduction section of most reports is often not specifically labeled "Introduction." The introduction immediately follows the abstract.

The Method Section

The method section describes the methods used to answer the research questions. In a quantitative study, the method section usually describes the following, which may be presented in labeled subsections:

- The research design
- The sampling plan
- Methods of measuring variables and collecting study data
- Study procedures, including procedures to protect human rights
- Data analysis methods

Qualitative researchers discuss many of the same issues, but with different emphases. For example, a qualitative study often provides more information about the research setting and the study context. Reports of qualitative studies also describe the researchers' efforts to enhance the integrity of the study.

The Results Section

The results section presents the **findings** that were obtained by analyzing the study data. The text presents a narrative summary of key findings, often accompanied by more detailed tables. Virtually all results sections contain descriptive information, including a description of the participants (e.g., average age, percent married or unmarried).

In quantitative studies, the results section usually reports the following information relating to **statistical tests** performed:

- *The names of statistical tests used*. Researchers test their hypotheses and assess the probability that the results are reliable using statistical tests. For example, if the researcher finds that the average birth weight of drug-exposed infants in the sample is lower than the birth weight of infants not exposed to drugs, how probable is it that the same would be true for the population of infants? A statistical test helps answer the question—Is the relationship between prenatal drug exposure and infant birth weight *real*, and would it likely be observed with a new sample from the same population? Statistical tests are based on common principles; you do not have to know the names of all statistical tests to comprehend the findings.
- *The value of the calculated statistic*. Computers are used to calculate a numeric value for the particular statistical test used. The value allows researchers to reach conclusions about their hypotheses. The *actual* value of the statistic, however, is not inherently meaningful and need not concern you.
- *Statistical significance*. A critical piece of information is whether the statistical tests were significant (not to be confused with clinically important). If a researcher reports that the results are statistically significant, it means the findings are probably true and replicable. Research reports also indicate the **level of significance**, which is an index of how *probable* it is that the findings are reliable. For example, if a report indicates that a finding was

significant at the .05 probability level (symbolized as *p*), this means that only five times out of 100 (5 ÷ 100 = .05) would the obtained result be spurious. In other words, 95 times out of 100, similar results would be obtained with a new sample. Readers can thus have a high degree of confidence—but not total assurance—that the results are accurate.

> **Example from the results section of a quantitative study**
> He and colleagues (2022) conducted a randomized clinical control trial in China to examine the effectiveness of a 16-week dance intervention to reduce the incidence of the fatigue–sleep disturbance–depression symptom cluster and improve the quality of life in patients with breast cancer who underwent *adjuvant chemotherapy*. Results indicated that at the completion of the intervention, those in the intervention group had a lower incidence of the symptom cluster ($p = .003$) and an increase in quality of life ($p = .001$) compared with the control group.

In this example, the researchers stated that the fatigue–sleep disturbance–depression symptom cluster and quality of life were significantly better among those who received the intervention. The differences between the groups were not likely to have been haphazard and probably would be replicated with a new sample. These findings are very reliable. For example, with regard to quality of life, it was found that a group difference of the magnitude obtained would occur just as a "fluke" less than 1 time in 1,000 ($p < .001$).

> **TIP** Results are *more* reliable if the *p* value is *smaller*. For example, there is a higher probability that the results are accurate when $p = .01$ (1 in 100 chance of a spurious result) than when $p = .05$ (5 in 100 chances of a spurious result). Researchers sometimes report an exact probability (e.g., $p = .03$) or a probability below conventional thresholds (e.g., $p < .05$—less than 5 in 100).

In qualitative reports, researchers often organize findings according to the major themes, processes, or categories that were identified in the data. The results section of qualitative reports sometimes has several subsections, the headings of which correspond to the researcher's labels for the themes. Excerpts from the *raw data* (the actual words of participants) are presented to support and provide a rich description of the thematic analysis. The results section of qualitative studies may also present the researcher's emerging theory about the phenomenon under study.

> **Example from the results section of a qualitative study**
> Weiss and colleagues (2024) used a qualitative descriptive design to explore the best practices for telehealth in nurse-led care settings in Colorado. They interviewed 18 providers and 30 patients and identified four themes: "(1) using multiple modalities, (2) tailoring triage and scheduling, (3) cultivating safety through boundaries and expectations, and (4) differentiating established versus new patient relationships" (p. 51).

The Discussion Section

In the discussion, the researcher presents conclusions about the meaning and implications of the findings, that is, what the results mean, why things turned out the way they did, how the findings fit with other evidence, and how the results can be used in practice. The discussion in both qualitative and quantitative reports may include the following elements:

- An interpretation of the results
- Clinical and research implications
- Study limitations and ramifications for the believability of the results

Researchers are in the best position to point out deficiencies in their studies. A discussion section that presents the researcher's grasp of study limitations demonstrates to readers that the authors were aware of the limitations and likely took them into account in interpreting the findings.

References

Research articles conclude with a list of the articles and books that were referenced. If you are interested in learning more about a topic, the reference list of a recent study is a good place to begin.

THE STYLE OF RESEARCH JOURNAL ARTICLES

Research reports tell a story. However, the style in which many research journal articles are written—especially for quantitative studies—makes it difficult for some readers to understand or become interested in the story.

Why Are Research Articles so Hard to Read?

To unaccustomed audiences, research reports may seem bewildering. Four factors contribute to this impression:

1. *Compactness.* Journal space is limited, so authors compress a lot of information into a small space. Interesting, personalized aspects of the investigation cannot be reported, and, in qualitative studies, only a handful of supporting quotes can be included.
2. *Jargon.* The authors of research articles use research terms that may seem esoteric.
3. *Objectivity.* Quantitative researchers tend to avoid any impression of subjectivity, and so they tell their research stories in a way that makes them sound impersonal. Most quantitative research articles are written in the passive voice, which tends to make the articles less inviting and lively. Qualitative reports are often written in a more conversational style.
4. *Statistical information.* In quantitative reports, numbers and statistical symbols may intimidate readers who do not have statistical training.

A goal of this textbook is to assist you in understanding the content of research reports and in overcoming anxieties about jargon and statistical information.

 HOW-TO-TELL TIP How can you tell if the voice is active or passive? In the active voice, the article would say what the researchers *did* (e.g., "We used a mercury sphygmomanometer to measure blood pressure"). In the passive voice, the article indicates what *was done*, without indicating who did it, although it is implied that the researchers were the agents (e.g., "A mercury sphygmomanometer *was used* to measure blood pressure").

Tips on Reading Research Articles

As you progress through this book, you will acquire skills for evaluating research articles, but the skills involved in critical appraisal take time to develop. The first step is to comprehend research articles. Here are some hints on digesting research reports.

- Grow accustomed to the style of research articles by reading them frequently, even though you may not yet understand the technical points.
- Read journal articles slowly. It may be useful to skim the article first to get the major points and then read the article more carefully a second time.

- On the second reading, train yourself to become an *active* reader. Reading actively means constantly monitoring yourself to verify that you understand what you are reading. If you have difficulty, you can ask someone for help. In most cases, that "someone" will be your instructor, but also consider contacting the researchers themselves.
- Keep this textbook with you as a reference when you read articles so that you can look up unfamiliar terms in the glossary or index.
- Try not to get bogged down in (or scared away by) statistical information. Try to grasp the gist of the story without letting symbols and numbers frustrate you.

CRITICALLY APPRAISING RESEARCH REPORTS

A critical reading of a research article involves a careful appraisal of the researcher's major conceptual and methodologic decisions. It would be difficult to assess these decisions at this point, but your skills will improve as you progress through this book.

Research Critiques and Critical Appraisals

A distinction is sometimes made between a research *critique* and a critical appraisal. The latter term is favored by those focusing on the evaluation of evidence for nursing practice. The term *critique* is more often used when individual studies are being evaluated for their scientific merit—for example, when a manuscript is reviewed by *peer reviewers* who make recommendations about publishing the paper in a journal. In both cases, the goal is to apply knowledge about research methods, theory, and substantive issues to draw conclusions about the validity and relevance of the findings.

Both critiques and critical appraisals involve objective assessments of a study's strengths and limitations, but they vary in scope and aims. Peer reviewers who are asked to prepare a written critique for a manuscript submitted to a journal may evaluate the strengths and weaknesses in terms of substantive issues (Was the research problem significant to nursing?), theoretical issues (Were the conceptual underpinnings sound?), methodologic decisions (Were the methods rigorous, yielding believable evidence?), interpretive (Did the researcher reach defensible conclusions?), ethics (Were participants' rights protected?), and style (Is the report clear, grammatical, and well organized?). In short, peer reviewers do a comprehensive review to provide feedback to the researchers and to journal editors about the merit of both the study and the report and typically offer suggestions for revisions.

Critical appraisals designed to inform evidence-based nursing practice are seldom comprehensive. For example, it is of little consequence to evidence-based practice (EBP) that an article is ungrammatical. An appraisal of the clinical utility of a study focuses on whether the evidence is accurate, sound, and clinically relevant—the focus is on appraising the research methods and the findings themselves.

Students taking a research methods course also may be asked to appraise a study. Such appraisals are often intended to cultivate critical thinking and to induce students to apply newly acquired skills in research methods.

Critical Appraisal Support in This Textbook

We provide a couple of types of support for the critical appraisal of individual studies. First, suggestions for appraising relevant aspects of a study are included at the end of each chapter.

Second, we offer key appraisal guidelines for quantitative and qualitative reports in this chapter, in Tables 3.1 and 3.2, respectively. The questions in the guidelines concern the rigor with which the researchers dealt with critical research challenges, some of which we describe in the next section.

TABLE 3.1 Guide to a Focused Critical Appraisal of Evidence Quality in a Quantitative Research Report

Aspect of the Report	Critical Appraisal Questions	Detailed Appraisal Guidelines
Method Research design	• What was the level of evidence for the study, and was the level the highest possible for the study purpose? • Were appropriate comparisons made to enhance interpretability of the findings? • Was the number of data collection points appropriate? Was the period of follow-up (if any) adequate? • Did the design minimize biases and threats to the validity of the study (e.g., was blinding used, was attrition low)?	Box 8.1 in Chapter 8
Population and sample	• Was the population of interest clearly identified? Was the sample adequately described? • Was the best possible sampling design used to enhance the sample's representativeness? Were sampling biases minimized? • Was the sample size adequate? Was a power analysis used to estimate sample size needs?	Box 9.1 in Chapter 9
Data collection and measurement	• Were key variables operationalized using the best possible method (e.g., interviews, observations, biomarkers)? • Were clinically important and patient-centered outcomes measured? Were the specific instruments adequately described? • Did the report provide evidence that the data collection methods yielded data that were reliable and valid?	Box 9.2 in Chapter 9
Procedures	• If there was an intervention, was it adequately described, and was it properly implemented? Did most participants allocated to the intervention group actually receive it? • Were data collected in a manner that minimized bias?	Box 8.1 in Chapter 8; Box 9.2 in Chapter 9
Results Data analysis	• Were appropriate statistical methods used? • Was the most powerful analytic method used (e.g., did the analysis control for confounding variables)? • Were Type I and Type II errors avoided or minimized?	Box 13.1 in Chapter 13
Findings and interpretation	• Was information about statistical significance presented? • Was information about effect size and precision of estimates (confidence intervals) presented? • Was the clinical significance of the findings discussed? • Did the design and analysis enhance the applicability of the study results?	Box 14.1 in Chapter 14
Summary assessment	• Despite any limitations, do the study findings appear to be valid—do you have confidence in the *truth* value of the results? • Does the study contribute any meaningful evidence that can be used in nursing practice or that is useful to the nursing discipline?	

TABLE 3.2 Guide to a Focused Critical Appraisal of Evidence Quality in a Qualitative Research Report

Aspect of the Report	Critical Appraisal Questions	Detailed Appraisal Guidelines
Method Research design and research tradition	• Is the identified research tradition (if any) congruent with the methods used to collect and analyze data? • Was an adequate amount of time spent in the field or with study participants? • Was there evidence of reflexivity in the design?	Box 10.1 in Chapter 10
Sample and setting	• Was the group or population of interest adequately described? • Were the setting and sample described in sufficient detail? • Was the best possible method of sampling used to enhance information richness? • Was the sample size adequate? Was saturation achieved?	Box 11.1 in Chapter 11
Data collection	• Were appropriate methods used to gather data? Were data gathered through two or more methods to achieve triangulation? • Were the data of sufficient depth and richness?	Box 11.2 in Chapter 11
Procedures	• Do data collection and recording procedures appear appropriate? • Were data collected in a manner that minimized bias?	Box 11.2 in Chapter 11
Enhancement of trustworthiness	• Did the researchers use effective strategies to enhance the trustworthiness/integrity of the study? • Was there "thick description" of the context, participants, and findings? • Do the researchers' clinical and methodologic experience enhance confidence in the findings and their interpretation?	Box 16.1 in Chapter 16
Results Data analysis	• Was the data analysis strategy compatible with the research tradition and with the nature and type of data gathered? • Did the analysis yield an appropriate "product" (e.g., a theory, taxonomy, thematic pattern)?	Box 15.1 in Chapter 15
Findings	• Were the findings effectively summarized, with good use of excerpts from the data and strong supporting arguments? • Did the analysis yield an insightful, provocative, authentic, and meaningful picture of the phenomenon under investigation? • Were the findings interpreted within an appropriate social or cultural context?	Box 15.1 in Chapter 15
Summary assessment	• Do the study findings appear to be trustworthy—do you have confidence in the *truth* value of the results? • Does the study contribute any meaningful evidence that can be used in nursing practice or that is useful to the nursing discipline?	

The second column of Tables 3.1 and 3.2 lists some important appraisal questions, and the third column cross-references the more detailed guidelines in the various chapters of the book. We know that most of the questions are too difficult for you to answer at this point, but your methodologic and appraisal skills will develop as you progress through this book.

The question wording in these guidelines calls for a yes or no answer (although it may well be that the answer sometimes will be "Yes, *but* …"). In all cases, the desirable answer is *yes*; a *no* suggests a possible limitation, and a *yes* suggests a strength. Therefore, the more *yeses* a study gets, the stronger it is likely to be. Cumulatively, then, these guidelines can suggest a global assessment—A study with 10 *yeses* is likely to be superior to one with only 2. However, these guidelines are not intended to yield a formal quality "score."

We acknowledge that our guidelines have shortcomings. In particular, they are generic even though appraisals cannot use a one-size-fits-all list of questions. Important questions that are relevant to certain studies (e.g., those that have a therapy purpose) do not fit into a set of general questions for all quantitative studies. Thus, you need to use some judgment about whether the guidelines are sufficiently comprehensive for the type of study you are appraising. We also note that there are questions in these guidelines for which there are no totally objective answers. Even experts sometimes disagree about methodologic strategies.

TIP Just as a careful clinician seeks research evidence that certain practices are or are not effective, you as a reader should demand evidence that the researchers' methodologic decisions were sound.

Critical Appraisal With Key Research Challenges in Mind

In appraising a study, it is useful to be aware of the challenges that confront researchers. For example, they face ethical challenges (e.g., Can the study achieve its goals without infringing on human rights?), practical challenges (Will I be able to recruit enough participants?), and methodologic challenges (Will the methods I use yield results that can be trusted?). Most of this book provides guidance relating to the last question, and this section highlights key methodologic challenges. This section offers us an opportunity to introduce important terms and concepts that are relevant in a critical appraisal. The worth of a study's evidence for nursing practice often relies on how well researchers deal with these challenges.

Inference

Inference is an integral part of doing and appraising research. An **inference** is a conclusion drawn from the study evidence using logical reasoning and taking into account the methods used to generate that evidence.

Inference is necessary because researchers use proxies that "stand in" for things that are fundamentally of interest. A sample of participants is a proxy for an entire population. A control group that does not receive an intervention is a proxy for what would happen to the people who received the intervention if they had *not* received it.

Researchers face the challenge of using methods that yield good and persuasive evidence in support of inferences that they wish to make. Readers must draw their own inferences based on an appraisal of methodologic decisions.

Reliability, Validity, and Trustworthiness

Researchers want their inferences to correspond to the truth. Research cannot contribute evidence to guide clinical practice if the findings are inaccurate, biased, or fail to represent the experiences of the target group.

Quantitative researchers use several criteria to assess the quality of a study, sometimes referred to as its **scientific merit**. Two especially important criteria are reliability and validity. **Reliability** refers to the accuracy and consistency of information obtained in a study.

The term is most often associated with the methods used to measure variables. For example, if a thermometer measures a patient's temperature first as 98.1°F and then as 102.5°F a minute later, the thermometer is not reliable.

Validity is a more complex concept that broadly concerns the *soundness* of the study's evidence. Like reliability, validity is an important criterion for evaluating methods to measure variables. In this context, the validity question is whether the methods are really measuring the concepts that they purport to measure. Is a paper-and-pencil measure of depression *really* measuring depression? Or is it measuring something else, such as loneliness or stress? Researchers strive for solid conceptual definitions of research variables and valid methods to operationalize them.

Another aspect of validity concerns the quality of evidence about the relationship between the independent variable and the dependent variable. Did a nursing intervention *really* bring about improvements in patients' outcomes—or were other factors responsible for patients' progress? Researchers make numerous methodologic decisions that can influence this type of study validity.

Qualitative researchers use different criteria and terminology in evaluating a study's integrity. In general, qualitative researchers pursue methods of enhancing the trustworthiness of the study's data and findings (Lincoln & Guba, 1985). **Trustworthiness** encompasses several different dimensions—credibility, transferability, confirmability, dependability, and authenticity—which are described in Chapter 16.

Credibility is an especially important aspect of trustworthiness. Credibility is achieved to the extent that the research methods inspire confidence that the results are truthful and accurate. Credibility in a qualitative study can be enhanced in several ways, but one strategy merits early discussion because it has implications for the design of all studies, including quantitative ones. **Triangulation** is the use of multiple sources or referents to draw conclusions about what constitutes the truth. In a quantitative study, this might mean having two ways to measure an outcome to assess whether results are consistent. In a qualitative study, triangulation might involve efforts to understand the complexity of a phenomenon by using multiple data collection methods to converge on the truth (e.g., having in-depth discussions with participants as well as watching their behavior in natural settings). Nurse researchers are also beginning to triangulate across paradigms—that is, to integrate both qualitative and quantitative data in a single study to enhance the validity of the conclusions in *mixed methods research* (see Chapter 12).

> **Example of triangulation**
> Nyhagen et al. (2023) conducted a case-oriented study using an exploratory interpretive design to explore communication between patients, family members, and nurses to investigate unidentified communication challenges. The authors achieved data triangulation by including three groups of participants: patients, family members, and clinicians. They did not aim to have the findings from the various participants to confirm or contradict one another, but rather provide a more complete answer to understanding the communication challenges in the intensive care setting.

Nurse researchers need to design their studies to minimize threats to the reliability, validity, and trustworthiness of their studies, and users of research must evaluate the extent to which they were successful.

 TIP In reading and appraising research articles, it is appropriate to have a "show me" attitude—that is, to expect researchers to build and present a solid case for the merit of their inferences. They do this by providing evidence that the findings are reliable and valid or trustworthy.

Bias

Bias can threaten a study's validity and trustworthiness. A **bias** is a distortion or influence that results in an error in inference. Bias can be caused by various factors, including researchers' preconceptions, faulty methods of collecting data, or participants' lack of candor.

Some bias is haphazard and affects only small segments of the data. As an example, a few study participants might provide inaccurate information because they were tired at the time of data collection. *Systematic bias* results when the bias is consistent or uniform. For example, if a scale consistently measured people's weight as being 2 lb heavier than their true weight, there would be systematic bias in the data on weight.

Rigorous research methods aim to eliminate or minimize bias, using a variety of strategies. Triangulation is one such approach, the idea being that multiple sources of information or points of view offer avenues to identify biases. In quantitative research, methods to combat bias often entail research control.

Research Control

In most quantitative studies, researchers strive to control aspects of the research. **Research control** usually involves holding constant influences on the outcome so that the relationship between the independent and dependent variables can be understood. In other words, research control attempts to eliminate contaminating factors that might cloud the relationship between the variables that are of central interest.

Contaminating factors, often called **confounding** (or *extraneous*) **variables**, can best be illustrated with an example—suppose we were studying whether urinary incontinence (UI) leads to depression. Prior evidence suggests that this might be the case, but previous studies have not clarified the nature of the relationship. The question is whether UI itself (the independent variable) contributes to higher levels of depression, or whether there are other factors that can account for the relationship between UI and depression. We need to design a study that controls other determinants of the outcome—determinants that are also related to the independent variable, UI.

One confounding variable here is age. Levels of depression tend to be higher in older people, and people with UI tend to be older than those without this problem. In other words, perhaps age is the real cause of higher depression in people with UI. If age is not controlled, then any observed relationship between UI and depression could be caused by UI, or by age.

Three possible explanations might be portrayed schematically as follows:

1. UI→depression
2. Age→UI→depression

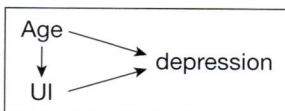

The arrows symbolize a causal mechanism or influence. In model 1, UI directly affects depression, independently of other factors. In model 2, UI is a *mediating variable*—the effect of age on depression is *mediated* by UI. According to this representation, age affects depression *through* the effect that age has on UI. In model 3, both age and UI have separate effects on depression, and age also increases the risk of UI. Some research is specifically designed to test paths of mediation and multiple causation, but in the present example, age is extraneous to the research question. We want to design a study that tests the first explanation. Age must be controlled if our goal is to explore the validity of model 1, which posits that, no matter what a person's age, having UI makes a person more vulnerable to depression.

How can we impose such control? There are a number of ways, as we discuss in Chapter 8, but the general principle underlying each alternative is that the confounding variable must be *held constant*. The confounding variable must somehow be handled so that, in the context of the study, it is not related to the independent variable or the outcome. As an example, let us say we wanted to compare the average scores on a depression scale for those with and without UI. We would want to design a study in such a way that the ages of those in the UI and non-UI groups are comparable, even though, in general, the groups are not comparable in terms of age.

By exercising control over age, we would be taking a step toward understanding the relationship between UI and depression. The world is complex, and many variables are interrelated in complicated ways. The evidence in quantitative studies is often affected by how well researchers controlled confounding influences.

Research rooted in the constructivist paradigm does not impose controls. With their emphasis on holism and individual human experience, qualitative researchers typically believe that imposing controls removes some of the meaning of reality.

Bias Reduction: Randomness and Blinding

For quantitative researchers, a powerful tool for eliminating bias involves **randomness**—having certain features of the study established by chance rather than by researcher preference. When people are selected *at random* to participate in a study, for example, each person in the initial pool has an equal chance of being selected. This in turn means that there are no systematic biases in the makeup of the sample. People of all genders have an equal chance of being selected, for example. Similarly, if participants are allocated *at random* to groups that will be compared (e.g., special intervention and "usual care" groups), then there are no biases in the groups' composition. Randomness is a compelling method of controlling confounding variables and reducing bias.

Another bias-reducing strategy is called **blinding** (or *masking*), which is used in some quantitative studies to prevent biases stemming from people's awareness. Blinding involves concealing information from participants, data collectors, or care providers to enhance objectivity. For example, if study participants are aware of whether they are getting an experimental drug or a sham drug (a **placebo**), then their outcomes could be influenced by their expectations of the new drug's efficacy. Blinding involves withholding information about participants' status in the study (e.g., whether they are in a certain group) or about study hypotheses.

> **Example of randomness**
> Krüger and colleagues (2023) described a study protocol for a pilot randomized controlled trial (RCT) to test the feasibility of the RCT comparing two units of a hospital in Germany: the intervention unit providing primary nursing as compared to a unit providing routine ICU nursing standard of care. A secondary aim plans to examine the incidence of delirium, anxiety, family satisfaction, and the effects of primary nursing. Randomization will be based on blocks with six patients in each block, generated by using the random function of Microsoft Excel software.

Qualitative researchers do not consider randomness or blinding desirable tools for understanding phenomena. A researcher's judgment is viewed as an indispensable vehicle for uncovering the complexities of the phenomena of interest.

Reflexivity

Qualitative researchers are also interested in discovering the truth about human experience. Qualitative researchers often rely on reflexivity to guard against personal bias and preconceptions. **Reflexivity** is the process of reflecting critically on the self and of analyzing and noting personal values and beliefs that could affect data collection and interpretation. Qualitative researchers are trained to explore these issues, to be reflective about decisions made during the inquiry, and to record their thoughts in personal diaries and memos. Researchers are beginning to include **positionality statements** in their manuscripts which describe how the researchers' identities, experiences, and beliefs are related to their study and to the participants (Beck, 2024). Positionality statements help to increase transparency regarding how researchers are positioned and their influence on the research process.

> **Example of reflexivity**
> Boakye and Prendergast (2024) described how they incorporated reflexivity in their study examining Black women's perceived sense of safety accessing pregnancy and intrapartum care. They reported the standpoint they hold as "Black scholars of African descent who have an explicit commitment to interrogate all forms of injustice that undermine the reproductive health of Black women" (p. 4). They also acknowledged the potential influence of their positionality that could have influenced their interpretation and reporting of the findings. However, to minimize potential bias, they also reported that they regularly debriefed with one another and invited colleagues with experience in Black scholarship who were not involved in the research to review the final draft of the paper.

TIP Reflexivity can be a useful tool in quantitative as well as qualitative research—self-awareness and introspection can enhance the quality of any study.

Generalizability and Transferability

Nurses increasingly rely on research evidence to guide their clinical practice. EBP is based on the assumption that study findings are not unique to the people, places, or circumstances of the original research.

As noted in Chapter 1, *generalizability* in quantitative studies refers to the extent to which the findings can be applied to other groups and settings. How do researchers enhance the generalizability of a study? First and foremost, they must design studies strong in reliability and validity. There is little point in wondering whether results are generalizable if they are not accurate or valid. In selecting participants, researchers must also give thought to the types of people to whom results might be generalized—and then select participants accordingly. If a study is intended to have implications for adult male and female patients, then men and women should be included in the sample.

Qualitative researchers do not specifically aim for generalizability, but they do want to generate knowledge that might be useful in other situations. Lincoln and Guba (1985), in their influential book on naturalistic inquiry, discuss the concept of **transferability**, the extent to which qualitative findings can be transferred to other settings, as another aspect of trustworthiness. An important mechanism for promoting transferability is the amount of rich descriptive information qualitative researchers provide about study contexts.

RESEARCH EXAMPLES WITH CRITICAL THINKING EXERCISES

Abstracts for a quantitative and a qualitative nursing study are presented in the following sections. Read the abstracts for Examples 1 and 2, and then answer the critical thinking questions that follow. The critical thinking questions for Examples 3 and 4 are based on the studies that appear in their entirety in Appendices A and B of this book.

EXAMPLE 1: QUANTITATIVE RESEARCH

Study: "Effects of a web-based pediatric oncology legacy intervention on the coping of children with cancer" (Cho et al., 2023)

Objective: The objective of this study was to examine the effects of a legacy intervention using digital storytelling on the coping strategies of children with recurrent or refractory cancer.

Background: Legacy interventions are evidence-based, family-centered palliative care strategies that help children with serious illness to cope. However, the impact of legacy interventions on coping in children with recurrent or refractory cancer is poorly understood.

Methods: This study used a two-arm randomized waitlist control clinical trial. Children with recurrent or refractory cancer and their parents were recruited via Facebook. They were randomly assigned to the intervention or control group through the use of a computer-generated permuted-block randomization sequence. The primary end point was the response to stress questionnaire (RSQ).

Results: The sample included 92 parent–child dyads (35—intervention group, 57—control group). Results indicate that the legacy intervention resulted in small and statistically nonsignificant effects on coping among children with recurrent or refractory cancer.

Conclusions: Although the findings indicated a small and statistically nonsignificant change in coping, this is the first RCT to test a legacy intervention in this population. More work is needed to understand if expanding the options for legacy interventions may yield better outcomes.

Critical Thinking Exercises

1. What were the independent and dependent variables in this study?
2. What are the PICO components?
3. Is this study experimental or nonexperimental?
4. How, if at all, was *randomness* used in this study?
5. How, if at all, was *blinding* used in this study?
6. Did the researchers use any statistical tests? If yes, were any of the results statistically significant?
7. If the results of this study are valid and generalizable, what might be some of the ways the findings could be used in clinical practice?

EXAMPLE 2: QUALITATIVE RESEARCH

Study: "Parents' shared experiences of separation from their newborns after birth in Denmark"

Objective: To explore parents' shared experiences of separation from their newborns after birth in Denmark

Design: Phenomenologic hermeneutic design

Setting: A NICU [neonatal intensive care unit] in the Capital Region of Denmark.

Participants: Four sets of parents ($N = 8$) with prematurely born neonates who were admitted to the NICU.

Methods: We used dyadic interviews for data collection. We applied a phenomenologic hermeneutic approach inspired by Ricoeur's theory of interpretation to analyze the data.

Results: Two overarching themes emerged that reflected two distinct temporal phases of separation. Initial separation caused an experience of becoming parents at different paces. Separation based on care needs (i.e., the NICU vs. maternity unit) left parents at the juncture between separation and closeness.

Conclusion: Separation from their newborns complicated parents' transitions into parenthood. Their sense of unity was undermined when different units assumed responsibility for the mother and the newborn. This challenged family-centered care. Our findings indicate the need to minimize separation through initiatives such as zero separation and couplet care.

Abstract reprinted from Brodsgaard, A., Bjerregaard, M., & Knudsen, J. B. (2024). Parents' shared experiences of separation from their newborns after birth in Denmark. *Journal of Obstetric, Gynecologic, and Neonatal Nursing, 53*(5), 534–542. https://doi.org/10.1016/j.jogn.2024.04.007. Copyright © 2024 AWHONN, the Association of Women's Health, Obstetric and Neonatal Nurses. With permission.

Critical Thinking Exercises

1. On which qualitative research tradition, if any, was this study based?
2. Is this study experimental or nonexperimental?
3. How, if at all, was *randomness* used in this study?
4. Is there any indication in the abstract that triangulation was used? Reflexivity?
5. If the results of this study are trustworthy and transferable, what might be some of the ways the findings could be used in clinical practice?

EXAMPLE 3: QUANTITATIVE RESEARCH IN APPENDIX A

Read the abstract and the introduction of Cheng and colleagues' (2024) study "Advance care planning affects end-of-life treatment preferences among patients with heart failure: A randomized controlled trial" in Appendix A of this book.

1. Did this article follow a traditional IMRAD format? Where does the introduction to this article begin and end?
2. How, if at all, was randomness used in this study?
3. How, if at all, was blinding used?
4. Comment on the possible generalizability of the study findings.

EXAMPLE 4: QUALITATIVE RESEARCH IN APPENDIX B

Read the abstract and the introduction of Morrison and colleagues' (2024) study "Lived experiences of fatherhood after infertility" in Appendix B of this book.

1. Where does the introduction to this article begin and end?
2. How, if at all, was randomness used in this study?
3. Is there any indication in the abstract that triangulation was used? Reflexivity?
4. Comment on the possible transferability of the study findings.

Summary Points

- Both qualitative and quantitative researchers disseminate their findings, most often by publishing reports of their research as **journal articles**, which concisely describe what researchers did and what they found.

- Journal articles often consist of an **abstract** (a synopsis of the study) and four major sections that often follow the **IMRAD format**: **I**ntroduction (the research problem and its context), **M**ethods (the strategies used to answer research questions), **R**esults (study findings), **a**nd **D**iscussion (interpretation and implications of the findings).

- Research reports are often difficult to read because they are dense, concise, and contain jargon. Quantitative research reports may be intimidating at first because, compared to qualitative reports, they are more impersonal and report on statistical tests.

- **Statistical tests** are used to test hypotheses and to evaluate the reliability of the findings. Findings that are **statistically significant** have a high probability of being "real."

- A goal of this book is to help students to prepare **critical appraisals** of the strengths and limitations of a study, to assess the worth of the evidence for nursing practice.

- Researchers face numerous challenges, the solutions to which must be appraised because they affect the inferences that can be made.

- An **inference** is a conclusion drawn from the study evidence, taking into account the methods used to generate that evidence. Researchers strive to have their inferences correspond to the *truth*.

- **Reliability** (a key challenge in quantitative research) refers to the accuracy of information obtained in a study. **Validity** broadly concerns the *soundness* and rigor of the study's methods—that is, whether the evidence is convincing and well grounded.

- **Trustworthiness** in qualitative research encompasses several different dimensions, including credibility, dependability, confirmability, transferability, and authenticity.

- **Credibility** is achieved to the extent that the methods engender confidence in the truth of the data and in the researchers' interpretations. **Triangulation**, the use of multiple sources to draw conclusions about the truth, is one approach to enhancing credibility.

- A **bias** is an influence that produces a distortion in the study results. In quantitative studies, research control is an approach to addressing bias. **Research control** is used to hold constant outside influences on the dependent variable so that the relationship between the independent and dependent variables can be better understood.

- Researchers seek to control **confounding** (or *extraneous*) **variables**—variables that are extraneous to the purpose of a specific study.

- For quantitative researchers, **randomness**—having certain features of the study established by chance—is a powerful tool to eliminate bias.

- **Blinding** (or *masking*) is sometimes used to avoid biases stemming from participants' or research agents' awareness of study hypotheses or research status.

- **Reflexivity**, the process of reflecting critically on the self and of scrutinizing personal values that could affect data collection and interpretation, is an important tool in qualitative research.

- A **positionality statement** describes how the researchers' identities, experiences, and beliefs are related to their study and to the participants.

- Generalizability in a quantitative study concerns the extent to which the findings can be applied to members of a population who were not included in the study sample.

- A similar concept in qualitative studies is **transferability**, the extent to which qualitative findings can be transferred to other settings. One mechanism for promoting transferability is a rich and thorough description of the research context so that others can make inferences about contextual similarities.

REFERENCES

Beck, C. T. (2024). Perspectives on positionality statements in scholarly discourse. *Journal of Obstetric, Gynecologic, and Neonatal Nursing*, 53(6), 581–584. https://doi.org/10.1016/j.jogn.2024.09.010

Boakye, P. N., & Prendergast, N. (2024). "There is nothing to protect us from dying": Black women's perceived sense of safety accessing pregnancy and intrapartum care. *Nursing Inquiry*, 31(3), e12638. https://doi.org/10.1111/nin.12638

Cheng, H. C., Wu, S. V., Chen, Y. H., Tsan, Y. H., Sung, S. H., & Ke, L. S. (2024). Advance care planning affects end-of-life treatment preferences among patients with heart failure: A randomized controlled trial. *Journal of Hospice and Palliative Nursing: JHPN: The Official Journal of the Hospice and Palliative Nurses Association*, 26(1), E13–E19. https://doi.org/10.1097/NJH.0000000000000988

Cho, E., Dietrich, M. S., Friedman, D. L., Gilmer, M. J., Gerhardt, C. A., Given, B. A., Hendricks-Ferguson, V. L., Hinds, P. S., & Akard, T. F. (2023). Effects of a web-based pediatric oncology legacy intervention on the coping of children with cancer. *The American Journal of Hospice & Palliative Care*, 40(1), 34–42. https://doi.org/10.1177/10499091221100809

He, X., Ng, M. S. N., Choi, K. C., & So, W. K. W. (2022). Effects of a 16-week dance intervention on the symptom cluster of fatigue-sleep disturbance-depression and quality of life among patients with breast cancer undergoing adjuvant chemotherapy: A randomized controlled trial. *International Journal of Nursing Studies*, 133, 104317. https://doi.org/10.1016/j.ijnurstu.2022.104317

Krüger, L., Mannebach, T., Zittermann, A., Wefer, F., von Dossow, V., Rojas Hernandez, S., Gummert, J., & Langer, G. (2023). Patientinnen- und patientenbezogene Auswirkungen von prozessverantwortlicher Pflege: Protokoll einer randomisierten kontrollierten Pilotstudie [Patient-related effects of primary nursing: Protocol of a pilot randomized controlled trial]. *Medical Clinic, Intensive Care Medicine and Emergency Medicine*, 118(4), 257–262. https://doi.org/10.1007/s00063-023-00998-w

Lee, C. S., Chu, S. H., Dunne, J., Spintzyk, E., Locatelli, G., Babicheva, V., Lam, L., Julio, K., Chen, S., & Jurgens, C. Y. (2024). Body listening in the link between symptoms and self-care management in cardiovascular disease: A cross-sectional correlational descriptive study. *International Journal of Nursing Studies*, 156, 104809. https://doi.org/10.1016/j.ijnurstu.2024.104809

Lincoln, Y. S., & Guba, E. G. (1985). *Naturalistic inquiry*. Sage.

Morrison, S., Bryanton, J., Murray, C., & Foley, V. (2024). Lived experiences of fatherhood after infertility. *Journal of Obstetric, Gynecologic, and Neonatal Nursing*, 53(3), 245–254. https://doi.org/10.1016/j.jogn.2023.12.002

Nyhagen, R., Egerod, I., Rustøen, T., Lerdal, A., & Kirkevold, M. (2023). Unidentified communication challenges in the intensive care unit: A qualitative study using multiple triangulations. *Australian Critical Care: Official Journal of the Confederation of Australian Critical Care Nurses*, 36(2), 215–222. https://doi.org/10.1016/j.aucc.2022.01.006

Weiss, C. R., Roberts, M., Florell, M., Wood, R., Johnson-Koenke, R., Amura, C. R., Kissler, K., Barton, A. J., & Jones, J. (2024). Best practices for telehealth in nurse-led care settings—A qualitative study. *Policy, Politics & Nursing Practice*, 25(1), 47–57. https://doi.org/10.1177/15271544231201417

4 Attending to Ethics in Research

Learning Objectives

On completing this chapter, you will be able to:

- Discuss the historical background that led to the creation of various codes of ethics
- Understand the potential for ethical dilemmas stemming from conflicts between ethical requirements and research goals
- Identify the three primary ethical principles articulated in the *Belmont Report* and the dimensions encompassed by each
- Identify procedures for adhering to ethical principles and protecting study participants
- Identify vulnerable groups who may require extra protection in participating in research
- Given sufficient information, evaluate the ethical dimensions of a research report
- Define new terms in the chapter

Key Terms

- Anonymity
- Assent
- *Belmont Report*
- Beneficence
- Certificate of Confidentiality
- Code of ethics
- Confidentiality
- Consent form
- Debriefing
- Ethical dilemma
- Full disclosure
- Informed consent
- Institutional Review Board (IRB)
- Minimal risk
- Risk/benefit assessment
- Stipend
- Vulnerable group

ETHICS AND RESEARCH

In research with humans or animals, researchers must take ethical issues into consideration. Ethical concerns are prominent in nursing research because the line between what constitutes the expected practice of nursing and the collection of research data sometimes gets blurred. This chapter discusses ethical principles that should be kept in mind when reading about a study.

Historical Background

We might like to think that violations of moral principles among researchers occurred centuries ago rather than recently, but this is not the case. The Nazi medical experiments of the 1930s and 1940s are the most famous examples of recent disregard for ethical conduct. The Nazi program of research involved using prisoners of war and "racial enemies" in medical experiments. The studies were unethical not only because they exposed people to harm but also because subjects could not refuse participation.

There are more recent examples. For instance, between 1932 and 1972, the Tuskegee Syphilis Study, sponsored by the U.S. Public Health Service, investigated the effects of syphilis among 400 poor African American men. Medical treatment was deliberately withheld to study the course of the untreated disease. It was revealed in 1993 that U.S. federal agencies had sponsored radiation experiments since the 1940s on hundreds of people, many of them were prisoners or older hospital patients. And, in 2010, it was revealed that a U.S. doctor who worked on the Tuskegee study inoculated prisoners in Guatemala with syphilis in the 1940s. Other examples of studies with ethical transgressions have emerged to give ethical concerns the high visibility they have today.

Codes of Ethics

In response to human rights violations, various codes of ethics have been developed. The ethical standards known as the Nuremberg Code were developed in 1949 in response to the Nazi atrocities. Several other international standards have been developed, including the Declaration of Helsinki, which was adopted in 1964 by the World Medical Association and was most recently revised in 2013.

Most disciplines, such as medicine and nursing, have established their own **code of ethics**. In the United States, the American Nurses Association (ANA) issued *Ethical Guidelines in the Conduct, Dissemination, and Implementation of Nursing Research* in 1995 (Silva, 1995). In 2025, the ANA published an updated *Code of Ethics for Nurses* that includes 10 provisions. While all the provisions are relevant to nursing, Provision 7 specifically addresses nursing knowledge development: "Nurses advance the profession through multiple approaches to knowledge development, professional standards, and the generation of policies for nursing, health, and social concerns" (ANA, 2025). The *Code* also specifically addresses areas of concern around the ethical pursuit of research and the implications for policy, education, and practice. The Canadian Nurses Association published a revised version of their *Code of Ethics for Registered Nurses* in 2017. The International Council of Nurses (ICN) revised the *ICN Code of Ethics for Nurses* in 2025.

Government Regulations for Protecting Study Participants

Governments throughout the world fund research and establish rules for adhering to ethical principles. In the United States, an important code of ethics was adopted by the National Commission for the Protection of Human Subjects of Biomedical and Behavioral Research. The commission issued a report in 1978, known as the *Belmont Report*, which provided a model for many guidelines adopted by disciplinary organizations in the United States. The *Belmont Report* also served as the basis for regulations affecting research sponsored by the U.S. government, including studies supported by National Institute of Nursing Research (NINR). The U.S. ethical regulations were codified in Title 45 Part 46 of the Code of Federal Regulations and were revised most recently in 2018.

Ethical Dilemmas in Conducting Research

Research that violates ethical principles typically occurs because a researcher believes that knowledge is potentially beneficial in the long run. For some research problems, participants' rights and study quality are put in direct conflict, posing **ethical dilemmas** for researchers. Here are examples of research problems in which the desire for rigor conflicts with ethical considerations:

1. *Research question:* Does a new medication prolong life in patients with AIDS?
   Ethical dilemma: The best way to test the effectiveness of an intervention is to administer the intervention to some participants but withhold it from others to see if the groups have

different outcomes. However, if the intervention is untested (e.g., a new drug), the group receiving the intervention may be exposed to potentially hazardous side effects. On the other hand, the group *not* receiving the drug may be denied a beneficial treatment.
2. *Research question:* Are nurses equally empathic in their care of male and female patients in the intensive care unit (ICU)?
Ethical dilemma: Ethics requires that participants be aware of their role in a study. Yet, if the researcher informs nurse participants that their empathy in caring for male and female ICU patients will be scrutinized, will their behavior be "normal?" If the nurses' usual behavior is altered because of the known presence of research observers, then the findings will be inaccurate.
3. *Research question:* How do parents cope when their children have a terminal illness?
Ethical dilemma: To answer this question, the researcher may need to probe into parents' psychological state at a vulnerable time; yet, knowledge of the parents' coping mechanisms might help to design effective ways of addressing parents' grief and stress.
4. *Research question:* What is the process by which adult children adapt to the day-to-day burden of caring for a parent with Alzheimer disease?
Ethical dilemma: Sometimes, especially in qualitative studies, a researcher may get so close to participants that they become willing to share "secrets" and privileged information. Interviews can become confessions—sometimes of unseemly or illegal behavior. In this example, suppose a person admitted to physically abusing their parent, how does the researcher respond to that information without undermining a pledge of confidentiality? If the researcher divulges the information to the authorities, how can a pledge of confidentiality be given in good faith to other participants?

As these examples suggest, researchers are sometimes in a bind. Their goal is to develop high-quality evidence for practice, but they must also protect human rights. Another dilemma may arise if nurse researchers face conflict-of-interest situations, in which their expected behavior as nurses conflicts with standard research behavior (e.g., deviating from a research protocol to assist a patient). It is precisely because of such dilemmas that codes of ethics are needed to guide researchers' efforts.

ETHICAL PRINCIPLES FOR PROTECTING STUDY PARTICIPANTS

The **Belmont Report** articulated three primary ethical principles on which standards of ethical research conduct are based: beneficence, respect for human dignity, and justice. We briefly discuss these principles and then describe methods researchers use to comply with them.

Beneficence

Beneficence imposes a duty on researchers to minimize harm and maximize benefits. Human research should be intended to produce benefits for participants, or—more typically—for others. This principle covers multiple aspects.

The Right to Freedom From Harm and Discomfort

Researchers have an obligation to prevent or minimize harm in studies with humans. Participants must not be subjected to unnecessary risks of harm or discomfort, and their participation in research must be necessary for achieving societally important aims. In research with humans, *harm* and *discomfort* can be physical (e.g., injury), emotional (e.g., stress), social (e.g., loss of social support), or financial (e.g., expenses incurred). Ethical researchers must use strategies to minimize all types of harm and discomfort, even temporary ones.

Protecting human beings from physical harm is often straightforward, but psychological consequences are often hard to discern. For example, participants may be asked questions about their personal lives that lead them to reveal deeply personal information. The need for sensitivity may be especially great in qualitative studies, which often involve in-depth exploration of highly personal experiences.

The Right to Protection From Exploitation

Involvement in a study should not place participants at a disadvantage. Participants need to be assured that their participation, or information they provide, will not be used against them. For example, people reporting illegal drug use should not fear of being reported for a crime.

Study participants enter into a special relationship with researchers, and this relationship should not be exploited. Nurse researchers may have a nurse–patient (in addition to a researcher–participant) relationship, so special care may be needed to avoid exploiting that bond. Patients' consent to participate in a study may result from their understanding of the researcher's role as *nurse*, not as *researcher*.

In qualitative research, psychological distance between researchers and participants often declines as the study progresses. The emergence of a pseudotherapeutic relationship is not uncommon, which could create additional risks that exploitation could inadvertently occur. On the other hand, qualitative researchers often are in a better position than quantitative researchers to *do good*, rather than just to avoid doing harm, because of the close relationships they develop with participants.

> **Example of therapeutic research experiences**
> One of the participants in Beck and Casavant's (2020) study on vicarious posttraumatic growth in the neonatal intensive care unit (NICU) nurses wrote the researchers the following: "Thank you for heading up this study and know that just acknowledging us and allowing this research to take place is healing and will help many nurses for futures to come."

Respect for Human Dignity

Respect for human dignity is the second ethical principle in the *Belmont Report*. This principle includes the right to self-determination and the right to full disclosure.

The Right to Self-Determination

The principle of *self-determination* means that prospective participants have the right to decide voluntarily whether to participate in a study without risk of prejudicial treatment. It also means that people have the right to ask questions, refuse to answer questions, and drop out of the study.

A person's right to self-determination includes freedom from coercion. *Coercion* involves explicit or implicit threats of penalty from failing to participate in a study or excessive rewards from agreeing to participate. The issue of coercion requires careful thought when researchers are in a position of authority or influence over potential participants, as might be the case in a nurse–patient relationship. Coercion can be subtle. For example, a generous monetary incentive (or **stipend**) to encourage the participation of a low-income group (e.g., individuals experiencing homelessness) might be considered mildly coercive because such an incentive might pressure prospective participants to cooperate.

The Right to Full Disclosure

Respect for human dignity encompasses people's right to make informed decisions about study participation, which requires full disclosure. **Full disclosure** means that the researcher has fully described the study, the person's right to refuse participation, and potential risks and benefits. The right to self-determination and the right to full disclosure are the two elements on which informed consent—discussed later in this chapter—is based.

Full disclosure is not always straightforward because it can result in biases and sample recruitment problems. Suppose we were testing the hypothesis that high school students with a high absentee rate are more likely to have substance use disorder than students with good attendance, and if we approached potential participants and fully explained the study's purpose, some students might refuse to participate, and nonparticipation would be selective; students with substance use disorder—the group of primary interest—might be least likely to participate. Moreover, by knowing the study purpose, those who participate might not give candid responses. In such a situation, full disclosure could undermine the study.

In such situations, researchers sometimes use *covert data collection* (*concealment*), which is collecting data without participants' knowledge and thus without their consent. This might happen if a researcher wanted to observe people's behavior and was worried that doing so openly would change the behavior of interest. Researchers might choose to obtain needed information through concealed methods, such as observing while pretending to be engaged in other activities.

A more controversial technique is the use of *deception*, which can involve deliberately withholding information about the study, or providing participants with false information. For example, in studying high school students' use of drugs, we might describe the research as a study of students' health practices, which is a mild form of misinformation.

Deception and concealment are problematic ethically because they interfere with people's right to make truly informed decisions about personal costs and benefits of participation. Some people think that deception is never justified, but others believe that if the study involves minimal risk yet offers benefits to society, then slight deceptiveness may be acceptable.

Full disclosure has emerged as a concern in connection with data collected from the internet (e.g., analyzing the content of messages posted to blogs or social media sites). The issue is whether such messages can be used as data without the authors' consent. Some researchers believe that anything posted electronically is in the public domain, but others feel that the same ethical standards must apply in cyberspace research and that researchers must carefully protect the rights of individuals who are participants in "virtual" communities.

Justice

The third principle articulated in the *Belmont Report* concerns justice, which includes participants' right to fair treatment and their right to privacy.

The Right to Fair Treatment

One aspect of justice concerns the equitable distribution of benefits and burdens of research. The selection of participants should be based on research requirements and not on people's vulnerabilities. For example, groups with lower social standing (e.g., individuals who are incarcerated) have sometimes been selected as study participants, raising ethical concerns.

Potential discrimination is another aspect of distributive justice. During the 1990s, it was found that women and other underrepresented groups were being *ex*cluded from many clinical studies. In the United States, this led to regulations requiring that researchers who seek funding from the National Institutes of Health (including NINR) include women and other underrepresented groups as study participants.

The right to fair treatment encompasses other obligations. For example, researchers must treat people who decline to participate in a study in a nonprejudicial manner, honor all agreements made with participants, show respect for the beliefs of people from different backgrounds, and treat participants courteously and tactfully at all times.

The Right to Privacy

Research with humans involves intrusions into people's lives. Researchers should ensure that their research is not more intrusive than it needs to be and that privacy is maintained. Participants have the right to expect that any data they provide will be kept in strict confidence.

Privacy issues have become even more salient in the U.S. health care community since the passage of the Health Insurance Portability and Accountability Act of 1996 (HIPAA), which articulates federal standards to protect patients' medical records and health information. For health care providers who transmit health information electronically, compliance with HIPAA regulations (the Privacy Rule) has been required since 2003.

PROCEDURES FOR PROTECTING STUDY PARTICIPANTS

Now that you are familiar with ethical principles for conducting research, you need to understand the procedures researchers use to adhere to them. It is adherence with these procedures that should be evaluated in critically appraising the ethical aspects of a study.

 TIP Information about ethical considerations is usually presented in the method section of a research report, often in a subsection labeled *procedures*.

Risk/Benefit Assessments

One strategy that researchers use to protect participants is to conduct a **risk/benefit assessment**. Such an assessment is designed to evaluate whether the benefits of participating in a study are in line with the costs—that is, whether the *risk/benefit ratio* is acceptable. Box 4.1 summarizes major costs and benefits of research participation to study participants. Benefits to society and to nursing should also be taken into account. The selection of a significant topic that has the potential to improve patient care is the first step in ensuring that research is ethical.

 TIP In evaluating the risk/benefit ratio of a study, you might want to consider how comfortable *you* would have felt about being a study participant.

Sometimes risks are negligible. **Minimal risk** is a risk expected to be no greater than those ordinarily encountered in daily life or during routine procedures. When the risks are not minimal, researchers must proceed with caution, taking every step possible to reduce risks and maximize benefits.

Informed Consent

An important procedure for safeguarding participants involves obtaining their informed consent. **Informed consent** means that participants have adequate information about the study, comprehend the information, and can consent to or decline participation voluntarily.

> **Box 4.1 Potential Benefits and Risks of Research to Participants**
>
> **Major Potential Benefits to Participants**
> - Access to a potentially beneficial intervention that might otherwise be unavailable
> - Relief in being able to discuss their situation or problem with a friendly, objective person
> - Increased knowledge about themselves or their conditions
> - Escape from normal routine
> - Satisfaction that information they provide may help others with similar problems
> - Direct gains through stipends or other incentives
>
> **Major Potential Risks to Participants**
> - Physical harm, including unanticipated side effects
> - Physical discomfort, fatigue, or boredom
> - Emotional distress from self-disclosure, discomfort with strangers, embarrassment relating to questions being asked
> - Social risks, such as the risk of stigma, negative effects on personal relationships
> - Loss of privacy
> - Loss of time
> - Monetary costs (e.g., for transportation, childcare, time lost from work)

Researchers usually document informed consent by having participants sign a **consent form**. This form includes information about the study purpose, specific expectations regarding participation (e.g., how much time will be required), the voluntary nature of participation, and potential costs and benefits.

> **Example of informed consent**
> Sun and colleagues (2024) aimed to assess the feasibility and acceptability of virtual programs to address issues of social connection and interaction for people with dementia and their informal caregivers. The facility stakeholders identified potential participants who met the inclusion criteria. Once identified, research assistants reached out either through telephone or e-mail and described the study details. If they expressed interest in participating, the researchers obtained written informed consent and scheduled an interview.

Researchers may not obtain written informed consent when data collection is through self-administered questionnaires. Researchers often assume *implied consent* (i.e., returning a completed questionnaire implies the person's consent to participate).

In qualitative studies that involve repeated data collection, it may be difficult to obtain meaningful consent at the outset. Because the design emerges during the study, researchers may not know what the risks and benefits will be. In such situations, consent may be an ongoing process, called *process consent*, in which consent is continuously renegotiated.

Confidentiality Procedures

Study participants have the right to expect that the data they provide will be kept in strict confidence. Participants' right to privacy is protected through confidentiality procedures.

Anonymity

Anonymity, the most secure means of protecting confidentiality, occurs when the researcher cannot link participants to their data. For example, if questionnaires were distributed to nursing home residents and were returned without identifying information, responses would be anonymous.

> **Example of anonymity**
> Petreca and colleagues (2024) conducted a hermeneutic phenomenologic study exploring men's reintegration into society after committing a sexual offense. To protect their anonymity, participants were assigned pseudonyms and all data were de-identified and coded.

Confidentiality in the Absence of Anonymity

When anonymity is not possible, other confidentiality procedures need to be implemented. A promise of **confidentiality** is a pledge that any information participants provide will not be publicly reported in a manner that identifies them and will not be made accessible to others.

Researchers can take a number of steps to ensure that a *breach of confidentiality* does not occur. These include maintaining identifying information in locked files, substituting *identification (ID) numbers* for participants' names on records, and reporting only aggregate data for groups of participants.

Confidentiality is especially salient in qualitative studies because of their in-depth nature: Anonymity is rarely possible. Qualitative researchers also face the challenge of adequately disguising participants in their reports. Because the number of respondents is small and because rich descriptive information is presented, qualitative researchers must be especially vigilant in safeguarding participants' identity.

> **TIP** As a means of enhancing individual and institutional privacy, researchers frequently avoid giving information about the study locale. For example, a report might say that data were collected in a 200-bed, private nursing home, without mentioning its name or location.

Confidentiality sometimes creates tension between researchers and legal authorities, especially if participants engage in criminal activity such as substance misuse. To avoid the forced disclosure of information (e.g., through a court order), researchers in the United States can apply for a **Certificate of Confidentiality** from the National Institutes of Health. The certificate allows researchers to refuse to disclose information on study participants in any legal proceeding.

> **Example of confidentiality procedures**
> Casey and colleagues (2024) conducted a qualitative study to describe the experiences of an intervention aimed at building resilience and strengthening the personal attributes of those experiencing dementia and their caregivers. Participants were assured that all information obtained for the study would be kept private and confidential.

Debriefings and Referrals

Researchers should show respect for participants during the interactions they have with them—they should be polite and make evident their tolerance of cultural, linguistic, and lifestyle diversity. Formal strategies for communicating respect are also available. For example, it is sometimes advisable to offer **debriefing** sessions following data collection so that participants can ask questions or express concerns. Researchers can also demonstrate their interest in participants by offering to share study findings with them after the data have been analyzed. Researchers also may need to assist participants by making referrals to appropriate health, social, or psychological services.

> **Example of referrals**
> Xu and colleagues (2024) explored the reproductive concerns experienced by young breast cancer survivors posttreatment. Because of the sensitivity of the information being obtained, the researchers sought to minimize the participants' emotional distress. Anyone displaying significant distress was referred to a psychiatric counselor.

Treatment of Vulnerable Groups

Adherence to ethical standards is often straightforward, but special **vulnerable groups** may need extra protection. Vulnerable populations may be incapable of giving fully informed consent (e.g., people with cognitive impairment) or may be at high risk of unintended side effects (e.g., pregnant people). You should pay particular attention to ethical aspects of a study when people who are vulnerable are involved. Among the groups that should be considered, vulnerable are the following:

- *Children*. Legally and ethically, children do not have the competence to give informed consent, so the consent of children's parents or guardians should be obtained. However, it is appropriate—especially if the child is at least 7 years of age—to obtain the child's assent as well. **Assent** refers to the child's affirmative agreement to participate.
- *People with mental or emotional impairment*. Individuals whose disability makes it impossible for them to make informed decisions (e.g., people in a coma) also cannot legally provide informed consent. In such cases, researchers should obtain the consent of a legal guardian.
- *People with severe illness or physical disability*. For patients who are very ill or undergoing certain treatments (e.g., mechanical ventilation), it might be necessary to assess their ability to make reasoned decisions about study participation.
- *People with terminal illness*. People with terminal illness seldom benefit personally from research, and thus, the risk/benefit ratio needs to be carefully assessed.
- *People who are institutionalized*. Nurses often conduct studies with hospitalized or institutionalized people (e.g., people who are incarcerated) who might feel that their care would be jeopardized by failure to cooperate. Researchers studying institutionalized groups need to emphasize the voluntary nature of participation.
- *Pregnant people*. The U.S. government has issued additional requirements governing research with pregnant people and fetuses. These requirements reflect a desire to safeguard both the pregnant person, who may be at heightened physical or psychological risk, and the fetus, who cannot give informed consent.

> **Example of research with a vulnerable group**
> Schmidt et al. (2023) explored the reproductive goals of women experiencing homelessness and substance use disorder in San Francisco. The researchers did not want to assume all potential participants had sufficient literacy, so they obtained verbal consent. Participants were asked to verbally repeat elements of the consent to ensure they understood the study and what was being asked of them as participants.

External Reviews and the Protection of Human Rights

Researchers may not be objective in developing procedures to protect participants' rights. Biases may arise from their commitment to an area of knowledge and their desire to conduct a rigorous study. Because a biased self-evaluation is possible, the ethical dimensions of a study are usually subjected to external review.

Most hospitals, universities, and other institutions where research is conducted have established formal committees for reviewing research plans. These committees are sometimes called *human subjects committees* or (in Canada) *Research Ethics Boards*. In the United States, the committee is often called an **Institutional Review Board (IRB)**. Before undertaking a study, researchers must submit research plans to the IRB and must also undergo formal IRB training. An IRB can approve the proposed plans, require modifications, or disapprove them.

> **Example of IRB approval**
> Hanan et al. (2024) conducted a study to describe long-term care health care professionals' perceptions of the barriers and facilitators to caring for residents experiencing serious persistent mental illness. The procedures and protocols for the study were approved by the IRB of Boston College.

Ethical Issues in Using Animals in Research

Some nurse researchers who focus on biophysiologic phenomena use animals as their subjects. Ethical considerations are clearly different for animals; for example, *informed consent* is not relevant. In the United States, the Public Health Service has issued a policy statement on the humane care and use of animals. The guidelines articulate principles for the proper care and treatment of animals used in research, covering such issues as the transport of research animals, pain and distress in animal subjects, the use of appropriate anesthesia, and euthanizing animals under certain conditions during or after the study.

> **Example of research with animals**
> Parra and colleagues (2022) conducted a study to determine the benefits of dog-assisted therapy on the emotional, behavioral, and cognitive function of people experiencing dementia who were in a nursing home in Azucaica, Toledo, Spain. The study was conducted per the Declaration of Helsinki and was approved by the Ethics Committee of the Catholic University of Murcia, approval (code CE031820).

CRITICALLY APPRAISING THE ETHICAL ASPECTS OF A STUDY

Guidelines for appraising the ethical aspects of a study are presented in Box 4.2. Members of an IRB or human subjects committee are provided with sufficient information to answer all these questions, but research articles do not always include detailed information about ethics because of space constraints in journals. Thus, it may be difficult to evaluate researchers' adherence to ethical guidelines. Nevertheless, we offer a few suggestions for considering ethical issues.

Many research reports do acknowledge that the study procedures were reviewed by an IRB or human subjects committee. When a report mentions a formal review, it is usually safe to assume that a panel of concerned people thoroughly reviewed ethical issues in a proposed study.

You can also come to some conclusions based on a description of the study methods. There may be sufficient information to judge, for example, whether study participants were subjected to harm or discomfort. Reports do not always state whether informed consent was secured, but you should be alert to situations in which the data could not have been gathered as described if participation had been purely voluntary (e.g., if data were gathered unobtrusively).

Box 4.2 Guidelines for Critically Appraising the Ethical Aspects of a Study

a. Was the study approved and monitored by an Institutional Review Board, Research Ethics Board, or other similar ethics review committee?
b. Were study participants subjected to any physical harm, discomfort, or psychological distress? Did the researchers take appropriate steps to remove or prevent harm?
c. Did the benefits to participants outweigh any potential risks or actual discomfort they experienced? Did the benefits to society outweigh the costs to participants?
d. Was any type of coercion or undue influence used to recruit participants? Did they have the right to refuse to participate or to withdraw without penalty?
e. Were participants deceived in any way? Were they fully aware of participating in a study, and did they understand the purpose and nature of the research?
f. Were appropriate informed consent procedures used with participants? If not, was there a justifiable rationale?
g. Were adequate steps taken to safeguard participants' privacy? How was confidentiality maintained? Was a Certificate of Confidentiality obtained, and, if not, should one have been obtained?
h. Were vulnerable groups involved in the research? If yes, were special precautions instituted because of their vulnerable status?
i. Were groups omitted from the inquiry without a justifiable rationale, such as a certain gender or underrepresented group?

In thinking about the ethical aspects of a study, you should also consider who the study participants were. For example, if the study involves vulnerable groups, there should be more information about protective procedures. You might also need to attend to who the study participants were *not*. For example, there has been considerable concern about the omission of underrepresented groups from clinical research.

RESEARCH EXAMPLES WITH CRITICAL THINKING EXERCISES

A brief summary focusing on the ethical aspects of a qualitative nursing study is presented in the following sections. Read the research summary for Example 1, and then answer the critical thinking questions that follow. The critical thinking questions for Examples 2 and 3 are based on the studies that appear in their entirety in Appendices A and B of this book.

EXAMPLE 1: ETHICAL ASPECTS OF A QUALITATIVE STUDY

Study: "The uncertainty in family caregivers of hospitalized persons with a stroke in Saudi Arabia: Unitary caring perspective" (Alselami et al., 2024)

Purpose: The purpose of this study was to explore how family caregivers described uncertainty while caring for a hospitalized family member who survived a stroke in light of the unitary caring theory of Smith.

Methods: This study used a unitary-caring-hermeneutic phenomenologic approach to conduct semi-structured interviews with 15 participants.

Ethics-Related Procedures: The study was approved by the Florida Atlantic University's IRB and the Research Ethical Committees of three hospitals in Saudi Arabia. Participants were assured confidentiality and that their responses would not interfere with their family member's care. Participants were also told that they could stop the interview at any time if they were not comfortable answering the questions. Written consent was obtained prior to the commencement of the interviews.

Key Findings: Five major themes and 16 subthemes were identified. The major themes include living in a dark reality, yearning for professional support, enduring a life full of tribulations, attempting resolution, and creating new patterns of living. The researchers further analyzed the findings in light of Smith's unitary caring theory.

Critical Thinking Exercises

1. Answer the relevant questions from Box 4.2 regarding this study.
2. The researchers offered a stipend—comment on whether you think this was ethically appropriate. Was it sufficiently large?
3. Comment on the appropriateness of the location of the interview.
4. If the results of this study are trustworthy and transferable, what might be some of the uses to which the findings could be put in clinical practice?

EXAMPLE 2: QUANTITATIVE STUDY IN APPENDIX A

Read the method section of Cheng and colleagues' (2024) study "Advance care planning affects end-of-life treatment preferences among patients with heart failure: A randomized controlled trial" in Appendix A of this book.

Critical Thinking Exercises

1. Answer the relevant questions from Box 4.2 regarding this study.
2. Where was the information about ethical issues located in this report?
3. What additional information regarding the ethical aspects of their study could the researchers have included in this article?

EXAMPLE 3: QUALITATIVE STUDY IN APPENDIX B

Read the method section from Morrison and colleagues' (2024) study "Lived experiences of fatherhood after infertility" in Appendix B of this book.

Critical Thinking Exercises

1. Answer the relevant questions from Box 4.2 regarding this study.
2. Where was the information about the ethical aspects of this study located in the report?
3. What additional information regarding the ethical aspects of Morrison et al.'s study could the researchers have included in this article?

Summary Points

- Because research has not always been conducted ethically and because of genuine **ethical dilemmas** that researchers face in designing studies that are both ethical and rigorous, **codes of ethics** have been developed to guide researchers.

- Three major ethical principles from the **Belmont Report** are incorporated into many ethical guidelines: beneficence, respect for human dignity, and justice.

- **Beneficence** involves the performance of some good and the protection of participants from physical and psychological harm and exploitation.

- Respect for human dignity involves the participants' right to self-determination, which includes participants' right to participate in a study voluntarily.

- **Full disclosure** means that researchers have fully described to prospective participants their rights and the study's costs and benefits. When full disclosure poses the risk of biased results, researchers sometimes use *concealment* (the collection of information without participants' knowledge) or *deception* (withholding information or providing false information).

- *Justice* includes the right to fair treatment and the right to privacy. In the United States, privacy has become a major issue because of the Privacy Rule regulations that resulted from the HIPAA.

- Procedures have been developed to safeguard study participants' rights, including the performance of a risk/benefit assessment, the implementation of informed consent procedures, and methods to safeguard participants' confidentiality.

- In a **risk/benefit assessment**, the potential benefits of the study to individual participants and to society are weighed against the costs to individuals.

- **Informed consent** procedures, which provide prospective participants with information needed to make a reasoned decision about participation, normally involve signing a consent form to document voluntary and informed participation.

- Privacy can be maintained through **anonymity** (wherein not even researchers know participants' identities) or through formal confidentiality procedures that safeguard the participants' data.

- Some U.S. researchers obtain a **Certificate of Confidentiality** that protects them against the forced disclosure of confidential information through a court order.

- Researchers sometimes offer **debriefing** sessions after data collection to provide participants with more information or an opportunity to air complaints.

- **Vulnerable groups** require additional protection. These people may be vulnerable because they are not able to make an informed decision about study participation (e.g., children), because of diminished autonomy (e.g., people who are incarcerated), or because their circumstances heighten the risk of harm (e.g., pregnant people, people with terminal illness).

- External review of the ethical aspects of a study by a human subjects committee or **IRB** is highly desirable and is often required by universities and organizations from which participants are recruited.

REFERENCES

Alselami, S., Butcher, H. K., & Longo, J. (2024). The uncertainty in family caregivers of hospitalized persons with a stroke in Saudi Arabia: Unitary caring perspective. *Advances in Nursing Science, 47*(1), 104–120. https://doi.org/10.1097/ANS.0000000000000519

American Nurses Association. (2025). *Code of ethics for nurses.* https://codeofethics.ana.org/home

Beck, C. T., & Casavant, S. (2020). Vicarious posttraumatic growth in NICU nurses. *Advances in Neonatal Care, 20*(4), 324–332. https://doi.org/10.1097/ANC.0000000000000689

Canadian Nurses Association. (2025). *Code of ethics for registered nurses.* Author.

Casey, D., Smyth, S., Doyle, P., Gallagher, N., O'Sullivan, G., Murphy, K., Dröes, R. M., & Whelan, B. (2024). An embedded qualitative study of the experiences of people with dementia, their caregivers and volunteer older adults who participated in the CREST resilience-building psychosocial intervention. *BMC Geriatrics, 24*(1), 780. https://doi.org/10.1186/s12877-024-05374-7

Cheng, H. C., Wu, S. V., Chen, Y. H., Tsan, Y. H., Sung, S. H., & Ke, L. S. (2024). Advance care planning affects end-of-life treatment preferences among patients with heart failure: A randomized controlled trial. *Journal of Hospice and Palliative Nursing, 26*(1), E13–E19. https://doi.org/10.1097/NJH.0000000000000988

Hanan, D. M., Lyons, K. S., Mahoney, E. K., Irwin, K. E., & Flanagan, J. M. (2024). Barriers and facilitators to caring for individuals with serious persistent mental illness in long-term care. *Archives of Psychiatric Nursing, 51*, 25–29. https://doi.org/10.1016/j.apnu.2024.05.006

Morrison, S., Bryanton, J., Murray, C., & Foley, V. (2024). Lived experiences of fatherhood after infertility. *Journal of Obstetric, Gynecologic, and Neonatal Nursing, 53*(3), 245–254. https://doi.org/10.1016/j.jogn.2023.12.002

Parra, E. V., Hernández Garre, J. M., & Pérez, P. E. (2022). Impact of dog-assisted therapy for institutionalized patients with dementia: A controlled clinical trial. *Alternative Therapies in Health and Medicine, 28*(1), 26–31. https://www.alternative-therapies.com/oa/6707.html

Petreca, V. G., Flanagan, J., Lyons, K. S., & Burgess, A. W. (2024). The reintegration of men into society after a sexual offense: A hermeneutic phenomenology study. *Issues in Mental Health Nursing, 45*(5), 453–467. https://doi.org/10.1080/01612840.2024.2322008

Schmidt, C. N., Wingo, E. E., Newmann, S. J., Borne, D. E., Shapiro, B. J., & Seidman, D. L. (2023). Patient and provider perspectives on barriers and facilitators to reproductive healthcare access for women experiencing homelessness with substance use disorders in San Francisco. *Women's Health (London, England), 19*, 17455057231152374. https://doi.org/10.1177/17455057231152374

Silva, M. C. (1995). *Ethical guidelines in the conduct, dissemination, and implementation of nursing research*. American Nurses Association.

Sun, W., Gabel, G., Akhter, R., Lawson, L., & Plishewsky, J. (2024). Feasibility and acceptability of virtual programs for people with dementia and their caregivers. *BMC Geriatrics, 24*(1), 783. https://doi.org/10.1186/s12877-024-05375-6

Xu, W., Liu, X., Zhang, C., Zhu, L., Zhao, Y., & Liao, C. (2024). Posttreatment experiences of reproductive concerns among young breast cancer survivors: A descriptive phenomenological study. *Asian Nursing Research, 18*(4), 331–340. https://doi.org/10.1016/j.anr.2024.09.003

Part 2: Preliminary Steps in Quantitative and Qualitative Research

5 Identifying Research Problems, Research Questions, and Hypotheses

Learning Objectives

On completing this chapter, you will be able to:

- Describe the process of developing and refining a research problem
- Distinguish the functions and forms of purpose statements and research questions for quantitative and qualitative studies
- Describe the purpose and characteristics of research hypotheses
- Critically appraise statements of purpose, research questions, and hypotheses in research reports with respect to their placement, clarity, wording, and relevance to nursing
- Define new terms in the chapter

Key Terms

- Complex hypothesis
- Directional hypothesis
- Hypothesis
- Nondirectional hypothesis
- Null hypothesis
- Problem statement
- Research hypothesis
- Research problem
- Research question
- Simple hypothesis
- Statement of purpose

OVERVIEW OF RESEARCH PROBLEMS

Studies begin in much the same fashion as an evidence-based practice (EBP) effort—as problems that need to be solved or questions that need to be answered. This chapter discusses research problems and research questions. We begin by clarifying some terms.

Basic Terminology

Researchers begin with a *topic* on which to focus. Claustrophobia during magnetic resonance imaging (MRI) tests and pain management for sickle cell disease are examples of research topics. Within broad topic areas are many possible research problems. In this section, we illustrate various terms using the topic *side effects of chemotherapy*.

TABLE 5.1 Terms Relating to Research Problems With Examples

Term	Example
Topic	Side effects of chemotherapy
Research problem (problem statement)	Nausea and vomiting are common side effects among patients on chemotherapy, and interventions to date have been only moderately successful in reducing these effects. New interventions that can reduce these side effects need to be identified.
Statement of purpose	The purpose of the study is to compare the effectiveness of patient-controlled vs. nurse-administered antiemetic therapy for controlling nausea and vomiting in patients on chemotherapy.
Research question	What is the relative effectiveness of patient-controlled antiemetic therapy vs. nurse-controlled antiemetic therapy with regard to (1) medication consumption and (2) control of nausea and vomiting in patients on chemotherapy?
Hypotheses	Patients receiving antiemetic therapy by a patient-controlled pump will (1) be less nauseous, (2) vomit less, and (3) consume less medication than patients receiving nurse-administered therapy.

A **research problem** is an enigmatic or troubling condition. The purpose of research is to "solve" the problem—or to contribute to its solution—by gathering relevant data. A **problem statement** articulates the problem and offers an *argument* explaining the need for a study. Table 5.1 presents a simplified problem statement related to the topic of side effects of chemotherapy.

Many reports provide a **statement of purpose** (or *purpose statement*), which summarizes an overall goal. **Research questions** are the specific queries researchers want to answer. Researchers who make specific predictions about the answers to research questions pose hypotheses that are then tested. These terms are not always consistently defined in research textbooks. Table 5.1 illustrates the interrelationships among terms as we define them.

Research Problems and Paradigms

Some research problems are better suited to qualitative versus quantitative inquiry. Quantitative studies usually involve concepts that are well developed and for which methods of measurement have been (or can be) developed. For example, a quantitative study might be undertaken to assess whether people with chronic illness are more likely to develop depression than people without a chronic illness. There are good measures of depression that would yield quantitative data about the level of depression in those with and without a chronic illness.

Qualitative studies are undertaken because a researcher wants to develop a rich, context-bound understanding of a poorly understood phenomenon. Qualitative methods would not be well suited to comparing levels of depression among those with and without chronic illness, but they would be ideal for exploring the *meaning* or *experience* of depression among people with chronic illness. In appraising a research report, one consideration is whether the research problem is suitable for the chosen paradigm.

Sources of Research Problems

Where do ideas for research problems come from? At the most basic level, research topics originate with researchers' interests. Because research is a time-consuming enterprise, curiosity about a topic that is appealing is essential to a project's success.

Research reports rarely indicate the origin of researchers' inspiration for a study, but a variety of sources can fuel their curiosity, such as their clinical experience or readings in the nursing literature. Also, topics are sometimes suggested by global social or political issues of relevance to the health care community (e.g., health disparities). Theories from nursing and other disciplines sometimes generate a research problem. Additionally, researchers who have developed a *program of research* may get inspiration for "next steps" from their own work or from discussions of their findings with others.

> **Example of a problem source for a quantitative study**
> Flanagan, one of the authors of this book, was working with a nursing research team from the Yvonne L. Munn Center for Nursing Research at the Massachusetts General Hospital in Boston Massachusetts, during the COVID-19 pandemic. The team had been deployed to several areas of the hospital. They noted that the usual nursing assessment had been replaced with an emergency assessment. Additionally, they noted that the patients being cared for were more socio-demographically diverse than patients who were typically cared for at the hospital. They discussed the need to explore this further to determine if the emergency documentation captured nurse-sensitive indicators, including social determinants of health (SDoH). The team led by Banister et al. (2022) found that SDoH were inconsistently documented, but 58.5% of the sample identified as belonging to an underrepresented racial or ethnic group and 34.4% required interpreter services. All but 3.2% of the sample was insured through private or public health insurance. Using a functional health pattern (FHP) framework, the team found that 9 of the 11 FHPs were reflected in nurse-sensitive indicators documented in the electronic health record (Banister et al., 2022).

Development and Refinement of Research Problems

Developing a research problem is a creative process. Researchers often begin with interests in a broad topic area and then develop a more specific researchable problem. For example, suppose a clinical nursing instructor wonders about secondary traumatic stress (the stress resulting from helping patients who have experienced trauma or suffering) in nursing students. The nurse has read that registered nurses report high levels of secondary traumatic stress and wonders if nursing students are also susceptible. This broad interest in secondary traumatic stress in students may lead to more specific musings, such as whether the students' type of nursing program is relevant to their secondary traumatic stress. The nurse also observes nursing students who have clinical rotations on their unit and may notice that students struggle caring for patients with certain conditions. These reflections may lead the nurse to have a discussion with colleagues, which may result in several research questions, such as the following:

- What is the experience of secondary traumatic stress like among nursing students?
- What are the frequency and intensity of secondary traumatic stress symptoms in nursing students?
- Do baccalaureate and associate degree nursing students differ in their level of secondary traumatic stress symptoms?
- What patient characteristics or clinical situations are most likely to provoke secondary traumatic stress in students?

These questions stem from the same broad problem, yet some suggest a qualitative approach and others suggest a quantitative one. Symptoms of secondary traumatic stress (Q2), type of nursing program (Q3), and patient characteristics (Q4) are all attributes that can be measured and suggest a quantitative inquiry. A qualitative researcher would be more interested in understanding the *essence* of students' stressful experiences or the *process* by which the stress was alleviated (Q1). These aspects of the problem would be difficult to measure. Researchers choose a problem to study based on its inherent interest to them and the fit with a paradigm of preference.

COMMUNICATING RESEARCH PROBLEMS AND QUESTIONS

Every study should have a problem statement that articulates clearly what is problematic and what must be solved. Most research reports also present either a statement of purpose, research questions, or hypotheses, and often, combinations of these three elements are included.

Many students do not understand problem statements and may have trouble identifying them in a research article. A problem statement is presented early in the report, whereas research questions, purpose statements, or hypotheses appear later in the introduction.

Problem Statements

A good problem statement is a declaration of what is problematic, what "needs fixing," or what is poorly understood. Problem statements, especially for quantitative studies, usually have most of the following six components:

1. *Problem identification:* What is wrong with the current situation?
2. *Background:* What is the nature of the problem, or the context of the situation, that readers need to understand?
3. *Scope of the problem:* How big a problem is it? How many people are affected?
4. *Consequences of the problem:* What is the cost of not fixing the problem?
5. *Knowledge gaps:* What information about the problem is lacking?
6. *Proposed solution:* How will the new study contribute to the solution of the problem?

Let us suppose that our topic was humor as a complementary therapy for reducing stress in hospitalized patients with cancer. One research question (discussed later in this section) might be, "What is the effect of nurses' use of humor on stress and natural killer cell activity in hospitalized cancer patients?" Box 5.1 presents a rough draft of a problem statement for such a study. This problem statement is a reasonable draft, but it can be improved.

Box 5.2 illustrates how the problem statement was strengthened by adding information about scope, long-term consequences, and possible solutions. This second draft builds a more compelling *argument* for new research: Millions of people are affected by cancer, and the disease has adverse consequences not only for patients and their families but also for society. The revised problem statement also suggests a possible solution that is the basis for the new study.

Box 5.1 Draft Problem Statement on Humor and Stress

A diagnosis of cancer is associated with high levels of stress. Sizable numbers of patients who receive a cancer diagnosis describe feelings of uncertainty, fear, anger, and loss of control. Interpersonal relationships, psychological functioning, and role performance have all been found to suffer following cancer diagnosis and treatment.

A variety of complementary and alternative therapies have been developed in efforts to decrease the harmful effects of cancer-related stress on psychological and physiologic functioning, and resources devoted to these therapies have increased in recent years. However, many of these therapies have not been carefully evaluated to assess their efficacy, safety, or cost-effectiveness. For example, the use of humor has been recommended as a therapeutic device to improve quality of life, decrease stress, and perhaps improve immune functioning, but the evidence to justify its advocacy is scant.

Box 5.2 Some Possible Improvements to Problem Statement on Humor and Stress

Each year, over 2 million people are diagnosed with cancer, which remains one of the top causes of death among adults (reference citations).[1] Numerous studies have documented that a diagnosis of cancer is associated with high levels of stress. Sizable numbers of patients who receive a cancer diagnosis describe feelings of uncertainty, fear, anger, and loss of control (citations). Interpersonal relationships, psychological functioning, and role performance have all been found to suffer following cancer diagnosis and treatment (citations). These stressful outcomes can, in turn, adversely affect health, long-term prognosis, and medical costs among cancer survivors (citations).

A variety of complementary and alternative therapies have been developed in efforts to decrease the harmful effects of cancer-related stress on psychological and physiologic functioning, and resources devoted to these therapies (money and staff) have increased in recent years (citations). However, many of these therapies have not been carefully evaluated to assess their efficacy, safety, or cost-effectiveness. For example, the use of humor has been recommended as a therapeutic device to improve quality of life, decrease stress, and perhaps improve immune functioning (citations), but the evidence to justify its advocacy is scant. Preliminary findings from a recent small-scale endocrinology study with a healthy sample exposed to a humorous intervention (citation) hold promise for further inquiry with immuno-compromised populations.

---

[1] Reference citations would be inserted to support the statements.

HOW-TO-TELL TIP How can you tell a problem statement? Problem statements are rarely explicitly labeled. The first sentence of a research report is often the starting point of a problem statement. The problem statement is usually interwoven with findings from the research literature, which provide supporting evidence and suggest gaps in knowledge. In many articles, it is difficult to disentangle the problem statement from the literature review, unless there is a subsection specifically labeled "Literature Review" or something similar.

Problem statements for a qualitative study similarly express the nature of the problem, its context, its scope, and information needed to address it. Qualitative studies embedded in a research tradition often incorporate terms and concepts that foreshadow the tradition in their problem statements. For example, a problem statement for a phenomenologic study might note the need to learn more about people's experiences or meanings they attribute to those experiences.

Statements of Purpose

Many researchers articulate their research goal as a statement of purpose. The purpose statement establishes the general direction of the inquiry and captures the study's substance. It is usually easy to identify a purpose statement because the word *purpose* is explicitly stated: "The purpose of this study was . . ."—although sometimes the words *aim*, *goal*, or *objective* are used instead, as in "The aim of this study was . . . ."

In a quantitative study, a statement of purpose identifies the key study variables and their possible interrelationships as well as the population of interest (i.e., all the PICO elements).

> **Example of a statement of purpose from a quantitative study**
> Lee and colleagues (2024) conducted a study to examine the patterns of self-care decision-making and associated factors in adults with chronic illness. One of the stated purposes was "to determine whether multiple patterns of self-care decision-making could be identified in the context of chronic illness" (Lee et al., 2024, p. 3).

This purpose statement indicates that the population (P) of interest is patients with chronic illness. The key study variables were the patients' status as having or not having chronic illness (the dependent variable [DV]) and the participants' pattern of self-care (the independent variable [IV]).

In qualitative studies, the statement of purpose indicates the nature of the inquiry; the key concept or phenomenon; and the group, community, or setting under study.

> **Example of a statement of purpose from a qualitative study**
> "The purpose of this study was to understand health care professionals' perceptions of the barriers and facilitators to caring for long-term care residents with serious persistent mental illness" (Hanan et al., 2024, p. 26).

This statement indicates that the population under study was health professionals caring for long-term care residents with serious, persistent mental illness, and the central phenomenon was the perceived barriers and facilitators of caring for these residents.

Researchers often communicate information about their approach through their choice of verbs. A study whose purpose is to *explore*, *investigate*, or *describe* some phenomenon is likely to be an investigation of a little-researched topic, often involving a qualitative approach such as phenomenology or ethnography. A statement of purpose for a qualitative study—especially a grounded theory study—may also use verbs such as *understand*, *discover*, or *generate*. Statements of purpose in qualitative studies also may "encode" the tradition of inquiry through certain terms or "buzz words" associated with those traditions, as follows:

- *Grounded theory*: processes; social structures; social interactions
- *Phenomenologic studies*: experience; lived experience; meaning; essence
- *Ethnographic studies*: culture; roles; lifeways; cultural behavior

Quantitative researchers also use verbs to communicate the nature of the inquiry. A statement indicating that the study purpose is to *test* or *evaluate* something (e.g., an intervention) suggests an experimental design, for example. A study whose purpose is to *examine* or *explore* the relationship between two variables is more likely to involve a nonexperimental design. Sometimes the verb is ambiguous: If a purpose statement states that the researcher's intent is to *compare* two things, the comparison could involve alternative treatments (using an experimental design) or two preexisting groups such as people who smoke tobacco and people who do not smoke tobacco (using a nonexperimental design). In any event, verbs such as *test*, *evaluate*, and *compare* suggest quantifiable variables and designs with scientific controls.

The verbs in a purpose statement should signal objectivity. A statement of purpose indicating that the study goal was to *prove*, *demonstrate*, or *show* something suggests a bias.

Research Questions

Research questions are, in some cases, direct rewordings of statements of purpose, phrased interrogatively rather than declaratively, as in the following example:

- *Purpose*: The purpose of this study is to assess the relationship between the functional dependence level of kidney transplant recipients and their rate of recovery.

- *Question*: Is the functional dependence level (I) of renal transplant recipients (P) related to their rate of recovery (O)?

Some research articles omit a statement of purpose and state only research questions—or vice versa. Some researchers use research questions to add greater specificity to a global purpose statement.

Research Questions in Quantitative Studies

In Chapter 1, we discussed questions to guide an EBP inquiry. The EBP question templates in Table 1.3 could yield questions to guide a research project as well, but *researchers* tend to conceptualize their questions in terms of their *variables*. Take, for example, the first question in Table 1.3: "In (population), what is the effect of (intervention) on (outcome)?" A researcher would be more likely to think of the question in these terms: "In (population), what is the effect of (independent variable) on (dependent variable)?" Thinking in terms of variables helps to guide researchers' decisions about how to operationalize them. Thus, in quantitative studies, research questions identify the population (P) under study, the key study variables (I, C, and O components), and relationships among the variables.

Most research questions concern relationships among variables, and thus, many quantitative research questions could be articulated using a general question template: "In (population), what is the relationship between (independent variable or IV) and (dependent variable or DV)?" Examples of variations include the following:

- *Therapy/intervention*: In (population), what is the effect of (IV: intervention vs. an alternative) on (DV)?
- *Prognosis*: In (population), does (IV: a disease or illness vs. its absence) affect or increase the risk of (DV)?
- *Etiology/harm*: In (population), does (IV: exposure vs. nonexposure) cause or increase the risk of (DV)?

Not all research questions are about relationships—some are descriptive. As examples, here are two descriptive questions that could be answered in a quantitative study on nurses' use of humor:

- What is the frequency with which nurses use humor as a complementary therapy with hospitalized patients with cancer?
- What are the characteristics of nurses who use humor as a complementary therapy with hospitalized patients with cancer?

Answers to such questions might be useful in developing effective strategies for reducing stress in patients with cancer.

> **Example of a research question from a quantitative study**
> Eroglu and Metin (2024) explored the experience of spiritual well-being in people experiencing heart failure and asked, does spiritual well-being increase with self-reported health perceptions in patients with heart failure?

In this example, the question asks about the relationship between an IV (spiritual well-being) and the DV (self-reported symptoms of heart failure).

Research Questions in Qualitative Studies

Research questions in qualitative studies stipulate the phenomenon and population of interest. Grounded theory researchers are likely to ask *process* questions, phenomenologists tend to ask *meaning* and *experience* questions, and ethnographers generally ask *descriptive* questions about cultures. The terms associated with the various traditions, discussed previously in connection with purpose statements, are likely to be incorporated into the research questions.

> **Example of research question from a phenomenologic study** • • • • • • • • • • •
> "What is the lived experience of parents and caregivers of children with medical complexity (CMC)?" (Holmes et al., 2024, p. 3).

Not all qualitative studies are rooted in a specific research tradition. Many researchers use constructivist approaches to describe or explore phenomena without focusing on cultures, meaning, or social processes.

> **Example of a research question from a descriptive qualitative study** • • • • • •
> In their descriptive qualitative study, Geyer and colleagues (2024) asked this question: "What was the experience of bringing your child home from the hospital for the first time?"

In qualitative studies, research questions sometimes evolve during the study. Researchers begin with a *focus* that defines the broad boundaries of the inquiry, but the boundaries are not cast in stone. Constructivists are often sufficiently flexible that the question can be modified as new information makes it relevant to do so.

 TIP Researchers most often state their purpose or research questions at the end of the introduction or immediately after the review of the literature. Sometimes, a separate section of a research article is devoted to formal statements about the research problem formally and might be labeled "Purpose," "Statement of Purpose," "Research Questions," or, in quantitative studies, "Hypotheses."

RESEARCH HYPOTHESES

A **hypothesis** is a prediction, usually involving a predicted relationship between two or more variables. Qualitative researchers do not have formal hypotheses because qualitative researchers want the inquiry to be guided by participants' viewpoints rather than by their own hunches. Thus, our discussion focuses on hypotheses in quantitative research.

Function of Hypotheses in Quantitative Research

Many research questions ask about relationships between variables, and hypotheses are predicted answers to these questions. For instance, the research question might ask: Does sexual abuse in childhood affect the development of irritable bowel syndrome (IBS) in women? The researcher might predict the following: Women (P) who suffered sexual abuse in childhood (I) have a higher incidence of IBS (O) than women who were not abused (C).

Hypotheses sometimes emerge from a theory. Scientists reason from theories to hypotheses and test those hypotheses in the real world (see Chapter 7). Even in the absence of a theory, hypotheses offer direction and suggest explanations. For example, suppose we hypothesized that the incidence of desaturation in low-birth-weight infants undergoing intubation and ventilation would be lower using the closed tracheal suction system (CTSS) than using partially ventilated endotracheal suction (PVETS). Our hypothesis might be based on prior studies or clinical observations.

Now let us suppose the hypothesis is not confirmed in a study; that is, we find that rates of desaturation are similar for both the PVETS and CTSS methods. The failure of data to support a prediction forces researchers to analyze theory or previous research critically, to scrutinize study limitations, and to explore alternative explanations for the findings. The use of hypotheses tends to promote critical thinking. Now, suppose we conducted the study guided only by the question, Is there a relationship between suction method and rates of desaturation? Without a hypothesis, the researcher is seemingly prepared to accept any results. The problem is that it is almost always possible to explain something superficially after the fact, no matter what the findings are. Hypotheses reduce the possibility that spurious results will be misconstrued.

TIP Some quantitative research articles explicitly state the hypotheses that guided the study, but many do not. The absence of a stated hypothesis often means that the researchers failed to disclose their hunches.

Characteristics of Testable Hypotheses

Research hypotheses usually state the expected relationship between the IV (the presumed cause or influence) and the DV (the presumed outcome or effect) within a population.

> **Example of a research hypothesis**
> Padilla and colleagues (2024) hypothesized that a prenatal education intervention aimed at reducing fear of childbirth (FOC) in conjunction with midwife-specific usual care during childbirth would significantly reduce fear levels in people with high levels of FOC to a greater extent than usual care.

In this example, the population is people with a FOC. The IV is participation versus nonparticipation in the prenatal education and midwife intervention, and the outcome or DV is fear. The hypothesis predicts that, in the population, participation in the program is related to less fear.

Hypotheses that do not make a relational statement are difficult to test. Take the following example: *Pregnant people who receive prenatal instruction about postpartum experiences are unlikely to experience postpartum depression.* This statement expresses no anticipated relationship and cannot be tested using standard statistical procedures. In our example, how would we decide whether to accept or reject the hypothesis?

We could, however, modify the hypothesis as follows: Pregnant people who receive prenatal instruction are less likely than those who do not to experience postpartum depression. Here, the outcome variable (O) is postpartum depression and the IV is receipt (I) versus nonreceipt (C) of prenatal instruction. The relational aspect of the prediction is embodied in the phrase *less . . . than*. If a hypothesis lacks a phrase such as *more than*, *less than*, *different from*, *related to*, or something similar, it is not testable. To test the revised hypothesis, we could ask two groups of people with different prenatal instruction experiences to respond to questions on depression and then compare the groups' responses.

TIP Hypotheses are typically fairly easy to identify because researchers make statements such as, "The study tested the hypothesis that . . ." or, "It was predicted that . . . ."

Wording of Hypotheses

Hypotheses can be stated in various ways, as in the following example:

1. Older patients are more likely to fall than younger patients.
2. There is a relationship between a patient's age and the likelihood of falling.
3. The risk of falling increases with the age of the patient.
4. Older patients differ from younger ones with respect to their risk of falling.

In each example, the hypothesis states the population (patients), the IV (age), the outcome variable (falling), and an anticipated relationship between them.

Hypotheses can be either directional or nondirectional. A **directional hypothesis** specifies the expected direction of the relationship between variables. In the four versions of the hypothesis, versions 1 and 3 are directional because they predict that older patients are more likely to fall than younger ones. A **nondirectional hypothesis** does not stipulate the direction of the relationship (versions 2 and 4). These versions predict that a patient's age and falling are related but do not specify whether *older* or *younger* patients are predicted to be at greater risk.

Types of Hypotheses

Hypotheses can be either **simple hypotheses** (with a single IV and DV) or **complex hypotheses** (multiple IVs or DVs). Many quantitative studies address questions about the relationship between two variables using simple hypotheses. For example, "What is the effect of a nursing intervention (the independent variable, IV) on pain (the dependent variable, DV)?" Most phenomena are affected by a multiplicity of factors. A person's weight, for example, is affected simultaneously by such factors as height, diet, bone structure, activity level, and metabolism. If the DV were weight, and the IV was a person's caloric intake, we would not be able to explain or understand individual variation in weight very well. For example, knowing that someone's daily caloric intake averages 2,000 calories would not permit a good prediction of their weight. The overlap in circles indicating the strength of the relationship between caloric intake and weight would likely be smaller than what is shown in Figure 5.1.

> **Nursing example of a simple hypothesis**
> In their study on factors impacting patients' responses to inflammatory bowel disease, Hu and Xu (2024) provide examples of varying types of hypotheses. An example of a simple hypothesis they tested was fear of disease progression (IV) had a negative and direct predictive effect on health-related quality of life (DV).

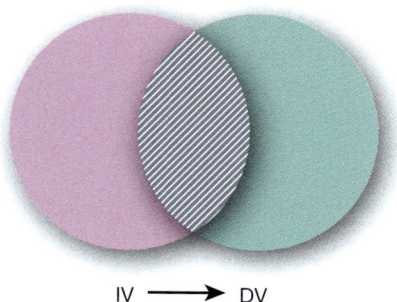

Figure 5.1 Schematic representation of a simple hypothesis. IV, independent variable; DV, dependent variable.

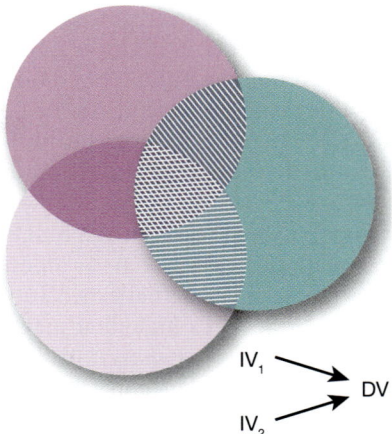

Figure 5.2 Schematic representation of a complex hypothesis with two independent variables. IV, independent variable; DV, dependent variable.

Many other factors are related to weight, and knowledge of those factors, such as height, would improve our ability to accurately understand and predict the person's weight. Figure 5.2 presents a schematic representation of a **complex hypothesis**, showing the prediction that the DV is influenced by two IVs, (IV_1 and IV_2). To pursue the preceding example, the hypothesis might be the following: Taller people (IV_1) and people with higher caloric intake (IV_2) weigh more (DV) than shorter people and those with lower caloric intake. In this example, we expect that caloric intake *and* height would do a better job in helping us explain variation in weight (DV) than caloric intake alone. Complex hypotheses have the advantage of allowing researchers to capture some of the complexity of the real world.

Just as a phenomenon can be caused or influenced by more than one IV, so a single IV can influence more than one phenomenon, as illustrated in Figure 5.3. A number of studies have found, for example, that cigarette smoking (the IV) can lead to both lung cancer (DV_1)

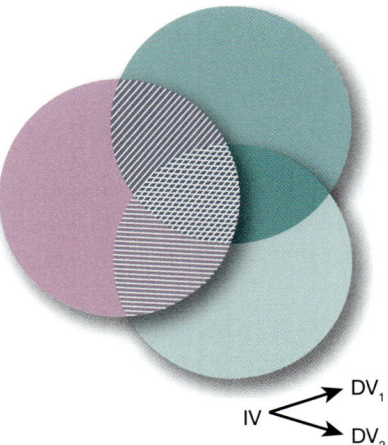

Figure 5.3 Schematic representation of a complex hypothesis with two dependent variables. IV, independent variable; DV, dependent variable.

and coronary disorders (DV_2). Complex hypotheses are common in studies that try to assess the impact of a nursing intervention on multiple outcomes.

Hypotheses can be even more complex (e.g., two IVs predicting two DVs). Hu and Xu (2024) in the same study referenced above provide an example of a complex hypothesis with multiple IVs and DVs. They hypothesize that health literacy and self-care (two IVs) jointly play a mediating role in the fear of progression and health-related quality of life (two DVs or outcomes).

Another distinction is between research and null hypotheses. **Research hypotheses** are statements of expected relationships between variables. All the hypotheses presented thus far are research hypotheses that indicate actual expectations.

Statistical inference operates on a logic that may be confusing. This logic requires that hypotheses be expressed as an expected *absence* of a relationship. **Null hypotheses** state that there is no relationship between the IVs and DVs. The null form of the first hypothesis in our example would be "Older patients and younger patients are equally likely to fall." The null hypothesis can be compared with the assumption of innocence in many systems of criminal justice: The variables are assumed to be "innocent" of a relationship until they can be shown "guilty" through statistical tests.

Research articles typically state research rather than null hypotheses. In statistical testing, underlying null hypotheses are assumed, without being stated.

TIP If a researcher uses statistical tests (which is true in most quantitative studies), it means that there are underlying hypotheses—regardless of whether the researcher explicitly stated them—because statistical tests are designed to test hypotheses.

Hypothesis Testing and Proof

Hypotheses are formally tested through statistical analysis. Researchers use statistics to test whether their hypotheses have a high probability of being correct (i.e., has a probability < .05). Statistical analysis does not offer proof; it only supports inferences that a hypothesis is *probably* correct (or not). Hypotheses are never *proved* or *disproved*; rather, they are *supported* or *rejected*. Hypotheses come to be increasingly supported with evidence from multiple studies.

To illustrate why this is so, suppose we hypothesized that height and weight are related. We predict that, on average, tall people weigh more than short people. Suppose we happened by chance to get a sample of short, heavy people and tall, thin people. Our results might indicate that there is no relationship between a person's height and weight. But we would not be justified in concluding that the study *proved* or *demonstrated* that height and weight are unrelated.

This example illustrates the difficulty of using observations from a sample to generalize to a population. Issues other than sampling, such as measurement flaws and the effects of confounding variables, prevent researchers from concluding that hypotheses are proved.

CRITICAL APPRAISAL OF RESEARCH PROBLEMS, RESEARCH QUESTIONS, AND HYPOTHESES

The problem statement, purpose, research questions, and hypotheses set the stage for describing what was done and what was learned. You should not have to dig too deeply to figure out the research problem or discover the questions.

A critical appraisal of the research problem involves multiple dimensions. Substantively, you need to consider whether the problem has significance for nursing. Studies that build

> **Box 5.3 Guidelines for Critically Appraising Research Problems, Research Questions, and Hypotheses**
>
> a. What was the research problem? Was the problem statement easy to locate and was it clearly stated? Did the problem statement build a coherent and persuasive argument for the new study?
> b. Does the problem have significance for nursing?
> c. Was there a good fit between the research problem and the paradigm (and tradition) within which the research was conducted?
> d. Did the report formally present a statement of purpose, research question, and/or hypotheses? Was this information communicated clearly and concisely, and was it placed in a logical and useful location?
> e. Were purpose statements or research questions worded appropriately (e.g., were key concepts/variables identified and the population specified)?
> f. If there were no formal hypotheses, was their absence justified? Were statistical tests used in analyzing the data despite the absence of stated hypotheses?
> g. Were hypotheses (if any) properly worded—did they state a predicted relationship between two or more variables? Were they presented as research or as null hypotheses?

on existing evidence in a meaningful way can make contributions to evidence-based nursing practice. Also, research problems stemming from research priorities (see Chapter 1) have a high likelihood of yielding important evidence for nurses.

Another dimension in appraising the research problem concerns methodologic issues—in particular, whether the research problem is compatible with the chosen research paradigm and its associated methods. You should also evaluate whether the statement of purpose or research questions lend themselves to research inquiry.

If an article describing a quantitative study does not state hypotheses, you should consider whether their absence is justified. If there are hypotheses, you should evaluate whether the hypotheses are sensible and consistent with existing evidence or relevant theory. Also, hypotheses are valid guideposts in scientific inquiry only if they are testable. To be testable, hypotheses must predict a relationship between two or more measurable variables.

Specific guidelines for appraising research problems, research questions, and hypotheses are presented in Box 5.3.

RESEARCH EXAMPLES WITH CRITICAL THINKING EXERCISES

This section describes how the research problem and research questions were communicated in two nursing studies—one quantitative and one qualitative. Read the summaries, and then answer the critical thinking questions that follow, referring to the full research report if necessary. The critical thinking questions for Examples 3 and 4 are based on the studies that appear in their entirety in Appendices A and B of this book.

EXAMPLE 1: QUANTITATIVE RESEARCH

Study: "Nurses' encounters with patients having end-of-life dreams and visions in an acute care setting—A cross-sectional survey study" (Hession et al., 2024)

Statement: End-of-life visions and dreams are experienced by patients nearing death and their families and loved ones. Patients report that these visions and dreams are comforting to them as do families, loved ones, and nurses who report bearing witness to these. While studies in palliative care or long-term care settings in Brazil and the United Kingdom have explored nurses' experiences of bearing witness to or discussing end-of-life visions and/or dreams with patients and families, there are no studies that have explored this phenomenon in other settings. Despite the comfort that patients, families, and loved ones may derive from discussing these experiences, nurses report not feeling prepared to do so.

Statement of Purpose: This study's purpose was to obtain an estimate of acute care nurses in acute care settings in Australia who either witnessed end-of-life dreams and/or visions or were told about one by a patient, family member, or loved one. A second objective of this study was to explore nurses' attitudes and beliefs about these experiences and to understand their perceived educational needs about how to address these experiences.

Hypothesis: This study was a descriptive exploratory study and did not include a hypothesis.

Methods: This study used a survey design to invite acute care nurses from medical and surgical units who provided care to patients receiving end-of-life care in the past 5 years. The survey was administered online and was also available or by paper-based questionnaires made available on various care units.

Key Findings: A total of 57 out of 169 nurses participated for a response rate of 34%. Findings indicate that 61% of respondents reported witnessing end-of-life dreams and visions. Nurses reported that these episodes were profoundly spiritual (74%) and meaningful (52.9%). While nurses reported feeling comfortable discussing these incidents with colleagues, nearly 28% reported discomfort discussing this with patients and 98% reported the need for further education about end-of-life dreams and visions.

Critical Thinking Exercises

1. Answer the relevant questions from Box 5.3 regarding this study.
2. Where in the research report do you think the researchers presented the hypotheses?
3. Were they presented as research or as null hypotheses?
4. Where in the report would the results of the hypothesis tests be placed?
5. Was the stated hypothesis directional or nondirectional?
6. Was the researchers' hypothesis supported in the statistical analysis?

EXAMPLE 2: QUALITATIVE RESEARCH

Study: "Caring touch as communication in intensive care nursing: A qualitative study"

Problem Statement (excerpt): "By touching a patient's skin in a comforting way, [the intensive care nurse (ICN)] non-verbally communicates to patients that they matter. Touching the patient's skin is a way of communicating safety and connection with the patient. Although caring is an important means of silent communication with critically ill patients, there is a scarcity of previous research on what ICNs communicate through their caring touch of patients' skin outside of procedural practice" (p. 2).

Statement of Purpose: To describe "intensive care nurses' experiences of using caring touch to communicate in a relationship with a critically ill patient" (p. 2).

Research Question: "What do intensive care nurses intend to communicate to patients through caring touch?" (p. 2)

Methods: Using a hermeneutic phenomenologic design, the researchers interviewed eight ICNs in two intensive care units at Norwegian hospitals. Nurses were asked several broad questions, such as "Could you talk about a situation where touch played an important role? What were your thoughts in that situation?" (p. 2)

Key Findings: The main theme was communicating safety and presence. This theme included four sub-themes: amplified presence; communicating security, trust, and care; creating and confirming relationships; and communicating openness to a deeper conversation.

Excerpt from Sandnes, L.., & Uhrenfeldt, L.. (2024). Caring touch as communication in intensive care nursing: A qualitative study. *International Journal of Qualitative Studies on Health and Well-Being, 19*, 2348891. https://doi.org/10.1080/17482631.2024.2348891. Reprinted by permission of Informa UK Limited, trading as Taylor & Francis Group, www.tandfonline.com

Critical Thinking Exercises

1. Answer the relevant questions from Box 5.3 regarding this study.
2. Where in the research report do you think the researchers presented the statement of purpose and research questions?
3. Does it appear that this study was conducted within one of the three main qualitative traditions? If so, which one?
4. If the results of this study are trustworthy, what are some of the uses to which the findings might be put in clinical practice?

EXAMPLE 3: QUANTITATIVE RESEARCH IN APPENDIX A

Read the abstract and the introduction of Cheng and colleagues' (2024) study "Advance care planning affects end-of-life treatment preferences among patients with heart failure: A randomized controlled trial" in Appendix A of this book.

Critical Thinking Exercises

1. Answer the relevant questions from Box 5.3 regarding this study.
2. What might a hypothesis for this study be? State it as a research hypothesis and as a null hypothesis.

EXAMPLE 4: QUALITATIVE RESEARCH IN APPENDIX B

Read the abstract and introduction from Morrison et al.'s (2024) study, "Lived experience of fatherhood after infertility," in Appendix B of this book.

Critical Thinking Exercises

1. Answer the relevant questions from Box 5.3 regarding this study.
2. Do you think that Morrison and colleagues provided a sufficient rationale for the significance of their research problem?

Summary Points

- A **research problem** is a perplexing or troubling situation that a researcher wants to address through disciplined inquiry.

- Researchers usually identify a broad *topic*, narrow the scope of the problem, and then identify research questions consistent with a paradigm of choice.

- Researchers communicate their aims in research articles as problem statements, statements of purpose, research questions, or hypotheses.

- A **problem statement** articulates the problem and an *argument* that explains the need for a study. Problem statements typically include several components: problem identification; background, scope, and consequences of the problem; knowledge gaps; and possible solutions to the problem.

- A **statement of purpose**, which summarizes the overall study goal, identifies the key concepts (variables) and the study group or population. Purpose statements often communicate, through the choice of verbs and other key terms, aspects of the study design, or the research tradition.

- **Research questions** are the specific queries researchers want to answer in addressing the research problem.

- A **hypothesis** states predicted relationships between two or more variables—that is, the anticipated association between IVs and DVs.

- **Directional hypotheses** predict the direction of a relationship; **nondirectional hypotheses** predict the existence of relationships, not their direction.

- **Research hypotheses** predict the existence of relationships; **null hypotheses**, which express the absence of relationships, are the hypotheses subjected to statistical testing.

- Hypotheses are never proved or disproved—they are accepted or rejected, supported or not supported by the data.

REFERENCES

Banister, G., Carroll, D. L., Dickins, K., Flanagan, J., Jones, D., Looby, S. E., & Cahill, J. E. (2022). Nurse-sensitive indicators during COVID-19. *International Journal of Nursing Knowledge*, *33*(3), 234–244. https://doi.org/10.1111/2047-3095.12372

Eroglu, H., & Metin, Z. G. (2024). Correlation between symptom status, health perception, and spiritual well-being in heart failure patients: A structural equation modeling approach. *Journal of Nursing Scholarship: An Official Publication of Sigma Theta Tau International Honor Society of Nursing*, *56*(4), 490–506. https://doi.org/10.1111/jnu.12961

Geyer, D., Flanagan, J. M., van de Water, B., McCarthy, S., & Vessey, J. A. (2024). A qualitative descriptive study exploring the systemic challenges of caring for children with medical complexity at home. *Journal of Pediatric Health Care: Official Publication of National Association of Pediatric Nurse Associates & Practitioners*, *39*, 24–32. https://doi.org/10.1016/j.pedhc.2024.08.010

Hanan, D. M., Lyons, K. S., Mahoney, E. K., Irwin, K. E., & Flanagan, J. M. (2024). Barriers and facilitators to caring for individuals with serious persistent mental illness in long-term care. *Archives of Psychiatric Nursing*, *51*, 25–29. https://doi.org/10.1016/j.apnu.2024.05.006

Hession, A., Luckett, T., Currow, D., & Barbato, M. (2024). Nurses' encounters with patients having end-of-life dreams and visions in an acute care setting—A cross-sectional survey study. *Journal of Advanced Nursing*, *80*(8), 3190–3198. https://doi.org/10.1111/jan.16079

Holmes, C., Zeleke, W., Sampath, S., & Kimbrough, T. (2024). "Hanging on by a Thread": The lived experience of parents of children with medical complexity. *Children (Basel, Switzerland)*, *11*(10), 1258. https://doi.org/10.3390/children11101258

Hu, X., & Xu, L. (2024). Relationship between fear of progression and quality of life in inflammatory bowel disease: Mediating role of health literacy and self-care. *Journal of Advanced Nursing*, *80*(10), 4147–4160. https://doi.org/10.1111/jan.16138

Lee, C. S., Freedland, K. E., Jaarsma, T., Strömberg, A., Vellone, E., Page, S. D., Westland, H., Pettersson, S., van Rijn, M., Aryal, S., Belfiglio, A., Wiebe, D., & Riegel, B. (2024). Patterns of self-care decision-making and associated factors: A cross-sectional observational study. *International Journal of Nursing Studies*, *150*, 104665. https://doi.org/10.1016/j.ijnurstu.2023.104665.

Padilla, S. M., González de la Torre, H., Alcaide, E. L., Verdú Soriano, J., & Martín Martínez, A. (2024). Randomized controlled trial of interventions used by midwives to treat fear of childbirth. *Nursing Research*, *73*, 221–231. https://doi.org/10.1097/NNR.0000000000000756

6 Finding and Reviewing Research Evidence in the Literature

Learning Objectives

On completing this chapter, you will be able to:

- Understand the steps involved in doing a literature review
- Identify bibliographic aids for retrieving research reports and locate references for a research topic
- Understand the process of screening, abstracting, appraising, and organizing research evidence
- Evaluate the style, content, and organization of a literature review
- Define new terms in the chapter

Key Terms

- Artificial intelligence
- Bibliographic database
- CINAHL
- Google Scholar
- Keyword
- Literature review
- MEDLINE
- MeSH
- Predatory journals
- Primary source
- PubMed
- Secondary source

A **literature review** is a written summary of the state of evidence on a research problem. It is useful for consumers of nursing research to acquire skills for reading, appraising, and preparing written evidence summaries.

BASIC ISSUES RELATING TO LITERATURE REVIEWS

Before discussing the activities involved in undertaking a research-based literature review, we briefly discuss some general issues. The first concerns the purposes of doing a literature review.

Purposes of Research Literature Reviews

The primary purpose of literature reviews is to summarize evidence on a topic—to sum up what is known and what is not known. Literature reviews are sometimes stand-alone reports intended to communicate the state of evidence to others, but reviews are also used to lay the foundation for new studies and to help researchers interpret their findings.

 TIP Sometimes, stand-alone reviews are called *integrative reviews*, a term that most often is used when a literature review integrates evidence from both qualitative and quantitative studies. Whittemore and Knafl (2005) and Knafl and Whittemore (2017) offer further guidance.

89

In qualitative research, opinions about doing an upfront literature review vary. Grounded theory researchers typically begin to collect data before examining the literature. As a theory takes shape, researchers turn to the literature, seeking to relate prior findings to the theory. Phenomenologists and ethnographers often undertake a literature search at the outset of a study.

Regardless of when they perform the review, researchers usually include a brief summary of relevant literature in the introductions of their reports. The literature review summarizes current evidence on a topic and illuminates the significance of the new study. Literature reviews are often intertwined with the problem statement as part of the argument for the new study.

Types of Information to Seek for a Research Review

Findings from prior studies are the "data" for a research review. If you are preparing a literature review, you should rely mostly on **primary sources**, which are descriptions of studies written by the researchers who conducted them. **Secondary sources** are descriptions of studies prepared by someone else. Literature reviews are secondary sources. Recent reviews are a good place to start because they offer overviews and valuable bibliographies. If you are doing your own literature review, however, secondary sources should not be considered substitutes for primary sources because secondary sources lack details and may not be completely objective.

 TIP For an evidence-based practice (EBP) project, a recent, high-quality systematic review may provide the needed information about the evidence base, although it is usually a good idea to search for studies published after the review.

A literature search may yield non-research references, such as case reports or clinical opinions. Such materials may broaden understanding of a problem or demonstrate a need for research. However, these writings have limited utility in research reviews, as they do not address the central question: What is the current state of *evidence* on this research problem?

Major Steps and Strategies in Doing a Literature Review

Conducting a literature review is an original study in its own right: A reviewer starts with a question and then must gather, analyze, and interpret the information. Figure 6.1 depicts the literature review process and shows that there are potential feedback loops, with opportunities to go back to earlier steps in search of more information.

Reviews should be unbiased, thorough, and up-to-date. Decision rules for including a study should be explicit—a good review should be reproducible. This means that another diligent reviewer would be able to apply the same decision rules and come to similar conclusions about the state of evidence on the topic.

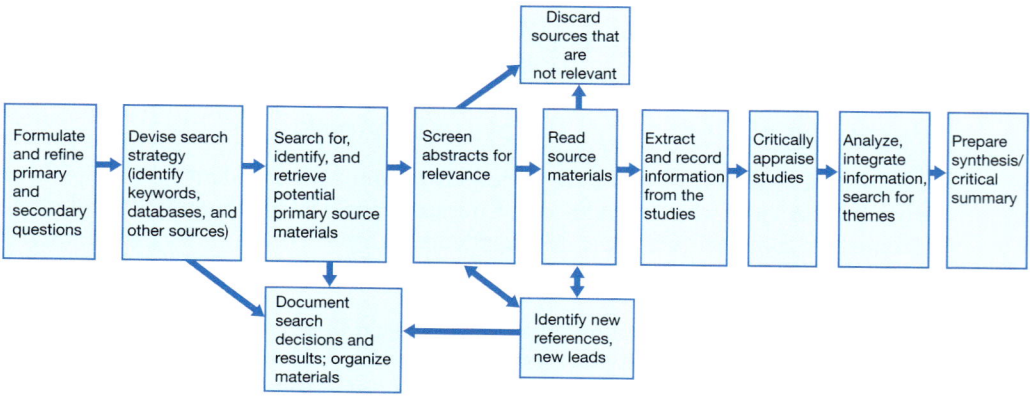

Figure 6.1 Flow of tasks in a literature review.

TIP Locating all relevant information on a research question is like being a detective. The literature retrieval tools we discuss in this chapter are helpful, but there inevitably needs to be some digging for, and sifting through, the clues to find evidence on a topic. Be prepared for sleuthing!

Doing a literature review is in some ways similar to undertaking a qualitative study. It is useful to have a flexible approach to "data collection" and to think creatively about opportunities for new sources of information.

LOCATING RELEVANT LITERATURE FOR A RESEARCH REVIEW

An early step in a literature review is devising a strategy to locate relevant studies. The ability to locate evidence on a topic is an important skill that requires adaptability—rapid technologic changes mean that new methods of searching the literature are introduced continuously. It is imperative that you consult with librarians and faculty at your institution for updated suggestions.

Developing a Search Strategy

A particularly productive approach to locating studies is to search for evidence in bibliographic databases, which we discuss next. Reviewers also use the *ancestry approach* ("footnote chasing"), in which citations from relevant studies are used to track down earlier research on which the studies are based (the "ancestors"). A third strategy, the *descendancy approach*, involves finding a pivotal early study and searching forward to find more recent studies ("descendants") that cited the key study.

TIP You may be tempted to begin a literature search through an internet search engine, such as Google. Such a search is likely to yield a lot of "hits" on your topic but is unlikely to give you full bibliographic information on *research* literature on your topic.

Decisions must also be made about limiting the search. For example, reviewers may restrict their search to reports written in one language. You may also want to limit your search to studies conducted within a certain time frame (e.g., within the past 10 years).

Searching Bibliographic Databases

Bibliographic databases are accessed by a computer. Most databases can be accessed through user-friendly software with menu-driven systems and on-screen support so that minimal instruction is needed to retrieve articles. Your university or hospital library probably has subscriptions to these services.

Getting Started With an Electronic Search

Before searching a bibliographic database, you should become familiar with the features of the software through which it is accessed. The software has options for restricting or expanding your search, for combining two searches, for saving your search, and so on. Most programs have tutorials, and most also have Help buttons.

An early task in an electronic search is identifying keywords to launch the search (an *author search* for prominent researchers in a field can also be done). A **keyword** is a word or phrase that captures key concepts in your review question. For quantitative studies, the keywords are usually the independent or dependent variables and perhaps the population.

For qualitative studies, the keywords are the central phenomenon and the population. If you use the question templates for asking clinical questions in Table 1.3, the words you enter in the blanks are likely to be good keywords.

 TIP If you want to identify all research reports on a topic, you need to be flexible and to think broadly about keywords. For example, if you are interested in anorexia, you might look up *anorexia*, *eating disorders*, and *weight loss* and perhaps *appetite*, *eating behavior*, *food habits*, *bulimia*, and *body weight changes*.

There are various approaches for a bibliographic search. All citations in a database are coded so they can be retrieved, and coders use database-specific systems of categorizing entries. The indexing systems have specific *subject headings* (subject codes).

You can undertake a *subject search* by entering a keyword into the search field. You do not have to worry about knowing the subject codes because most software has mapping capabilities. *Mapping* is a feature that allows you to search for topics using your own keywords rather than the exact subject heading used in the database. The software translates ("maps") your keywords into the most plausible subject heading and then retrieves citation records that have been coded with that subject heading.

When you enter a keyword into the search field, the program likely will launch both a subject search and a textword search. A *textword search* looks for your keyword in the text fields of the records—in the title and the abstract. Thus, if you searched for *cancer* in the MEDLINE (**Med**ical Literature On-**Line**) database (described in a subsequent section), the search would retrieve citations coded for the MEDLINE subject code of *neoplasms* as well as any entries in which the phrase *cancer* appeared in text fields even if it had not been coded for the *neoplasm* subject heading.

Some features of an electronic search are similar across databases, such as the use of *Boolean operators* to expand or delimit a search. Three widely used Boolean operators are AND, OR, and NOT (in all caps). The operator *AND* delimits a search. If we searched for *pain AND children*, the software would retrieve only records that have both terms. The operator *OR* expands the search: *pain OR children* could be used in a search to retrieve records with either term. Finally, *NOT* narrows a search: *pain NOT children* would retrieve all records with pain that did not include the term *children*.

Truncation symbols are another useful tool. A *truncation symbol* (often an asterisk, *) expands a search term to include all forms of a root. For example, a search for *child** would instruct the computer to search for any word that begins with "child," such as children, childhood, or childbearing. For each database, it is important to learn what the special symbols are and how they work. The use of special symbols, while useful, may turn off a software's mapping feature.

One way to force a textword search in some databases is to use quotation marks around a phrase to retrieve citations in which the exact phrase appears in text fields. In other words, searches for *lung cancer* and "lung cancer" might yield different results. A thorough search strategy might entail doing a search with and without quotation marks.

Two especially useful electronic databases for nurses are CINAHL (**C**umulative **I**ndex to **N**ursing and **A**llied **H**ealth **L**iterature) and MEDLINE, which we discuss in the next sections. We also briefly discuss Google Scholar (GS). Other useful bibliographic databases for nurses include the Cochrane Database of Systematic Reviews, Web of Knowledge, Scopus, and Embase (the Excerpta Medica database). The Web of Science database is useful for a descendancy search strategy because of its strong citation indexes.

 TIP If your goal is to conduct a *systematic* review, you will need to establish an explicit formal plan about your search strategy and keywords, as discussed in Chapter 17.

The CINAHL Database

CINAHL is an important electronic database for nurses. It covers references to thousands of nursing and allied health journals as well as to books and dissertations. CINAHL contains more than 6 million records.

CINAHL provides information for locating references (i.e., the author, title, journal, year of publication, volume, and page numbers) and abstracts for most citations. We illustrate features of CINAHL but note that some features may be different at your institution, and changes are introduced regularly.

A "basic search" in CINAHL involves entering keywords in the search field (more options for expanding and limiting the search are available in the "Advanced Search" mode). You can restrict your search to records with certain features (e.g., only ones with abstracts), to specific publication dates (e.g., only those after 2015), and to those with certain attributes (e.g., those published in English or those from specific countries).

To illustrate with a concrete example, suppose we were interested in research on pain management in people with dementia. We entered these terms in the search field and placed a limit on the search—only records written in English: "pain management" AND "people with dementia."

By clicking the Search button, 145 citations were retrieved. Note that we used one Boolean operator. The use of "AND" ensured that the retrieved records had to include both of the two keywords.

By clicking the Search button, all of the identified references would be displayed on the monitor, and we could view and print full information for ones that seemed promising. An example of a CINAHL record entry for a report identified through this search is presented in Box 6.1. The title of the article and author information are displayed, followed by source information. The source indicates the following:

- Name of the journal (*International Journal of Older People Nursing*)
- Year of publication (2022)
- Volume (17)
- Issue (6)
- Page numbers (1–10)

The abstract for the study is then presented; based on the abstract, we would decide whether this reference was pertinent to our inquiry. Note that there is also a sidebar link in each record, labeled *Find Similar Results*, that can be used to identify other relevant references.

The MEDLINE Database

The **MEDLINE** database, developed by the U.S. National Library of Medicine, is the premier source for bibliographic coverage of the biomedical literature. MEDLINE covers about 5,250 medical, nursing, and health journals and has more than 34 million records. MEDLINE can be accessed for free on the internet at the **PubMed** website. PubMed is a lifelong resource regardless of your institution's access to bibliographic databases.

MEDLINE uses a controlled vocabulary called **MeSH** (Medical Subject Headings) to code and index articles. MeSH terminology provides a consistent way to retrieve information that may use different terminology for the same concepts. Once you have begun a search, a field on the right side of the screen labeled "Search Details" lets you see how the search terms you entered mapped onto MeSH terms, which might lead you to pursue other leads.

When we did a PubMed search of MEDLINE analogous to the one described earlier for CINAHL, using the same keywords and restrictions, 95 records were retrieved. The list of records in the PubMed and CINAHL searches did overlap, but some unique references were found in each search. Both searches, however, retrieved the study by Harkin

Box 6.1 Example of a Record From a CINAHL Search

Exploring ways to enhance pain management for older people With dementia in acute care settings using a Participatory Action Research approach.

Authors:	Harkin, Deirdre;[1] Coates, Vivien;[2] Brown, Donna[1]
Affiliation:	[1]Ulster University, Londonderry, UK [2]Florence Nightingale Foundation Professor of Clinical Nursing Practice Research, Ulster University & Western Health & Social Care Trust, Londonderry, UK
Source:	International Journal of Older **People** Nursing (INT J OLDER PEOPLE NURS), Nov2022; 17(6): 1–10. (10p)
Publication Type:	Journal Article—research, tables/charts
Language:	**English**
Major Subjects:	**Pain Management** **Dementia** Patients—In Old Age Quality Improvement Hospitalization of Older Persons
Minor Subjects:	Human; Action Research; Audit; Focus Groups; Thematic Analysis; Conceptual Framework; Acute Care; United Kingdom: Semi-Structured Interview; Convenience Sample; Case Studies; Professional Knowledge; Aged
Abstract:	Background: **Dementia** is a progressive condition that leads to reduced cognition, deteriorating communication and is a risk factor for other acute and chronic health problems. The rise in the prevalence of **dementia** means untreated pain is becoming increasingly common with healthcare staff being challenged to provide optimal **pain management**. This negatively impacts the person living with **dementia** and their carers. There is minimal evidence that explores the **pain management** experience of patients as they move through acute care settings. Objective: To understand the complexities of managing the pain of older people with **dementia** as they progress through acute care settings, with the view of assisting staff to improve practice. Method: A Participatory Action Research approach, guided by the Promoting Action Research in Health Services framework, was used. Three Action Cycles were completed comprising of an exploratory audit and two case studies (Action Cycle One), three focus groups with a total of 14 participants (Action Cycle Two) and the development and implementation of immediate and long-term actions (Action Cycle Three). Results: Thematic analysis identified four themes that affected **pain management** practices. These were not knowing the patient; balancing competing priorities; knowledge and understanding of pain and **dementia** and not assimilating available information. Conclusion: **Pain management** practices for patient living with **dementia**, across acute care settings, was influenced by shared ways of thinking and working. Not knowing the patient, fragmentation of information and having insufficient knowledge of the subtleties of **dementia** led participants to deliver task-focused, target and policy-driven care that was not person-centred in its approach. Facilitated reflection enabled acute care teams to actively participate in identifying problems and finding solutions to enhance practice.

Box 6.1 Example of a Record From a CINAHL Search (*continued*)

Journal Subset:	Core Nursing; Europe; Nursing; Peer Reviewed; UK & Ireland
Special Interest:	**Pain** and **Pain Management**
ISSN:	1748-3735
MEDLINE Info:	*NLM U/O:* 101267281
Entry Date:	20221118
Revision Date:	20231101
DOI:	10.1111/opn.12487
Accession Number:	160148822
Publisher Logo:	WILEY Blackwell

Abstract reprinted with permission from Harkin, D., Coates, V., & Brown, D. (2022). Exploring ways to enhance pain management for older people with dementia in acute care settings using a Participatory Action Research approach. *International Journal of Older People Nursing, 17*(6), e12487. https://doi.org/10.1111/opn.12487

et al. (2022)—the CINAHL record in Box 6.1. Box 6.2, the PubMed record for this study, provides similar information. Box 6.3 shows how the PubMed record also lists the MeSH terms that were indexed for this study at the bottom. In PubMed, after identifying a relevant study, you could review the list of "similar articles" that appear beneath the abstract to locate additional studies.

 TIP Note that in both the CINAHL and PubMed records, the authors' names are hyperlinks that can be clicked on to retrieve other articles written by these authors.

Google Scholar

Google Scholar (GS) is a bibliographic search engine that was launched in 2004. GS includes articles in journals from scholarly publishers in all disciplines as well as books, technical reports, and other documents. GS is accessible free of charge over the internet. Like other bibliographic search engines, GS allows users to search by topic, by a title, and by author and uses Boolean operators and other search conventions. Because of its expanded coverage of material, GS can provide greater access to free full-text publications.

In the field of medicine, GS has generated controversy, with some arguing that it is of similar utility and quality to popular medical databases and others urging caution in depending primarily on GS. The capabilities and features of GS may improve in the years ahead, but at the moment, it is risky to depend on GS exclusively. We note that a GS search with the same search terms used in CINAHL and PubMed may not retrieve all the studies retrieved through CINAHL and PubMed.

Example of a bibliographic search
In their literature review, Dickins and colleagues (2021) explored the physical and behavioral health characteristics of women aged 50 years or more who were unhoused in the United States. They searched six databases, including (1) MEDLINE (via Ovid); (2) Embase; (3) Ovid Nursing Database; (4) Cochrane Library (via Ovid); (5) CINAHL (via EBSCOhost); and (6) Web of Science. A total of 3,177 articles were initially included in the title and abstract screening. They found that 3,089 records did not meet the eligibility criteria. They reviewed 88 articles for full-text screening, and of those, 78 did not meet the eligibility criteria. As a result, 10 articles were included in the review.

Box 6.2 Example of a Record From a PubMed Search

> Int J Older People Nurs. 2022 Nov;17(6):e12487. doi: 10.1111/opn.12487. Epub 2022 Jun 27.

Exploring ways to enhance pain management for older people With dementia in acute care settings using a Participatory Action Research approach

Deirdre Harkin[1], Vivien Coates[2], Donna Brown[1]

Affiliations + expand
PMID: 35761509   PMCID: PMC9787744   DOI: 10.1111/opn.12487

Abstract

Background: Dementia is a progressive condition that leads to reduced cognition, deteriorating communication and is a risk factor for other acute and chronic health problems. The rise in the prevalence of dementia means untreated pain is becoming increasingly common with healthcare staff being challenged to provide optimal pain management. This negatively impacts the person living with dementia and their carers. There is minimal evidence that explores the pain management experience of patients as they move through acute care settings.

Objective: To understand the complexities of managing the pain of older people with dementia as they progress through acute care settings, with the view of assisting staff to improve practice.

Method: A Participatory Action Research approach, guided by the Promoting Action Research in Health Services framework, was used. Three Action Cycles were completed comprising of an exploratory audit and two case studies (Action Cycle One), three focus groups with a total of 14 participants (Action Cycle Two) and the development and implementation of immediate and long-term actions (Action Cycle Three).

Results: Thematic analysis identified four themes that affected pain management practices. These were not knowing the patient; balancing competing priorities; knowledge and understanding of pain and dementia and not assimilating available information.

Conclusion: Pain management practices for patient living with dementia, across acute care settings, was influenced by shared ways of thinking and working. Not knowing the patient, fragmentation of information and having insufficient knowledge of the subtleties of dementia led participants to deliver task-focused, target and policy-driven care that was not person-centred in its approach. Facilitated reflection enabled acute care teams to actively participate in identifying problems and finding solutions to enhance practice.

Keywords: Participatory Action Research; acute care; context; dementia; older people; pain management.

© 2022 The Authors. International Journal of Older People Nursing published by John Wiley & Sons Ltd.

PubMed Disclaimer

Conflict of interest statement
No conflict of interest has been declared by the authors.

Abstract reprinted with permission from Harkin, D., Coates, V., & Brown, D. (2022). Exploring ways to enhance pain management for older people with dementia in acute care settings using a Participatory Action Research approach. *International Journal of Older People Nursing, 17*(6), e12487. https://doi.org/10.1111/opn.12487

> **Box 6.3 Example of List of MeSH Terms Associated With the PubMed Search Record for Harkin et al. (2022)**
>
> **MeSH Terms**
> - Aged
> - Caregivers
> - Dementia*
> - Health services research
> - Humans
> - Pain
> - Pain management*

Use of Artificial Intelligence in Searches

Artificial intelligence (AI) is a strategy used in some systematic reviews. It is an attractive tool because of the potential time saved (Ge et al., 2024). Typical systematic reviews from the time of protocol registration to publication can take approximately 12 to 18 months to complete, but AI can shorten this timeframe to 2 weeks (Fabiano et al., 2024; Tufanaru et al., 2024). This ability to have new evidence readily available was critical during the COVID-19 pandemic. The reduced timeframe allowed scientists and clinicians to address this public health crisis by expediting the dissemination of information needed to slow the spread of the disease and treat those impacted by it (Comito & Pizzuti, 2022).

The use of AI will continue to grow in light of the continued refinement of AI and the number of new tools being developed. However, while the advantage of AI in systematic reviews is the expeditious availability of evidence to the practice setting, it does raise quality concerns. Danler et al. (2024) cautioned that the use of freely available AI resulted in variation in the information retrieved, including material that was outdated and from nonacademic sources. They also noted a lack of transparency in reporting of sources for the information retrieved; it was not clear if the sources were trusted bibliographic sources such as MEDLINE. For these reasons, AI is not yet widely accepted in some scholarly journals, although this landscape is likely to change as AI improves.

Those using AI must acknowledge its use and outline the processes for how it was used, as with other search engines. Researchers must disclose the type of AI use; how AI was used in each step of the systematic process, from asking the original questions, obtaining and screening the information, to the quality rating of the evidence and synthesis of information; and how potential bias was addressed (Fabiano et al., 2024; Ge et al., 2024). AI requires content expertise throughout the process to reduce the possibility of misinformation being reported through nonacademic sources or predatory journal sources (Fabiano et al., 2024).

Further, it is important to know the requirements of the journal in which you choose to publish. The International Committee of Medical Journal Editors (ICMJE) offers guidance on publication in medical (and nursing) journals. The guidelines were updated in 2024 to include the topic of AI use and authorship. Some scholarly journals may not allow the use of AI, while others require that authors report its use not only in the process of a systematic review but also in writing the abstract or any part of the paper. Despite current variations in the application and extent of AI use in the scientific community, with continued refinement AI will become more popular. Keeping abreast of the rapidly changing environment of this technology and its use in scholarly work is critical.

Screening, Documentation, and Abstracting

After searching for and retrieving references, several important steps remain before a synthesis can begin.

Screening and Gathering References

References that have been identified in the search need to be screened for relevance. You can usually surmise relevance by reading the abstract. When you find a relevant article, you should obtain a full copy rather than relying on information in the abstract only.

TIP One way to retrieve an article that is not available online or through your library resources is by communicating with the lead author, either directly through an email or through scholarly collaboration networks such as *Research Gate* (www.researchgate.net). Papers retrieved this way must be indexed in appropriate bibliographic sources such as CINAHL or PubMed due to predatory publication issues.

Predatory journals have been an unfortunate outcome of the open-access journal movement. Open-access journals provide articles free of charge online, which helps to disseminate research findings much sooner and to a larger audience than traditional print publications. There is typically a fee of around $3,000 for the author to submit a paper through this format. Predatory journals take advantage of this model, offering the same expedited process for a fee, but without meeting publishing standards as outlined by the ICMJE. The critical scholarly peer review process is either nonexistent or conducted by unqualified reviewers. Further, after paying to have the paper published, authors find their paper either is posted for a limited time or vanishes altogether. As a result of this trend, nursing editors of scholarly journals have provided guidance via a series of editorials since 2015 through the International Academy of Nursing Editors (INANE). For more information, refer to https://nursingeditors.com/workgroups-initiatives/workgroup-history/open-access-editorial-standards. Oermann et al. (2022) provide further guidance on how to detect predatory journals.

Documentation in Literature Retrieval

Search strategies are often complex, so it is wise to document your search actions and results. You should make note of databases searched, keywords used, limits instituted, and any other information that would help you keep track of what you did. Part of your strategy can be documented by printing your search history from the electronic databases. Documentation will promote efficiency by preventing unintended duplication and will also help you to assess what else needs to be tried.

Extracting and Recording Information

Once you have retrieved useful articles, you need a strategy to organize the information in the articles. For simple reviews, it may be sufficient to make notes about key features of the retrieved studies and to base your review on these notes. When a literature review involves a large number of studies, a formal system of recording information from each study may be needed. One mechanism that we recommend for complex reviews is to *code* the characteristics of each study and then record codes in matrices, a system that we describe in detail elsewhere (Flanagan & Beck, 2025). Another approach is to use a form that allows you to record systematically important features of the study (e.g., number of study participants, type of design, and main findings).

CRITICAL APPRAISAL OF THE EVIDENCE

In drawing conclusions about a body of evidence, reviewers must make judgments about the worth of the studies. Thus, an important part of doing a literature review is evaluating the body of completed research and integrating the evidence across studies.

Appraising Studies for a Review

In reviewing the literature, you would not undertake a comprehensive critique of every study, but you would need to assess the quality of each study so that you could draw conclusions about the overall body of evidence and about gaps in the evidence. Appraisals for a literature review tend to focus on study methods, so the guidelines in Tables 3.1 and 3.2 might be useful.

In literature reviews, methodologic features of the studies under review need to be assessed with an eye to answering a broad question: To what extent do the findings reflect the *truth* (the true state of affairs) or, conversely, to what extent do flaws undermine the believability of the evidence? The "truth" is most likely to be discovered when researchers use powerful designs, good sampling plans, high-quality data collection procedures, and appropriate analyses.

Analyzing and Synthesizing Evidence

Once relevant studies have been retrieved and appraised, the information has to be analyzed and synthesized. We find the analogy between doing a literature review and doing a qualitative study useful: In both, the focus is on the identification of important *themes*.

A thematic analysis essentially involves detecting patterns and regularities—as well as inconsistencies. Several different types of themes can be identified for a literature review, three of which are as follows:

- *Substantive themes*: What is the pattern of evidence—what findings predominate? How much evidence is there? How consistent is the body of evidence? What gaps are there in the evidence?
- *Methodologic themes*: What methods have been used to address the question? What are major methodologic deficiencies and strengths?
- *Generalizability/transferability themes*: To what population does the evidence apply? Do the findings vary for different types of people (e.g., men vs. women) or setting (e.g., urban vs. rural)?

In preparing a review, you would need to determine which themes are most relevant for the purpose at hand. Substantive themes usually are of greatest interest.

PREPARING A WRITTEN LITERATURE REVIEW

Writing a literature review can be challenging, especially when voluminous information and thematic analyses must be condensed into a few pages. We offer some suggestions, but we note that skills in writing literature reviews develop over time.

Organizing a Written Review

Organization is crucial in preparing a written review. When literature on a topic is extensive, it is useful to summarize the retrieved information in a table. The table could include columns with headings such as Author and Year, Sample, Design, and Key Findings. Such a table provides a quick overview that allows you to make sense of a mass of information.

Most writers find an outline helpful. Unless the review is simple, it is important to have an organizational plan so that the review has a meaningful and understandable flow. Although the specifics of the organization differ from topic to topic, the goal is to structure the review to lead logically to a conclusion about the state of evidence on the topic. After finalizing an organizing structure, you should review your notes or protocols to decide where a particular reference fits in the outline. If some references do not seem to fit anywhere, they may need to be omitted. Remember that the number of references is less important than their relevance.

Writing a Literature Review

It is beyond the scope of this textbook to offer detailed guidance on writing research reviews, but we offer a few comments on their content and style. Additional assistance is provided in books such as those by Fink (2020) and Garrard (2020).

Content of the Written Literature Review

A written research review should provide readers with an objective synthesis of current evidence on a topic. Although key studies may be described in detail, it is not necessary to provide particulars for every reference. Studies with similar findings often can be summarized together—for example, "Several studies have found ... (Forbes, 2020; Lowe, 2019; Rivera, 2021)."

Findings should be summarized in your own words. The review should demonstrate that you have considered the cumulative worth of the body of research. Stringing together quotes from articles fails to show that previous research has been assimilated and understood.

The review should be as unbiased as possible. The review should not omit a study because its findings contradict those of other studies or conflict with your ideas. Inconsistent results should be analyzed objectively.

A literature review typically concludes with a summary of current evidence on the topic. When the literature review is conducted for a new study, the summary should demonstrate the need for the research.

As you read this book, you will become increasingly proficient in critically evaluating the research literature. We hope you will understand the mechanics of doing a research review once you have completed this chapter, but we do not expect that you will be in a position to write a state-of-the-art review until you have acquired more skills in research methods.

Style of a Research Review

Students preparing research reviews often have trouble writing in an acceptable style. Remember that hypotheses cannot be proved or disproved by statistical testing, and no question can be definitely answered in a single study. The problem is partly semantic: Hypotheses are not proved or verified, they are *supported* by research findings.

TIP Phrases indicating the tentativeness of research results, such as the following, are appropriate:

- Several studies have *found* ...
- Findings thus far *suggest* ...
- The results *are consistent* with the conclusion that ...
- There *appears* to be evidence that ...

Also, a literature review should include opinions sparingly and should explicitly reference the source. Reviewers' own opinions do not belong in a review, with the exception of assessments of study quality.

CRITICAL APPRAISAL OF RESEARCH LITERATURE REVIEWS

Some nurses never prepare a written research review, and perhaps you will never be required to do one. Most nurses, however, do *read* research reviews (including the literature review sections of research reports), and they should be prepared to evaluate such reviews critically.

It is often difficult to appraise a research review if you are not familiar with the topic. You may not be able to judge whether the review includes all relevant literature and is an adequate summary of knowledge on that topic. Some aspects of a research review, however, are amenable to evaluation by readers who are not experts on the topic. A few suggestions for appraising research reviews are presented in Box 6.4. Additional appraisal questions relevant for systematic reviews are presented in Chapter 17.

In assessing a literature review, the overarching question is whether it summarizes the current state of research evidence. If the review is written as part of an original research report, an equally important question is whether the review lays a solid foundation for the new study.

TIP Literature reviews in the introductions of research articles are almost always very brief and are unlikely to present a thorough critique of existing evidence. Gaps in what has been studied, however, should be identified.

Box 6.4 Guidelines for Critically Appraising Literature Reviews

a. Does the review seem thorough and up-to-date? Did it include major studies on the topic? Did it include recent research?
b. Did the review rely mainly on research reports, using primary sources?
c. Did the review critically appraise and compare key studies? Did it identify important gaps in the literature?
d. Was the review well organized? Is the development of ideas clear?
e. Did the review use appropriate language, suggesting the tentativeness of prior findings? Is the review objective?
f. If the review was in the introduction for a new study, did the review support the need for the study?
g. If the review was designed to summarize evidence for clinical practice, did it draw appropriate conclusions about practice implications?

RESEARCH EXAMPLES WITH CRITICAL THINKING EXERCISES

The best way to learn about the style, content, and organization of a research literature review is to read reviews that appear in the nursing literature. In Example 1, we present an excerpt from a review for a quantitative study. The excerpt is followed by some questions to guide critical thinking—you can refer to the entire report if needed. The critical thinking questions for Examples 2 and 3 are based on the studies that appear in their entirety in Appendices A and B of this book.

EXAMPLE 1: EXAMPLE OF A LITERATURE REVIEW FROM A QUANTITATIVE STUDY

Study: "Psychosocial interventions aimed at family members caring for patients with cancer in the palliative period: A systematic review"

Statement of Purpose: The purpose of this study "was to examine the results of randomized controlled studies and meta-analyses, including such studies involving psychosocial interventions for family members providing care for patients with cancer during the palliative period" (Yıldız et al., 2024, p. 137).

Literature Review[1]**:** "According to International Agency for Research on Cancer data for 2020, there are approximately 19 million patients with cancer world-wide (Ferlay et al., 2020; Sung et al., 2021).

---
[1] References within this literature review are not provided.

Being diagnosed with cancer affects not only the patient, but also the entire family and its dynamics. In particular, family members providing primary care for an individual diagnosed with cancer have to reorganize their roles and responsibilities and review their priorities (Zaider & Kissane, 2015). The US National Alliance for Caregiving reports that 53 million individuals care for patients with cancer free of charge. More than 24% of caregivers care for more than one individual, and 26% find it difficult to coordinate care. Seventeen percent of caregivers report a high level of financial difficulty as a result of their caring duties, 36% think that their caregiving is highly stressful, whereas 28% report moderate emotional stress (AARP and National Alliance for Caregiving, 2020).

Palliative Care: It aims to alleviate the suffering of both patients and their families through the management and treatment of the physical, psychosocial, and spiritual symptoms of patients with cancer. After the death of the patient, it focuses on supporting the family and mourning (Kabalak et al., 2013). Palliative care services are provided by nurses who have completed basic training in managing cancer and its treatment-related symptoms such as pain and providing psychosocial support (Sahan Uslu & Terzioğlu, 2015).

Palliative care requirements among individuals diagnosed with cancer increase with the course of the disease, and various psychosocial needs arise in both the patient and the caregiver, such as planning the future, managing uncertainty, and existential distress (Zaider & Kissane, 2015). The presence of such psychosocial problems in the patient and the caregiver gradually makes it difficult for patients with cancer to adapt to the disease and to their experiencing even more problems (Northouse & McCorkle, 2015). As patients' symptoms and period of care increase, this causes greater difficulties for the caregiver, and the caregiver burden grows in the face of these needs (von Heymann-Horan et al., 2018; Vrettos et al., 2023). The risk of developing psychological problems (Northouse & McCorkle, 2015; Petursdottir & Svavarsdottir, 2019) such as high anxiety and depression (Chong et al., 2022; von Heymann-Horan et al., 2018) increases as a result. In addition, their increased anxiety is likely to cause caregivers to feel guilt (Chong et al., 2022).

The psychological problems experienced by caregivers must not be overlooked by health professionals, the caregiver burden and the factors exacerbating it must be evaluated, and the requisite psychosocial support must be provided. Psychosocial interventions, including psychoeducation (Bakitas et al., 2009), coping skills training (McMillan et al., 2006), art therapy (Kaimal et al., 2019), may be beneficial in reducing the caregiver burden and increasing their well-being (Petursdottir & Svavarsdottir, 2019). It can also include supporting the caregiver and indirectly the patient to cope with death and grief (Chong et al., 2022). In its report titled 'Cancer Care for the Whole Patient: Meeting Psychosocial Health Needs,' the US Institute of Medicine referred to the importance of finding ways of providing psychosocial care for patients with cancer and their families. However, there is no widely recognized clinical guideline in the national or international sphere that health professionals can use to provide caregiver support (Northouse & McCorkle, 2015). Although there have been many studies of the caregiver burden and the factors affecting it (Cochrane et al., 2021; Ochoa et al., 2020), the emphasis in the international literature has been on a family-focused approach in the treatment of cancer (Caruso et al., 2017; Petursdottir & Svavarsdottir, 2019). In Turkey, deficiencies have been identified in the implementation of psychosocial interventions for family members who care for patients with cancer (Toptaş Kılıç & Öz, 2019). Due to the absence of a guideline intervention and the lack of practical interventions in this area in our country, this study is required. The purpose of this systematic review was to examine the results of randomized controlled studies and meta-analyses, including such studies involving psychosocial interventions for family members providing care for patients with cancer during the palliative period" (pp. 136–137).

Excerpt from Yıldız, M., Terzioğlu, C., & Ayhan, F. (2024). Psychosocial interventions aimed at family members caring for patients with cancer in the palliative period: A systematic review. *International Journal of Nursing Knowledge*, 35(2), 136–151. https://doi.org/10.1111/2047-3095.12423. Copyright © 2023 NANDA International, Inc. Reprinted by permission of John Wiley & Sons, Inc.

Critical Thinking Exercises

1. Answer the relevant questions from Box 6.4 regarding this literature review.
2. In performing the literature review, what keywords might the researchers have used to search for prior studies?
3. Using the keywords, perform a search of a bibliographic database to see if you can find a recent relevant study to augment the review.

EXAMPLE 2: QUANTITATIVE RESEARCH IN APPENDIX A

Read the introduction to Cheng and colleagues' (2024) "Advance care planning affects end-of-life treatment preferences among patients with heart failure: A randomized controlled trial" in Appendix A of this book.

1. Answer the relevant questions in Box 6.4 regarding this study.
2. In performing the literature review, what keywords might have been used to search for prior studies?
3. Using the keywords, perform a search of a bibliographic database to see if you can find a recent relevant study to augment the review.

EXAMPLE 3: QUALITATIVE RESEARCH IN APPENDIX B

Read the abstract and introduction from Morrison et al.'s (2024) study "Lived experiences of fatherhood after infertility" in Appendix B of this book.

1. Answer the relevant questions in Box 6.4 regarding this study.
2. What was the central phenomenon in this study? Was that phenomenon adequately covered in the literature review?
3. In performing their literature review, what keywords might Morrison and colleagues have used to search for prior studies?

Summary Points

- A research **literature review** is a written summary of the state of evidence on a research problem.
- The major steps in preparing a written research review include formulating a question, devising a search strategy, searching and retrieving relevant sources, abstracting and encoding information, appraising studies, analyzing and integrating the information, and preparing a written synthesis.
- Research reviews rely primarily on findings in research reports. Information in nonresearch references (e.g., opinion articles, case reports) may broaden understanding of a problem but has limited utility in summarizing evidence.
- A **primary source** is the original description of a study prepared by the researcher who conducted it; a **secondary source** is a description of a study by another person. Literature reviews should rely mostly on primary source material.
- Strategies for finding studies on a topic not only include electronic searches of **bibliographic databases** but also include the *ancestry*

- *approach* (tracking down earlier studies cited in a reference list) and the *descendancy approach* (using a pivotal study to search forward to subsequent studies that cited it).

- The bibliographic databases that are especially useful for nurses are **CINAHL** and **MEDLINE. Google Scholar** and **PubMed** (for the MEDLINE database) are free bibliographic resources. **Artificial intelligence (AI)** is being used by some scholars in searches. However, the technology is new and evolving and comes with potential pitfalls. It is important to follow the standards of the journal you wish to publish in if you use AI.

- In searching a bibliographic database, users can do a **keyword** search that looks for terms in *text fields* of a database record (or that *maps* keywords onto the database's subject codes), or they can search according to the *subject heading* codes themselves. References identified in the search must be retrieved and screened for relevance; then, pertinent information can be extracted and encoded for subsequent analysis. Studies must also be appraised for the quality of the evidence.

- When retrieving publications, it is important to be aware of **predatory journals**. The literature from these journals does not undergo a rigorous peer review and as a result may be a source of misinformation.

- The analysis of information from a literature search essentially involves the identification of important *themes*—regularities and patterns in the information.

- In preparing a written review, it is important to organize materials coherently. Preparation of an outline is recommended. The reviewers' role is to point out what has been studied, how adequate and dependable the studies are, and what gaps exist in the body of research.

REFERENCES

Comito, C., & Pizzuti, C. (2022). Artificial intelligence for forecasting and diagnosing COVID-19 pandemic: A focused review. *Artificial Intelligence in Medicine, 128*, 102286. https://doi.org/10.1016/j.artmed.2022.102286

Danler, M., Hackl, W. O., Neururer, S. B., & Pfeifer, B. (2024). Quality and effectiveness of AI tools for students and researchers for scientific literature review and analysis. *Studies in Health Technology and Informatics, 313*, 203–208. https://doi.org/10.3233/SHTI240038

Dickins, K. A., Philpotts, L. L., Flanagan, J., Bartels, S. J., Baggett, T. P., & Looby, S. E. (2021). Physical and behavioral health characteristics of aging homeless women in the United States: An integrative review. *Journal of Women's Health (2002), 30*(10), 1493–1507. https://doi.org/10.1089/jwh.2020.8557

Fabiano, N., Gupta, A., Bhambra, N., Luu, B., Wong, S., Maaz, M., Fiedorowicz, J. G., Smith, A. L., & Solmi, M. (2024). How to optimize the systematic review process using AI tools. *JCPP Advances, 4*(2), e12234. https://doi.org/10.1002/jcv2.12234

Fink, A. (2020). *Conducting research literature reviews: From the Internet to paper* (5th ed.). Sage.

Flanagan, J., & Beck, C. (2025). *Nursing research: Generating and assessing evidence for nursing practice* (12th ed.). Wolters Kluwer.

Garrard, J. (2020). *Health sciences literature review made easy: The matrix method* (6th ed.). Jones & Bartlett Learning.

Ge, L., Agrawal, R., Singer, M., Kannapiran, P., De Castro Molina, J. A., Teow, K. L., Yap, C. W., & Abisheganaden, J. A. (2024). Leveraging artificial intelligence to enhance systematic reviews in health research: Advanced tools and challenges. *Systematic Reviews, 13*(1), 269. https://doi.org/10.1186/s13643-024-02682-2

Harkin, D., Coates, V., & Brown, D. (2022). Exploring ways to enhance pain management for older people with dementia in acute care settings using a participatory action research approach. *International Journal of Older People Nursing, 17*(6), e12487. https://doi.org/10.1111/opn.12487

International Committee of Medical Journal Editors. *Recommendations for the conduct, reporting, editing, and publication of scholarly work in medical journals*. Updated January 2024. https://www.icmje.org/news-and-editorials/updated_recommendations_jan2024.html

Knafl, K., & Whittemore, R. (2017). Top 10 tips for undertaking synthesis research. *Research in Nursing & Health, 40*(3), 189–193. https://doi.org/10.1002/nur.21790

Oermann, M. H., Nicoll, L. H., Carter-Templeton, H., Owens, J. K., Wrigley, J., Ledbetter, L. S., & Chinn, P. L. (2022). How to identify predatory journals in a search: Precautions for nurses. *Nursing, 52*(4), 41–45. https://doi.org/10.1097/01.NURSE.0000823280.93554.1a

Tufanaru, C., Surian, D., Scott, A. M., Glasziou, P., & Coiera, E. (2024). The 2-week systematic review (2weekSR) method was successfully blind-replicated by another team: A case study. *Journal of Clinical Epidemiology, 165*, 111197. https://doi.org/10.1016/j.jclinepi.2023.10.013

Whittemore, R., & Knafl, K. (2005). The integrative review: Updated methodology. *Journal of Advanced Nursing, 52*(5), 546–553. https://doi.org/10.1111/j.1365-2648.2005.03621.x

7 Understanding Theoretical and Conceptual Frameworks

Learning Objectives

On completing this chapter, you will be able to:

- Identify major characteristics of theories, conceptual models, and frameworks
- Identify several conceptual models or theories frequently used by nurse researchers
- Describe how theory and research are linked in quantitative and qualitative studies
- Appraise the appropriateness of a conceptual/theoretical framework—or its absence—in a study
- Define new terms in the chapter

Key Terms

- Conceptual framework
- Conceptual map
- Conceptual model
- Descriptive theory
- Framework
- Middle-range theory
- Model
- Schematic model
- Theoretical framework
- Theory

High-quality studies typically achieve a high level of *conceptual integration*. This happens when the research questions fit the chosen methods, when the questions are consistent with existing evidence, and when there is a conceptual rationale for expected outcomes—including a rationale for any hypotheses or interventions. For example, suppose a research team hypothesized that a nurse-led smoking cessation intervention would reduce smoking among patients with cardiovascular disease. Why would they make this prediction—what is the "theory" about how the intervention might change people's behavior? Do the researchers predict that the intervention will change patients' knowledge? their attitudes? their motivation? The researchers' theoretical expectations about how the intervention would "work" should drive the design of the intervention and the study.

Studies are not developed in a vacuum—researchers have an underlying conceptualization of people's behaviors and characteristics. In some studies, the conceptualization is vague or unstated, but in well-designed research, it is made explicit. This chapter discusses theoretical and conceptual contexts for nursing research problems.

THEORIES, MODELS, AND FRAMEWORKS

Many terms are used in connection with conceptual contexts for research, such as theories, models, frameworks, schemes, and maps. We offer guidance in distinguishing these terms.

Theories

In nursing education, the term *theory* is used to refer to content covered in classrooms, as opposed to actual nursing practice. In both lay and scientific language, *theory* connotes an abstraction.

Theory is often defined as an abstract generalization that explains how phenomena are interrelated. As classically defined, theories consist of two or more concepts and a set of propositions that form a logically interrelated system, providing a mechanism for deducing hypotheses. To illustrate, consider *reinforcement theory*, which posits that behavior that is reinforced (i.e., rewarded) tends to be repeated and learned. The proposition lends itself to hypothesis generation. For example, we could deduce from the theory that children who are hyperactive are rewarded when they engage in quiet play will exhibit less acting-out behavior than unrewarded children. This prediction, as well as others based on reinforcement theory, could be tested in a study.

The term *theory* is also used less restrictively to refer to a broad characterization of a phenomenon. A **descriptive theory** accounts for and thoroughly describes a phenomenon. Descriptive theories are inductive, observation-based abstractions that describe or classify characteristics of individuals, groups, or situations by summarizing their commonalities. Such theories play an important role in qualitative studies.

Theories can help to make research findings interpretable. Theories may guide researchers' understanding not only of the "what" of natural phenomena but also of the "why" of their occurrence. Theories can also help to stimulate research by providing direction and impetus.

Theories vary in their level of generality. *Grand theories* (or *macrotheories*) claim to explain large segments of human experience. In nursing, there are grand theories that offer explanations of the whole of nursing and characterize the nature and mission of nursing practice, as distinct from other disciplines. An example of a nursing theory that has been described as a grand theory is Parse's Humanbecoming Paradigm (Parse, 2014). Theories of relevance to researchers are often less abstract than grand theories. **Middle-range theories** attempt to explain such phenomena as stress, comfort, and health promotion. Middle-range theories, compared to grand theories, are more specific and more amenable to empirical testing.

Nursology.net (https://nursology.net/about/) is a website managed by several nurse scholars, including Jane Flanagan, one of the authors of this book. The site is freely available. It provides up-to-date and accurate information about many nursing conceptual models, grand theories, middle-range theories, and situation-specific theories, philosophies, and associated methodologies.

Models

A **conceptual model** deals with abstractions (concepts) that are assembled because of their relevance to a common theme. Conceptual models provide a conceptual perspective on interrelated phenomena, but they are more loosely structured than theories and do not link concepts in a logical deductive system. A conceptual model broadly presents an understanding of a phenomenon and reflects the assumptions of the model's designer. Conceptual models can serve as springboards for generating hypotheses.

Some writers use the term **model** to designate a method of representing phenomena with a minimal use of words. Two types of models used in research contexts are schematic models and statistical models. *Statistical models*, not discussed here, are equations that mathematically express relationships among a set of variables and are tested statistically.

Schematic models (or conceptual maps) visually represent relationships among phenomena and are used in both qualitative and quantitative research. Concepts and linkages between them are depicted graphically through boxes, arrows, or other symbols. An example of a schematic model is Roy's Adaptation Model (RAM), initially developed in 1970 for the purpose of explaining and predicting the adaptation process. Sister Callista Roy provides an overview of this model and its evolution at https://nursology.net/nurse-theories/roys-adaptation-model.

Frameworks

A **framework** is the conceptual underpinning of a study. Not every study is based on a theory or model, but every study has a framework. In a study based on a theory, the framework is called the **theoretical framework**; in a study that has its roots in a conceptual model, the framework may be called the **conceptual framework**. However, the terms *conceptual framework*, *conceptual model*, and *theoretical framework* are often used interchangeably.

A study's framework is often implicit (i.e., not formally stated). Worldviews shape how concepts are defined, but researchers often fail to clarify the conceptual foundations of their concepts. Researchers who clarify conceptual definitions of key variables provide important information about the study's framework.

In recent years, *concept analysis* has become an important enterprise among students and nurse scholars. Several methods have been proposed for undertaking a concept analysis and clarifying conceptual definitions (e.g., Walker & Avant, 2021). Efforts to analyze concepts of relevance to nursing should facilitate greater conceptual clarity among nurse researchers.

> **Example of developing a conceptual definition**
> Ventura and colleagues (2024) used Walker and Avant's (2021) eight-step concept analysis approach to conceptually define *neonatal near miss*. They performed a literature search that yielded 43 relevant articles. They proposed the following definition: "a serious complication in the first days of life that could have led to the death of the newborn" (p. 417).

The Nature of Theories and Conceptual Models

Theories, conceptual frameworks, and models are not *discovered*; they are created. Theory building depends not only on observable evidence but also on a theorist's ingenuity in pulling evidence together and making sense of it. Because theories are not just "out there" waiting to be discovered, it follows that theories are tentative. A theory cannot be proved—a theory represents a theorist's best efforts to describe and explain phenomena. Through research, theories evolve and are sometimes discarded. This may happen if new evidence undermines a previously accepted theory. Or, a new theory might integrate new observations with an existing theory to yield a more parsimonious explanation of a phenomenon.

Theory and research have a reciprocal relationship. Theories are built inductively from observations, and research is an excellent source for those observations. The theory, in turn, must be tested by subjecting deductions from it (hypotheses) to systematic inquiry. Thus, research plays a dual and continuing role in theory building and testing.

CONCEPTUAL MODELS AND THEORIES USED IN NURSING RESEARCH

Nurse researchers have used both nursing and nonnursing frameworks as conceptual contexts for their studies. This section briefly discusses several frameworks that nurse researchers have found useful.

Conceptual Models of Nursing

Several nurses have formulated conceptual models representing explanations of what the nursing discipline is and what the nursing process entails. As Fawcett (2023) has noted, four concepts are central to models of nursing: *human beings*, *global environment*, *planetary health*, and *nursologists' activities*. The various conceptual models define these concepts differently, link them in diverse ways, and emphasize different relationships among them. Moreover, the models emphasize different processes as being central to nursing.

The conceptual models were not developed primarily as a base for nursing research. Indeed, most models have had more impact on nursing education and clinical practice than on research. Nevertheless, some nurse researchers have turned to these conceptual frameworks for inspiration in formulating research questions and hypotheses.

Let us consider one conceptual model of nursing that has received research attention, RAM. In this model, humans are viewed as biopsychosocial adaptive systems who cope with environmental change through the process of adaptation (Roy & Andrews, 2009). Within the human system, there are four subsystems: physiologic/physical, self-concept/group identity, role function, and interdependence. These subsystems constitute adaptive modes that provide mechanisms for coping with environmental stimuli and change. Health is viewed as both a state and a process of becoming integrated and whole that reflects the mutuality of persons and environment. The goal of nursing, according to this model, is to promote client adaptation. Nursing interventions usually take the form of increasing, decreasing, modifying, removing, or maintaining internal and external stimuli that affect adaptation. RAM has been the basis for several middle-range theories and dozens of studies.

> **Example using Roy's Adaptation Model**
> Based on RAM, Aydogdu and colleagues (2023) studied the effects of instrumental reminiscence therapy on adaptation, life satisfaction, and happiness in older people. This study is described in greater detail at the end of the chapter.

Middle-Range Theories Developed by Nurses

In addition to conceptual models that describe and characterize the nursing process, nurses have developed middle-range theories and models that focus on more specific phenomena of interest to nurses. Examples of middle-range theories that have been used in research include Beck's (2015) Theory of Traumatic Childbirth, Barrett's (2010) Theory of Power as Knowing Participation in Change, Kolcaba's (2003) Comfort Theory, Pender's Health Promotion Model (Murdaugh et al., 2019), and Mishel's (1990) Uncertainty in Illness Theory. The latter two are briefly described here.

Nola Pender's Health Promotion Model (HPM) focuses on explaining health-promoting behaviors, using a wellness orientation (Murdaugh et al., 2019). According to the model, *health promotion* entails activities directed toward developing resources that maintain or enhance a person's well-being. The model embodies several propositions that can be used to develop interventions and to understand health behaviors. For example, one HPM proposition is that people engage in behaviors from which they anticipate deriving valued benefits and another is that perceived competence (or *self-efficacy*) relating to a given behavior increases the likelihood of performing it.

> **Example using the Health Promotion Model**
> Choi and colleagues (2024) conducted a systematic review and meta-analysis to identify the effect sizes between the health-promoting behaviors as described in Pender's HPM and related variables in nurses working in Korea.

Mishel's Uncertainty in Illness Theory (Mishel, 1990) focuses on the concept of uncertainty—a person's inability to determine the meaning of illness-related events. According to this theory, people develop subjective appraisals to assist them in interpreting the experience of illness and treatment. Uncertainty occurs when people are unable to recognize and categorize stimuli. Uncertainty results in the inability to obtain a clear conception of the situation, but a situation appraised as uncertain will mobilize individuals to use their resources to adapt to the situation. Many nursing studies have used Mishel's conceptualization of uncertainty and her Uncertainty in Illness Scale.

> **Example using uncertainty in illness theory**
> Lin et al. (2023) evaluated the efficacy of a mobile app for patients with gynecologic cancer receiving chemotherapy in China. The app was developed based on Mishel's Uncertainty in Illness Theory.

Other Models Used by Nurse Researchers

Many concepts in which nurse researchers are interested are not unique to nursing, and so their studies are sometimes linked to frameworks that are not models from nursing. Several alternative models have gained prominence in the development of nursing interventions to promote health-enhancing behaviors and life choices. Four nonnursing theories have frequently been used in nursing studies: Social Cognitive Theory, the Transtheoretical (Stages of Change) Model, the Health Belief Model, and the Theory of Planned Behavior.

Social Cognitive Theory (Bandura, 2001), which is sometimes called *self-efficacy theory*, offers an explanation of human behavior using the concepts of self-efficacy, outcome expectations, and incentives. Self-efficacy concerns people's belief in their own ability to carry out certain behaviors (e.g., smoking cessation). Self-efficacy expectations determine the behaviors people choose to perform, their degree of perseverance, and the quality of the performance.

> **Example using Social Cognitive Theory**
> Brown and colleagues (2023) conducted a secondary analysis to examine the associations between obesity, exercise preferences, and related Social Cognitive Theory constructs such as self-efficacy, exercise barriers, and social support among breast cancer survivors enrolled in a physical activity clinical trial.

TIP Self-efficacy is a key construct in several models. Self-efficacy has repeatedly been found to affect people's behaviors *and* to be amenable to change. Self-efficacy enhancement is often a goal in interventions designed to change people's health-related behavior.

In the Transtheoretical Model (Prochaska et al., 2002), the core construct is *stages of change*, which conceptualizes a continuum of motivational readiness to change problem behavior. The five stages of change are precontemplation, contemplation, preparation, action, and maintenance. Studies have found that successful self-changers use different processes at each stage, thus suggesting the desirability of interventions that are individualized to the person's stage of readiness for change.

> **Example using the transtheoretical model**
> Cevik and Kocatas (2024) tested the effect of an online individual motivational interviewing program guided by the Transtheoretical Model on pregnant people's smoking cessation behavior.

The Theory of Planned Behavior (TPB) (Ajzen, 2005), which is an extension of another theory called the Theory of Reasoned Action, offers a framework for understanding people's behavior and its psychological determinants. According to the theory, behavior that is volitional is determined by people's *intention* to perform that behavior. Intentions, in turn, are affected by attitudes toward the behavior, subjective norms (i.e., perceived social pressure to perform or not perform the behavior), and perceived behavioral control (i.e., anticipated ease or difficulty of engaging in the behavior).

> **Example using the Theory of Planned Behavior**
> Ding and colleagues (2023) examined the impact of the anticoagulation programs based on the TPB and nudge strategy among patients with nonvalvular atrial fibrillation.

As nurses increasingly collaborate with other disciplines through team science, it stands to reason that they develop theories reflecting this interdisciplinary perspective. One example is the Theory of Dyadic Illness Management (Lyons & Lee, 2018). Lyons (a family and human development scientist) and Lee (a nurse scientist) have collaborated on many studies over several years, specifically focusing on older adults and chronic disease self-management. The Theory of Dyadic Illness Management considers the dyad of the individual and care partner as an interdependent team. The theory suggests that the way the dyad appraises the illness influences how the dyad manages the illness together, ultimately influencing the health of the dyad. The goal of this theory is to optimize the health of the dyad. Lyons et al. (2024) conducted a study aimed at understanding the dyadic benefits of dyadic family care behavioral interventions on the person with Parkinson disease and their care partner.

USING A THEORY OR FRAMEWORK IN RESEARCH

The ways in which theory is used by qualitative and quantitative researchers is elaborated on in this section. The term *theory* is used in its broadest sense to include conceptual models, formal theories, and frameworks.

Theories and Qualitative Research

Theory is almost always present in studies that are embedded in a qualitative research tradition such as ethnography or phenomenology. However, different traditions involve theory in different ways.

Some nursing researchers insist that qualitative researchers adopt an atheoretical stance vis-à-vis the phenomenon of interest, with the goal of suspending prior conceptualizations (theories) that might bias their inquiry. For example, some descriptive phenomenologists are committed to theoretical naiveté and bracket preconceived views of the phenomenon. Nevertheless, all phenomenologists are guided by a philosophical framework that focuses their inquiry on certain aspects of a person's lifeworld—that is, lived experiences. Glasdam et al. (2024) suggest theoretical and philosophical perspectives inform the interpretation of data and that stating one's perspective is critical to being transparent in the reporting of the findings. Others suggest that qualitative nursing research must flow from nursing's philosophical, theoretical, and disciplinary epistemologic positionings and must add to nursing knowledge and inform practice in cyclical and meaningful ways (Chiu et al., 2022; Thorne, 2020; Thorne et al., 2016).

Ethnographers bring a cultural perspective to their studies, and this perspective shapes their fieldwork. Cultural theories include *ideational theories*, which suggest that cultural conditions stem from mental activity and ideas, and *materialistic theories*, which view material conditions (e.g., resources, production) as the source of cultural developments (Fetterman, 2019).

The theoretical underpinning of grounded theory is a melding of sociologic formulations, the most prominent of which is *symbolic interaction*. Three underlying premises include (1) humans act toward things based on the meanings that the things have for them; (2) the meaning of things is derived from the human interactions; and (3) meanings are handled in, and modified through, an interpretive process (Blumer, 1986).

Despite this theoretical perspective, grounded theory researchers, like some phenomenologists, try to hold prior substantive theory about the phenomenon in abeyance until their own substantive theory emerges. The goal of grounded theory is to develop a conceptually dense understanding of a phenomenon that is *grounded* in actual observations. Grounded theory researchers, who focus on social or psychological processes, often develop conceptual maps to illustrate how a process works or unfolds. Figure 7.1 illustrates such a conceptual map for a study of the process of self-management of opioid recovery through pregnancy and early parenting (Mattson et al., 2024). The central process, growing as a healthy dyad,

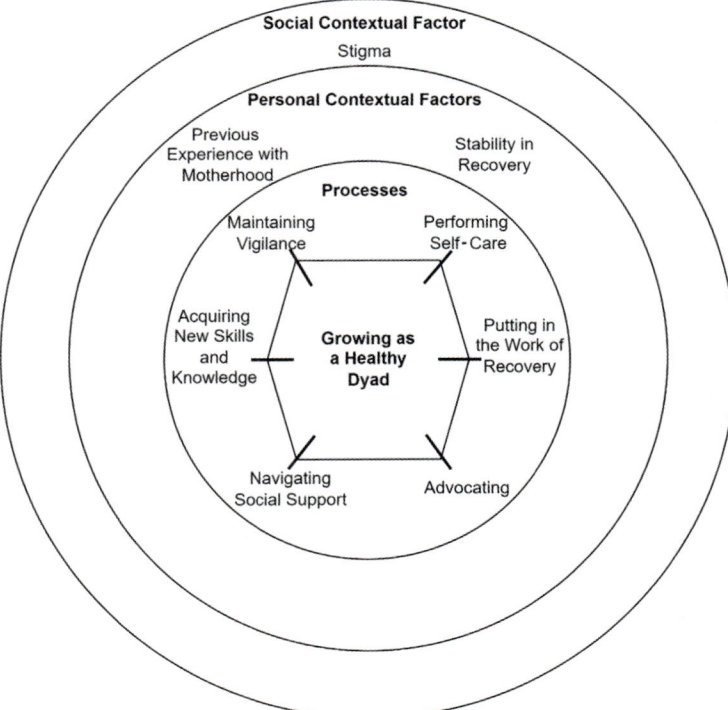

Figure 7.1 The self-management of opioid recovery through pregnancy and early parenting grounded theory. (Reprinted with permission from Mattson, N. M., Ohlendorf, J. M., & Haglund, K. [2024]. Grounded theory approach to understand self-management of opioid recovery through pregnancy and early parenting. *Journal of Obstetric, Gynecologic and Neonatal Nursing, 53*, 34–45. https://doi.org/10.1016/j.jogn.2023.09.001. Copyright © 2023 AWHONN, the Association of Women's Health, Obstetric and Neonatal Nurses. With permission.)

consisted of six processes birthing parents used to self-manage their recovery: maintaining vigilance, performing self-care, putting in the work of recovery, advocating, navigating social support, and acquiring skills and knowledge.

> **Example of a grounded theory study**
> Sun et al. (2024) conducted a qualitative study using grounded theory to develop a theoretical understanding of the factors that influence the public's willingness and attitudes to perform cardiopulmonary resuscitation.

In recent years, some qualitative nurse researchers have used *critical theory* as a framework in their research. Critical theory is a paradigm that involves a critique of society and societal structures, as we discuss in Chapter 10.

Qualitative researchers sometimes use conceptual models of nursing or other theories as interpretive frameworks. For example, a number of qualitative nurse researchers acknowledge that the philosophic roots of their studies lie in conceptual models of nursing such as those developed by Roy (Roy & Andrews, 2009), Rogers (1992; 1994), or Newman (1999; 2007).

 TIP Systematic reviews of qualitative studies on a specific topic can lead to substantive theory development. In metasyntheses, qualitative studies are combined to identify their essential elements used for theory building.

Theories in Quantitative Research

Quantitative researchers link research to theory or models in various ways. The classic approach is to test hypotheses deduced from an existing theory. For example, a nurse might read about Pender's Health Promotion Model and might reason as follows: If the HPM is valid, then I would expect that patients with osteoporosis who perceive the benefit of a calcium-enriched diet would be more likely to alter their eating patterns than those who perceive no benefits. This hypothesis could be tested through statistical analysis of data on patients' perceptions in relation to their eating habits. Repeated acceptance of hypotheses derived from a theory lends support to the theory.

 TIP When a quantitative study is based on a theory or model, the research article typically states this fact early—often in the abstract or the title. Some reports also have a subsection of the introduction called "Theoretical Framework." The report usually includes a brief overview of the theory so that all readers can understand, in a broad way, the conceptual context of the study.

Some researchers test theory-based interventions. Theories have implications for modifying people's attitudes or behavior and hence their health outcomes. Interventions based on an explicit conceptualization of human behavior have a better chance of being effective than ones developed in a conceptual vacuum. Interventions rarely affect outcomes directly—there are mediating factors that play a role in the pathway between the intervention and desired outcomes. For example, researchers developing interventions based on Social Cognitive Theory posit that improvements to a person's self-efficacy will result in positive changes in health behaviors or health outcomes.

Many researchers who cite a theory or model as their framework are not directly *testing* the theory but using the theory to provide an *organizing structure*. In such an approach, researchers *assume* that the model they adopt is valid and then use its constructs to provide an interpretive context.

CRITICAL APPRAISAL OF FRAMEWORKS IN RESEARCH REPORTS

It is often challenging to critically appraise the theoretical context of a research report—or its absence—but we offer a few suggestions.

In a qualitative study in which a grounded theory is developed, you may not be given enough information to refute the proposed theory because only evidence supporting the theory is presented. You can, however, assess whether conceptualizations are insightful and whether the evidence is convincing. In a phenomenologic study, you should look for a discussion of the study's philosophical underpinnings, that is, the philosophy of phenomenology.

For quantitative studies, the first task is to see whether the study has an explicit conceptual framework. If there is no mention of a theory, model, or framework (and often there is not), you should consider whether this absence diminishes the value of the study. Research often benefits from an explicit conceptual context, but some studies are so pragmatic that the lack of a theory has no effect on its utility. If, however, the study involves the test of a hypothesis or a complex intervention, the absence of a formal framework suggests conceptual fuzziness.

If the study does have an explicit framework, you can reflect on its appropriateness. You may not be able to challenge the researcher's use of a particular theory, but you can assess whether the link between the problem and the theory is genuine. Did the researcher present a convincing rationale for the framework used? In quantitative studies, did the hypotheses *flow* from the theory? Did the researcher interpret the findings within the context of the framework? If the answer to such questions is no, you may have grounds for criticizing the study's framework, even though you may not be able to suggest ways to improve the conceptual basis of the study. Some suggestions for evaluating the conceptual basis of a quantitative study are offered in Box 7.1.

 TIP Some studies claim theoretical linkages that are contrived. This is most likely to occur when researchers first formulate the research problem and then later find a theoretical context to fit it. An after-the-fact linkage of theory to a research question is often artificial. If a research problem is truly linked to a conceptual framework, then the design of the study, the measurement of key constructs, and the analysis and interpretation of data will *flow* from that conceptualization.

Box 7.1 Guidelines for Critically Appraising Theoretical/Conceptual Frameworks in a Research Report

a. Did the report describe an explicit theoretical or conceptual framework for the study? If not, does the absence of a framework detract from the study's conceptual integration?
b. Did the report adequately describe the major features of the theory or model so that readers could understand the conceptual basis of the study?
c. Is the theory or model appropriate for the research problem? Does the purported link between the problem and the framework seem contrived?
d. Was the theory or model used for generating hypotheses, or is it used as an organizational or interpretive framework? Do the hypotheses (if any) naturally flow from the framework?
e. Were concepts defined in a way that is consistent with the theory? If there was an intervention, were intervention components consistent with the theory?
f. Did the framework guide the study methods? For example, was the appropriate research tradition used if the study was qualitative? If quantitative, do the operational definitions correspond to the conceptual definitions?
g. Did the researcher tie the study findings back to the framework at the end of the report? Were the findings interpreted within the context of the framework?

RESEARCH EXAMPLES WITH CRITICAL THINKING EXERCISES

This section presents an example of a study that described its theoretical links. Read the summary, and then answer the critical thinking questions, referring to the full research report if necessary. The critical thinking questions for Examples 2 and 3 are based on the studies that appear in their entirety in Appendices A and B of this book.

EXAMPLE 1: ROY'S ADAPTATION MODEL IN A QUANTITATIVE STUDY

Study: "The effects of the instrumental reminiscence therapy based on RAM on adaptation, life satisfaction, and happiness in older people: A randomized controlled trial" (Aydogdu et al., 2023).

Statement of Purpose: The purpose of this study was to evaluate the effects of instrumental reminiscence therapy based on RAM on older people's adaptation, life satisfaction, and happiness.

Theoretical Framework: RAM served as the theoretical basis of this study. It was used to develop theory-based nursing interventions. The four adaptive modes of RAM, specifically the physiological, self-concept, role function, and interdependence modes, were considered to categorize the sessions of instrumental reminiscence therapy. It was suggested that RAM may facilitate the systematic planning of the sessions and group activities of the instrumental reminiscence therapy according to each adaptive mode.

Method: This experimental quantitative study utilized a pretest–posttest randomized control trial design. The study was conducted in two nursing homes in Cyprus. A total of 34 people participated in the study. Using block randomization, 17 participants were randomized to the control group and 17 were randomized to the intervention group. Measures included a demographic descriptive form, the Assessment Scale of Adaptation Difficulty for the Elderly, Life Satisfaction Index A, and the Oxford Happiness Questionnaire-Short Form.

Key Findings: The researchers observed that there was no statistically significant difference between the intervention and control groups in terms of the sociodemographic characteristics of participants ($p > .05$). They did find a statistically significant increase in the mean posttest scores of the Assessment Scale of Adaptation Difficulty for the Elderly, Life Satisfaction Index A, and Oxford Happiness Questionnaire—Short Form ($p < .05$) in the intervention group.

1. Answer the relevant questions from Box 7.1 regarding this study.
2. Is there another model or theory that was described in this chapter that could have been used to study the effect of this intervention?
3. If the results of this study are valid and generalizable, what might be some of the uses to which the findings could be put in clinical practice?

EXAMPLE 2: QUANTITATIVE RESEARCH IN APPENDIX A

Read the introduction to Cheng and colleagues (2024) "Advance care planning affects end-of-life treatment preferences among patients with heart failure: A randomized controlled trial" in Appendix A of this book,

1. Answer the relevant questions from Box 7.1 regarding this study.
2. Would any of the other theories or models described in this chapter have provided an appropriate conceptual context for this study?

EXAMPLE 3: QUALITATIVE RESEARCH IN APPENDIX B

Read the introduction of Morrison and colleagues (2024) "Lived experiences of fathers after infertility" in Appendix B of this book.
1. Answer the relevant questions from Box 7.1 regarding this study.
2. Do you think that a schematic model would have helped to summarize the findings in this report?
3. Did Morrison et al. resent convincing evidence to support their use of the philosophy of phenomenology?

Summary Points

- High-quality research requires *conceptual integration*, one aspect of which is having a defensible theoretical rationale for the study.

- As classically defined, a **theory** consists of two or more concepts and propositions that form a logically interrelated system, providing a mechanism for deducing hypotheses. **Descriptive theory** thoroughly describes a phenomenon.

- *Grand theories* (or *macrotheories*) attempt to describe or explain large segments of the human experience. **Middle-range theories** are specific to certain phenomena; examples include Pender's HPM and Mishel's Uncertainty in Illness Theory.

- Concepts are also the basic elements in **conceptual models**, but concepts are not linked in a logically ordered, deductive system.

- In research, the goals of theories and models are to make findings meaningful, to integrate knowledge into coherent systems, to stimulate new research, and to explain phenomena and relationships among them.

- **Schematic models** (or **conceptual maps**) are graphic representations of phenomena and their interrelationships using symbols or diagrams and a minimal use of words.

- A **framework** is the conceptual underpinning of a study, including an overall rationale and conceptual definitions of key concepts. In qualitative studies, the framework often springs from distinct research traditions.

- Several conceptual models of nursing have been used in nursing research. The concepts central to models of nursing are *human beings*, *environment*, *health*, and *nursing*. An example of a model of nursing used by nurse researchers is RAM. Nonnursing models are also used by nurse researchers (e.g., Bandura's Social Cognitive Theory).

- In some qualitative research traditions (e.g., phenomenology), the researcher strives to suspend previously held *substantive theories* of the specific phenomena under study, but each tradition has rich theoretical underpinnings.

- Some qualitative researchers seek to develop *grounded theories*, data-driven explanations to account for phenomena under study through inductive processes.

- In the classical use of theory, researchers test hypotheses deduced from an existing theory. An emerging trend is the testing of theory-based interventions.

- In both qualitative and quantitative studies, researchers sometimes use a theory or model as an organizing framework or as an interpretive tool.

REFERENCES

Ajzen, I. (2005). *Attitudes, personality and behavior* (2nd ed.). Open University Press/McGraw Hill.

Aydogdu, O., Tastan, S., & Kublay, G. (2023). The effects of the instrumental reminiscence therapy based on Roy's adaptation model on adaptation, life satisfaction, and happiness in older people: A randomized controlled trial. *International Journal of Nursing Practice*, 29(3), e13101. https://doi.org/10.1111/ijn.13101

Bandura, A. (2001). Social cognitive theory: An agentic perspective. *Annual Review of Psychology*, 52, 1–26.

Barrett, E. (2010). Power as knowing participation in change: What's new and what's next. *Nursing Science Quarterly*, 23, 47–54.

Beck, C. T. (2015). Middle-range theory of traumatic childbirth: The ever-widening ripple effect. *Global Qualitative Nursing Research*, 2, 1–13.

Blumer, H. (1986). *Symbolic interactionism: Perspective and method*. University of California Press.

Brown, N. I., Pekmezi, D. W., Oster, R. A., Courneya, K. S., McAuley, E., Ehlers, D. K., Phillips, S. M., Anton, P., & Rogers, L. Q. (2023). Relationships between obesity, exercise preferences, and related social cognitive theory variables among breast cancer survivors. *Nutrients*, 15(5), 1286. https://doi.org/10.3390/nu15051286

Cevik, B. E., & Kocatas, S. (2024). The effect of online motivational interviewing on pregnant women's smoking cessation behaviour: A randomized controlled trial. *International Journal of Nursing Practice*, 30(6), e13303. https://doi.org/10.1111/ijn.13303

Chiu, P., Thorne, S., Schick-Makaroff, K., & Cummings, G. G. (2022). Theory utilization in applied qualitative nursing research. *Journal of Advanced Nursing*, 78(12), 4034–4041. https://doi.org/10.1111/jan.15456

Choi, M. J., Kim, S., & Jeong, S. H. (2024). Factors associated with health-promoting behaviors among nurses in South Korea: Systematic review and meta-analysis based on Pender's health promotion model. *Asian Nursing Research*, 18(2), 188–202. https://doi.org/10.1016/j.anr.2024.04.007

Chong, H. J., Jang, M. K., Lockwood, M. B., & Park, C. (2023). Health belief model constructs affect influenza vaccine uptake in kidney transplant recipients. *Western Journal of Nursing Research*, 45(5), 395–401. https://doi.org/10.1177/01939459221136354

Ding, Y., Jiang, H., Liu, J., Chen, D., & Yang, F. (2023). Effects of the theory of planned behavior and nudge strategy-based intervention on the adherence to anticoagulation treatment in patients with non-valvular atrial fibrillation. *Geriatric Nursing*, 51, 17–24. https://doi.org/10.1016/j.gerinurse.2023.01.023

Fawcett, J. (2023, January 17). *Evolution of one version of our disciplinary metaparadigm*. Nursology. https://nursology.net/2023/01/17/evolution-of-one-version-of-our-disciplinary-metaparadigm/

Fetterman, D. M. (2019). *Ethnography: Step by step* (4th ed.). Sage.

Glasdam, S., Xu, H., & Gulestø, R. J. A. (2024). A call for theory-inspired analysis in qualitative research: Ways to construct different truths in and about healthcare. *Nursing Inquiry*, 31(3), e12642. https://doi.org/10.1111/nin.12642

Kolcaba, K. (2003). *Comfort theory and practice: A vision for holistic health care and research*. Springer Publishing.

Lin, H., Ye, M., Lin, Y., Chen, F., Chan, S., Cai, H., & Zhu, J. (2023). Mobile app for gynecologic cancer support for patients with gynecologic cancer receiving chemotherapy in China: Multicenter randomized controlled trial. *Journal of Medical Internet Research*, 25, e49939. https://doi.org/10.2196/49939

Lyons, K. S., & Lee, C. S. (2018). The theory of dyadic illness management. *Journal of Family Nursing*, 24(1), 8–28. https://doi.org/10.1177/1074840717745669

Lyons, K. S., Russell, L. T., Bonds Johnson, K., Brewster, G. S., Carter, J. H., & Miller, L. M. (2024). Evaluating the dyadic benefits of early-phase behavioral interventions: An exemplar using data from couples living with Parkinson's disease. *The Gerontologist*, 64(7), gnad172. https://doi.org/10.1093/geront/gnad172

Mattson, N. M., Ohlendorf, J. M., & Haglund, K. (2024). Grounded theory approach to understand self-management of opioid recovery through pregnancy and early parenting. *Journal of Obstetric, Gynecologic and Neonatal Nursing*, 53, 34–45. https://doi.org/10.1016/j.jogn.2023.09.001

Mishel, M. H. (1990). Reconceptualization of the uncertainty in illness theory. *Image—The Journal of Nursing Scholarship*, 22(4), 256–262.

Murdaugh, C., Parsons, M. A., & Pender, N. J., (2019). *Health promotion in nursing practice* (8th ed.). Pearson.

Newman, M. A. (1999). *Health as expanding consciousness*. National League for Nursing.

Newman, M. A. (2007). *Transforming presence: The difference that nursing makes*. F.A. Davis.

Parse, R. R. (2014). *The humanbecoming Paradigm: A transformational worldview*. Discovery International Publication.

Prochaska, J. O., Redding, C. A., & Evers, K. E. (2002). The Transtheoretical Model and stages of changes. In K. Glanz, B. K. Rimer, & F. M. Lewis (Eds.), *Health behavior and health education: Theory, research, and practice* (3rd ed., pp. 99–120). Jossey-Bass.

Rogers, M. E. (1992). Nursing science and the space age. *Nursing Science Quarterly*, 5(1), 27–34. https://doi.org/10.1177/089431849200500108

Rogers, M. E. (1994). The science of unitary human beings: Current perspectives. *Nursing Science Quarterly*, 7, 33–35.

Roy, C., & Andrews, H. (2009). *The Roy adaptation model* (3rd ed.). Pearson.

Sun, M., Waters, C. M., & Zhu, A. (2024). Public willingness, attitudes and related factors toward cardiopulmonary resuscitation: A grounded theory study. *Public Health*, 41(2), 233–244. https://doi.org/10.1111/phn.13271

Thorne, S. (2020). Beyond theming: Making qualitative studies matter. *Nursing Inquiry*, 27(1), e12343. https://doi.org/10.1111/nin.12343

Thorne, S., Stephens, J., & Truant, T. (2016). Building qualitative study design using nursing's disciplinary epistemology. *Journal of Advanced Nursing*, 72(2), 451–460. https://doi.org/10.1111/jan.12822

Ventura, M. W. S., Lima, G. A., da Silva, V. M., Lopes, M. V. O., & Lima, F. E. T. (2024). Concept analysis of neonatal near miss. *Journal of Pediatric Nursing*, 77, e411–e419. https://doi.org/10.1016/j.pedn.2024.05.004

Walker, L., & Avant, K. (2021). *Strategies for theory construction in nursing* (6th ed.). Pearson.

Part 3: Designs and Methods for Quantitative and Qualitative Nursing Research

8 Appraising Quantitative Research Design

Learning Objectives

On completing this chapter, you will be able to:

- Discuss key research design decisions for a quantitative study
- Discuss the concept of causality and identify criteria for causal relationships
- Describe and identify experimental, quasi-experimental, and nonexperimental designs
- Distinguish between cross-sectional and longitudinal designs
- Identify and evaluate alternative methods of controlling confounding variables
- Understand various threats to the validity of quantitative studies
- Evaluate a quantitative study in terms of its research design and methods of controlling confounding variables
- Define new terms in the chapter

Key Terms

- Attrition
- Baseline data
- Blinding
- Case-control design
- Cause
- Cohort design
- Comparison group
- Construct validity
- Control group
- Correlation
- Correlational research
- Correlational studies
- Crossover design
- Cross-sectional design
- Descriptive research
- Effect
- Experiment
- Experimental group
- External validity
- History threat
- Homogeneity
- Internal validity
- Intervention
- Longitudinal design
- Matching
- Maturation threat
- Mortality threat
- Nonequivalent control group
- Nonexperimental study
- Placebo
- Posttest data
- Pretest–posttest design
- Prospective (cohort) designs Prospective design
- Quasi-experiment
- Randomization
- Randomized controlled trial (RCT)
- Research design
- Retrospective design
- Selection threat
- Statistical conclusion validity
- Statistical power
- Threats to validity
- Time-series design
- Validity

For quantitative studies, no aspect of a study's methods has a bigger impact on the validity of the results than the research design—particularly if the inquiry is *cause-probing*. This chapter has information about how you can draw conclusions about key aspects of evidence quality in a quantitative study.

OVERVIEW OF RESEARCH DESIGN ISSUES

The research design of a study encompasses the strategies that researchers adopt to answer their questions and test their hypotheses. This section describes some basic design issues.

Key Research Design Features

Table 8.1 describes seven key features that are typically addressed in the design of a quantitative study. Design decisions that researchers must make include the following:

- *Will there be an intervention?* A basic design issue is whether researchers will introduce an intervention and test its effects—the distinction between experimental and nonexperimental research.
- *What types of comparisons will be made?* Quantitative researchers often make comparisons to provide an interpretive context. Sometimes, the *same* people are compared at different points in time (e.g., preoperatively vs. postoperatively), but often, different people are compared (e.g., those getting vs. not getting an intervention).
- *How will confounding variables be controlled?* In quantitative research, efforts are often made to control factors extraneous to the research question.
- *Will blinding be used?* Researchers must decide if information about the study (e.g., who is getting an intervention) will be withheld from data collectors, study participants, or others to minimize the risk of *expectation bias*, that is, the risk that such knowledge could influence study outcomes.

TABLE 8.1 Key Design Features

Feature	Key Questions	Design Options
Intervention	Will there be an intervention?	Experimental (RCT), quasi-experimental, nonexperimental/observational design
Comparisons	What type of comparisons will be made to illuminate relationships?	Same participants at different times or conditions OR different participants
Control over confounding variables	How will confounding variables be controlled? Which confounding variables will be controlled?	Randomization, crossover, homogeneity, matching, statistical control
Blinding	From whom will critical information be withheld to avoid bias?	Blinding of participants, interventionists, other staff, data collectors
Time frames	How often will data be collected? When, relative to other events, will data be collected?	Cross-sectional, longitudinal design
Relative timing	When will information on independent and dependent variables be collected—looking backward or forward?	Retrospective (case control), prospective (cohort) design
Location	Where will the study take place?	Setting selection; single site versus multisite

- *How often will data be collected?* Data sometimes are collected from participants at a single point in time (*cross-sectionally*), but other studies involve multiple points of data collection (*longitudinally*).
- *When will "effects" be measured, relative to potential causes?* Some studies collect information about outcomes and then look back *retrospectively* for potential causes. Other studies begin with a potential cause and then see what outcomes ensue, in a *prospective* fashion.
- *Where will the study take place?* Data for quantitative studies are collected in various settings, such as in hospitals or people's homes. Researchers must also decide how many sites will be involved in the study—a decision that could affect the generalizability of the results.

Many design decisions are independent of the others. For example, both experimental and nonexperimental studies can compare different people or the same people at different times.

 TIP Information about a study's research design usually appears early in the method section of a research article.

Causality

Many research questions are about *causes* and *effects*. For example, does turning patients cause reductions in pressure ulcers? Does exercise cause improvements in heart function? Causality is a hotly debated issue, but we all understand the general concept of a cause. For example, we understand that failure to sleep *causes* fatigue and that higher caloric intake than output *causes* weight gain. Most phenomena are multiply determined. Fatigue, for example, can reflect poor sleep *or* other factors. Causes are seldom *deterministic*—they only increase the likelihood that an effect will occur. For example, smoking is a cause of lung cancer, but not everyone who smokes develops lung cancer, and not everyone with lung cancer smoked.

While it might be easy to grasp what researchers mean when they talk about a *cause*, what exactly is an **effect?** One way to understand an effect is by conceptualizing a counterfactual (Shadish et al., 2002). A *counterfactual* is what would happen to people if they were exposed to a causal influence and were simultaneously *not* exposed to it. An effect represents the difference between what actually did happen with the exposure and what would have happened without it. A counterfactual clearly can never be realized, but it is a good model to keep in mind in thinking about research design.

Three criteria for establishing causal relationships are attributed to John Stuart Mill (1859).

1. *Temporal*: A cause must precede an effect in time. If we test the hypothesis that smoking causes lung cancer, we need to show that cancer occurred *after* smoking began.
2. *Relationship*: There must be an association between the presumed cause and the effect. In our example, we have to demonstrate an association between smoking and cancer—that is, that a higher percentage of smokers than nonsmokers get lung cancer.
3. *Confounders*: The relationship cannot be explained as being *caused by a third variable*. Suppose that smokers tended to live predominantly in urban environments. There would then be a possibility that the relationship between smoking and lung cancer reflects an underlying causal connection between the environment and lung cancer.

Other criteria for causality have been proposed. One important criterion in health research is *biologic plausibility*—evidence from basic physiologic studies that a causal pathway is credible. Researchers investigating casual relationships must provide persuasive evidence regarding these criteria through their research design.

TABLE 8.2 Hierarchy of Designs for Different Cause-Probing Research Questions

Type of Question	Hierarchy of Designs
Therapy/intervention	RCT/Experimental > Quasi-experimental > Cohort > Case control > Descriptive correlational
Prognosis	Cohort > Case control > Descriptive correlational
Etiology (causation)/prevention of harm	RCT/Experimental > Quasi-experimental > Cohort > Case control > Descriptive correlational

Research Questions and Research Design

Different quantitative designs are appropriate for different types of question. In this chapter, we focus primarily on designs for therapy, prognosis, etiology/harm, and description questions; meaning questions require a qualitative approach and are discussed in Chapter 10.

Except for description questions, those that call for a quantitative approach usually concern causal relationships:

- Does a telephone counseling intervention (I) for patients with prostate cancer (P) *cause* improvements in their psychological distress (O)? (therapy question)
- Do birth weights under 1,500 g (I) *cause* developmental delays (O) in children (P)? (prognosis question)
- Does salt (I) *cause* high blood pressure (O) in adults (P)? (etiology/harm question)

Some designs are better at revealing cause-and-effect relationships than others. In particular, experimental designs (**randomized controlled trials [RCTs]**) are the best possible designs for illuminating causal relationships—but using such designs is not always possible. Table 8.2 summarizes a "hierarchy" of designs for answering different types of causal questions and augments the evidence hierarchy presented in Figure 1.2 (Chapter 1).

EXPERIMENTAL, QUASI-EXPERIMENTAL, AND NONEXPERIMENTAL DESIGNS

This section describes designs that differ with regard to whether or not there is an intervention.

Experimental Design: Randomized Controlled Trials

Early scientists learned that complexities occurring in nature can make it difficult to understand relationships through pure observation. This problem was addressed by isolating phenomena and controlling the conditions under which they occurred. These experimental procedures have been adopted by researchers interested in human physiology and behavior.

Characteristics of True Experiments

A true **experiment** is characterized by the following properties:

- *Intervention*—The experimenter *does* something to some participants by manipulating the independent variable.
- *Control*—The experimenter introduces controls into the study, including devising an approximation to a counterfactual—usually a *control group* that does not receive the intervention.
- *Randomization*—The experimenter assigns participants to a control or experimental condition on a random basis.

By introducing an **intervention**, experimenters consciously vary the independent variable and then observe its effect on the outcome. To illustrate, suppose we were investigating the effect of gentle massage (I), compared to no massage (C), on pain (O) in nursing home residents (P). One experimental design for this question is a **pretest–posttest design**, which involves observing the outcome (pain levels) before and after the intervention. Participants in the experimental group receive a gentle massage, whereas those in the control group do not. This design permits us to see whether changes in pain were *caused* by the massage because only some people received it, providing an important comparison. In this example, we met the first criterion of a true experiment by varying massage receipt, the independent variable.

This example also meets the second requirement for experiments, use of a control group. Inferences about causality require a comparison, but not all comparisons yield equally persuasive evidence. For example, if we were to supplement the diet of premature babies (P) with special nutrients (I) for 2 weeks, their weight (O) at the end of 2 weeks would tell us nothing about the intervention's effectiveness. At a minimum, we would need to compare posttreatment weight with pretreatment weight to see if weight had increased. But suppose we find an average weight gain of 1 lb. Does this finding support an inference of a causal connection between the nutritional intervention (the independent variable) and weight gain (the outcome)? No, because infants normally gain weight as they mature. Without a control group—a group that does not receive the supplements (C)—it is impossible to separate the effects of maturation from those of the treatment. The term **control group** refers to a group of participants whose performance on an outcome is used to evaluate the performance of the **experimental group** (the group getting the intervention) on the same outcome.

Experimental designs also involve placing participants in groups at random. Through **randomization** (also called *random assignment*), every participant has an equal chance of being included in any group. If people are randomly assigned, there is no systematic bias in the groups with regard to attributes that may affect the outcome. Randomly assigned groups are expected to be comparable, on average, with respect to an infinite number of biologic, psychological, and social traits at the outset of the study. Group differences on outcomes observed after randomization can therefore be inferred as being caused by the intervention.

Random assignment can be accomplished by flipping a coin or pulling names from a hat. Researchers typically use computers to perform the randomization.

TIP There is a lot of confusion about random assignment versus random sampling. Random assignment is a signature of an experimental design (RCT). If subjects are not randomly assigned to treatment groups, then the design is not a true experiment. Random *sampling*, by contrast, refers to a method of selecting people for a study, as we discuss in Chapter 9. Random sampling is *not* a signature of an experimental design. In fact, random sampling is seldom used in RCTs.

Experimental Designs

The most basic experimental design involves randomizing people to different groups and then measuring outcomes. This design is sometimes called a *posttest-only design*. A more widely used design is the pretest–posttest design, which involves collecting **baseline** (pretest) **data** on the dependent variable before the intervention and **posttest** (outcome) **data** after it.

Example of a pretest–posttest design
Uslu and Arslan (2023) conducted a randomized control trial to test the effect of using virtual reality glasses on anxiety and fatigue in women with breast cancer who were receiving adjuvant chemotherapy. The control group received the usual care, whereas

the intervention group wore virtual reality glasses and listened to nature sounds for 30 minutes. Researchers administered measures before the intervention or standard of care and post the intervention.

 TIP Experimental designs can be depicted graphically using symbols to represent design features. Some diagrams of these designs are presented in Table 8.3.

TABLE 8.3 Selected Experimental (Randomized) Designs

Type of Design	Schematic Diagram	Situations That Are Best Suited	Drawbacks
Basic posttest-only experimental design	R X O R X_A O_1 R O_1 or R X_B O_1	When the outcome is not relevant until after the intervention is complete (e.g., length of stay in hospital)	Does not permit evaluation of whether the two groups were comparable at the outset on the outcome of interest—not a major concern if randomization done properly
Basic pretest–posttest experimental design	R O X O_2 R O_1 O_2	When the focus of the intervention is on *changes in* outcomes	Sometimes the pretest itself can affect the outcomes of interest.
Multiple treatment design	R O_1 X_A O_2 R O_1 X_B O_2 R O_1 O_2	Can be used to disentangle effects of different components of a complex intervention ("black box" issue) or to test competing interventions	Requires larger sample than basic designs; may be at risk of threats to statistical conclusion validity if A and B are not very different (small effects)
Wait-list (delay of treatment) design	R O_1 X O_2 O_3 R O_1 O_2 X O_3	Attractive when there is patient preference for the innovative treatment; can strengthen inferences by virtue of replication aspect for the second group	Controls may be inclined to drop out of study before they get deferred treatment; not suitable if key outcomes are measured long after treatment (e.g., mortality) or if there is interest in assessing long-term effects (wait-list period is then too long); history threat a possibility
Crossover design—participants serve as their own controls	R O_1 X_A O_2 X_B O_3 R O_1 X_B O_2 X_A O_3	Appropriate only if no possibility of carryover effects from one period to the next (effects should have rapid onset, short half-life); useful when recruitment is difficult (i.e., smaller sample needed); excellent for controlling confounding variables	Often cannot assume there are no carryover effects; if the first treatment received "fixes" a problem for participants, they may not remain in the study for the second one
Factorial design	R O_1 X_{A1B1} O_2 R O_1 X_{A1B2} O_2 R O_1 X_{A2B1} O_2 R O_1 X_{A2B2} O_2	Efficient for testing two interventions simultaneously; most useful when strong synergistic/additive effects or no interaction effects are expected	Power needed to detect interactions could require larger sample size than when testing each intervention separately

O, observation or measurement of the outcome; R, randomization; X, intervention (XA, one treatment; XB, alternative treatment or dose).

The people who are randomly assigned to different conditions usually are different people. For example, if we were testing the effect of music on agitation (O) in patients with dementia (P), we could give some patients music (I) and others no music (C). A crossover design, by contrast, involves exposing people to more than one treatment. Such studies are true experiments only if people are randomly assigned to different orderings of treatment. For example, if a crossover design were used to compare the effects of music on patients with dementia, some would be randomly assigned to receive music first followed by a period of no music, and others would receive no music first. In such a study, the three conditions for an experiment have been met: There is intervention, randomization, and control—with participants serving as their own control group.

A crossover design has the advantage of ensuring the highest possible equivalence among the people exposed to different conditions. Such designs are sometimes inappropriate, however, because of possible *carryover effects*. When participants are exposed to two different treatments, they may be influenced in the second condition by their experience in the first. However, when carryover effects are implausible, as when intervention effects are immediate and short-lived, a crossover design is powerful.

Example of a crossover design
Ulger and colleagues (2023) used a crossover design to test the impact of spinal stabilization exercises and yoga exercises on sleep, kinesiophobia, pain, functional status, and metabolic capacity in individuals with chronic low back pain. One group of participants was initially assigned to stabilization exercises and then added yoga, whereas the second group was assigned to yoga and then added the stabilization exercises.

Experimental and Control Conditions

To give an intervention a fair test, researchers need to design one of sufficient intensity and duration that effects on the outcome might reasonably be expected. Researchers describe the intervention in formal *protocols* that stipulate exactly what the treatment is.

Researchers have choices about what to use as the control condition, and the decision affects the interpretation of the findings. Among the possibilities for the control condition are the following:

- "Usual care"—standard or normal procedures
- An alternative treatment (e.g., music vs. massage)
- A **placebo** or pseudointervention presumed to have no therapeutic value
- An *attention control condition* (the control group gets attention but not the intervention's active ingredients)
- Delayed treatment, that is, control group members are *wait-listed* and exposed to the intervention after outcomes are assessed

Example of a wait-listed control group
Low and colleagues (2023) conducted a randomized controlled pilot study using a wait-list control group to determine the feasibility of an individual coaching and counseling program for people recently diagnosed with dementia to help them adjust to the diagnosis and live well. The study, conducted in Australia, enrolled 11 participants. While the intervention group ($n = 6$) received the coaching and counseling immediately, the control group ($n = 5$) did not receive the intervention until 6 months later.

Ethically, the delayed treatment design is attractive but is not always feasible. Testing two alternative interventions is also appealing ethically and clinically, but a risk is that the results will be inconclusive if differential effects of two good treatments cannot be detected.

However, there is growing interest in such *comparative effectiveness research*, which we will discuss at greater length in subsequent chapters.

Researchers must also consider possibilities for **blinding**. There are several types of blinding, including single, double and triple. Single blinding means the participants are not aware if they are receiving the intervention or not. Double blinding means neither the participant nor those interacting with the participant are aware of who is receiving the intervention. Lastly, triple blinding means all the above is true and in addition, those doing the data analysis are also blinded as to who was in the intervention or control group. Many nursing interventions do not lend themselves easily to blinding. For example, if the intervention were a smoking cessation program, participants would know whether they were receiving the intervention, and the intervener would know who was in the program. It is usually possible and desirable, however, to blind the participants' group status from the people collecting outcome data.

> **Example of a randomized controlled trial with blinding**
> Aoki and Nakayama (2023) describe a RCT study protocol in which they plan to evaluate the impact of decision-aid use on decision-making participation and conflict regarding the selection of postdischarge care locations for older adult stroke survivors and their families. The study will take place in Japan. They plan to blind the units and allocate the participants according to their rooms.

TIP The term *double blind* is widely used when more than one group is blinded (e.g., participants and interventionists). However, this term is falling into disfavor because of its ambiguity, in favor of clear specifications about exactly who was blinded and who was not.

Advantages and Disadvantages of Experiments

RCTs are the "gold standard" for therapy questions because they yield the most persuasive evidence about the effects of an intervention. Through randomization to groups, researchers come as close as possible to attaining an ideal counterfactual.

The great strength of experiments lies in the confidence with which causal relationships can be inferred. Through the controls imposed by intervening, comparing, and—especially—randomizing, alternative explanations can often be ruled out. For this reason, meta-analyses of RCTs, which integrate evidence from multiple experimental studies, are at the pinnacle of evidence hierarchies for cause-and-effect questions (Fig. 1.2 in Chapter 1).

Despite the advantages of experiments, they have limitations. First, many interesting variables simply are not amenable to intervention. A large number of human traits, such as disease or health habits, cannot be randomly conferred. That is why RCTs are not at the top of the hierarchy for prognosis questions (Table 8.2), which concern the consequences of health problems. For example, infants could not be randomly assigned to having or not having cystic fibrosis to see if this disease causes poor psychosocial adjustment.

Second, many variables could technically—but not ethically—be experimentally varied. For example, there have been no RCTs to study the effect of cigarette smoking on lung cancer. Such a study would require people to be assigned randomly to a smoking group (people forced to smoke) or a nonsmoking group (people prohibited from smoking). Thus, although RCTs are technically at the top of the evidence hierarchy for etiology/harm questions (Table 8.2), many etiology questions cannot be answered using an experimental design.

Sometimes, RCTs are not feasible because of practical issues. It may, for instance, be impossible to secure administrative approval to randomize people to groups. In summary, experimental designs have some limitations that restrict their use for some real-world problems; nevertheless, RCTs have a clear superiority to other designs for testing causal hypotheses.

HOW-TO-TELL TIP How can you tell if a study is experimental? Researchers usually indicate in the method section of their reports that they used an experimental or randomized design (RCT). If such terms are missing, you can conclude that a study is experimental if the article says that the study purpose was to test the effects of an intervention AND if participants were put into groups at random.

Quasi-Experiments

Quasi-experiments (called *trials without randomization* in the medical literature) also involve an intervention; however, quasi-experimental designs lack randomization, the signature of a true experiment. Some quasi-experiments even lack a control group. The signature of a quasi-experimental design is the testing of an intervention in the absence of randomization.

Quasi-Experimental Designs

A frequently used quasi-experimental design is the **nonequivalent control group** pretest–posttest design, which involves comparing two or more groups of people before and after implementing an intervention. For example, suppose we wished to study the effect of a chair yoga intervention (I) for older people (P) on quality of life (O). The intervention is being offered to everyone at a community senior center, and randomization is not possible. For comparative purposes, we collect outcome data at a different senior center that is not instituting the intervention (C). Data on quality of life (QOL) are collected from both groups at baseline and 10 weeks later.

This quasi-experimental design is identical to a pretest–posttest experimental design, except people were not randomized to groups. The quasi-experimental design is weaker because, without randomization, it cannot be assumed that the experimental and comparison groups are equivalent at the outset. The design is, nevertheless, strong because the baseline data allow us to see whether older adults in the two senior centers had similar QOL scores, on average, before the intervention. If the groups are comparable at baseline, we could be relatively confident in inferring that posttest differences in QOL are the result of the yoga intervention. If QOL scores are different initially, however, postintervention differences are hard to interpret. Note that in quasi-experiments, the term **comparison group** is often used in lieu of *control group* to refer to the group against which outcomes in the treatment group are evaluated.

Now suppose we had been unable to collect baseline data. Such a design (*nonequivalent control group posttest-only*) has a flaw that is hard to remedy. We no longer have information about initial equivalence. If QOL in the experimental group is higher than that in the control group at the posttest, can we conclude that the intervention *caused* improved QOL? There could be other explanations for the differences. In particular, the QOL of people in the two centers might have differed initially. The hallmark of strong quasi-experiments is the effort to introduce control mechanisms, such as baseline measurements.

> **Example of a nonequivalent control group design**
> Lee and Noh (2023) used a nonequivalent control group pretest–posttest design to determine the effectiveness of simulation-based education provided to nursing students in Korea to help them learn how to care for patients with COVID-19. Through convenience sampling, 79 participants were included with 37 in the intervention group and 42 in the control group.

Some quasi-experiments have neither randomization nor a comparison group. Suppose a hospital implemented rapid response teams (RRTs) in its acute care units and wanted to learn the effects on patient outcomes (e.g., mortality). For the purposes of this example, assume no other hospital would be a good comparison, so the only possible comparison is a before–after contrast. If RRTs were implemented in January, we could compare the mortality rate, for example, during the 3 months before RRTs with the mortality rate in the subsequent 3-month period.

This *one-group pretest–posttest design* seems logical, but it has weaknesses. What if one of the 3-month periods is atypical, apart from the RRTs? What about the effect of other changes instituted during the same period? What about the effects of external factors, such as seasonal morbidity? The design in question offers no way to control these factors.

However, the design could be modified so that some alternative explanations for changes in mortality could be ruled out. For example, **time-series designs** involve collecting data over an extended time period and introducing the treatment during that period. Our study could be designed with four observations before the RRTs are introduced (e.g., four quarters of mortality data for the prior year) and four observations after it (mortality for the next four quarters). Although a time-series design does not eliminate all interpretive problems, the extended time perspective strengthens the ability to attribute improvements to the intervention.

> **Example of a time-series design**
> Bogh and colleagues (2023) used a time-series design to examine how the reconfiguration of the Danish public hospital system emergency care into extensive and specialized emergency departments affected patient readmission rates.

Advantages and Disadvantages of Quasi-Experiments

One strength of quasi-experiments is their practicality. Nursing research often occurs in natural settings, where it is difficult to deliver an innovative treatment randomly to some people but not to others. Strong quasi-experimental designs introduce some research control when full experimental rigor is not possible.

Another issue is that people are not always willing to be randomized. Quasi-experimental designs, because they do not involve random assignment, are likely to be acceptable to more people. This, in turn, has implications for the generalizability of the results—but the problem is that the results are less conclusive.

The major disadvantage of quasi-experiments is that causal inferences cannot be made as readily as with RCTs. Alternative explanations for results abound with quasi-experiments. For example, suppose we administered a special diet to a group of frail nursing home residents to assess its impact on weight gain. If we use a nonequivalent control group and then observe a weight gain, we must ask: Is it *plausible* that some other factor caused the gain? Is it *plausible* that pretreatment differences in weight or diet between the groups resulted in differential gain? Is it *plausible* that there was an average weight gain simply because the most frail died or were transferred to a hospital? If the answer to any of these *rival hypotheses* is yes, then inferences about the causal effect of the intervention are weakened. With quasi-experiments, there is almost always at least one plausible rival explanation.

 HOW-TO-TELL TIP How can you tell if a study is quasi-experimental? Researchers do not always identify their designs as quasi-experimental. If a study involves the testing of an intervention and if the report does not explicitly mention random assignment, it is probably safe to conclude that the design is quasi-experimental.

Nonexperimental Studies

Many cause-probing questions cannot be addressed with an RCT or quasi-experiment. For example, take this prognosis question: Do birth weights under 1,500 g *cause* developmental delays in children? Clearly, we cannot manipulate birth weight, the independent variable. When researchers do not intervene by controlling the independent variable, the study is **nonexperimental**, or, in the medical literature, *observational*.

There are various reasons for doing a nonexperimental study. In some situations, the independent variable inherently cannot be manipulated (prognosis questions); in others, it would be unethical to manipulate the independent variable (some etiology questions). Experimental designs are also not appropriate for description questions.

Types of Nonexperimental/Observational Studies

When researchers study the effect of a cause they cannot manipulate, they undertake **correlational research** to examine relationships between variables. A **correlation** is an association between two variables, that is, a tendency for variation in one variable (e.g., weight) to be related to variation in another (e.g., height). Correlations can be detected through statistical analysis.

It is risky to infer causal relationships in correlational research. In RCTs, investigators predict that deliberate variation of the independent variable will result in a change to the outcome variable. In correlational research, investigators do not control the independent variable, which often has already occurred. A famous research dictum is relevant: *Correlation does not prove causation*. The mere existence of a relationship between variables is not enough to conclude that one variable caused the other, even if the relationship is strong.

Correlational studies are weaker than RCTs for cause-probing questions, but different designs offer varying degrees of supportive evidence. The strongest design for prognosis questions, and for etiology questions when randomization is impossible, is a cohort design (Table 8.2). Observational studies with a **cohort design** (sometimes called a **prospective design**) start with a presumed cause and then go forward to the presumed effect. For example, in prospective lung cancer studies, researchers start with a cohort of adults (P) that includes smokers (I) and nonsmokers (C) and then compare subsequent lung cancer incidence (O) in the two groups.

> **Example of a cohort (prospective) design**
> Caumette et al. (2023) conducted a study using a prospective cohort design to examine data collected in a large multicenter cohort of breast cancer survivors in France. They aimed to assess the shift in life priorities, quantify the magnitude of the change in the work-life value compared to private life value, and identify the clinical, demographic, work-related, and psychosocial factors associated with this change.

> **TIP** RCTs are inherently prospective because the researcher institutes the intervention and subsequently examines its effect.

In correlational studies with **a retrospective design**, an effect (outcome) observed in the present is linked to a potential cause occurring in the past. For example, in retrospective lung cancer research, researchers begin with some people who have lung cancer and others who do not and then look for differences in antecedent behaviors or conditions, such as smoking habits. This type of study uses a **case-control design**—*cases* with a certain condition such as lung cancer are compared to *controls* without it. In designing a case-control study, researchers try to identify controls who are as similar as possible to cases with regard to confounding variables (e.g., age, gender). The difficulty, however, is that the two groups are almost never comparable with respect to *all* factors influencing the outcome.

> **Example of a case-control design**
> Dykes et al. (2023) used a matched case-control design to assess changes in fall rates in two U.S. health care systems following the implementation of an evidence-based fall prevention program. They then conducted an economic analysis to assess the cost benefits associated with program implementation.

Prospective studies are more costly, but stronger, than retrospective studies. For one thing, any ambiguity about the temporal sequence of phenomena is resolved in prospective research (i.e., smoking is known to precede the lung cancer). In addition, samples are more likely to be representative of smokers and nonsmokers.

A second broad class of nonexperimental studies is **descriptive research**. The purpose of descriptive studies is to observe, describe, and document aspects of a situation. For example, an investigator may wish to discover the percentage of teenagers who smoke—that is, the *prevalence* of certain behaviors. Sometimes a study design is *descriptive correlational*, meaning that researchers seek to describe relationships among variables, without inferring causal connections. For example, researchers might be interested in describing the relationship between fatigue and psychological distress in patients with HIV. In such situations, a descriptive nonexperimental design is appropriate.

> **Example of a descriptive correlational study**
> Gürler et al. (2022) used a descriptive, correlational, cross-sectional design to assess the preoperative anxiety level and to evaluate the fears associated with surgery and anesthesia in surgical patients in Turkey.

 TIP For description questions, the strongest design is a nonexperimental study that relies on random sampling of participants. Random sampling is discussed in Chapter 9.

Advantages and Disadvantages of Nonexperimental Research

The major disadvantage of nonexperimental studies is that they yield weak evidence for causal inferences. This is not a problem when the aim is description, but correlational studies are often undertaken to explore causes. Yet, correlational studies are susceptible to faulty interpretation because groups being compared have formed through **self-selection**. A researcher doing a correlational study cannot assume that any groups being compared were similar before the occurrence of the independent variable.

As an example of such interpretive problems, suppose we studied differences in depression (O) of patients with cancer (P) who do (I) or do not (C) have good social support. Suppose we found a correlation, that is, that patients without social support were more depressed than patients with social support. We could interpret this to mean that patients' emotional state is influenced by the adequacy of their social support, as diagrammed in Figure 8.1A. There are, however, alternative interpretations. Maybe a third variable influences *both* social support and depression, such as whether the patients are married. Having a spouse may influence patients' depression *and* the quality of their social support (Fig. 8.1B). A third possibility is reversed causality (Fig. 8.1C). Depressed cancer patients may find it more difficult to elicit social support than patients who are cheerful. In this interpretation, the person's depression causes the amount of received social support, not the other way around. The point is that correlational results should be interpreted cautiously.

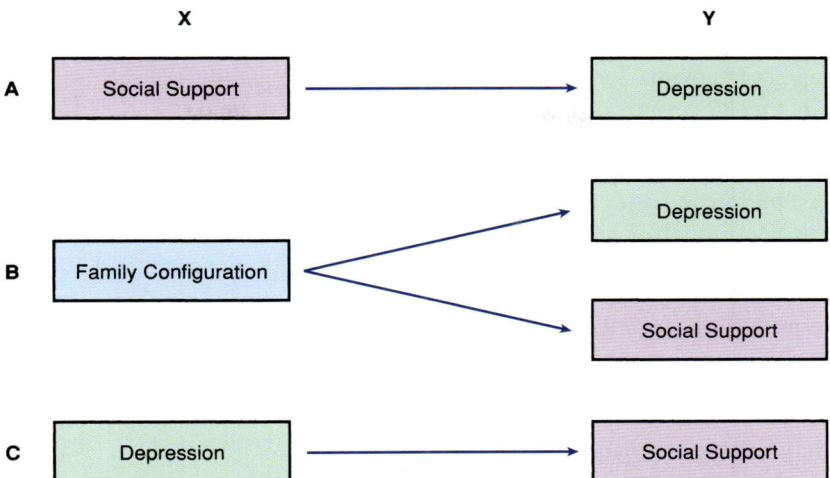

Figure 8.1 Alternative explanations for correlation between depression and social support in patients with cancer.

 TIP Be prepared to think critically when a researcher claims to be studying the "effects" of one variable on another in a nonexperimental study. For example, if a report title were "The Effects of Eating Disorders on Depression," the study would be nonexperimental (i.e., participants were not randomly assigned to an eating disorder). In such a situation, you might ask, did the eating disorder have an effect on depression or did depression have an effect on eating patterns? Or did a third variable (e.g., childhood abuse) have an effect on both?

Nevertheless, nonexperimental studies play a big role in nursing because many important problems are not amenable to intervention. An example is whether smoking causes lung cancer. Despite the absence of any RCTs with humans, few people doubt that this causal connection exists. There is ample evidence of a relationship between smoking and lung cancer and, through prospective studies, that smoking precedes lung cancer. In numerous replications, researchers have been able to control for, and thus rule out, other possible "causes" of lung cancer.

Correlational research offers an efficient way to collect large amounts of data about a problem. For example, it would be possible to collect information about people's health problems and their diet. Researchers could then examine which problems correlate with which dietary patterns. By doing this, many relationships could be discovered in a short time. By contrast, an experimenter looks at only a few variables at a time. For example, one RCT might manipulate cholesterol, whereas another might manipulate protein. Nonexperimental work is often necessary before interventions can be justified.

THE TIME DIMENSION IN RESEARCH DESIGN

Research designs incorporate decisions about when and how often data will be collected. A major distinction is between cross-sectional and longitudinal designs.

Cross-Sectional Designs

In **cross-sectional designs**, data are collected at one point in time. For example, a researcher might study whether psychological symptoms in menopausal people are correlated contemporaneously with physiologic symptoms. Retrospective studies are usually cross-sectional: Data on the independent and outcome variables are collected concurrently (e.g., participants' lung cancer status and smoking habits), but the independent variable usually involves events or behaviors occurring in the past.

Cross-sectional designs can be used to study time-related phenomena, but they are less persuasive than longitudinal designs. Suppose we were studying changes in children's health promotion activities between ages 8 and 10 years. One way to investigate this would be to interview children at 8 years of age and then 2 years later at the age of 10—a longitudinal design. Or, we could question two groups of children, ages 8 and 10 years, at one point in time and then compare responses—a cross-sectional design. If 10-year-olds are engaged in more health-promoting activities than 8-year-olds, it might be inferred that children made healthier choices as they aged. To make this inference, we have to assume that the older children would have responded as the younger ones did had they been questioned 2 years earlier or, conversely, that 8-year-olds would report more health-promoting activities if they were questioned again 2 years later.

Cross-sectional designs are economical, but they pose problems for inferring changes over time. The amount of social and technologic change that characterizes our society makes it questionable to assume that differences in the behaviors or characteristics of different age groups are the result of the passage through time rather than cohort differences.

Example of a cross-sectional study
Ma (2023) conducted a study using a cross-sectional descriptive design to explore the perceived levels of self-leadership among nurse managers in the United States. Findings indicate that participants identified moderate levels of self-leadership, which is the ability to influence and engage oneself to be self-aware and responsible and to leverage strengths to perform.

Longitudinal Designs

Longitudinal designs involve collecting data multiple times over an extended period. Such designs are useful for studying changes over time and for establishing the sequencing of phenomena, which is a criterion for inferring causality.

In nursing research, longitudinal studies are often *follow-up studies* of a clinical population, undertaken to assess the subsequent status of people with a specified condition or who received an intervention. For example, patients who received a smoking cessation intervention could be followed up to assess its long-term effectiveness. As a nonexperimental example, samples of premature infants could be followed up to assess subsequent motor development.

Example of a longitudinal study
Chen et al. (2023) conducted a longitudinal study from August 2020 to June 2021 to explore changes in the symptom clusters of older adults in China with lung cancer at different time points in the perioperative period. Data were collected on the day of admission, 2 to 4 days after surgery, 1 month after discharge, and 3 months after discharge.

In longitudinal studies, researchers must decide the number of data collection points and the time intervals between them. When change is rapid, numerous data collection points at relatively short intervals may be required to understand transitions. By convention, however, the term *longitudinal* implies multiple data collection points over an extended period of time.

A challenge in longitudinal studies is the loss of participants (**attrition**) over time. Attrition is problematic because those who drop out of a study usually differ in important ways from those who continue to participate, resulting in potential biases and problems with generalizability.

> **TIP** Not all longitudinal studies are prospective because sometimes the independent variable occurred even before the initial wave of data collection. And not all prospective studies are longitudinal in the classic sense. For example, an experimental study that collects data at 1, 2, and 4 hours after an intervention would be prospective but not longitudinal (i.e., data are not collected over a long time period).

TECHNIQUES OF RESEARCH CONTROL

A major goal of research design in quantitative studies is to maximize researchers' control over confounding variables. Two broad categories of confounders need to be controlled—those that are intrinsic to study participants and those that are situational factors.

Controlling the Study Context

External factors, such as the research context, can affect outcomes. In well-controlled quantitative research, steps are taken to achieve *constancy of conditions* so that researchers can be confident that outcomes reflect the effect of the independent variable and not the study context.

Researchers cannot totally control study contexts, but some opportunities exist. For example, blinding is a way to control bias. By keeping data collectors and others unaware of group allocation, researchers minimize the risk that other people involved in the study will influence the results.

Most quantitative studies also standardize communications to participants. Formal scripts are often prepared to inform participants about the study purpose and methods. In intervention studies, researchers develop formal intervention protocols. Careful researchers pay attention to *intervention fidelity*—that is, they monitor whether an intervention is faithfully delivered in accordance with its plan and that the intended treatment was actually received.

> **Example of attention to intervention fidelity**
> Newman and colleagues (2024) described their extensive efforts to ensure intervention fidelity in the control arm of a pediatric palliative care randomized control study. The attention control arm was structured using National Institutes of Health guidelines for assessing and implementing strategies to promote intervention fidelity, including designing the attention control arm of the study, providing training, and monitoring for quality assurance.

Controlling Participant Factors

Outcomes of interest to nurse researchers are affected by dozens of attributes, and most are irrelevant to the research question. For example, suppose we were investigating the effects of a physical fitness program on the physical functioning of nursing home residents. In this study, variables such as the participants' age, sex, and smoking history would be confounding variables; each is likely to be related to the outcome variable (physical functioning), independent of the program. In other words, the effects that these variables have on the outcome are extraneous to the study. In this section, we review strategies researchers can use to control confounding variables.

Randomization

Randomization is the most effective way to control participants' characteristics. A critical advantage of randomization, compared with other control strategies, is that it controls *all* possible sources of extraneous variation, without any conscious decision about which variables should be controlled. In our example of a physical fitness intervention, random assignment of older adults to an intervention or control group would yield groups presumably comparable in terms of age, sex, smoking history, and dozens of other characteristics that could affect the outcome. Randomization to different treatment orderings in a crossover design is especially powerful: Participants serve as their own controls, thereby controlling all confounding characteristics.

Homogeneity

When randomization is not feasible, other methods of controlling extraneous characteristics can be used. One alternative is **homogeneity**, in which only people who are similar with respect to confounding variables are included in the study. In the physical fitness example, if age was considered a confounding variable, participation could be limited to a specified age range. Using a homogeneous sample is easy, but a consequence is limits to generalizability.

> **Example of control through homogeneity**
> Salamanca-Sanabria and colleagues (2024) describe a study protocol that aims to assess the effectiveness of a mobile holistic lifestyle intervention in people with a history of gestational diabetes mellitus (GDM) to prevent the onset of type 2 diabetes mellitus and common mental disorders in Singapore. Several variables will be controlled through homogeneity including age, history of GDM at least 1 year and no more than 10 years, ethnicity, and a body mass index between 18.5 and 35 kg/m^2.

Matching

A third method of controlling confounding variables is **matching**, which involves consciously forming comparable groups. For example, suppose we began with a group of nursing home residents who agreed to participate in the physical fitness program. A comparison group of nonparticipating residents could be created by matching participants on the basis of important confounding variables (e.g., age and sex). This procedure results in groups known to be similar on specific confounding variables. Matching is often used to form comparable groups in case-control designs.

Matching has some drawbacks, however. To match effectively, researchers must know what the relevant confounders are. Also, after two or three variables, it becomes difficult to match. Suppose we wanted to control age, sex, and length of nursing home stay. In this situation, if a program participant were an 85-year-old female whose length of stay was 5 years, we would have to seek another female with these characteristics as a comparison group counterpart. With more than three variables, matching may not be possible. Thus, matching is a control method used primarily when more powerful procedures are not feasible.

> **Example of control through matching**
> Singh and colleagues (2024) used data from three national surveys in the United States to examine social determinants of health and disease outcomes for Native Americans including Alaska Natives and tribal communities. This group was matched to other racial/ethnic groups in the United States and the general population for socioeconomic, health, healthcare, disability, disease, and mortality patterns.

Statistical Control

Researchers can also control confounding variables statistically. Methods of statistical control are complex, so a detailed description of powerful statistical control mechanisms, such as *analysis of covariance*, will not be attempted. You should recognize, however, that nurse researchers are increasingly using powerful statistical techniques to control confounding variables. A brief description of statistical control methods is presented in Chapter 13.

Evaluation of Control Methods

Random assignment is the most effective approach to controlling confounding variables because randomization tends to control individual variation on all possible confounders. Crossover designs are especially powerful, but they cannot be used in many situations because of the risk of carryover effects. The alternatives described here share two disadvantages. First, researchers must decide in advance which variables to control. To select homogeneous samples, match, or use statistical control, researchers must identify which variables to control. Second, these methods control only the specified characteristics, leaving others uncontrolled.

Although randomization is an excellent tool, it is not always feasible. It is better to use matching or statistical control than to ignore the problem of confounding variables.

CHARACTERISTICS OF GOOD DESIGN

An important question in critically appraising a quantitative study is whether the research design yielded valid evidence. Four key questions regarding research design, particularly in cause-probing studies, are as follows:

1. What is the strength of evidence that a relationship between variables really exists?
2. If a relationship exists, what is the strength of evidence that the independent variable (e.g., an intervention), rather than other factors, *caused* the outcome?
3. What is the strength of evidence that observed relationships are generalizable across people, settings, and time?
4. What are the theoretical constructs underlying the study variables, and are those constructs adequately captured?

These questions, respectively, correspond to four aspects of a study's validity: (1) statistical conclusion validity, (2) internal validity, (3) external validity, and (4) construct validity (Shadish et al., 2002).

Statistical Conclusion Validity

A criterion for establishing causality is a demonstrated relationship between the independent and dependent variable. Statistical tests are used to support inferences about whether such a relationship exists. Several threats can undermine a study's **statistical conclusion validity**.

Statistical power, the capacity to detect true relationships, affects statistical conclusion validity. The most straightforward way to achieve adequate statistical power is to use a sufficiently large sample. With small samples, the analyses may fail to show that the independent variable and the outcome are related—even when they are. Power and sample size are discussed in Chapter 9.

Researchers can also enhance power by strengthening differences on the independent variable (i.e., making the *cause* powerful) so as to maximize differences on the outcome (the effect). If the groups or treatments are not very different, the statistical analysis might not be sufficiently sensitive to detect effects that actually exist. Intervention fidelity can enhance the power of an intervention.

Thus, if you are appraising a study in which outcomes for the groups being compared were not significantly different, one possibility is that the study had low statistical conclusion validity. The report might give clues about this possibility (e.g., too small a sample or substantial attrition) that should be taken into consideration in interpreting what the results mean.

Internal Validity

Internal validity is the extent to which it can be inferred that the independent variable is causing the outcome. RCTs tend to have high internal validity because randomization enables researchers to rule out competing explanations for group differences in outcomes. With quasi-experiments and correlational studies, there are rival explanations, which are sometimes called threats to internal validity. Evidence hierarchies rank study designs mainly in terms of internal validity.

Threats to Internal Validity

Temporal Ambiguity

In a causal relationship, the cause precedes the effect. In RCTs, researchers create the independent variable and then observe the outcome, so establishing a temporal sequence is never a problem. In correlational studies, however—especially ones using a cross-sectional design—it may be unclear whether the independent variable preceded the dependent variable, or vice versa, as illustrated in Figure 8.1.

Selection

The **selection threat** (*self-selection*) reflects biases stemming from preexisting differences between groups. When people are not assigned randomly to groups, the groups being compared may not be equivalent; group differences in the outcome may be caused by extraneous factors rather than by the independent variable. Selection bias is the most challenging threat to the internal validity of studies not using an experimental design, but it can be partially addressed using control strategies described in the previous section.

History

The **history threat** is the occurrence of events concurrent with the independent variable that can affect the outcome. For example, suppose we were studying the effectiveness of a community program to encourage flu shots among older adults. Now suppose a story about a flu epidemic was aired in the national media at about the same time. Our outcome variable, number of flu shots administered, is now influenced by at least two forces, and it would be hard to disentangle the two effects. In RCTs, history is not typically a threat because external events are as likely to affect one randomized group as another. The designs most likely to be affected by the history threat are one-group pretest–posttest designs and time-series designs.

Maturation

The **maturation threat** arises from processes occurring as a result of time (e.g., growth, fatigue) rather than the independent variable. For example, if we were studying the effect of an intervention for children with developmental delays, our design would have to deal with the fact that progress would occur without an intervention. *Maturation* does not refer only to developmental changes but to any change that occurs as a function of time. Phenomena such as wound healing or postoperative recovery occur with little intervention, so maturation may be a rival explanation for favorable posttreatment outcomes if the design does not include a comparison group. One-group pretest–posttest designs are especially vulnerable to the maturation threat.

Mortality threat/Attrition

Mortality threat arises from attrition in groups being compared. If different kinds of people remain in the study in one group versus another, then these differences, rather than the independent variable, could account for group differences in outcomes. The most severely ill patients might drop out of an experimental condition because it is too demanding, for example. Attrition bias essentially is a selection bias that occurs after the study unfolds: Groups initially equivalent can lose comparability because of attrition, and differential group composition, rather than the independent variable, could be the "cause" of any group differences on outcomes.

TIP If attrition is random (i.e., those dropping out of a study are similar to those remaining in it), then there would not be bias. However, attrition is rarely random. In general, the higher the rate of attrition, the greater the risk of bias. Biases are usually of concern if the rate exceeds 10% to 15%.

Internal Validity and Research Design

Quasi-experimental and correlational studies are especially susceptible to internal validity threats, which compete with the independent variable as a cause of the outcome. The aim of a good quantitative research design is to rule out these competing explanations. The control mechanisms previously described are strategies for improving internal validity—and thus for strengthening the quality of evidence that studies yield.

An experimental design often, but not always, eliminates competing explanations. Attrition is a particularly salient threat. Because researchers do different things with the groups, members may drop out of the study for different reasons. This is particularly likely to happen if the intervention is stressful or time-consuming or if the control condition is boring or disappointing. Participants remaining in a study may differ from those who left, nullifying the initial equivalence of the groups.

You should carefully consider possible rival explanations for study results, especially in non-RCT studies. When researchers do not have control over critical confounding variables, caution in drawing conclusions about causal relationships is appropriate.

External Validity

External validity concerns inferences about whether relationships observed for study participants might hold true for different people and settings. External validity is critical to evidence-based practice (EBP) because it is important to generalize evidence from controlled research settings to real-world practice settings.

External validity questions can take several different forms. For example, we may ask whether relationships observed with a study sample can be generalized to a larger population—for example, whether results about rates of postpartum depression in Boston can be generalized to birthing parents in northeastern United States. Thus, one aspect of a study's external validity concerns sampling. If the sample is representative of the population, generalizing results to the population is safer (Chapter 9).

Other external validity questions are about generalizing to different types of people, settings, or situations. For example, can findings about a pain reduction treatment in Norway be generalized to people in the United States? New studies are often needed to answer questions about generalizability. *Replication* is an important concept. Multisite studies are powerful because generalizability of the results can be enhanced if the results have been replicated in several sites—particularly if the sites differ on important dimensions (e.g., size). In studies with a diverse sample of participants, researchers can assess whether results are replicated for various subgroups—for example, whether an intervention benefits older and younger people. Systematic reviews represent a crucial aid to external validity precisely because they explore consistency in results based on replications across time, space, people, and settings.

The demands for internal and external validity may conflict. If a researcher exercises tight control to maximize internal validity, the setting may become too artificial to generalize to more natural environments. We discuss this issue in Chapter 18.

Construct Validity

Research involves constructs. Researchers conduct a study with specific exemplars of treatments, outcomes, settings, and people, but these are all stand-ins for broad constructs. **Construct validity** involves inferences from the particulars of the study to the higher order constructs they are intended to represent. If studies contain construct errors, the evidence could be misleading. One aspect of construct validity concerns the degree to which an intervention is a good representation of the construct that was theorized as having the potential to cause beneficial outcomes. Lack of blinding can be a threat to construct validity: Is it the intervention, or *awareness* of the intervention, that resulted in benefits? Another issue is whether the measures used to represent the research variables are good operationalizations of constructs. This aspect of construct validity is discussed in Chapter 9.

CRITICAL APPRAISAL OF QUANTITATIVE RESEARCH DESIGNS

A key evaluative question is whether the research design enabled researchers to get good answers to the research question. This question has both substantive and methodologic facets.

> **Box 8.1 Guidelines for Critically Appraising Research Design in a Quantitative Study**
>
> a. Was the design experimental, quasi-experimental, or nonexperimental? What specific design was used? Was this a cause-probing study? Given the type of question (therapy, prognosis, etc.), was the most rigorous possible design used?
> b. What type of comparison was called for in the research design? Was the comparison strategy effective in illuminating key relationships?
> c. If the study involved an intervention, were the intervention and control conditions adequately described? Was blinding used, and if so, who was blinded? If not, is there a good rationale for failure to use blinding?
> d. If the study was nonexperimental, why did the researcher opt not to intervene? If the study was cause-probing, which criteria for inferring causality were potentially compromised? Was a retrospective or prospective design used, and was such a design appropriate?
> e. Was the study longitudinal or cross-sectional? Were the number and timing of data collection points appropriate?
> f. What did the researcher do to control confounding participant characteristics, and were the procedures effective? What are the threats to the study's internal validity? Did the design enable the researcher to draw causal inferences about the relationship between the independent variable and the outcome?
> g. What are the major limitations of the design used? Were these limitations acknowledged by the researcher and taken into account in interpreting results? What can be said about the study's external validity?

Substantively, the issue is whether the design matches the aims of the research. If the research purpose is descriptive or exploratory, an experimental design is not appropriate. If the researcher is searching to understand the full nature of a phenomenon about which little is known, a structured design that allows little flexibility might block insights (flexible designs are discussed in Chapter 10). We have discussed research control as a bias-reducing strategy, but too much control can introduce bias—for example, when a researcher tightly controls how a phenomenon under study can be manifested and so obscures its true nature.

Methodologically, the main design issue in quantitative studies is whether the research design provides the most valid, unbiased, and interpretable evidence possible. Indeed, there usually is no other aspect of a quantitative study that affects the quality of evidence as much as research design. Box 8.1 provides questions to assist you in appraising research designs.

RESEARCH EXAMPLES WITH CRITICAL THINKING EXERCISES

This section presents examples of studies with different research designs. Read these summaries, and then answer the critical thinking questions, referring to the full research report if necessary.

EXAMPLE 1: EXAMPLE OF A QUASI-EXPERIMENT

Study: "A quasi-experimental study to assess the effect of Benson's relaxation on anxiety and depression among patients with heart failure in Jordan" (Aloran et al., 2024).

Purpose: The purpose of this study was to test the effectiveness of a relaxation intervention in reducing anxiety and depression among patients with heart failure in Jordan.

Treatment Groups: This study utilized a quasi-experimental pre- and post-study design. Participants were recruited from four hospitals in Jordan. The relaxation intervention was delivered to the intervention group in 10-minute sessions repeated twice daily for 8 weeks. The control group received usual care.

Methods: To estimate their sample size needs, the researchers undertook a power analysis (see Chapter 9) that suggested that a sample of 204 participants per group would be needed to achieve statistical conclusion validity. A total of 204 patients (100 in the intervention group and 104 in the comparison group) participated in the research. Patient-reported assessment data for the primary outcomes (e.g., anxiety, depression) were gathered at baseline and at the end of the intervention.

Key Findings: The intervention and comparison group members were similar demographically and clinically. The analysis of program effects revealed statistically significant improvements for those in the intervention group, compared to those in the comparison group, with respect to depression and anxiety.

Critical Thinking Exercises

1. Answer the relevant questions from Box 8.1 regarding this study.
2. What can be inferred about the statistical conclusion validity of the study?

EXAMPLE 2: RANDOMIZED CONTROLLED TRIAL IN APPENDIX A

Read the method section from Cheng et al. (2024) "Advance care planning affects end-of-life treatment preferences among patients with heart failure: A randomized controlled trial" in Appendix A of this book.

1. Answer the relevant questions from Box 8.1 regarding this study.
2. Could a crossover design have been used in this study?

Summary Points

- A **research design** is the overall plan for answering research questions. In quantitative studies, the design designates whether there is an intervention, the nature of any comparisons, methods for controlling confounding variables, whether there will be **blinding**, and the timing and location of data collection.

- Therapy, prognosis, and etiology questions are cause-probing; the challenge of research design is to facilitate causal inferences.

- Key criteria for inferring causality include the following: (1) a **cause** (the independent variable) must precede an **effect** (the outcome), (2) there must be a detectable relationship between a cause and an effect, and (3) the relationship between the two does not reflect the influence of a third (confounding) variable.

- A *counterfactual* is what would have happened to the same people simultaneously exposed *and* not exposed to a causal factor. The *effect* is the difference between the two. A good research design for cause-probing questions entails finding a good approximation to the idealized counterfactual.

- **Experiments** (or **randomized controlled trials [RCTs]**) involve an **intervention** (the researcher manipulates the independent variable by introducing an intervention), control (including the use of a **control group** that does not receive the intervention), and **randomization/random assignment** (with participants allocated to experimental and control conditions at random to achieve group comparability at the outset).

- RCTs are considered the gold standard for therapy questions because they come closer than any other design to meeting the criteria for inferring causal relationships.

- In **pretest–posttest designs**, data are collected both before the intervention (at baseline) and after it.

- In **crossover designs**, people are exposed to more than one condition in random order and serve as their own controls. Crossover designs are inappropriate if there is a risk of *carryover effects*.

- Possible control group conditions include standard treatment ("usual care"), an alternative treatment, a **placebo** (a pseudointervention), an *attention control* condition, or a *wait-list* (*delayed treatment*) condition.

- **Quasi-experiments** (trials without randomization) involve an intervention but lack a comparison group or randomization. Strong quasi-experimental designs introduce features to compensate for these missing components.

- The **nonequivalent control group** in a **pretest–posttest design** involves a **comparison group** that was not created through randomization and the collection of pretreatment data from both groups to assess initial group equivalence.

- In a **time-series design**, outcome data are collected over a period of time before and after the intervention, usually for a single group.

- **Nonexperimental** (*observational*) **studies** include **descriptive research**—studies that summarize the status of phenomena—and **correlational studies** that examine relationships among variables but do not involve an intervention.

- In **prospective (cohort) designs**, researchers begin with a possible cause and then subsequently collect data about outcomes.

- **Retrospective designs** (**case-control designs**) involve collecting data about an outcome in the present and then looking back in time for possible causes.

- Making causal inferences in correlational studies is risky; a basic research dictum is that *correlation does not prove causation*.

- **Cross-sectional designs** involve the collection of data at one time period, whereas longitudinal designs involve data collection at two or more times over an extended period. In nursing, longitudinal studies often are *follow-up studies* of clinical populations.

- Longitudinal studies are typically expensive, time-consuming, and subject to the risk of **attrition** (loss of participants over time), but they yield valuable information about time-related phenomena.

- Quantitative researchers strive to control external factors that could affect study outcomes and participant characteristics that are extraneous to the research question.

- Researchers delineate the intervention in formal *protocols* that stipulate exactly what the treatment is. Careful researchers attend to *intervention fidelity*—whether the intervention was properly implemented as planned and actually received.

- Techniques for controlling participant characteristics include **homogeneity** (restricting the sample to reduce variability on confounding variables), **matching** (deliberately making groups comparable on some extraneous variables), statistical procedures, and randomization—the most effective method because it controls all possible confounding variables without researchers having to identify them.

- Study **validity** concerns the extent to which appropriate inferences can be made. **Threats to validity** are reasons that an inference could be wrong. A key function of quantitative research design is to rule out validity threats.

- **Statistical conclusion validity** concerns the strength of evidence that a relationship exists between two variables. One threat to statistical conclusion validity is low statistical power (the ability to detect true relationships among variables).

- **Internal validity** concerns inferences that outcomes were caused by the independent variable, rather than by extraneous factors. Threats to internal validity include temporal ambiguity (uncertainty about whether the presumed cause preceded the outcome), selection (preexisting group differences), history (external events that could affect outcomes), maturation (changes due to the passage of time), and **mortality** (effects attributable to attrition).

- **External validity** concerns inferences about generalizability—whether findings hold true over variations in people, conditions, and settings.

REFERENCES

Aloran, A. A. M., Jarrah, S. S., Ahmed, F. R., & AbuRuz, M. E. (2024). A quasi-experimental study to assess the effect of Benson's relaxation on anxiety and depression among patients with heart failure in Jordan. *Acute and Critical Care*, *39*(3), 430–438. https://doi.org/10.4266/acc.2023.01053

Aoki, Y., & Nakayama, K. (2023). Improving older adults stroke survivors' decision-making when selecting a discharge location: A randomized controlled trial protocol. *International Journal of Nursing Knowledge*, *34*(3), 185–192. https://doi.org/10.1111/2047-3095.12393

Bogh, S. B., Fløjstrup, M., Möller, S., Bech, M., Lassen, A. T., Brabrand, M., & Mogensen, C. B. (2023). Readmission trends before and after a national reconfiguration of emergency departments in Denmark. *Journal of Health Services Research & Policy*, *28*(1), 42–49. https://doi.org/10.1177/13558196221108894

Caumette, E., Di Meglio, A., Vaz-Luis, I., Charles, C., Havas, J., de Azua, G. R., Martin, E., Vanlemmens, L., Delaloge, S., Everhard, S., Martin, A. L., Merimeche, A. D., Rigal, O., Coutant, C., Fournier, M., Jouannaud, C., Soulie, P., Cottu, P. H., Tredan, O., ... Dumas, A. (2023). Change in the value of work after breast cancer: Evidence from a prospective cohort. *Journal of Cancer Survivorship: Research and Practice*, *17*(3), 694–705. https://doi.org/10.1007/s11764-022-01197-w

Chen, K., Yang, D., Li, F., Gao, L., Tian, Y., Xu, B., Xu, X., Xu, Q., & Cao, J. (2023). Changes in the symptom clusters of elderly patients with lung cancer over the course of postoperative rehabilitation and their correlation with frailty and quality of life: A longitudinal study. *European Journal of Oncology Nursing: The Official Journal of European Oncology Nursing Society*, *67*, 102388. https://doi.org/10.1016/j.ejon.2023.102388

Dykes, P. C., Curtin-Bowen, M., Lipsitz, S., Franz, C., Adelman, J., Adkison, L., Bogaisky, M., Carroll, D., Carter, E., Herlihy, L., Lindros, M. E., Ryan, V., Scanlan, M., Walsh, M. A., Wien, M., & Bates, D. W. (2023). Cost of inpatient falls and cost-benefit analysis of implementation of an evidence-based fall prevention program. *JAMA Health Forum*, *4*(1), e225125. https://doi.org/10.1001/jamahealthforum.2022.5125

Gürler, H., Yılmaz, M., & Türk, K. E. (2022). Preoperative anxiety levels in surgical patients: A comparison of three different scale scores. *Journal of Perianesthesia Nursing: Official Journal of the American Society of PeriAnesthesia Nurses*, *37*(1), 69–74. https://doi.org/10.1016/j.jopan.2021.05.013

Lee, M. H., & Noh, E. Y. (2023). Effectiveness of Simulation-based education for caring patients with COVID-19. *Journal of Korean Academy of Nursing*, *53*(4), 397–411. https://doi.org/10.4040/jkan.22151

Low, L. F., Barcenilla-Wong, A., Fitzpatrick, M., Swaffer, K., Brodaty, H., Hancock, N., McLoughlin, J., & Naismith, S. (2023). Dementia lifestyle coach pilot program. *Australasian Journal on Ageing*, *42*(3), 508–516. https://doi.org/10.1111/ajag.13169

Ma, H. (2023). Nurse managers' perceived self-leadership levels: A cross-sectional study. *JONA: The Journal of Nursing Administration*, *53*(12), 634–640. https://doi.org/10.1097/NNA.0000000000001359

Mill, J. S. (1859). *A system of logic: Ratiocinative and inductive, being a connected view of the principles of evidence and the methods of scientific investigation*. Harper and Brothers.

Newman, A. R., Moody, K. M., Becktell, K., Connelly, E., Holladay, C., Parisio, K., Powell, J. L., Steineck, A., & Hendricks-Ferguson, V. L. (2024). Ensuring intervention fidelity of an attention control arm in a multisite randomized controlled trial. *Nursing Research*, *73*(2), 166–171. https://doi.org/10.1097/NNR.0000000000000710

Salamanca-Sanabria, A., Liew, S. J., Mair, J., De Iorio, M., Ling, Y. D. Y., Tint, M. T., Wei, Y. T., Lim, K., Ong, D., Chooi, Y. C., Tay, V., & Eriksson, J. G. (2024). A holistic lifestyle mobile health intervention for the prevention of type 2 diabetes and common mental disorders in Asian women with a history of gestational diabetes: A randomised control trial with 3-year follow-up protocol. *Trials*, *25*(1), 443. https://doi.org/10.1186/s13063-024-08247-x

Shadish, W. R., Cook, T. D., & Campbell, D. T. (2002). *Experimental and quasi-experimental designs for generalized causal inference*. Houghton Mifflin.

Singh, G. K., Lee, H., Kim, L. H., & Williams, S. D. (2024). Social determinants of health among American Indians and Alaska Natives and tribal communities: Comparison with other major racial and ethnic groups in the United States, 1990–2022. *International Journal of MCH and AIDS*, *13*, e010. https://doi.org/10.25259/IJMA_10_2024

Ulger, O., Oz, M., & Ozel Asliyuce, Y. (2023). The effects of yoga and stabilization exercises in patients with chronic low back pain: A randomized crossover study. *Holistic Nursing Practice*, *37*(4), E59–E68. https://doi.org/10.1097/HNP.0000000000000593

Uslu, A., & Arslan, S. (2023). The effect of using virtual reality glasses on anxiety and fatigue in women with breast cancer receiving adjuvant chemotherapy: A pretest-posttest randomized controlled study. *Seminars in Oncology Nursing*, *39*(5), 151503. https://doi.org/10.1016/j.soncn.2023.151503

9 Appraising Sampling and Data Collection in Quantitative Studies

Learning Objectives

On completing this chapter, you will be able to:

- Distinguish nonprobability and probability samples and compare their advantages and disadvantages
- Identify and describe several sampling designs in quantitative studies
- Evaluate the appropriateness of the sampling method and sample size used in a study
- Discuss dimensions along which data collection approaches vary
- Identify phenomena that lend themselves to self-reports, observation, and physiologic measurement
- Describe various approaches for collecting self-report data (e.g., interviews, questionnaires, composite scales)
- Describe methods of collecting and recording observational data
- Describe the major features and advantages of biomarkers
- Critically appraise researchers' decisions about a data collection plan
- Describe approaches for assessing the reliability and validity of measures
- Define new terms in the chapter

Key Terms

- Biomarker
- Biophysiologic measure
- Category system
- Checklist
- Closed-ended question
- Consecutive sampling
- Construct validity
- Content validity
- Convenience sampling
- Criterion validity
- Eligibility criteria
- Face validity
- Internal consistency
- Interrater reliability
- Interview schedule
- Likert scale
- Measurement
- Measurement property
- Nonprobability sampling
- Observation
- Observational methods
- Open-ended question
- Patient-reported outcome (PRO)
- Population
- Power analysis
- Probability sampling
- Psychometric assessment
- Purposive sampling
- Questionnaire
- Quota sampling
- Rating scale
- Reliability
- Respondents' response
- Response options
- Response rate
- Response set bias
- Sample
- Sample size
- Sampling bias
- Sampling plan
- Scale
- Self-reports
- Simple random sampling
- Strata
- Stratified random sampling
- Summated rating scale
- Test–retest reliability
- Validity

141

This chapter covers two important research topics—how quantitative researchers select study participants and how they collect data from them.

SAMPLING IN QUANTITATIVE RESEARCH

Researchers answer research questions using data from a sample of participants. In testing the effects of an intervention for pregnant people, nurse researchers reach conclusions without testing it with all pregnant people. Quantitative researchers develop a **sampling plan** that specifies in advance how—and how many—participants will be selected.

Basic Sampling Concepts

Let us begin by considering some terms associated with sampling.

Populations

A **population** ("P" in PICO questions) is the entire group of interest. For instance, if a researcher were studying U.S. nurses with doctoral degrees, the population could be defined as all registered nurses (RNs) in the United States with a doctoral-level degree. Other populations might be all patients who had cardiac surgery in St. Peter's Hospital in 2021 or all Australian children younger than age 10 years with cystic fibrosis. Populations are not restricted to people. A population might be all patient records in Memorial Hospital. A population is an entire aggregate of elements.

Researchers specify population characteristics through **eligibility criteria**. For example, consider the population of U.S. nursing students. Does the population include part-time students? Are RNs returning to school for a bachelor's degree included? Researchers establish criteria to determine whether a person qualifies as a member of the population (*inclusion* criteria) or should be excluded (*exclusion* criteria). For example, patients who are severely ill might be excluded. However, exclusion criteria should not be listed as the mere opposite of the inclusion criteria. In some cases, there may not be clear reasons for exclusion, and this should be stated as such.

> **Example of eligibility criteria** •
> Martins et al. (2024) conducted a longitudinal study over a 15-month period to determine the trajectories of spiritual distress and religious involvement among patients with cancer. To be eligible for the study, the participants were required to meet the following inclusion criteria: age ≥18 years and starting chemotherapy in an outpatient setting in Portugal for any stage of cancer. No exclusion criteria were anticipated.

Quantitative researchers sample from an accessible population in the hope of generalizing to a target population. The *target population* is the entire population of interest. The *accessible population* is the portion of the target population that is accessible to the researcher. For example, a researcher's target population might be all patients with diabetes in the United States, but, in reality, the population that is accessible might be patients with diabetes in a particular city.

Samples and Sampling

Sampling involves selecting cases to represent the population—a **sample** is a subset of population elements. In nursing research, the *elements* (basic units) are usually humans. Researchers work with samples rather than populations for practical reasons.

Information from samples can, however, lead to faulty conclusions. In quantitative studies, a criterion for judging a sample is its representativeness. A *representative sample* is one whose characteristics closely approximate those of the population. Some sampling plans are more likely to yield biased samples than others. **Sampling bias** is the systematic overrepresentation or underrepresentation of a population segment on a characteristic relevant to the research question (e.g., too few or too many men in the sample).

Strata

Populations consist of subpopulations, or **strata**. Strata are mutually exclusive segments of a population based on a specific characteristic. For instance, a population consisting of all RNs in the United States could be divided into two strata based on attainment or nonattainment of a bachelor's degree. Strata can be designated in sample selection to enhance the sample's representativeness—elements in each stratum can be sampled in the correct proportions.

> **TIP** The sampling plan is usually discussed in a report's method section, sometimes in a subsection labeled "Sample" or "Study participants." Sample characteristics (e.g., average age) are often described in the results section.

Sampling Designs in Quantitative Studies

The two broad classes of sampling designs in quantitative research are nonprobability sampling and probability sampling.

Nonprobability Sampling

In **nonprobability sampling**, researchers select elements by nonrandom methods in which every element does not have a chance to be included. Nonprobability sampling is less likely than probability sampling to produce representative samples—and yet, *most* research samples in nursing and other disciplines are nonprobability samples.

Convenience sampling entails selecting the most conveniently available people as participants. A nurse who distributes questionnaires about vitamin use to college students leaving the library is sampling by convenience, for example. The problem with convenience sampling is that people who are readily available might be atypical of the population. The price of convenience is the risk of bias. Convenience sampling is the weakest form of sampling, but it is also the most commonly used method.

> **Example of a convenience sample**
> Zeleníková et al. (2025) aimed to determine the effect of group reminiscent therapy on the assessment of depression, anxiety, and self-esteem in older adults living in the community. They used convenience sampling to obtain a sample of 31 participants enrolled in a reminiscent therapy group in the Czech Republic.

In **quota sampling**, researchers identify population strata and figure out how many people are needed from each stratum. By using information about the population, researchers can ensure that diverse segments are represented in the sample. For example, if the population is known to have 48% men, 48% women, and 4% other gender, then the sample should have similar percentages. Procedurally, quota sampling is similar to convenience sampling: Participants are a convenience sample from each stratum. Because of this fact, quota sampling shares some weaknesses of convenience sampling. Nevertheless, quota sampling is a big improvement over convenience sampling and does not require sophisticated skills or a lot of effort. Surprisingly, few researchers use this strategy.

> **Example of a quota sample**
> Kim and colleagues (2025) conducted an online cross-sectional study to examine the association between positive psychological capital, social support, illness attitudes toward COVID-19, and health-promoting behaviors in Korean adults. Participants were recruited through quota sampling and included 820 South Korean adults aged 19 to 64 years.

Consecutive sampling is a nonprobability sampling method that involves recruiting *all* people from an accessible population over a specific time interval or for a specified sample size. For example, in a study of ventilator-associated pneumonia in intensive care unit (ICU) patients, a consecutive sample might consist of all eligible patients who were admitted to an ICU over a 6-month period. Or it might be the first 250 eligible patients admitted to the ICU, if 250 were the targeted sample size. Consecutive sampling is often the best possible choice when there is "rolling enrollment" into an accessible population.

> **Example of a consecutive sample**
> Albaqawi and Alshammari (2024) aimed to study the mediating impact of resilience on compassion fatigue, moral distress, and moral injury among nurses. They used consecutive sampling to select 511 staff nurses from three government hospitals in Saudi Arabia.

Purposive sampling involves using researchers' knowledge about the population to handpick sample members. Researchers might decide purposely to select people judged to be knowledgeable about the issues under study. This method can lead to bias but can be a useful approach when researchers want a sample of experts.

> **Example of purposive sampling**
> Schwanda et al. (2024) conducted a quantitative descriptive study to refine and validate the NANDA-I nursing diagnosis risk for perioperative hypothermia. Purposive sampling was used to recruit a panel that included 92 nurse experts from seven countries and three continents.

 HOW-TO-TELL TIP   How can you tell what type of sampling design was used in a quantitative study? If the report does not explicitly mention or describe the sampling design, it is usually safe to assume that a convenience sample was used.

Probability Sampling

Probability sampling involves random selection of elements from a population. With random sampling, each element in the population has an equal, independent chance of being selected. Random selection should not be (although it often is) confused with random assignment, which is a signature of a randomized controlled trial (RCT; see Chapter 8). Random *assignment* to different treatment conditions has no bearing on how participants in the RCT were selected.

The most basic probability sampling is **simple random sampling**. Researchers using simple random sampling often establish a *sampling frame*—a list of population elements. If nursing students at the University of Connecticut were the population, a student roster would be the sampling frame. Elements in a sampling frame are numbered; then, a table of random numbers or an online randomizer is used to draw a random sample of the desired size. Samples selected randomly are unlikely to be biased. There is no *guarantee* of a representative sample, but random selection guarantees that differences between the sample and the population are purely a function of chance. The probability of selecting a markedly atypical sample through random sampling is low and decreases as sample size increases.

> **Example of a simple random sample**
> Menevşe and Yayla (2024) aimed to determine the effect of the emotional freedom technique on participants' anxiety and fear before undergoing laparoscopic cholecystectomy. They used a simple randomization method to enroll participants into the control and intervention groups.

In **stratified random sampling**, the population is first divided into two or more strata, from which elements are randomly selected. As with quota sampling, the aim of stratified sampling is to enhance representativeness.

> **Example of stratified random sampling**
> Riegel et al. (2024) tested the efficacy of a virtual health coaching intervention, compared with health information alone, on the self-care, stress, coping, and health status of heart failure caregivers. They used stratified random sampling by sex and relationship to the care recipient to enroll 250 caregivers.

 TIP Many large national studies use *multistage sampling*, in which large units are first randomly sampled (e.g., census tracts, hospitals), then smaller units are selected (e.g., individual people). Another type of sampling used by some researchers is *systematic sampling*, which involves the selection of every *k*th person on a list, such as every 10th person. If the first person is chosen at random, systematic sampling is essentially the same as simple random sampling.

Evaluation of Nonprobability and Probability Sampling

Probability sampling is the only viable method of obtaining representative samples. If all elements in a population have an equal chance of being selected, then the resulting sample is likely to do a good job of representing the population. Probability sampling also allows researchers to estimate the magnitude of *sampling error*, which is the difference between population values (e.g., the average age of the population) and sample values (e.g., the average age of the sample).

Nonprobability samples are rarely representative of the population—some segment of the population is likely to be underrepresented. When there is sampling bias, there is a chance that the results could be misleading. Why, then, are nonprobability samples used in most studies? Clearly, the advantage lies in their ease and expediency. Quantitative researchers using nonprobability samples must be cautious about the inferences drawn from the data, and consumers should be alert to possible sampling biases.

 TIP The quality of the sampling plan is of particular importance when the focus of the research is to obtain descriptive information about prevalence or average values for a population. For quantitative studies whose purpose is primarily description, data from a probability sample would be high on an evidence hierarchy for individual studies.

Sample Size in Quantitative Studies

Sample size—the number of study participants—is a major concern in quantitative research. There is no simple formula to determine how large a sample should be, but larger is usually better than smaller. When researchers calculate a percentage or an average using sample data, the purpose is to estimate a population value, and larger samples have less sampling error.

Researchers can estimate how large their samples should be for testing hypotheses through **power analysis**. An example can illustrate basic principles of power analysis. Suppose we were testing effectiveness of an intervention to help people quit smoking; people who smoke would be randomized to an intervention group or a control group. How many people should be in the sample? When using power analysis, researchers must estimate how large the group difference will be on a key outcome (e.g., daily number of cigarettes smoked). The estimate is often based on prior research. When differences are expected to be sizable, a large sample is not needed to reveal group differences statistically, but when small differences are predicted, large samples are necessary. In our example, if a small-to-moderate group difference in postintervention smoking were expected, the sample size needed to test group differences in smoking, with standard statistical criteria, would be about 250 people who smoke (125 per group).

The risk of "getting it wrong" (i.e., failing to achieve statistical conclusion validity) increases when samples are too small: Researchers risk gathering data that will not support their hypotheses *even when those hypotheses are correct*. Large samples are no assurance of accuracy, though: With nonprobability sampling, even a large sample can harbor bias. A famous illustration of this point is the 1936 U.S. presidential poll conducted by the magazine *Literary Digest*, which predicted that Alfred Landon would defeat Franklin Roosevelt by a landslide. A sample of about 2.5 million people was polled, but biases arose because the sample was drawn from telephone directories and auto registrations during a Depression year when only the well-to-do (who favored Landon) had a car or telephone.

A large sample cannot correct for a faulty sampling design; nevertheless, a large nonprobability sample is better than a small one. When appraising quantitative studies, you must assess both the sample size and the sample selection method to judge how good the sample was.

 TIP The sampling plan is often one of the weakest aspects of quantitative studies. Most nursing studies use samples of convenience, and many are based on small samples that risk disappointing results.

Critical Appraisal of Sampling Plans

In coming to conclusions about the quality of evidence that a study yields, the sampling plan merits special scrutiny. If the sample is seriously biased or too small, the findings may be misleading or just plain wrong. In appraising the description of a sampling plan, consider whether the researcher has adequately explained the sampling strategy. Ideally, research reports should describe the following:

- The type of sampling approach used (e.g., convenience, consecutive, random)
- The population and eligibility criteria for sample selection
- The sample size, with a rationale
- A description of the sample's main characteristics (e.g., age, gender, clinical status)

A second issue is whether the researcher made good sampling decisions. We have stressed that a key criterion for assessing a sampling plan in quantitative research is whether the sample is representative of the population. You will never know for sure, of course, but if the sampling strategy is weak or if the sample size is small, there is reason to suspect some bias.

Even with a rigorous sampling plan, the sample may be biased if not all people invited to participate in a study agree to do so. If certain subgroups in the population decline to participate, then a biased sample can result, even when probability sampling is used. Research reports ideally should provide information about **response rates** (i.e., the number of people actually participating in a study relative to the number of people sampled) and about possible *nonresponse bias*—differences between participants and those who declined to participate (also sometimes referred to as *response bias*).

Your job as reviewer is to come to conclusions about the reasonableness of generalizing the findings from the researcher's sample to the accessible population and a broader target population. If the sampling plan is flawed, it is risky to generalize the findings at all without replicating the study with another sample. Replication is, in any event, always desirable.

Box 9.1 presents some guiding questions for appraising the sampling plan of a quantitative research report.

DATA COLLECTION IN QUANTITATIVE RESEARCH

Phenomena in which researchers are interested must be translated into data that can be analyzed. This section discusses the challenging task of collecting quantitative research data.

Overview of Data Collection and Data Sources

Data collection methods vary along several dimensions. One issue is whether the researcher collects original data or uses existing data. Existing *records*, for example, are an important data source for nurse researchers. A wealth of clinical data gathered for nonresearch purposes can be fruitfully analyzed to answer research questions.

> **Example of a study using records** •
> Rossi and colleagues (2023) conducted a retrospective review to examine documentation in the electronic health records (EHR) of hospitalized patients requiring cardiac surgery to explore the extent to which nursing assessment data were present in the EHR and linked to the classifications of North American Nursing *Diagnosis* Association International (NANDA-I), Nursing *Interventions* Classification (NIC), and Nursing *Outcomes* Classification (NOC).

> **Box 9.1 Guidelines for Critically Appraising Quantitative Sampling Plans**
>
> a. Was the population identified? Were eligibility criteria specified?
> b. What type of sampling design was used? Was the sampling plan one that could be expected to yield a representative sample?
> c. How many participants were in the sample? Was the sample size affected by high rates of refusals or attrition? Was the sample size large enough to support statistical conclusion validity? Was the sample size justified on the basis of a power analysis or other rationale?
> d. Were key characteristics of the sample described (e.g., mean age, percentage of females)?
> e. To whom can the study results reasonably be generalized?

Researchers usually collect new data and must decide the type of data to gather. Three types have been frequently used by nurse researchers: self-reports, observations, and biomarkers. **Self-report** data—also called **patient-reported outcome (PRO)** data—are participants' responses to researchers' questions, such as in an interview. In nursing studies, self-reports are the most common data collection approach. Direct **observation** of people's behaviors and characteristics can be used for certain questions. Nurses also use **biomarkers** (biophysiologic measures) to assess important clinical variables.

Regardless of type of data collected in a study, data collection methods vary along several dimensions, including degree of structure, quantifiability, and objectivity. Data for quantitative studies tend to be quantifiable and structured, with the same information gathered from all participants in a comparable, prespecified way. Quantitative researchers generally strive for methods that are as objective as possible.

Self-Reports/Patient-Reported Outcomes

Structured self-report methods are used when researchers know in advance exactly what they need to know and can frame appropriate questions to obtain the desired information. Structured self-report data are collected with a formal, written document—an *instrument*. The instrument is known as an **interview schedule** when the questions are asked orally face-to-face or by telephone and as a **questionnaire** when respondents complete the instrument themselves.

Question Form and Wording

In a totally structured instrument, participants are asked to respond to the same questions in the same order. **Closed-ended questions** are ones in which the **response options** are prespecified. The options may range from a simple yes or no to complex expressions of opinion. Such questions ensure comparability of responses and facilitate analysis. Some examples of closed-ended questions are presented in Table 9.1.

Some structured instruments also include **open-ended questions**, which allow participants to respond to questions in their own words (e.g., Why did you stop smoking?). When open-ended questions are included in questionnaires, respondents must write out their responses. In interviews, the interviewer records responses verbatim.

If participants are verbally expressive and cooperative, open-ended questions provide richer information than closed-ended questions. However, responses to closed-ended

TABLE 9.1 Examples of Closed-Ended Questions

Question Type	Example
1. Dichotomous question	Have you ever been pregnant? Yes No
2. Multiple-choice question	How important is it to you to avoid a pregnancy at this time? Extremely important Very important Somewhat important Not important
3. Forced-choice question	Which statement most closely represents your point of view? What happens to me is my own doing. Sometimes I feel I don't have enough control over my life.
4. Rating question	On a scale from 0 to 10, where 0 means "extremely dissatisfied" and 10 means "extremely satisfied," how satisfied were you with the nursing care you received during your hospitalization?

questions are easier to analyze, and people may be unwilling to compose lengthy written responses to open-ended questions in questionnaires. A major drawback of closed-ended questions is that researchers might fail to include important responses, and some respondents may object to choosing from alternatives that do not reflect their opinions precisely.

In drafting questions for a structured instrument, researchers must carefully monitor the wording of each question for clarity, absence of bias, and (in questionnaires) reading level. Questions must be sequenced in a psychologically meaningful order that encourages cooperation and candor. Developing, pretesting, and refining a self-report instrument can take months.

Interviews Versus Questionnaires

Researchers using structured self-reports must decide whether to use interviews or self-administered questionnaires. Questionnaires have the following advantages:

- Questionnaires are less costly and are advantageous for geographically dispersed samples. Internet questionnaires are especially economical and are an increasingly important means of gathering self-report data, although response rates to internet questionnaires tend to be low.
- Questionnaires offer the possibility of anonymity, which may be crucial in obtaining information about certain opinions or traits.

> **Example of internet questionnaires**
> Hale et al. (2024) conducted an online survey among university employees to examine predictors of subjective happiness. They sent the online surveys to 30% of faculty/staff and received responses from 85 people, reflecting a 20% response rate.

The strengths of interviews outweigh those of questionnaires. Among the advantages are the following:

- Response rates tend to be high in face-to-face interviews. Respondents are less likely to refuse to talk to an interviewer than to ignore a questionnaire. Low response rates can lead to bias because respondents are rarely a random subset of the original sample. Hale and colleagues (2024) noted that their 20% response rate is typical for online surveys.
- Some people cannot fill out a questionnaire (e.g., young children). Interviews are feasible with most people.

Some advantages of face-to-face interviews also apply to telephone interviews. Long or complex instruments are not well suited to telephone administration, but for relatively brief instruments, telephone interviews combine relatively low costs with high response rates.

> **Example of telephone interviews**
> Lemons and colleagues (2024) compared data on the prevalence of adverse childhood events (ACE) from two publicly available surveys conducted on the same population of children's caregivers. One was a web- or mail-based survey and the other was a telephone-based one. Interestingly, they found a greater amount of ACE disclosure in the telephone interview survey format.

Summated Rating Scales

Psychosocial scales are often incorporated into self-report instruments. A **scale** is a device that assigns a numeric score to people along a continuum, like a scale for measuring weight. Psychosocial scales are used to measure attitudes, perceptions, and psychological traits such as anxiety or depression.

TABLE 9.2 Example of a Likert Scale to Measure Attitudes Toward Using Condoms

Direction of Scoring[a]	Item	Responses[b]					Score	
		SA	A	?	D	SD	Person 1 (✓)	Person 2 (X)
+	1. Using a condom shows you care about your partner.		✓			X	4	1
−	2. My partner would be angry if I talked about using condoms.			X		✓	5	3
−	3. I wouldn't enjoy sex as much if my partner and I used condoms.		X		✓		4	2
+	4. Condoms are a good protection against AIDS and other sexually transmitted infections.				✓	X	3	2
+	5. My partner would respect me if I insisted on using condoms.	✓				X	5	1
−	6. I would be too embarrassed to ask my partner about using a condom.		X			✓	5	2
	Total score						26	11

[a]Researchers would not indicate the direction of scoring on a Likert scale administered to participants. The scoring direction is indicated in this table for illustrative purposes only.
[b]SA, strongly agree; A, agree; ?, uncertain; D, disagree; SD, strongly disagree.

One technique is the **Likert scale**, which traditionally consists of several declarative statements (*items*) that express a viewpoint on a topic. Respondents are asked to indicate how much they agree or disagree with the statement. Table 9.2 presents a six-item Likert scale for measuring attitudes toward condom use. In this example, agreement with positively worded statements is assigned a higher score. The first statement is positively worded; agreement indicates a favorable attitude toward condom use. Because there are five response alternatives, a score of 5 would be given for *strongly agree*, 4 for *agree*, and so on. Responses of two hypothetical participants are shown by a check or an X and their item scores are shown in the right-hand columns. Person 1, who agreed with the first statement, has a score of 4, whereas person 2, who strongly disagreed, got a score of 1. The second statement is negatively worded, so scoring is reversed—a score of 1 is assigned for *strongly agree*, and so forth. *Item reversals* ensure that a high score consistently reflects positive attitudes toward condom use.

A person's total score is the sum of item scores—hence, such scales are often called **summated rating scales** or *composite scales*. In our example, person 1 has a more positive attitude toward condoms (total score = 26) than person 2 (total score = 11). Summing item scores makes it possible to finely discriminate among people with different opinions. Composite scales are often composed of two or more *subscales* that measure different aspects of a construct. Developing high-quality scales requires a lot of skill and effort.

 TIP Summated rating scales can be used to measure a wide array of attributes. The bipolar scale is not always on an agree/disagree continuum—it might be always/never, likely/unlikely, and so on.

> **Example of a summated rating scale**
> Feng and colleagues (2024) developed and validated the Nurse–Patient Relationship Scale in China, a 23-item scale with five dimensions. Each item of the scale is rated on a five-point Likert scale. A summed score is calculated for each domain and then the entire scale, with a higher score indicating a more positive nurse–patient relationship.

Scales permit researchers to efficiently quantify subtle gradations in the intensity of individual characteristics. Scales can be administered either verbally or in writing, so they can be used with most people. Scales are susceptible to several common problems, however, referred to as **response set biases**, which include the following:

- *Social desirability response set bias*—a tendency to misrepresent oneself by giving answers that are consistent with prevailing social views
- *Extreme response set bias*—a tendency to consistently select extreme alternatives (e.g., strongly agree), leading to distortions if the extreme responses reflect a personality trait and not intense feelings about the phenomenon under study
- *Acquiescence response set bias*—a tendency of some people to agree with statements regardless of their content (*yea-sayers*); the opposite tendency to disagree with statements independently of the question content (*naysayers*) is less common.

Researchers can reduce these biases by developing sensitively worded questions, creating a nonjudgmental atmosphere, and guaranteeing the confidentiality of responses.

> **TIP** Other self-report approaches include vignettes, visual analog scales, and *Q*-sorts. *Vignettes* are brief descriptions of situations to which respondents are asked to react. *Visual analog scales* are used to measure subjective experiences (e.g., fatigue) on a bipolar continuum. *Q-sorts* present participants with a set of cards on which statements are written. Participants are asked to sort the cards along a specified dimension, such as most helpful/least helpful.

Evaluation of Self-Report Methods

If researchers want to know how people feel or what they believe, the most direct approach is to ask them. Self-reports frequently yield information that would be difficult or impossible to gather by other means. Behaviors can be *observed* but only if people are willing to engage in them publicly—and engage in them at the time of data collection.

Nevertheless, self-reports have some weaknesses. The most serious issue concerns the validity and accuracy of self-reports: How can we be sure that participants feel or act the way they say they do? Investigators usually have no choice but to assume that most respondents have been frank. Yet, we all have a tendency to present ourselves in the best light, and this may conflict with the truth. When reading research reports, you should be alert to potential biases in self-reported data.

Observational Methods

For some research questions, direct observation of people's behavior is an alternative to self-reports, especially in clinical settings. Observational methods can be used to gather such information as patients' conditions (e.g., their sleep–wake state), verbal communication (e.g., exchange of information at discharge), nonverbal communication (e.g., body language), activities (e.g., geriatric patients' self-grooming activities), and environmental conditions (e.g., noise levels).

In studies that use observation, researchers have flexibility on several dimensions. For example, the focus of the observation can be on broadly defined events (e.g., patient mood swings) or on small, specific behaviors (e.g., facial expressions). Observations can be made through the human senses and then recorded manually, but they can also be done with equipment such as video recorders.

 TIP Researchers often use structured observations when participants cannot be asked questions or cannot be expected to provide reliable answers. Many observational instruments are designed to capture the behaviors of infants, children, or people whose communication skills are impaired.

Structured observation involves the use of formal instruments and protocols that dictate what to observe, how long to observe it, and how to record the data. Structured observation is not intended to capture a broad slice of life but rather to document specific behaviors, actions, and events. Structured observation requires the formulation of a system for accurately categorizing, recording, and encoding the observations.

Methods of Structured Observation

The most common approach to making structured observations is to use a category system for classifying observed phenomena. A category system represents a method of recording in a systematic fashion the behaviors and events of interest that transpire within a setting.

Some category systems require that *all* observed behaviors in a specified domain (e.g., body positions) be classified. A contrasting technique is a system in which only particular types of behavior (which may or may not occur) are categorized. For example, if we were studying children's aggressive behavior, we might develop such categories as "strikes another child" or "throws objects." In this category system, many behaviors—all that are nonaggressive—would not be classified; some children may exhibit *no* aggressive actions.

Example of nonexhaustive categories for observation
Cohen and colleagues (2024) conducted an observational study to examine the prevalence and outcomes of restraint use in a general ICU in Israel. They retrospectively reviewed the records of 647 patients over 1 year. The data they collected included demographics, reason for admission, medical history, medication use including anti-psychotics, length of stay, need for physical restraint, need for mechanical ventilation, number of ventilation days, treatments such as dialysis, 28-day mortality, and agitation and sedation assessments.

Category systems must have careful, explicit definitions of the behaviors and characteristics to be observed. Each category must be explained, and observers must be given clear-cut criteria for assessing the occurrence of the phenomenon.

Category systems are the basis for constructing a **checklist**—the instrument observers use to record observations. The checklist is usually formatted with a list of behaviors from the category system on the left and space for tallying the frequency or duration on the right. Observers using an exhaustive category system must place *all* observed behaviors in one category for each "unit" of behavior (e.g., a time interval). With nonexhaustive category systems, categories of behaviors that may or may not be manifested are listed. The observer watches for instances of these behaviors and records their occurrence.

Another approach to structured observations is to use a **rating scale**, an instrument that requires observers to rate phenomena along a continuum. The observer may be required to make ratings at intervals throughout the observation or to summarize an entire episode after observation is completed.

> **Example of observational ratings**
> Otani and colleagues (2024) conducted a cross-sectional study in a 27-bed palliative care unit of a 940-bed cancer hospital in Japan to examine whether an objective measure of activity scores via a non-wearable sensor correlated with agitation levels measured using the modified Richmond Agitation-Sedation Scale (RASS) in terminally ill patients with cancer. They found that the non-wearable sensor significantly correlated with the RASS.

Observational Sampling

Researchers must decide when, and for how long, structured observations will be undertaken. Observational sampling methods are a means of obtaining representative examples of the behaviors being observed. One system is *time sampling*, which involves selecting time periods during which observations will occur. Time frames may be selected systematically (e.g., for 30 seconds at 5-minute intervals) or at random.

With *event sampling*, researchers select integral events to observe. Event sampling requires researchers to either know when events will occur (e.g., nursing shift changes) or wait for their occurrence. Event sampling is a good choice when events of interest are infrequent and may be missed if time sampling is used. When behaviors and events are frequent, however, time sampling enhances the representativeness of the observed behaviors.

> **Example of observational sampling**
> White-Traut and colleagues (2022) conducted a prospective study to describe the change in feeding behaviors in 35 preterm infants who received extended tube feedings during hospitalization in a neonatal ICU in the midwestern United States. The feeding behaviors they evaluated using weekly recorded videos included infant state, social interactive behaviors, orally directed behaviors, and hunger/satiation cues.

Evaluation of Observational Methods

Certain research questions are better suited to observation than to self-reports, such as when people cannot describe their own behaviors. This may be the case when people are unaware of their behavior (e.g., stress-induced behavior), when behaviors are emotionally laden (e.g., grieving), or when people are not capable of reporting their actions (e.g., young children). Observational methods have an intrinsic appeal for directly capturing behaviors. Nurses are often in a position to watch people's behaviors and may, by training, be especially sensitive observers.

Shortcomings of observational methods include possible *reactivity* (behavioral distortions resulting from being observed) when the observer is conspicuous and the vulnerability of observations to bias. For example, the observer's values and prejudices may lead to faulty inference. Observational biases probably cannot be eliminated, but they can be minimized by training and monitoring observers.

Biomarkers

Nurse researchers have used biomarkers (**biophysiologic measures**) for a wide variety of purposes. Examples include studies of basic biophysiologic processes, explorations of the ways in which nursing actions and interventions affect physiologic outcomes, product assessments, studies to evaluate the accuracy of biophysiologic information gathered by nurses, and studies of the correlates of physiologic functioning in patients with health problems.

Both in vivo and in vitro measurements are used in research. In vivo measurements are those performed directly within or on living organisms, such as blood pressure and body temperature measurement. Technologic advances continue to improve the ability to measure biophysiologic phenomena accurately and conveniently. With in vitro measures, data are gathered from participants by extracting biophysiologic material from them and subjecting it to laboratory analysis. In vitro measures include chemical measures (e.g., hormone levels), microbiologic measures (e.g., bacterial counts and identification), and cytologic or histologic measures (e.g., tissue biopsies). Recently, there has been a growing interest among nurse researchers about microbiomes, especially gut microbiomes. Nurse researchers also use *anthropomorphic measures*, such as waist circumference.

> **Example of a study with in vivo and in vitro measures**
> Cetinbas et al. (2023) studied the impact of antibiotic use in preterm infants on the microbiome over the course of hospitalization. In vivo measures included birth weight and breast milk intake in the first 28 days, and an in vitro measure included 363 stool samples from 65 preterm infants treated with antibiotics and 52 samples from 14 preterm infants not treated with antibiotics.

Biomarkers are relatively accurate and precise, especially compared to psychological measures, such as self-report measures of anxiety or pain. Biophysiologic measures are also objective. Two nurses reading from the same spirometer output are likely to record identical tidal volume measurements, and two spirometers are likely to produce the same readouts. Patients cannot easily distort measurements of biophysiologic functioning. Finally, biophysiologic instruments provide valid measures of targeted variables: Thermometers can be relied on to measure temperature and not blood volume, and so forth. For nonbiophysiologic measures, there are often concerns about whether an instrument is really measuring the target concept.

Data Quality in Quantitative Research

In developing a data collection plan, researchers must strive for the highest possible quality data. One aspect of data quality concerns the procedures used to collect the data. For example, the people who collect and record the data must be properly trained to ensure that procedures are diligently followed. Another aspect concerns the circumstances of data collection. For example, it is important to ensure privacy and to create an atmosphere that encourages participant candor.

A crucial issue for data quality concerns the adequacy of the *measures* used to operationalize constructs. **Measurement** involves assigning numbers to represent the amount of an attribute present in a person or object. When a new measure of a construct (e.g., anxiety) is developed, rules for assigning numerical values (*scores*) need to be established. Then, the rules must be evaluated to see if they are good rules—they must yield numbers that accurately correspond to different amounts of the targeted trait.

Measures that are not perfectly accurate yield measurements that contain some error. Many factors contribute to *measurement error*, including personal states (e.g., fatigue), response set biases, and situational factors (e.g., temperature). In self-report measures, measurement errors can result from question wording.

Careful researchers select measures that are known to be psychometrically sound. *Psychometrics* is the branch of psychology concerned with the theory and methods of measurements of psychosocial phenomena, such as depression, pain, or anxiety. When a new measure is developed, the developers undertake a **psychometric assessment**, which involves an evaluation of the measure's **measurement properties**.

Psychometricians (and most nurse researchers) have traditionally focused on two measurement properties when assessing the quality of a measure: reliability and validity. Measurement experts in medicine have advocated attending to additional measurement properties that concern the measurement of change (Polit & Yang, 2016). Here, we describe the two properties that you are most likely to encounter in reading articles in the nursing literature. Methods used to assess these properties are briefly described in the chapter on statistical analysis (see Chapter 13).

Reliability

Reliability, broadly speaking, is the extent to which scores are free from measurement error. Reliability can also be defined as the extent to which scores for people *who have not changed* are the same for repeated measurements. In other words, reliability concerns consistency—the *absence* of variation—in measuring a stable attribute. In all types of assessments, reliability involves a *replication* to evaluate the extent to which scores for a stable trait are the same.

In **test–retest reliability**, replication takes the form of administering a measure to the same people on two occasions (e.g., 1 week apart). The assumption is that for traits that have not changed, any differences in people's scores on the two tests are the result of measurement error. When score differences across waves are small, reliability is high. Except for highly volatile constructs (e.g., mood), test–retest reliability can be assessed for most measures, including biophysiologic ones.

When measurements involve people who make scoring judgments, a key source of measurement error stems from the person making the measurements. This is the situation for observational measures (e.g., ratings of agitation) and for some biophysiologic measurements (e.g., skinfold measurement). In such situations, it is important to evaluate how reliably the measurements reflect attributes of the person being rated rather than attributes of the raters. The most typical approach is to undertake an **interrater** (or *interobserver*) **reliability** assessment, which involves having two or more observers independently applying the measure with the same people to see if the scores are consistent across raters.

Another aspect of reliability is **internal consistency**. In responding to a self-report item, people are influenced not only by the underlying construct but also by idiosyncratic reactions to item wording. By combining multiple items with various wordings, item irrelevancies are expected to cancel each other out. An instrument is said to be internally consistent to the extent that its items measure the same trait. For internal consistency, replication involves people's responses to multiple items during a single administration. Whereas other reliability estimates assess a measure's degree of consistency across time or raters, internal consistency captures consistency across items.

As we explain in Chapter 13, assessments of reliability yield coefficients that summarize how reliable a measure is. *Reliability coefficients* range in value from .00 to 1.00, with higher values being desirable. Coefficients of .80 or higher usually are considered acceptable. Researchers should select instruments with demonstrated reliability and should document this in their reports. Researchers undertaking a study often compute internal consistency reliability coefficients with their own data.

> **Example of internal consistency reliability**
> Curcio and colleagues (2024) assessed the psychometric properties of the Italian version of the Neonatal Skin Risk Assessment Scale. They reported that the internal consistency reliability was .86, which was similar to the value (.85) reported by researchers who assessed the Spanish version of this scale.

Validity

Validity in a measurement context is the degree to which an instrument is measuring the construct it purports to measure. When researchers develop a scale to measure *resilience*, they need to be sure that the resulting scores validly reflect this construct and not something else, such as self-efficacy or perseverance. Assessing the validity of abstract constructs requires a careful conceptualization of the construct—as well as a conceptualization of what the construct is *not*. Like reliability, measurement validity has different aspects: face validity, content validity, criterion validity, and construct validity.

Face validity refers to whether the instrument *looks* like it is measuring the target construct. Although face validity is not considered good evidence of validity, it is helpful for a measure to have face validity. If patients' resistance to being measured reflects the view that the scale is not relevant to their problems or situations, then face validity is an issue.

Content validity may be defined as the extent to which an instrument's content adequately captures the construct—that is, whether a composite instrument (e.g., a multi-item scale) has an appropriate sample of items for the construct being measured. Content validity is assessed by having a panel of experts rate the scale items for relevance to the construct and comment on the need for revisions.

Criterion validity is the extent to which the scores on a measure are a good reflection of a "gold standard"—that is, a criterion considered an ideal measure of the construct. Not all measures can be validated using a criterion approach because there is not always a "gold standard" criterion. As an example, scores on a self-report scale to measure stress could be compared to wake-up salivary free cortisol levels (a *concurrent* criterion). Screening scales are often tested against some future criterion—namely, the occurrence of the phenomenon for which a screening tool is sought (e.g., a patient fall). This is called *predictive validity*.

For many abstract, unobservable human attributes (constructs), no gold standard criterion exists, so other validation avenues must be pursued. **Construct validity** is the degree to which evidence about a measure's scores in relation to other variables supports the inference that the construct has been well represented. Construct validity typically involves hypothesis testing, which follows a similar path: Hypotheses are developed about a relationship between scores on the focal measure and values on other constructs, data are collected to test the hypotheses, and then validity conclusions are reached based on the results of the hypothesis tests.

One approach to construct validity is called *known-groups validity*, which tests hypotheses about a measure's ability to discriminate between two or more groups known (or expected) to differ with regard to the construct of interest. For instance, in validating a measure of anxiety about the labor experience, the scores of primiparas and multiparas could be contrasted. Evidence suggests that, on average, people who have never given birth experience more anxiety than people who already have children; one might question the validity of the instrument if such differences did not emerge.

> **Example of known-groups validity** •
> Keymeulen et al. (2023) evaluated the known-groups validity of the Structured Problem Analysis of Raising Kids aged 36 months (SPARK36) by conducting a cross-sectional analysis in two groups in Flanders: parents with lower socioeconomic status and families with ≥4 risk factors for child maltreatment.

TIP Another aspect of construct validity is called cross-cultural validity, which is relevant for measures that have been translated or adapted for use with a different cultural group than that for the original instrument. *Cross-cultural validity* is the degree to which the components (e.g., items) of a translated or culturally adapted measure perform adequately and equivalently relative to their performance on the original instrument.

An instrument does not possess or lack validity; it is a question of degree. An instrument's validity is not proved, demonstrated, or verified but rather is supported to a greater or lesser extent by evidence. Researchers strive to select measures for which good validity information is available.

Critical Appraisal of Data Collection Methods

The goal of a data collection plan is to produce data that are of excellent quality. Decisions that researchers make about their data collection methods and procedures can affect data quality and hence the quality of the study.

It may, however, be difficult to critically appraise data collection methods in studies reported in journals because researchers' descriptions are seldom detailed. However, researchers do have a responsibility to communicate basic information about their approach so that readers can assess the quality of evidence that the study yields.

Information about data quality (reliability and validity of the measures) should be provided in quantitative research reports. Ideally—especially for composite scales—the report should provide internal consistency coefficients based on data from the study itself, not just from previous research. Interrater or interobserver reliability is especially crucial for assessing data quality in studies that use observational methods. The values of the reliability coefficients should be sufficiently high to support confidence in the findings.

Validity is more difficult to document than reliability. At a minimum, researchers should defend their choice of existing measures based on validity information from the developers, and they should cite the relevant publication. Guidelines for appraising data collection methods are presented in Box 9.2.

Box 9.2 Guidelines for Critically Appraising Quantitative Data Collection Plans

a. Did the researchers use the best method of capturing study phenomena (i.e., self-reports, observation, biomarkers)?
b. If self-report methods were used, did the researchers make good decisions about the specific methods used to solicit information (e.g., in-person interviews, Internet questionnaires)? Were composite scales used? If not, should they have been?
c. If observational methods were used, did the report adequately describe what the observations entailed and how observations were sampled? Were risks of observational bias addressed? Were biomarkers used in the study, and was this appropriate?
d. Did the report provide adequate information about data collection procedures (e.g., the training of the data collectors)?
e. Did the report offer evidence of the reliability of measures? Did the evidence come from the research sample itself, or was it based on other studies? If reliability was reported, which estimation method was used? Was the reliability sufficiently high?
f. Did the report offer evidence of the validity of the measures? If validity information was reported, which validity approach was used?
g. If there was no reliability or validity information, what conclusion can you reach about the quality of the data in the study?

RESEARCH EXAMPLES WITH CRITICAL THINKING EXERCISES

In this section, we describe the sampling and data collection plan of a quantitative nursing study. For Example 1, read the summary, and then answer the critical thinking questions that follow. The critical thinking questions for Example 2 are based on the study that appears in its entirety in Appendix A of this book.

EXAMPLE 1: SAMPLING AND DATA COLLECTION IN A QUANTITATIVE STUDY

Study: "Effect of a hydration game-based learning program in improving fluid intake and hydration status in institutional residents" (Lin et al., 2024)

Statement of Purpose: The purpose of this study was to explore the effects of a hydration game-based learning program on the fluid intake and hydration status of institutional residents in Taiwan.

Design: The research team enrolled participants from five long-term care facilities in northern Taiwan in a single-blind, cluster, randomized control trial.

Sampling: The inclusion criteria included current resident of a long-term care facility, able to orally hydrate independently, able to use at least one hand, ≥18 on the Mini-Mental State Examination (MMSE), and plasma osmolality >290 mOsm/kg. Exclusion criteria were nasogastric tube feeding, disease requiring fluid restriction, and history of head or neck radiotherapy or chemotherapy. The team used a generalized estimating equation method to determine the minimum sample size of 70. Initially, 67 participants met inclusion criteria; three were unable to remain in the study due to issues such as hospitalization. The final sample included 64 participants. The experimental group ($N = 33$) received a 40-minute game-based hydration and education intervention twice weekly for 8 weeks, and the control group ($N = 31$) received routine care.

Data Collection: Measures of mental status, independent activities of daily living, fluid intake via a diary, body composition analyzer, urine specific gravity, and urine leukocytes and nitrites were taken at 4 and 8 weeks of the study period.

Key Findings: The sample included mostly males (61.3% in the control group and 69.7% in the experimental group) with a mean age of 81.7 years in the control group and 86 years in the experimental group. Findings indicated that the experimental group had a significant improvement in fluid intake at 4 and 8 weeks ($p = .002$ and $p < .001$, respectively). At 8 weeks, the experimental group had a significantly improved total body water ($p = .009$), urine leukocytes ($p = .029$), and nitrites ($p = .004$). However, there was no significant improvement in urine specific gravity.

Critical Thinking Exercises

1. Answer the relevant questions from Box 9.1 regarding this study.
2. Answer the relevant questions from Box 9.2 regarding this study.
3. Are there variables in this study that could have been measured through self-report but were not?
4. If the results of this study are valid and reliable, what might be some of the uses to which the findings could be put in clinical practice?

EXAMPLE 2: SAMPLING AND DATA COLLECTION IN THE STUDY IN APPENDIX A

Read the method section of Cheng et al.'s (2024) "Advance care planning affects end-of-life treatment preferences among patients with heart failure: A randomized controlled trial" in Appendix A of this book.
1. Answer the relevant questions from Box 9.1 regarding this study.
2. Answer the relevant questions from Box 9.2 regarding this study.

Summary Points

- **Sampling** is the process of selecting elements from a **population**, which is an entire aggregate. An *element* is the basic unit of a population—usually humans in nursing research.

- **Eligibility criteria** (including both *inclusion criteria* and *exclusion criteria*) are used to define population characteristics.

- A key criterion in assessing a sample in a quantitative study is its *representativeness*—the extent to which the sample is similar to the population and avoids bias. **Sampling bias** is the systematic overrepresentation or underrepresentation of some segment of the population.

- **Nonprobability sampling** (in which elements are selected by nonrandom methods) includes convenience, quota, consecutive, and purposive sampling. Nonprobability sampling is convenient and economical; a major disadvantage is its potential for bias.

- **Convenience sampling** uses the most readily available or convenient people.

- **Quota sampling** divides the population into homogeneous **strata** (subpopulations) to ensure representation of the subgroups in the sample; within each stratum, people are sampled by convenience.

- **Consecutive sampling** involves taking *all* of the people from an accessible population who meet the eligibility criteria over a specific time interval or for a specified sample size.

- In **purposive sampling**, participants are handpicked to be included in the sample based on the researcher's knowledge about the population.

- **Probability sampling** designs, which involve the random selection of elements from the population, yield more representative samples than nonprobability designs and permit estimates of the magnitude of *sampling error*.

- **Simple random sampling** involves the random selection of elements from a *sampling frame* that enumerates all the elements; **stratified random sampling** divides the population into homogeneous subgroups from which elements are selected at random.

- In quantitative studies, researchers can use a **power analysis** to estimate **sample size** needs. Large samples are preferable because they enhance statistical conclusion validity and tend to be more representative, but large samples do not *guarantee* representativeness.

- The three principal data collection methods for nurse researchers are self-reports, observations, and biomarkers.

- **Self-reports**, which are also called **patient-reported outcomes** or PROs, involve directly questioning study participants and are the most widely used method of collecting data for nursing studies.

- Structured self-reports for quantitative studies involve a formal instrument—a **questionnaire** or **interview schedule**—that may contain **open-ended questions** (which permit respondents to respond in their own words) and multiple **closed-ended questions** (which

- offer respondents response options from which to choose).

- Questionnaires are less costly than interviews and offer the possibility of anonymity, but interviews yield higher response rates and are suitable for a wider variety of people.

- Social psychological **scales** are self-report instruments for measuring such characteristics as attitudes and psychological attributes. **Summated rating scales** such as **Likert scales** present respondents with a series of *items*; each item is scored on a continuum (e.g., from strongly agree to strongly disagree) and then summed into a composite score.

- Scales are versatile and powerful but are susceptible to **response set biases**—the tendency of some people to respond to items in characteristic ways, independently of item content.

- **Observational methods** are techniques for acquiring data through the direct observation of phenomena.

- Structured observations dictate what the observer should observe; they often involve **checklists**—instruments based on **category systems** for recording the appearance, frequency, or duration of behaviors or events. Observers may also use **rating scales** to rate phenomena along a dimension of interest (e.g., lethargic/energetic).

- Structured observations often involve a sampling plan (such as *time sampling* or *event sampling*) for selecting the behaviors, events, and conditions to be observed. When observers are conspicuous, *reactivity* (behavioral distortions) can affect data quality.

- Data may also be derived from biophysiologic measures (**biomarkers**), which include in vivo measurements (those performed within or on living organisms) and in vitro measurements (those performed outside the organism's body, such as blood tests). Biomarkers have the advantage of being objective, accurate, and precise.

- In quantitative studies, variables are measured. **Measurement** involves assigning numbers to represent the amount of an attribute present in a person, using a set of rules; researchers strive to use measures that have good rules that minimize *measurement error*.

- *Measures* (and the quality of the data that the measures yield) can be evaluated in a **psychometric assessment** in terms of several **measurement properties**, most often reliability and validity.

- **Reliability** is the extent to which scores for people *who have not changed* are the same for repeated measurements. A reliable measure minimizes measurement error.

- Methods of assessing reliability include **test–retest reliability** (administering a measure twice in a short period to see if the measure yields consistent scores), **interrater reliability** (assessing whether two raters or observers independently assign similar scores), and **internal consistency** (assessing whether there is consistency across items in a composite scale in measuring a trait).

- Reliability is assessed statistically by computing coefficients that range from .00 to 1.00; higher values indicate greater reliability.

- **Validity** is the degree to which an instrument measures what it is supposed to measure.

- Aspects of validity include **face validity** (the extent to which a measure looks like it is measuring the target construct), **content validity** (in composite scales, the extent to which an instrument's content adequately captures the construct), **criterion validity** (the extent to which scores on a measure are a good reflection of a "gold standard"), and **construct validity** (the extent to which an instrument adequately measures the targeted construct, as assessed mainly by testing hypotheses).

- A measure's validity is not proved or established but rather is supported to a greater or lesser extent by evidence.

REFERENCES

Albaqawi, H. M., & Alshammari, M. H. (2024). Resilience, compassion fatigue, moral distress and moral injury of nurses. *Nursing Ethics, 32*(3), 798–813. https://doi.org/10.1177/09697330241287862

Cetinbas, M., Thai, J., Filatava, E., Gregory, K. E., & Sadreyev, R. I. (2023). Long-term dysbiosis and fluctuations of gut microbiome in antibiotic treated preterm infants. *iScience, 26*(10), 107995. https://doi.org/10.1016/j.isci.2023.107995

Cohen, S., Meyer, A., Ifrach, N., & Dichtwald, S. (2024). Physical restraint and associated agitation. *Nursing in Critical Care, 29*(5), 1132–1141. https://doi.org/10.1111/nicc.13130

Curcio, F., Vaquero Abellán, M., Dioni, E., de Lima, M. M., Ez Zinabi, O., & Romero Saldaña, M. (2024). Validity and reliability of the Italian-Neonatal Skin Risk Assessment Scale (i-NSRAS). *Intensive and Critical Care Nursing, 80*, 103561. https://doi.org/10.1016/j.iccn.2023.103561

Feng, Y., Liu, C., Tao, S., Wang, C., Zhang, H., Liu, X., Liu, Z., Liu, W., Zhao, J., Zou, D., Liu, Z., Liu, J., Wang, N., Wu, L., Wu, Q., Hao, Y., Xu, W., & Liang, L. (2024). Developing and validating the Nurse-Patient Relationship Scale (NPRS) in China. *BMC Nursing, 23*(1), 255. https://doi.org/10.1186/s12912-024-01941-w

Hale, F. B., Fontenot, H. B., Davis, J. W., & Albright, C. L. (2024). Mental illness as a predictor of subjective happiness among university employees working in Hawai'i. *Journal of Psychosocial Nursing and Mental Health Services, 62*(5), 39–48. https://doi.org/10.3928/02793695-20231017-01

Keymeulen, A., Staal, I. I. E., de Kroon, M. L. A., & van Achterberg, T. (2023). Known groups validity of the SPARK36: To guide nurse-led consultations for the early detection of child developmental and parenting problems. *Journal of Advanced Nursing, 79*(10), 3997–4007. https://doi.org/10.1111/jan.15711

Kim, Y., Chae, H., Kwak, Y. H., & Kim, J. S. (2025). Factors associated with health-promoting behaviors among South Korean adults: A cross-sectional study. *Public Health Nursing, 42*(1), 265–274. https://doi.org/10.1111/phn.13474

Lemons, J., Saravanan, M., Tumin, D., & Anyigbo, C. (2024). Caregiver report of adverse childhood events: Comparison of self-administered and telephone questionnaires. *Children and Youth Services Review, 163*, 107758. https://doi.org/10.1016/j.childyouth.2024.107758

Lin, L. C., Chen, T. W., Chen, Y. H., & Wu, S. C. (2024). Effect of a hydration game-based learning program in improving fluid intake and hydration status in institutional residents. *The Journal of Nursing Research: JNR, 32*(6), e365. https://doi.org/10.1097/jnr.0000000000000650

Martins, H., Domingues, T. D., & Caldeira, S. (2024). Spiritual distress and religious involvement among cancer patients receiving chemotherapy: A longitudinal study. *International Journal of Nursing Knowledge, 35*(3), 272–280. https://doi.org/10.1111/2047-3095.12442

Menevşe, Ş., & Yayla, A. (2024). Effect of emotional freedom technique applied to patients before laparoscopic cholecystectomy on surgical fear and anxiety: A randomized controlled trial. *Journal of Perianesthesia Nursing: Official Journal of the American Society of PeriAnesthesia Nurses, 39*(1), 93–100. https://doi.org/10.1016/j.jopan.2023.07.006

Otani, H., Yokomichi, N., Imai, K., Toyota, S., Yamauchi, T., Miwa, S., Yuasa, M., Okamoto, S., Kogure, T., Inoue, S., & Morita, T. (2024). A novel objective measure for terminal delirium: Activity scores measured by a sheet-type sensor. *Journal of Pain and Symptom Management, 68*(3), 246–254. https://doi.org/10.1016/j.jpainsymman.2024.05.024

Polit, D. F., & Yang, F. M. (2016). *Measurement and the measurement of change: A primer for health professionals.* Lippincott.

Riegel, B., Quinn, R., Hirschman, K. B., Thomas, G., Ashare, R., Stawnychy, M. A., Bowles, K. H., Aryal, S., & Wald, J. W. (2024). Health coaching improves outcomes of informal caregivers of adults with chronic heart failure: A randomized controlled trial. *Circulation: Heart Failure, 17*(7), e011475. https://doi.org/10.1161/CIRCHEARTFAILURE.123.011475

Rossi, L., Butler, S., Coakley, A., & Flanagan, J. (2023). Nursing knowledge captured in electronic health records. *International Journal of Nursing Knowledge, 34*(1), 72–84. https://doi.org/10.1111/2047-3095.12365

Schwanda, M., Brunner, S., Abreu Almeida, M., Koller, M., Müller Staub, M., & Ewers, A. (2024). Content validation of the NANDA-I nursing diagnosis risk for perioperative hypothermia (00254). *International Journal of Nursing Knowledge*, Online ahead of print. https://doi.org/10.1111/2047-3095.12491

White-Traut, R., Griffith, T., Zheng, C., Lagatta, J., Rigby-McCotter, C., Walsh, C., & Gralton, K. (2022). Descriptive longitudinal pilot study: Behaviors surrounding feeding of preterm infants who received extended tube feedings. *Herald Scholarly Open Access Journal Neonatology & Clinical Pediatrics, 9*(1), 092. https://doi.org/10.24966/ncp-878x/100092

Zeleníková, R., Hosáková, J., Kozáková, R., Bobčíková, K., & Bužgová, R. (2025). The effect of reminiscence therapy on the assessment of depression, anxiety and self-esteem in community-dwelling older adults: An intervention study. *International Journal of Older People Nursing, 20*(1), e70004. https://doi.org/10.1111/opn.70004

10 Appraising Qualitative Designs and Approaches

Learning Objectives

On completing this chapter, you will be able to:

- Discuss the rationale for an emergent design in qualitative research and describe qualitative design features
- Identify the major research traditions for qualitative research and describe the domain of inquiry of each
- Describe the main features and methods associated with ethnographic, phenomenologic, and grounded theory studies
- Describe key features of case studies, narrative analyses, and descriptive qualitative studies
- Discuss the goals and features of research with ideologic perspectives
- Define new terms in the chapter

Key Terms

- Autoethnography
- Basic social process (BSP)
- Bracketing
- Case study
- Constant comparison
- Constructivist grounded theory
- Core variable
- Critical ethnography
- Critical theory
- Descriptive phenomenology
- Descriptive qualitative study
- Emergent design
- Ethnonursing research
- Feminist research
- Grounded theory
- Hermeneutics
- Historical research
- Institutional ethnography
- Interpretive phenomenology
- Narrative analysis
- Netnography
- Participant observation
- Participatory action research (PAR)
- Reflexive journal
- Situational analysis

THE DESIGN OF QUALITATIVE STUDIES

Quantitative researchers develop a research design before collecting their data and rarely depart from that design once the study is underway: They design and *then* they do. In qualitative research, by contrast, the study design often evolves during the project: Qualitative researchers design *as* they do. Qualitative studies use an emergent design that evolves as researchers make ongoing decisions about their data needs based on what they have already learned. An emergent design supports the researchers' desire to have the inquiry reflect the realities and viewpoints of those under study—realities and viewpoints that are not known at the outset.

Characteristics of Qualitative Research Design

Qualitative inquiry has been guided by different disciplines with distinct methods and approaches. Some characteristics of qualitative research design are broadly applicable, however. In general, qualitative design:

- Is flexible, capable of adjusting to what is learned during data collection
- Benefits from ongoing data analysis to guide subsequent strategies
- Often involves triangulating various data sources
- Tends to be holistic, aimed at understanding the whole
- Requires researchers to become intensely involved and reflexive

Although design decisions are not finalized beforehand, qualitative researchers typically do advance planning that supports their flexibility. For example, qualitative researchers make advance decisions with regard to the study site, a broad data collection strategy, and the equipment they will need in the field. Qualitative researchers plan for a variety of circumstances, but decisions about how to deal with them are resolved when the social context is better understood.

Qualitative Design Features

Some of the design features discussed in Chapter 8 apply to qualitative studies. To contrast qualitative and quantitative research design, we consider the elements identified in Table 8.1 in Chapter 8.

Intervention, Control, and Blinding

Qualitative research is almost always nonexperimental—although a qualitative component may be embedded in an experiment (see Chapter 12). Qualitative researchers do not conceptualize their studies as having independent and dependent variables and rarely control the people or environment under study. Blinding is rarely used by qualitative researchers. The goal is to develop a rich understanding of a phenomenon as it exists and as it is constructed by individuals within their own context.

Comparisons

Qualitative researchers typically do not plan to make group comparisons because the intent is to thoroughly describe or explain a phenomenon. Yet, patterns emerging in the data sometimes suggest illuminating comparisons. Indeed, as Morse (2004) noted in an editorial in *Qualitative Health Research*, "All description requires comparisons" (p. 1323). In analyzing qualitative data and in determining whether categories are saturated, there is a need to compare "this" to "that."

> **Example of qualitative comparisons**
> Jenkins and Astroth (2024) explored the intergenerational differences in perceptions related to civility among nursing students and nurse educators. The faculty described civil nursing students as open to learning, polite, appreciative, and gracious. Students explained that civil faculty listened without judgment and were supportive and respectful. Faculty described uncivil students as being disrespectful and entitled, and improperly using social media. Nursing students noted that uncivil faculty as belittling, impatient, and failing to listen.

Research Settings

Qualitative researchers usually collect their data in naturalistic settings. And, whereas quantitative researchers usually strive to collect data in one type of setting to maintain constancy of conditions (e.g., conducting all interviews in participants' homes), qualitative researchers may deliberately study phenomena in various natural contexts, especially in ethnographic research.

Time Frames

Qualitative research, like quantitative research, can be either cross-sectional, with one data collection point, or longitudinal, with multiple data collection points designed to observe the evolution of a phenomenon.

> **Example of a longitudinal qualitative study**
> Monaro et al. (2024) conducted a longitudinal qualitative study in Australia to understand patient and family experiences of making decisions for amputation for chronic limb-threatening ischemia. The researchers conducted interviews with the patients and their families at two points in time. The first occurred soon after advice was given to consider major amputation as a possible treatment. Then, for those who did choose amputation, the next occurred at 6 months postoperation.

Causality and Qualitative Research

In evidence hierarchies that rank evidence in terms of support of causal inferences (e.g., see Fig. 1.2 in Chapter 1), qualitative research is often near the base, which has led some to criticize evidence-based initiatives. The issue of causality, which has been controversial throughout the history of science, is especially contentious in qualitative research.

Some believe that causality is an inappropriate construct within the naturalistic paradigm. For example, Lincoln and Guba (1985) devoted an entire chapter of their book to a critique of causality and argued that it should be replaced with a concept that they called *mutual shaping*. According to their view, "Everything influences everything else, in the here and now" (p. 151).

QUALITATIVE RESEARCH TRADITIONS

There is a wide variety of qualitative approaches. One classification system involves categorizing qualitative research according to disciplinary traditions. These traditions vary in their conceptualization of the types of questions that are important to ask and in the methods considered appropriate for answering them. This section describes traditions that have been prominent in nursing research.

Ethnography

Ethnography, the research tradition of anthropologists, involves the description and interpretation of a culture and cultural behavior. *Culture* refers to the way a group of people live—the patterns of human activity and the values and norms that give activity significance. Ethnographies typically involve extensive *fieldwork*, which is the process by which the ethnographer comes to understand a culture. Because culture is, in itself, not visible or tangible, it must be inferred from the words, actions, and products of members of a group.

Ethnographic research sometimes concerns broadly defined cultures (e.g., the Maori culture of New Zealand) in a *macroethnography*. However, ethnographers sometimes focus on more narrowly defined cultures in a *focused ethnography*. Focused ethnographies are studies of small units in a group or culture (e.g., the culture of an intensive care unit). An underlying assumption of the ethnographer is that every human group eventually evolves a culture that guides the members' view of the world and the way they structure their experiences.

> **Example of a focused ethnography**
> Sheen et al. (2024) used a focused ethnographic approach to study diabetes self-management among 21 first-generation Vietnamese Americans using participant observation and interviews.

Ethnographers seek to learn from (rather than to study) members of a cultural group—to understand their world view. Ethnographers distinguish "emic" and "etic" perspectives. An *emic perspective* refers to the way the members of the culture regard their world—the insiders' view. The emic is the local concepts or means of expression used by members of the group under study to characterize their experiences. The *etic perspective*, by contrast, is the outsiders' interpretation of the culture's experiences—the words and concepts they use to refer to the same phenomena. Ethnographers strive to acquire an emic perspective of a culture and to reveal *tacit knowledge*—information about the culture that is so deeply embedded in cultural experiences that members do not talk about it or may not even be consciously aware of it.

Three broad types of information are usually sought by ethnographers: cultural behavior (what members of the culture do), cultural artifacts (what members make and use), and cultural speech (what they say). Ethnographers rely on a wide variety of data sources, including observations, in-depth interviews, records, and other types of physical evidence (e.g., photographs, diaries). Ethnographers typically use a strategy called **participant observation** in which they make observations of the culture under study while participating in its activities. Ethnographers also enlist *key informants* to help them understand and interpret the events and activities being observed.

Ethnographic research is time-consuming—months and even years of fieldwork may be required to learn about a culture. Ethnography requires a certain level of intimacy with members of the cultural group that can be developed only over time and by working with those members as active participants.

The products of ethnographies are rich, holistic descriptions and interpretations of the culture under study. Among health care researchers, ethnography provides access to the health beliefs and health practices of a culture. Ethnographic inquiry can thus help to foster understanding of behaviors affecting health and illness. Leininger (1985) coined the phrase **ethnonursing research**, which she defined as "the study and analysis of the local or indigenous people's viewpoints, beliefs, and practices about nursing care behavior and processes of designated cultures" (p. 38).

> **Example of an ethnonursing study**
> Strange and colleagues (2024) conducted an ethnonursing study to discover the influences of faith on rural Appalachian older adult health. Interviews were conducted with 12 key and 20 general informants.

Ethnographers are often, but not always, "outsiders" to the culture under study. A type of ethnography that involves the scrutiny of groups or cultures to which researchers themselves belong is called **autoethnography** or *insider research*. Autoethnography has several advantages, including ease of recruitment and the ability to get candid data based on preestablished trust. The drawback is that an "insider" may have biases about certain issues or may be so entrenched in the culture that valuable data get overlooked.

Other types of ethnography are institutional ethnography and netnography. **Institutional ethnography** was founded by Dorothy Smith, a Canadian sociologist. Institutional ethnography seeks to understand the social determinants of people's everyday experiences in institutional settings. The focus is on social organization and institutional processes.

Netnography, sometimes called *online ethnography*, focuses on cultural experiences of data from social media environments such as Facebook, Instagram, and blogs (Kozinets, 2020). In netnography, online traces are studied, which are what people leave behind online when they post text, images, blogs, etc.

Phenomenology

Phenomenology is an approach to understanding people's everyday life experiences. Phenomenologic researchers ask: What is the *essence* of this phenomenon as experienced by people and what does it *mean?* Phenomenologists assume there is an *essence*—an essential structure—that can be understood, much as ethnographers assume that cultures exist. Essence is what makes a phenomenon what it is, and without which it would not be what it is. Phenomenologists investigate subjective phenomena in the belief that critical truths about reality are grounded in people's lived experiences. The topics appropriate to phenomenology are ones that are fundamental to the life experiences of humans, such as the meaning of suffering or the grief of losing a child to cancer.

In phenomenologic studies, the main data source is in-depth conversations. Through these conversations, researchers strive to gain entrance into the informants' world and to have access to their experiences as lived. Phenomenologic studies usually involve a small number of participants—often fewer than 15. For some phenomenologic researchers, the inquiry includes gathering not only information from informants but also efforts to experience the phenomenon, through participation, observation, and reflection. Phenomenologists share their insights in rich, vivid reports that describe key *themes*. The results section in a phenomenologic report should help readers "see" something in a different way that enriches their understanding of experiences.

Phenomenology has two main variants: descriptive phenomenology and interpretive phenomenology (hermeneutics).

Descriptive Phenomenology

Descriptive phenomenology was developed first by Husserl, who was primarily interested in the question: *What do we know as persons?* Descriptive phenomenologists insist on the careful portrayal of ordinary conscious experience of everyday life—a depiction of "things" as people experience them to understand the *essence* of the experience. These "things" include hearing, seeing, believing, feeling, remembering, deciding, and evaluating.

Descriptive phenomenologic studies often involve the following four steps: bracketing, intuiting, analyzing, and describing. **Bracketing** refers to the process of identifying and holding in abeyance preconceived beliefs and opinions about the phenomenon under study. Researchers strive to bracket out presuppositions in an effort to confront the data in pure form. Phenomenologic researchers (and other qualitative researchers) often maintain a **reflexive journal** in their efforts to bracket.

Intuiting, the second step in descriptive phenomenology, occurs when researchers remain open to the meanings attributed to the phenomenon by those who have experienced it. Phenomenologic researchers then proceed to an analysis (i.e., extracting significant statements, categorizing, and making sense of essential meanings). Finally, the descriptive phase occurs when researchers come to understand and define the phenomenon.

> **Example of a descriptive phenomenologic study**
> Bennett et al. (2024) used a descriptive phenomenologic approach in their study of the experience of hope in adolescents and young adults living with advanced cancer. The researchers discovered that music played a role in helping adolescents cope. The main theme identified was *Simple Supports of Hope* with a subtheme of *Diversion*.

Interpretive Phenomenology

Heidegger, a student of Husserl, is the founder of **interpretive phenomenology** or **hermeneutics**. Heidegger stressed interpreting—not just describing—human experience. He believed that lived experience is inherently an interpretive process and argued that **hermeneutics** ("understanding") is a basic characteristic of human existence. (The term *hermeneutics* refers to the art and philosophy of interpreting the meaning of an object such as a *text* or work of art.) The goals of interpretive phenomenologic research are to enter another's world and to discover the understandings found there.

Gadamer, another interpretive phenomenologist, described the interpretive process as a circular relationship—the *hermeneutic circle*—where one understands the whole of a text (e.g., an interview transcript) in terms of its parts and the parts in terms of the whole. Researchers continually question the meanings of the text.

Heidegger believed it is impossible to bracket one's being-in-the-world, so bracketing does not occur in interpretive phenomenology. Hermeneutics presupposes prior understanding on the part of the researcher. Interpretive phenomenologists ideally approach each interview text with openness—they must be open to hearing what it is the text is saying.

Interpretive phenomenologists, like descriptive phenomenologists, rely primarily on in-depth interviews with individuals who have experienced the phenomenon of interest, but they may go beyond a traditional approach to gathering and analyzing data. For example, interpretive phenomenologists sometimes augment their understandings of the phenomenon through an analysis of relevant supplementary texts, such as novels, poetry, or other artistic expressions.

> **Example of a hermeneutic study**
> In Denmark, Soegaard et al. (2024) used a hermeneutic approach to explore the experiences of 10 people with spinal cord injuries who were affected with pressure injuries. Participants revealed that they had difficulty balancing their active, redefined daily lives with having a strict pressure relief protocol.

HOW-TO-TELL TIP How can you tell if a phenomenologic study is descriptive or interpretive? Phenomenologists often use terms that can help you make this determination. In a descriptive phenomenologic study, such terms may be bracketing, description, or essence. The names Colaizzi, van Kaam, or Giorgi may be mentioned in the method section. In an interpretive phenomenologic study, key terms can include being-in-the-world, hermeneutics, and understanding. The names van Manen or Benner may appear in the method section, as we discuss in Chapter 15 on qualitative data analysis.

Grounded Theory

Grounded theory research has contributed to the development of many middle-range theories of phenomena relevant to nurses. Grounded theory was developed in the 1960s by two sociologists, Glaser (1978) and Strauss (1967), whose theoretical roots were in *symbolic interaction*, which focuses on the manner in which people make sense of social interactions.

Grounded theory tries to account for people's actions from the perspective of those involved. Grounded theory researchers seek to identify a main concern or problem and then to understand the behavior designed to resolve it—the **core variable**. One type of core variable is a **basic social process (BSP)**. Grounded theory researchers generate conceptual categories and integrate them into a substantive theory, grounded in the data.

Grounded Theory Methods

Grounded theory methods constitute an entire approach to the conduct of field research. A study that truly follows Glaser and Strauss's precepts does not begin with a focused research problem. The problem and the process used to resolve it emerge from the data and are discovered during the study. In grounded theory research, data collection, data analysis, and sampling of participants occur simultaneously. The grounded theory process is recursive: Researchers collect data, categorize them, describe the emerging central phenomenon, and then recycle earlier steps. Two main types of coding are used in Glaser and Strauss's grounded theory: substantive and theoretical. Substantive codes include the empirical substance of the topic under study being conceptualized and often are the actual words of the participants. There are two types of substantive codes: open and selective, which are described in greater detail in Chapter 15. Theoretical codes provide insight into how the substantive codes are related to each other.

A procedure called **constant comparison** is used to develop and refine theoretically relevant concepts and categories. Categories elicited from the data are constantly compared with data obtained earlier so that commonalities and variations can be detected. As data collection proceeds, the inquiry becomes increasingly focused on the emerging theory.

In-depth interviews and participant observation are common data sources in grounded theory studies, but existing documents and other data may also be used. Typically, a grounded theory study involves interviews with a sample of about 20 to 30 people.

Alternate Views of Grounded Theory

In 1990, Strauss and Corbin published a controversial book, *Basics of Qualitative Research: Grounded Theory Procedures and Techniques*. The book's stated purpose was to provide beginning grounded theory researchers with basic procedures for building a grounded theory. The book is currently in its fourth edition (Corbin & Strauss, 2015).

Glaser, however, disagreed with some procedures advocated by Strauss (his original co-author) and Corbin (a nurse researcher). Glaser (1992) believed that Strauss and Corbin (1990) developed a method that is not grounded theory but rather what he called "full conceptual description." According to Glaser, the purpose of grounded theory is to generate concepts and theories that explain and account for variation in behavior in the substantive area under study. *Conceptual description*, by contrast, is aimed at describing the full range of behavior of what is occurring in the substantive area.

Some students of Glaser and Strauss have gone on to develop other approaches to grounded theory. These researchers are called second-generation grounded theorists.

Charmaz (2025) regarded Glaser and Strauss's grounded theory as having positivist roots. In Charmaz's **constructivist grounded theory**, she chose the term constructivist to highlight the researcher's involvement in the construction and interpretation of data. The data collected and analyzed are acknowledged to be constructed from shared experiences and relationships between the researcher and the participants. Data and analyses are viewed as social constructions. Reflexivity of both the researcher's own interpretations and the interpretations of the participants is important. Charmaz's grounded theory turns toward social justice inquiry.

Clarke's **situational analysis** (2021) focuses on the situation under study as the key unit of analysis and not on discovering one BSP. Several kinds of analytic maps are made to help understand the complexities of a situation. Situational maps identify human and nonhuman elements in the situation under study. Relational maps focus on the relations among the various elements in the situational maps. In social worlds/arenas maps, the different social groups and sites are identified. Positional maps are used to analyze discursive materials in the situation.

> **Example of a constructivist grounded theory study**
> Mattson and colleagues (2024) used constructivist grounded theory methods to explore the process women used to self-manage recovery from opioid use disorder during pregnancy, the postpartum period, and parenting. The participants described a central process of Growing as a Healthy Dyad, which included six processes to self-manage recovery: maintaining vigilance, performing self-care, pulling in the work of recovery, advocating, navigating social support, and acquiring skills and knowledge.

OTHER TYPES OF QUALITATIVE RESEARCH

Qualitative studies often can be characterized and described in terms of the disciplinary research traditions discussed in the previous section. However, several other important types of qualitative research that are not associated with a particular discipline also deserve mention.

Case Studies

Case studies are in-depth investigations of a single entity or small number of entities. The entity may be an individual, family, institution, or other social unit. Case study researchers attempt to understand issues that are important to the circumstances of the focal entity.

In most studies, whether qualitative or quantitative, certain phenomena or variables are the core of the inquiry. In a case study, the *case* itself is at "center stage." The focus of case studies is typically on understanding *why* a person thinks, behaves, or develops in a particular manner rather than on *what* their status or actions are. Probing research of this type may require study over a considerable period. Data are often collected not only about the person's present state but also about past experiences relevant to the problem being examined.

The greatest strength of case studies is the depth that is possible when a small number of entities are being investigated. Case study researchers can gain an intimate knowledge of a person's feelings, actions, and intentions. Yet, this same strength is a potential weakness: Researchers' familiarity with the case may make objectivity more difficult. Another limitation concerns generalizability: If researchers discover important relationships, it is difficult to know whether the same relationships would occur with others. However, case studies can play a role in challenging generalizations from other types of research.

> **Example of a case study**
> Keefner and colleagues (2024) explored young adults' experiences of suicide attempts during adolescence in the context of spirituality. The researchers used a multiple case study approach with six participants to help understand how they used emotional pain resulting from life challenges to experience self-transcendence.

Narrative Analyses

Narrative analysis focuses on *story* as the object of inquiry to understand how individuals make sense of events in their lives. A basic premise of narrative research is that people most effectively make sense of their world—and communicate these meanings—by narrating stories. Individuals construct stories when they wish to understand specific events and situations that require linking an inner world of needs to an external world of observable actions. Analyzing stories opens up *forms* of telling about experience and is more than just content. Narrative analysts ask, *Why did the story get told that way?* A number of structural approaches can be used to analyze stories, including ones based in literary analysis and linguistics.

> **Example of a narrative analysis**
> Prendergast et al. (2024) conducted a narrative analysis to gain insight into racism experienced by Black nurses in Canada. Personal narratives of 12 Black nurses were gathered and analyzed. The researchers learned that the participants had idealistic beliefs about nursing when they began their professional careers. However, they experienced working in a toxic environment where they felt devalued and treated unfairly by managers, colleagues, and patients.

Historical Research

Historical research is the systematic collection, critical evaluation, and interpretation of historical evidence, or data relating to past occurrences. In general, historical research is undertaken to answer questions about causes, effects, or trends in past events that may shed light on present behaviors or practices. Historical research can take many forms. For example, many nurse researchers have undertaken biographical histories that focus on the lives and contributions of individuals such as nursing leaders. Others undertake social histories that focus on a particular period in attempts to understand prevailing values that may have helped to shape subsequent developments. Still others undertake intellectual or technologic histories.

> **Example of nursing archives**
> The Archives of Nursing Leadership are housed in the Thomas J. Dodd Research Center at the University of Connecticut. The archives include papers and records of Connecticut organizations that support nursing and personal papers of people who contributed significantly to nursing in Connecticut. Letters written by Ella Lousie Wolcott, a Connecticut native who was a nurse during the Civil War, are in the Josephine Dolan Collection within the archive.

> **Example of historical research**
> Larkin and colleagues (2024) investigated the origins of the Boston Training School for Nurses (1873), which was later named the Massachusetts General Hospital (MGH) School of Nursing, and the role played by the Boston civic group Woman's Education Association in its founding. Primary sources of data included the minutes, memoirs, letters, journals, and diary entries from the MGH archives, the Sherwin Collection of the MGH School of Nursing Archives, and the Massachusetts Historical Society.

Descriptive Qualitative Studies

Many qualitative studies claim no particular disciplinary or methodologic roots. The researchers may simply indicate that they have conducted a qualitative study, a naturalistic inquiry, or a *content analysis* or *thematic analysis* of qualitative data (i.e., an analysis of themes and patterns that emerge in the narrative content). Thus, some qualitative studies do not have a formal name or do not fit into the typology we have presented in this chapter. We refer to these as **descriptive qualitative studies**.

Descriptive qualitative studies tend to be eclectic in their methods and are based on the general premises of constructivist inquiry. In descriptive studies, researchers tend not to penetrate their data in any interpretive depth. Descriptive qualitative studies produce findings closer to the data than studies within traditions such as grounded theory or phenomenology (Sandelowski, 2010).

> **Example of a descriptive qualitative study** •
> Baker and colleagues (2024) conducted a qualitative descriptive study to explore the postinjury lives of Black men with disabilities resulting from violent injuries in a hospital-based violence intervention program. Analysis of 10 interviews revealed three themes: perceptions of manhood, loss of independence and burden on others, and mobility.

Research With Ideologic Perspectives

Some qualitative researchers conduct inquiries within an ideologic framework, typically to draw attention to social problems or the needs of certain groups and to bring about change. These approaches represent important investigative avenues.

Critical Theory

Critical theory originated with a group of Marxist-oriented German scholars in the 1920s. Essentially, a critical researcher is concerned with a critique of society and with envisioning new possibilities. Critical research is action oriented. Its aim is to make people aware of contradictions and disparities in social practices and to inspire them to make changes. Critical theory calls for inquiries that foster enlightened self-knowledge and sociopolitical action.

Critical researchers often triangulate methods and emphasize multiple perspectives (e.g., alternative racial or social class perspectives) on problems. Critical researchers typically interact with participants in ways that emphasize participants' expertise.

Critical theory has been applied in several disciplines but has played an especially important role in ethnography. **Critical ethnography** focuses on raising consciousness in the hope of effecting social change. Critical ethnographers attempt to increase the political dimensions of cultural research and undermine oppressive systems.

> **Example of critical ethnography** •
> Hirani (2024) undertook a critical ethnography designed to uncover barriers affecting breastfeeding practices of 27 refugee mothers with young children in Canada. Multiple data collection methods included in-depth interviews, field observations of community-based services/facilities available to refugees, and a review of medical communications. The researcher learned that psychosocial, health care, and environmental barriers led to physiologic challenges and mental health issues that negatively affected breastfeeding practices.

Feminist Research

Feminist research is similar to critical theory research, but the focus is on gender domination and discrimination within patriarchal societies. Similar to critical researchers, feminist researchers seek to establish collaborative and nonexploitative relationships with their informants and to conduct research that is transformative. Feminist investigators seek to understand how gender and a gendered social order have shaped women's lives. The aim is to facilitate change in ways relevant to ending women's unequal social position.

Feminist research methods typically include in-depth, interactive, and collaborative individual or group interviews that offer the possibility of reciprocally educational encounters. Feminists usually seek to negotiate the meanings of the results with those participating in the study and to be self-reflective about what they themselves are learning.

> **Example of feminist research**
> Graf and colleagues (2024) used a Chicana, postcolonial, and Black feminist lens in their study of 34 Latina migrant farmworkers' perception of mental health and their mental health–seeking experiences. Overarching themes included "Mental health is everything," "It is in your mind," "It is when you are like crazy," "It was a problem that had to be suffered alone," and "Praying helped my mental health."

Participatory Action Research

Participatory action research (PAR) is based on the view that the production of knowledge can be used to exert power. PAR researchers typically work with groups or communities that are vulnerable to the control or oppression of a dominant group.

The PAR tradition has as its starting point a concern for the powerlessness of the group under study. In PAR, researchers and participants collaborate in defining the problem, selecting research methods, analyzing the data, and deciding how the findings will be used. The aim of PAR is to produce not only knowledge but also action, empowerment, and consciousness raising.

In PAR, the research methods are designed to facilitate processes of collaboration that can motivate and generate community solidarity. Thus, "data-gathering" strategies are not only the traditional methods of interview and observation but may include storytelling, sociodrama, photography, and other activities designed to encourage people to find creative ways to explore their lives, tell their stories, and recognize their own strengths.

> **Example of participatory action research**
> Nguyen-Truong and coresearchers (2024) used community-based PAR in an effort to examine the readiness of older Asian American immigrants to use a web-based senior center and identify the psychosocial health impacts that this type of senior center could be in a position to meet.

CRITICAL APPRAISAL OF QUALITATIVE DESIGNS

Evaluating a qualitative design is often difficult. Qualitative researchers do not always describe design decisions or the process by which such decisions were made. Researchers often do, however, indicate whether the study was conducted within a specific qualitative tradition. This information can be used to come to some conclusions about the study design. For example, if a report indicated that the researcher conducted 2 months of fieldwork for an ethnographic study, you might suspect that insufficient time had been spent in the field to obtain an emic perspective of the culture under study. Ethnographic studies may also be critiqued if their only source of information was from interviews, rather than from a broader range of data sources, particularly observations.

In a grounded theory study, look for evidence about when the data were collected and analyzed. If the researcher collected all the data before analyzing any of it, you might question whether the constant comparative method was used correctly.

In appraising a phenomenologic study, you should first determine if the study is descriptive or interpretive. This will help you to assess how closely the researcher kept to the basic tenets of that qualitative research tradition. For example, in a descriptive phenomenologic study, did the researcher bracket? When appraising a phenomenologic study, you should also look at its power in capturing the meaning of the phenomena being studied.

No matter what qualitative design is identified in a study, look to see if the researchers stayed true to a single qualitative tradition throughout the study or if they mixed qualitative traditions. For example, did the researcher state that grounded theory was used but then present results that described *themes* instead of a substantive theory?

The guidelines in Box 10.1 are designed to assist you in appraising the design of qualitative studies.

> **Box 10.1 Guidelines for Critically Appraising Qualitative Designs**
>
> a. Was the research tradition for the qualitative study identified? If none was identified, can one be inferred?
> b. Is the research question congruent with a specific research tradition? Are the data sources and research methods congruent with the research tradition?
> c. How well was the research design described? Are design decisions explained and justified? Does it appear that the design emerged during data collection, allowing researchers to capitalize on early information?
> d. Did the design lend itself to a thorough, in-depth examination of the focal phenomenon? Was there evidence of reflexivity? What design elements might have strengthened the study (e.g., a longitudinal perspective rather than a cross-sectional one)?
> e. Was the study undertaken with an ideologic perspective? If so, is there evidence that ideologic goals were achieved (e.g., Was there full collaboration between researchers and participants? Did the research have the power to be transformative?)?

RESEARCH EXAMPLES WITH CRITICAL THINKING EXERCISES

This section presents examples of qualitative studies. Read about the studies and then answer the critical thinking questions, referring to the full research report if necessary. The critical thinking questions for Example 2 are based on the phenomenologic study that appears in its entirety in Appendix B of this book.

EXAMPLE 1: A GROUNDED THEORY STUDY

Study: "Reclaiming self-balancing on a tightrope across time: A grounded theory of transition to survivorship in older adult blood cancer survivors" (Wood, 2025)

Statement of Purpose: The purpose of the study was to develop a theoretical understanding of the process of transition to survivorship for older adult blood cancer survivors.

Method: Classic Glaserian grounded theory was the chosen research design to explain participants' main concern and how they sought to resolve it. Seventeen participants were recruited from the Leukemia and Lymphoma Society community group web pages. Each participant completed an in-depth interview via Zoom. The researcher used theoretical sampling. For example, after the 13th interview, Wood identified that the transition to survivorship process could not be completely understood within the original time span of the first 12 months from diagnosis, so she sought participants beyond 12 months from diagnosis. The constant comparison method was used to analyze the data. First, Wood used open coding until the core category was discovered. Then, she used selective coding to focus only on the core category. Theoretical coding was also used to connect the conceptual categories and the core category.

Key Findings: The main concern identified was the depersonalized experience of diagnosis and surviving a blood cancer that was disruptive and traumatic to one's sense of self. The core category discovered was "reclaiming self-balancing on a tightrope across time." This process involved six phases: receiving a blood cancer diagnosis, finding bearings, reclaiming self, persevering through, realizing a transition, and living in a new reality.

Critical Thinking Exercises

1. Answer the relevant questions from Box 10.1 regarding this study.
2. Comment on the amount of time spent in the field in this study.
3. Could this study have been undertaken as a phenomenologic inquiry?
4. If the results of this study are trustworthy, what are some of the uses to which the findings might be put in clinical practice?

EXAMPLE 2: PHENOMENOLOGIC STUDY IN APPENDIX B

Read the method section from trauma Morrison et al.'s (2024) study, "Lived experiences of fatherhood after infertility," in Appendix B of this book.

Critical Thinking Exercises

1. Answer the relevant questions in Box 10.1 regarding this study.
2. Was this study a descriptive or interpretive phenomenology?
3. Could this study have been conducted as a grounded theory study? As an ethnographic study? Why or why not?
4. Could this study have been conducted as a feminist inquiry? If yes, what might Morrison and colleagues have done differently?

Summary Points

- Qualitative research involves an **emergent design** that develops in the field as the study unfolds. Qualitative studies can be either cross-sectional or longitudinal.

- Ethnography focuses on the culture of a group of people and relies on extensive fieldwork that usually includes **participant observation** and in-depth interviews with *key informants*. Ethnographers strive to acquire an *emic* (insider's) *perspective* of a culture rather than an *etic* (outsider's) *perspective*.

- Nurses sometimes refer to their ethnographic studies as **ethnonursing research**.

- **Autoethnography** is a type of ethnography where researchers study their own culture or group. The focus of **institutional ethnography** is on social organization and institutional processes. **Netnography** focuses on cultural experiences of data from social media environments such as blogs or Facebook.

- Phenomenologists seek to discover the *essence* and *meaning* of a phenomenon as it is experienced by people, mainly through in-depth interviews with people who have had the relevant experience.

- In **descriptive phenomenology**, which seeks to describe lived experiences, researchers **bracketing** out preconceived views and *intuiting* the essence of the phenomenon remain open to meanings attributed to them by those who have experienced them.

- **Interpretive phenomenology (hermeneutics)** focuses on interpreting the meaning of experiences rather than just describing them.

- **Grounded theory** researchers try to account for people's actions by focusing on the main concern that their behavior is designed to resolve. The manner in which people resolve this main concern is the core variable. A prominent type of **core variable** is called a **basic social process (BSP)** that explains the processes of resolving the problem.

- Grounded theory uses **constant comparison**: Categories elicited from the data are constantly compared with data obtained earlier.

- Grounded theory researchers opt to follow either the original approach of Glaser and Strauss (1967) or to use procedures adapted by Corbin and Strauss (2015). Glaser (1992) argued that the latter approach does not result in *grounded theories* but rather in *conceptual descriptions*. More recently, Charmaz's (2025) **constructivist grounded theory** has emerged, emphasizing interpretive aspects in which the grounded theory is constructed from relationships between the researcher and participants. In **situational analysis**, relational maps, social worlds/arenas maps, positional maps, and situational maps are created that identify human and nonhuman elements in the situation under study.

- **Case studies** are intensive investigations of a single entity or a small number of entities, such as individuals, groups, families, or communities.

- **Narrative analysis** focuses on *story* in studies in which the purpose is to determine how individuals make sense of events in their lives.

- **Historical research** is the systematic collection, critical evaluation, and interpretation of historical evidence.

- **Descriptive qualitative studies** are not embedded in a disciplinary tradition. Such studies may be referred to as qualitative studies, naturalistic inquiries, or as qualitative content analyses.

- Research is sometimes conducted within an ideologic perspective. **Critical theory** is concerned with a critique of existing social structures; critical researchers conduct studies in collaboration with participants in an effort to foster self-knowledge and transformation. **Critical ethnography** uses the principles of critical theory in the study of cultures.

- **Feminist research**, like critical research, aims at being transformative, but the focus is on how gender domination and discrimination shape women's lives.

- **Participatory action research (PAR)** produces knowledge through close collaboration with groups that are vulnerable to oppression by a dominant culture; in PAR, a goal is to develop processes that can motivate people and generate community solidarity.

REFERENCES

Baker, N. S., VanHook, C., Ricks, T., St Vil, C., Lassiter, T., & Bonne, S. (2024). Protect and provide: Perceptions of manhood and masculinities among disabled violently injured Black men in a hospital-based violence intervention program. *American Journal of Men's Health*, 18(1), 15579883231221390. https://doi.org/10.1177/15579883231221390

Bennett, C. R., Weaver, C., Coats, H. L., & Hendricks-Ferguson, V. L. (2024). "Music played a role in saving my life and getting me through all of this": A descriptive qualitative study of hope in adolescents and young adults living with advanced cancer. *Journal of Pediatric Hematology/Oncology Nursing*, 41(6), 399–407. https://doi.org/10.1177/27527530241286008

Charmaz, K. (2025). *Constructing grounded theory* (3rd ed.). Sage.

Clarke, A. E. (2021). From grounded theory to situational analysis: What's new? Why? How? In J. M. Morse, B. J. Bowers, K. Charmaz, A. E. Clarke, J. Corbin, & P. N. Stern (Eds.), *Developing grounded theory: The second generation revisited* (pp. 223–266). Routledge.

Corbin, J., & Strauss, A. (2015). *Basics of qualitative research: Techniques and procedures for developing grounded theory* (4th ed.). Sage.

Glaser, B. G. (1978). *Theoretical sensitivity*. Sociology Press.

Glaser, B. G. (1992). *Emergence versus forcing: Basics of grounded theory analysis*. Sociology Press.

Glaser, B. G., & Strauss, A. L. (1967). *The discovery of grounded theory: Strategies for qualitative research*. Aldine.

Graf, M. D. C., Bullis, M. M., Lopez, A. A., Snethen, J., Silvstre, E., & Mikandawire-Valhmu, L. (2024). A qualitative analysis of Latina migrant farmworkers' perception of mental health: Voices from Wisconsin. *Journal of Transcultural Nursing*, 35(1), 11–20. https://doi.org/10.1177/10436596231207490

Hirani, S. A. A. (2024). Barriers affecting breastfeeding practices of refuge mothers: A critical ethnography in Saskatchewan, Canada. *International Journal of Environmental Research and Public Health*, 21, 398. https://doi.org/10.3390/ijerph21040398

Jenkins, S. H., & Astroth, K. S. (2024). An intergenerational comparison of civility: Nursing students and nurse educators. *Journal of Nursing Education*, 63(2), 86–92. https://doi.org/10.3928/01484834-20231205-03

Keefner, T., Minton, M., & Antonen, K. (2024). Embracing emotional pain: A case study of adolescent suicidality and spirituality. *Journal of the American Psychiatric Nurses Association*, 30(2), 397–408. https://doi.org/10.1177/10783903221118932

Kozinets, R. V. (2020). *Netnography: The essential guide to qualitative social media research* (3rd ed.). Sage.

Larkin, M. E., Fisher, S. L., & White, K. R. (2024). Post-civil war maternity and the nurse training movement: The "experiment" of the Boston Training School for Nurses. *Nursing Outlook*, 72, 102148. https://doi.org/10.1016/j.outlook.2024.102148

Leininger, M. M. (Ed.). (1985). *Qualitative research methods in nursing*. Grune and Stratton.

Lincoln, Y. S., & Guba, E. G. (1985). *Naturalistic inquiry*. Sage.

Mattson, N. M., Ohlendork, J. M., & Haglund, K. (2024). Grounded theory approach to understand self-management of opioid recovery though pregnancy and early parenting. *Journal of Obstetric, Gynecologic, and Neonatal Nursing*, 53(1), 34–45. https://doi.org/10.1016/j.jogn.2023.09.001

Monaro, S., West, S., & Gullick, J. (2024). Making decisions about amputation for chronic limb threatening ischaemia. *Journal of Vascular Nursing*, 42, 65–73. https://doi.org/10.1016/j.jvn.2023.11.011

Morse, J. M. (2004). Qualitative comparison: Appropriateness, equivalence, and fit. *Qualitative Health Research*, 14, 1323–1325. https://doi.org/10.1177/1049732304270426

Nguyen-Truong, C. K. Y., Wuestney, K., Leung, H., Chiu, C., Park, M., Chac, C., & Fritz, R. L. (2024). Toward sustaining web-based senior center programming accessibility with and for older adult immigrants: Community-based participatory research cross-sectional study. *Asian/Pacific Island Nursing Journal*, 8, e49493. https://doi.org/10.2196/49493

Prendergast, N., Boakye, P., Bailey, A., & Igwenagu, H. (2024). Anti-Black racism: Gaining insight into the experiences of Black nurses in Canada. *Nursing Inquiry*, 31, e12604. https://doi.org/10.1111/nin.12604

Sandelowski, M. (2010). What's in a name? Qualitative description revisited. *Research in Nursing and Health*, 23, 334–340. https://doi.org/10.1002/nur.20362

Sheen, L. H., Casarez, R., Gallagher, M. R., Hayes, A. E., Diep, C. S., & Engebretson. J. (2024). Understanding diabetes self-management among Vietnamese Americans: A focus ethnography. *Journal of Transcultural Nursing*, 35(2), 142–150. https://doi.org/10.1177/10436596231217698

Soegaard, K., Sig, J. R., Nielsen, C., Verhaeghe, S., Beeckman, D., Biering-Sørensen, F., & Sørensen, J. A. (2024). "I am just trying to live a life!"—A qualitative study of the lived experience of pressure ulcers in people with spinal cord injuries. *Journal of Tissue Viability*, 33(1), 50–59. https://doi.org/10.1016/j.jtv.2023.11.009

Strange, K. E., Mixer, S. J., Embler, P., Smith, J. L., & Troutman-Jordan, M. (2024). Influences of faith on rural Appalachian older adult health: An ethnonursing study. *Journal of Transcultural Nursing*, 35(2), 112–124. https://doi.org/10.1177/10436596231213343

Strauss, A., & Corbin, J. (1990). *Basics of qualitative research: Grounded theory procedures and techniques*. Sage.

Wood, S. K. (2025). Reclaiming self-balancing on a tightrope across time: A grounded theory of transition to survivorship in older adult blood cancer survivors. *Journal of Advanced Nursing*, 81, 366–382. https://doi.org/10.1111/jan.16200

11 Appraising Sampling and Data Collection in Qualitative Studies

Learning Objectives

On completing this chapter, you will be able to:

- Describe the logic of sampling for qualitative studies
- Identify and describe several types of sampling approaches in qualitative studies
- Evaluate the appropriateness of the sampling method and sample size used in a qualitative study
- Identify and describe methods of collecting unstructured self-report data
- Identify and describe methods of collecting and recording unstructured observational data
- Critically appraise a qualitative researcher's decisions regarding the data collection plan
- Define new terms in the chapter

Key Terms

- Data saturation
- Diary
- Field notes
- Focus group interview
- Key informant
- Log
- Maximum variation sampling
- Participant observation
- Photo elicitation
- Photovoice
- Purposive (purposeful) sampling
- Semi-structured interview
- Snowball sampling
- Theoretical sampling
- Think-aloud method
- Topic guide
- Unstructured interview

This chapter covers two important aspects of qualitative studies—sampling (selecting informative study participants) and data collection (gathering the right types and amount of information to address the research question).

SAMPLING IN QUALITATIVE RESEARCH

Qualitative studies typically rely on small nonprobability samples. Qualitative researchers are as concerned as quantitative researchers with the quality of their samples, but they use different considerations in selecting study participants.

The Logic of Qualitative Sampling

Quantitative researchers measure attributes and identify relationships in a population; they desire a representative sample so that findings can be generalized. The aim of most qualitative studies is to discover *meaning* and to uncover multiple realities, not to generalize to a population.

Qualitative researchers ask such sampling questions as, Who would be an *information-rich* data source for my study? Whom should I talk to, or what should I observe, to maximize my understanding of the phenomenon? A first step in qualitative sampling is selecting settings with potential for information richness.

As the study progresses, new sampling questions emerge, such as Whom can I talk to or observe who would confirm, challenge, or enrich my understandings? As with the overall design, sampling design in qualitative studies tends to be an emergent one that capitalizes on early information to guide subsequent action.

 TIP Like quantitative researchers, qualitative researchers identify eligibility criteria for their studies. Although they do not specify an explicit population to whom results could be generalized, they do establish the kinds of people who are eligible to participate in their research.

Types of Qualitative Sampling

Qualitative researchers avoid random samples because they are not the best method of selecting people who are knowledgeable, articulate, reflective, and willing to talk at length with researchers. Qualitative researchers use various nonprobability sampling designs.

Convenience and Snowball Sampling

Qualitative researchers often begin with a *volunteer* (convenience) *sample*. Volunteer samples are often used when researchers want participants to come forward and identify themselves. For example, if we wanted to study the experiences of people with frequent nightmares, we might recruit them by placing a notice on the internet on a relevant website. We would be less interested in obtaining a representative sample of people with nightmares than in recruiting a group with diverse nightmare experiences.

Sampling by convenience is efficient but is not a preferred approach. The aim in qualitative studies is to extract the greatest possible information from a small number of people, and a convenience sample may not provide the most information-rich sources. However, a convenience sample may be an economical way to begin the sampling process.

> **Example of a convenience sample**
> In Sweden, Patriksson and coresearchers (2024) explored midwives' experiences of intact cord resuscitation in nonvigorous neonates after vaginal birth. They used a convenience sample of 13 midwives who had experience with neonatal resuscitation while keeping the umbilical cord intact as they worked close to the birthing parent.

Qualitative researchers also use **snowball sampling** (or *network sampling*), asking early informants to make referrals. A weakness of this approach is that the eventual sample might be restricted to a small network of acquaintances. Also, the quality of the referrals may be affected by whether the referring sample member trusted the researcher and truly wanted to cooperate.

> **Example of a snowball sample**
> In their phenomenologic study, Pekyiğit and colleagues (2024) explored the experiences and needs of parents after perinatal loss in Turkey. Participants were recruited using snowball sampling and resulted in a sample of six mothers and six fathers who had suffered at least one perinatal loss.

Purposive Sampling

Qualitative sampling may begin with volunteer informants and may be supplemented with new participants through snowballing. Many qualitative studies, however, evolve to a **purposive** (or **purposeful**) **sampling** strategy in which researchers deliberately choose the cases or types of cases that will best contribute to the study.

Dozens of purposive sampling strategies have been identified (Patton, 2015), only some of which are mentioned here. Researchers do not necessarily refer to their sampling plans with Patton's labels; his classification shows the diverse strategies qualitative researchers have adopted to meet the conceptual needs of their research:

- **Maximum variation sampling** involves deliberately selecting cases with a range of variation on dimensions of interest.
- *Extreme (deviant) case sampling* provides opportunities for learning from the most unusual and extreme informants (e.g., outstanding successes and notable failures).
- *Typical case sampling* involves the selection of participants who illustrate or highlight what is typical or average.
- *Criterion sampling* involves studying cases who meet a predetermined criterion of importance.

Maximum variation sampling is often the sampling mode of choice in qualitative research because it is useful in illuminating the scope of a phenomenon and in identifying important patterns that cut across variations. Other strategies can also be used advantageously, however, depending on the nature of the research question.

> **Example of maximum variation sampling**
> George et al. (2024) investigated the physical and psychological burden experienced by 12 women on maintenance hemodialysis in India. Maximum variation sampling was used to recruit participants with end-stage renal disease undergoing hemodialysis to facilitate a diverse group in regards to age, marital status, employment, and length of time on hemodialysis.

Sampling confirming and disconfirming cases is another purposive strategy used toward the end of data collection. As researchers analyze their data, emerging conceptualizations sometimes need to be checked. *Confirming cases* are additional cases that fit researchers' conceptualizations and strengthen credibility. *Disconfirming cases* are new cases that do not fit and serve to challenge researchers' interpretations. These "negative" cases may offer insights about how the original conceptualization needs to be revised.

TIP Some qualitative researchers call their sample *purposive* simply because they "purposely" selected people who experienced the phenomenon of interest. Exposure to the phenomenon is, however, an eligibility criterion. If the researcher then recruits *any* person with the desired experience, the sample is selected by convenience, not purposively. Purposive sampling implies an intent to choose *particular* exemplars or *types* of people who can best enhance the researcher's understanding of the phenomenon.

Theoretical Sampling

Theoretical sampling is used in grounded theory studies. Theoretical sampling involves decisions about where to find data to develop an emerging theory. The basic question in theoretical sampling is "What types of people should the researcher turn to next to further the theoretical development of the emerging conceptualization?"

> **Example of a theoretical sampling**
> Ruan and colleagues (2024) used theoretical sampling in their grounded theory study of the process of coping with financial toxicity among 29 young women with breast cancer in China. Purposive sampling was used at the initial state of recruitment, but theoretical sampling was used as the study progressed.

Sample Size in Qualitative Research

Sample size in qualitative research is usually based on informational needs. **Data saturation** involves sampling until no new information is obtained and redundancy is achieved. Data saturation relates to the degree to which new data repeat what was expressed in previous data. Morse (2015) warned that saturation doesn't indicate a researcher saturated the specific details of a participant or individual event but, instead, saturated characteristics within themes or categories.

The number of participants needed to reach saturation depends on various factors. For example, the broader the scope of the research question, the more participants will likely be needed. Data quality can affect sample size: If participants are insightful and can communicate effectively, saturation can be achieved with a relatively small sample. Also, a larger sample is likely to be needed with maximum variation sampling than with typical case sampling.

Depending on which qualitative method a researcher uses, saturation is viewed differently. For example, Dahlberg et al. (2008) stated that data saturation is not part of their phenomenologic research because meanings are viewed as infinite, always expanding so meaning saturation cannot exist. In their thematic analysis, Braun and Clarke (2022) explained that the concept of data saturation is problematic and recommend instead to avoid claiming data are saturated. They prefer the concept of information power (Malterud et al., 2016), which has the researcher reflect on the richness of their data set and how it fits with the aims of their study.

> **Example of data saturation**
> Mage et al.'s (2024) study focused on 14 Latino family caregivers' experiences covering out-of-pocket costs when caring for someone living with dementia. The researchers determined data saturation was met after completion of the ninth interview, as the next two interviews did not provide any new data.

> **TIP** Sample size adequacy in a qualitative study is difficult to evaluate because the main criterion is information redundancy, which consumers cannot judge. Some (but not all) reports explicitly mention that saturation was achieved.

Sampling in the Three Main Qualitative Traditions

There are similarities among the main qualitative traditions with regard to sampling: Small samples and nonrandom methods are used, and final sampling decisions usually take place during data collection. However, there are some differences as well.

Sampling in Ethnography

Ethnographers often begin with a "big net" approach—they mingle and converse with many members of the culture. However, they usually rely heavily on a smaller number of **key informants**, who are knowledgeable about the culture and serve as the researcher's main link to the "inside." Ethnographers may use an initial framework to develop a pool of potential key informants. For example, an ethnographer might decide to recruit different types of key informants based on their *roles* (e.g., nurses, advocates). Once potential key informants are identified, key considerations for final selection are their level of knowledge about the culture and willingness to collaborate with the ethnographer in revealing and interpreting the culture.

Sampling in ethnography typically involves sampling *things* as well as people. For example, ethnographers make decisions about observing *events* and *activities*, about examining *records* and *artifacts*, and about exploring *places* that provide clues about the culture. Key informants often help ethnographers decide what to sample.

> **Example of an ethnographic sample**
> Kaldal and colleagues (2024) conducted an ethnographic study in Denmark of newly graduated nurses' commitment to the nursing profession and their workplace during their first year of employment. In-depth interviews were conducted with 10 newly graduated nurses working in acute care settings along with 94 hours of participant observations.

Sampling in Phenomenologic Studies

Phenomenologists tend to rely on very small samples of participants—typically 15 or fewer. Two principles guide the selection of a sample for a phenomenologic study: (1) All participants must have experienced the phenomenon, and (2) they must be able to articulate what it is like to have lived that experience. Phenomenologic researchers often want to explore diversity of individual experiences, so they may specifically look for people with demographic or other differences who have shared a common experience.

> **Example of a sample in a phenomenologic study**
> In their phenomenologic study, Srichalerm et al. (2024) examined Thai novice nurses' experiences of breastfeeding and human milk in a neonatal intensive care unit (NICU). The researchers recruited a purposive sample of 13 novice nurses working in NICUs in Thailand who had provided breastfeeding support to NICU mothers.

Interpretive phenomenologists may, in addition to sampling people, sample artistic or literary sources. Experiential descriptions of a phenomenon may be selected from literature, such as poetry, novels, or autobiographies. These sources can help increase phenomenologists' insights into the phenomena under study.

Sampling in Grounded Theory Studies

Grounded theory research is typically done with samples of about 20 to 30 people, using theoretical sampling. The goal in a grounded theory study is to select informants who can best contribute to the evolving theory. Sampling, data collection, data analysis, and theory construction occur concurrently, so study participants are selected serially and contingently (i.e., contingent on the emerging conceptualization). Sampling might evolve as follows:

1. The researcher begins with a general notion of where and with whom to start. The first few cases may be sampled by convenience.
2. Maximum variation sampling might be used next to gain insights into the range and complexity of the phenomenon.
3. The sample is continually adjusted: Emerging conceptualizations inform the theoretical sampling process.

4. Sampling continues until saturation is achieved.
5. Final sampling may include a search for confirming and disconfirming cases to test, refine, and strengthen the theory.

Critically Appraising Qualitative Sampling Plans

Qualitative sampling plans can be evaluated in terms of their adequacy and appropriateness (Morse, 1991). *Adequacy* refers to the sufficiency and quality of the data the sample yielded. An adequate sample provides data without "thin" spots. When researchers have truly obtained saturation, informational adequacy has been achieved, and the resulting description or theory is richly textured and complete.

Appropriateness concerns the methods used to select a sample. An appropriate sample results from the selection of participants who can best supply information that meets the study's conceptual requirements. The sampling strategy must yield a full understanding of the phenomenon of interest. A sampling approach that excludes negative cases or that fails to include people with unusual experiences may not fully address the study's information needs.

Another important issue concerns the potential for transferability of the findings. The transferability of study findings is a function of the similarity between the study sample and other people to whom the findings might be applied. Thus, in appraising a report, you should assess whether the researcher provided an adequately *thick description* of the sample and the study context so that someone interested in transferring the findings could make an informed decision. Further guidance in critically appraising qualitative sampling is presented in Box 11.1.

DATA COLLECTION IN QUALITATIVE STUDIES

In-depth interviews are the most common method of collecting qualitative data. Observation is used in some qualitative studies as well. Physiologic data are rarely collected in a constructivist inquiry. Table 11.1 compares the types of data and aspects of data collection used by researchers in the three main qualitative traditions. Ethnographers typically collect a wide array of data, with observation and interviews being the primary methods. Ethnographers also gather or examine products of the culture under study, such as documents, artifacts, photographs, and so on. Phenomenologists and grounded theory researchers rely primarily on in-depth interviews, although observation sometimes plays a role.

Box 11.1 Guidelines for Critically Appraising Qualitative Sampling Plans

a. Was the setting appropriate for addressing the research question, and was it adequately described?
b. What type of sampling strategy was used?
c. Were the eligibility criteria for the study specified? How were participants recruited into the study?
d. Given the information needs of the study—and, if applicable, its qualitative tradition—was the sampling approach effective?
e. Was the sample size adequate and appropriate? Did the researcher indicate that saturation had been achieved? Do the findings suggest a richly textured and comprehensive set of data without any apparent "holes" or thin areas?
f. Were key characteristics of the sample described (e.g., age, gender)? Was a rich description of participants and context provided, allowing for an assessment of the transferability of the findings?

TABLE 11.1 Comparison of Data Collection in Three Qualitative Traditions

Issue	Ethnography	Phenomenology	Grounded Theory
Types of data	Primarily observation and interviews plus artifacts, documents, photographs, social network diagrams	Primarily in-depth interviews, sometimes diaries, other written materials, observations	Primarily individual interviews, sometimes group interviews, observation, diaries, documents
Unit of data collection	Cultural systems	Individuals	Individuals
Data collection points	Cross-sectional or longitudinal	Mainly cross-sectional	Cross-sectional or longitudinal
Length of time for data collection	Typically long, several months or years	Typically moderate	Typically moderate
Data recording	Field notes/logs, interview notes or recordings	Interview notes or recordings	Interview notes or recordings, memos, observational notes
Salient field issues	Gaining entrée, determining a role, learning how to participate, encouraging candor, loss of objectivity, premature exit, reflexivity	Bracketing one's views, building rapport, encouraging candor, listening while preparing what to ask next, keeping "on track," handling emotionality	Building rapport, encouraging candor, listening while preparing what to ask next, keeping "on track," handling emotionality

Qualitative Self-Report Techniques

Qualitative researchers do not have a set of questions that must be asked in a specific order and worded in a given way. Instead, they start with general questions and allow respondents to tell their narratives in a naturalistic fashion. Qualitative interviews tend to be conversational. Interviewers encourage respondents to define the important dimensions of a phenomenon and to elaborate on what is relevant to them.

Types of Qualitative Self-Reports

Researchers use completely **unstructured interviews** when they have no preconceived view of the information to be gathered. Researchers begin by asking a *grand tour question*, such as "What happened when you first learned that you had AIDS?" Subsequent questions are guided by initial responses. Ethnographic and phenomenologic studies often gather data through unstructured interviews.

Semi-structured (or *focused*) interviews are used when researchers have a list of topics or broad questions that must be covered in an interview. Interviewers use a written **topic guide** to ensure that all question areas are addressed. The interviewer's function is to encourage participants to talk freely about all the topics on the guide.

> **Example of a semi-structured interview**
> Ollivier and coresearchers (2024) studied how 11 postpartum individuals understood and made meaning of their experiences surrounding postpartum sexual activities. In their semi-structured interview, the researchers asked questions such as "What emotions do you experience when you think of your sexuality or sexual relationships after having a baby?" Or "Tell me about a time when you thought about your sexual health and sexuality after giving birth."

Focus group interviews involve groups of about 5 to 10 people whose opinions and experiences are solicited simultaneously. The interviewer (or *moderator*) guides the discussion using a topic guide. A group format is efficient and can generate a lot of dialogue, but not everyone is comfortable sharing their views or experiences in front of a group.

Joint interviews involve two or more people being simultaneously questioned (Brown & Gale, 2022). Joint (dyadic) interviews can be helpful when researchers want to observe the dynamics between two participants. A disadvantage is that there may be issues that one person in the dyad does not want to discuss in front of the other person.

> **Example of focus group interviews**
> Missel et al. (2024) explored nursing care practices for patients who underwent thoracic surgery for non-small-cell lung cancer and remained hospitalized despite having recovered somatically. The researchers conducted four focus groups with 16 nurses in Denmark. Two of the researchers led the focus groups, with one as the moderator and the other as assistant moderator in charge of logistics.

Personal **diaries** are a standard data source in historical research. It is also possible to generate new data for a study by asking participants to maintain a diary over a specified period. Diaries can be useful in providing an intimate description of a person's everyday life. The diaries may be completely unstructured; for example, individuals who had an organ transplantation could be asked to spend 15 minutes a day jotting down their thoughts. Frequently, however, people are asked to make diary entries regarding some specific aspect of their lives.

> **Example of diaries**
> In Norway, Daltviet and colleagues (2024) explored burn patients' and burn intensive care nurses' experiences of the photos included in patient diaries written by the nurses. The researchers interviewed six former burn patients and held two focus groups with 11 burn intensive care nurses. The photos in the diaries filled in gaps in patients' memories and told more than words alone could.

Photo elicitation involves an interview guided by photographic images. This procedure, most often used in ethnographies and participatory action research, can help to promote a collaborative discussion. The photographs sometimes are ones that researchers have made of the participants' world, but photo elicitation can also be used with photos in participants' homes. Researchers have also used the technique of asking participants to take photographs themselves and then interpret them, a method sometimes called **photovoice**. Photovoice can be used as a strategy to promote empowerment and give voice to participants to help bring about change at community and policy levels (Kyololo et al., 2023).

> **Example of a photovoice study**
> Photovoice was used by Hladek and colleagues (2024) to explore the living conditions and experiences of 16 older adults with frailty on their kidney transplant journey. Photovoice was used to prompt discussions in individual interviews and also in two focus groups. The visual data helped to clarify the interpretations of the text alone.

The **think-aloud method** is a technique for collecting data about cognitive processes, such as thinking, problem-solving, and decision making (Fonteyn et al., 1993). Think-aloud is essentially designed to "eavesdrop" on a person's thinking. This method involves having people use recording devices to discuss decisions as they are being made or while problems are being solved.

Gathering Qualitative Self-Report Data

Researchers gather narrative self-report data to develop a construction of a phenomenon that is consistent with that of participants. This goal requires researchers to overcome communication barriers and to enhance the flow of information. Although qualitative interviews are conversational, the conversations are purposeful ones that require preparation. For example, the wording of questions should reflect the participants' worldview and language. In addition to being good questioners, researchers must be good listeners. Only by attending carefully to what respondents are saying can in-depth interviewers develop useful follow-up questions.

Unstructured interviews are typically long, sometimes lasting an hour or more, so an important issue is how to record such abundant information. Some researchers take notes during the interview, but this is risky in terms of data accuracy. Most researchers record the interviews for later transcription. Although some respondents are self-conscious when their conversation is recorded, they typically forget about the presence of recording equipment (often a cell phone) after a few minutes.

In addition to the possibility of soliciting narrative data on the internet through structured and semi-structured interview methods, a potential rich data source for qualitative researchers involves narrative self-reports available directly on the internet. Some data that can be analyzed qualitatively are simply "out there" in social media posts, blogs, or online forums.

Using the internet to access narrative data has obvious advantages. This approach is economical and allows researchers to obtain information from geographically dispersed and perhaps remote internet users. However, a number of ethical concerns have been raised, and authenticity and other methodologic challenges need to be considered. Kristiansen (2022) suggested a tentative framework of ethical decision making when using internet-mediated data collection methods.

> **Example of blog analysis** •
> Beck (2025), one of the authors of this textbook, conducted a qualitative study to describe the experiences of survivors of placenta accreta as written in their blogs. Content analysis of 22 blogs identified seven themes that provided an insider's view of placenta accreta: "the shock of it all," "living in constant fear," "advocate for yourself to get some sense of control," "my mental health is deteriorating," "you saved our lives," "recommendations," and "posttraumatic growth."

 TIP Although qualitative self-report data are often gathered in face-to-face interviews, they can also be collected in writing. Internet "interviews" are also possible.

Evaluation of Qualitative Self-Report Methods

In-depth interviews are a flexible approach to gathering data and, in many research contexts, offer distinct advantages. In clinical situations, for example, it is often appropriate to let people talk freely about their problems and concerns, allowing them to take the initiative in directing the flow of conversation. Unstructured self-reports may allow investigators to ascertain what the basic issues or problems are, how sensitive or controversial the topic is, how individuals conceptualize and talk about the problems, and what range of opinions or behaviors exist relevant to the topic. In-depth interviews may also help elucidate the underlying meaning of a relationship repeatedly observed in more structured research. On the other hand, qualitative methods are very time-consuming and demanding of researchers' skills in gathering, analyzing, and interpreting the resulting data.

Qualitative Observational Methods

Qualitative researchers sometimes collect loosely structured observational data, often as a supplement to self-report data. The aim of qualitative observation is to understand the behaviors and experiences of people as they occur in naturalistic settings. Skillful observation permits researchers to see the world as participants see it, to develop a rich understanding of the focal phenomenon, and to grasp subtleties of cultural variation.

Unstructured observational data are often gathered through **participant observation**. Participant observers take part in the functioning of the group under study and strive to observe, ask questions, and record information within the contexts and structures that are relevant to group members. Participant observation is characterized by prolonged periods of social interaction between researchers and participants. By assuming a participating role, observers often have insights that would have eluded more passive or concealed observers.

 TIP Not all qualitative observational research is *participant* observation (i.e., with observations occurring from *within* the group). Some unstructured observations involve watching and recording behaviors without the observers' active participation in activities. Be on the alert for the misuse of the term "participant observation." Some researchers use the term inappropriately to refer to all unstructured observations conducted in the field.

The Observer–Participant Role in Participant Observation

In participant observation, the role that observers play in the group is important because their social position determines what they are likely to see. The extent of the observers' actual participation in a group is best thought of as a continuum. At one extreme is complete immersion in the setting, with researchers assuming full participant status; at the other extreme is complete separation, with researchers as onlookers. Researchers may in some cases assume a fixed position on this continuum throughout the study, but often researchers' role evolves toward increasing participation over the course of the fieldwork.

Observers must overcome two major hurdles in assuming a satisfactory role in the group. The first is to gain entrée into the group under study; the second is to establish rapport and trust within that group. Without gaining entrée, the study cannot proceed, but without the group's trust, the researcher will be restricted to "front stage" knowledge—information distorted by the group's protective facades. The goal of participant observers is to "get backstage"—to learn the true realities of the group's experiences. On the other hand, being a fully participating member does not *necessarily* offer the best perspective for studying a phenomenon—just as being an actor in a play does not offer the most advantageous view of the performance.

Gathering Participant Observation Data

Participant observers typically place few restrictions on the nature of the data collected, but they often have a broad plan for types of information desired. Among the aspects of an observed activity likely to be considered relevant are the following:

1. *The physical setting—Where questions.* What are the main features of the setting?
2. *The participants—Who questions.* Who is present and what are their characteristics?
3. *Activities—What questions.* What is going on? What are participants doing?
4. *Frequency and duration—When questions.* When did the activity begin and end? Is the activity a recurring one?
5. *Process—How questions.* How is the activity organized? How does it unfold?
6. *Outcomes—Why questions.* Why is the activity happening? What did not happen (especially if it ought to have happened) and why?

Participant observers must decide how to sample events and select observational locations. They often use a variety of positioning approaches—staying in a single location to observe activities in that location (*single positioning*), moving around to observe behaviors from different locations (*multiple positioning*), or following a person around (*mobile positioning*).

Direct observation is usually supplemented with information from interviews. For example, key informants may be asked to describe what went on in a meeting the observer was unable to attend or to describe an event that occurred before the study began. In such cases, the informant functions as the observer's observer.

Recording Observations

The most common forms of record keeping for participant observation are logs and field notes, but photographs and video recordings may also be used. A **log** (or *field diary*) is a daily record of events and conversations. **Field notes** are broader and more interpretive. Field notes represent the observer's efforts to record information and to synthesize and understand the data.

Field notes serve multiple purposes. *Descriptive notes* are objective descriptions of events and conversations that were observed. *Reflective notes* document researchers' personal experiences, reflections, and progress in the field. For example, some notes document the observers' interpretations; others are reminders about how future observations should be made. Observers often record personal notes, which are comments about their own feelings during the research process.

The success of participant observation depends on the quality of the logs and field notes. It is essential to record observations as quickly as possible, but participant observers cannot usually record information by openly carrying a clipboard or a recording device because this would undermine their role as ordinary participants. Observers must develop skills in making detailed mental notes that can later be written or recorded.

Evaluation of Unstructured Observational Methods

Qualitative observational methods—especially participant observation—can provide a deeper understanding of human behaviors and social situations than is possible with structured methods. Participant observation offers opportunities to delve deeply into a situation and illuminate its complexities. Participant observation can answer questions about phenomena that are difficult for insiders themselves to explain because these phenomena are taken for granted.

Like all research methods, however, participant observation faces potential problems. Observers may lose objectivity in sampling, viewing, and interpreting observations. Once they begin to participate in a group's activities, emotional involvement might become a concern. Researchers in their member role may develop a myopic view on issues of importance to the group. Finally, the success of participant observation depends on the observer's observational and interpersonal skills—skills that may be difficult to cultivate.

> **Example of participant observation**
> Thiengtham and coresearchers (2024) conducted an ethnographic study in Thailand to examine the experiences of Thai-Isan older stroke survivors and their family caregivers across different points in the transition from hospital to home. In addition to semi-structured interviews with 15 dyads, the researchers used participant observation in their study. The researchers observed the participants' activities, conversations, and interactions during hospitalization and during home care.

Critical Appraisal of Unstructured Data Collection

It is often difficult to critically appraise the decisions that researchers made in collecting qualitative data because details about those decisions are seldom spelled out. In particular, there is often scant information about participant observation. It is not uncommon for a report to simply say that the researcher undertook participant observation, without descriptions of how much time was spent in the field, what exactly was observed, how observations were recorded, and what level of participation was involved. Thus, one aspect of an appraisal is likely to involve an evaluation of how much information the article provided about the data collection methods. Even though space constraints in journals make it impossible for researchers to fully elaborate their methods, researchers have a responsibility to communicate basic information about their approach so that readers can assess the quality of evidence that the study yields. Researchers should provide examples of questions asked and types of observations made.

Triangulation of methods provides important opportunities for qualitative researchers to enhance the integrity of their data. Thus, an important issue to consider in evaluating unstructured data is whether the types and amount of data collected are sufficiently rich to support an in-depth, holistic understanding of the phenomena under study. Box 11.2 provides guidelines for appraising the collection of unstructured data.

Box 11.2 Guidelines for Critically Appraising Data Collection Methods in Qualitative Studies

a. Given the research question and the characteristics of study participants, did the researcher use the best method of capturing study phenomena (i.e., self-reports, observation)? Should supplementary methods have been used to enrich the data available for analysis?
b. If self-report methods were used, did the researcher make good decisions about the specific method used to solicit information (e.g., unstructured interviews, focus group interviews, and so on)?
c. If a topic guide was used, did the report present examples of specific questions? Did the wording of questions encourage rich responses?
d. Were interviews recorded and transcribed? If interviews were not recorded, what steps were taken to ensure data accuracy?
e. If observational methods were used, did the report adequately describe what the observations entailed? What did the researcher actually observe, in what types of setting did the observations occur, and how often and over how long a period were observations made?
f. What role did the researcher assume in terms of being an observer and a participant? Was this role appropriate?
g. How were observational data recorded? Did the recording method maximize data quality?

RESEARCH EXAMPLES WITH CRITICAL THINKING EXERCISES

In this section, we describe the sampling plan and data collection strategies used in a qualitative nursing study. For Example 1, read the summary and then answer the critical thinking questions that follow, referring to the full research report if necessary. The critical thinking questions for Example 2 are based on the study that appears in its entirety in Appendix B of this book.

EXAMPLE 1: SAMPLING AND DATA COLLECTION IN A QUALITATIVE STUDY

Study: "The relationship between urban greenspace perception and use within the adolescent population: A focused ethnography" (Lyons et al., 2024)

Statement of Purpose: The aim of the study was threefold: to understand why adolescents use greenspace, to identify how they use greenspace, and to explore how they feel when they are in greenspace.

Design: The researchers used a focus ethnography method to identify new concepts from the participants' emic perspective. Culture in ethnography included a population of adolescents in a natural setting where they lived and where greenspace was available or used.

Sampling Strategy: A purposive sampling strategy was used to obtain 11 adolescents aged 12 to 18 years who lived in Newark, New Jersey. Recruitment occurred near a youth program that focused on developing critical workface skills and helping adolescents develop stewardship in greenspace as park ambassadors. The gatekeeper was a horticulturist and chief operating officer of the regional youth program. He helped to identify potential participants.

Data Collection: Photo elicitation, semi-structured interviews, and observation were the three primary modes of data collection. The researcher collected data over a 5-week period in the summer. Participants were asked to take photographs of what they perceived as greenspace and how they used it. Participants also kept a journal to record any events or reminders about when and why they took the photographs. In-person semi-structured interviews were conducted with the adolescents once their photos were developed. The questions in the interview focused on asking the adolescents to discuss their photographs. The researcher also observed participants in greenspace 3 to 4 days a week for 6 hours per day. Fieldnotes were kept to record the observations.

Key Findings: The researchers identified three themes: (1) tranquil space in an unsafe place, (2) parks mean family connection with burgeoning independence, and (3) my park: sense of ownership and responsibility.

Critical Thinking Exercises

1. Answer the relevant questions from Box 11.1 regarding this study.
2. Answer the relevant questions from Box 11.2 regarding this study.
3. Comment on the researchers' overall data collection plan in terms of the amount of information gathered.
4. If the results of this study are valid and trustworthy, what might be some of the uses to which the findings could be put in clinical practice?

EXAMPLE 2: SAMPLING AND DATA COLLECTION IN THE STUDY IN APPENDIX B

Read the method section from Morrison et al.'s (2024) study, "Lived experience of fatherhood after infertility" in Appendix B of this book.

1. Answer the relevant questions in Box 11.1 regarding this study.
2. Answer the relevant questions in Box 11.2 regarding this study.
3. Comment on the characteristics of the participants, given the purpose of the study.
4. Do you think that Morrison and colleagues should have limited their sample to women from one country only? Provide a rationale for your answer.
5. Did Morrison et al.'s study involve a "grand tour" question?

Summary Points

- Qualitative researchers typically select articulate and reflective informants with relevant experiences in an emergent way, capitalizing on early learning to guide subsequent sampling decisions.

- Qualitative researchers may start with convenience or **snowball sampling** but usually rely eventually on **purposive sampling** to guide them in selecting data sources that maximize information richness.

- One purposive strategy is **maximum variation sampling**, which entails purposely selecting cases that are diverse on key traits. Another important strategy is *sampling confirming and disconfirming cases*—that is, selecting cases that enrich and challenge the researchers' conceptualizations.

- Samples in qualitative studies are typically small and based on information needs. A guiding principle is **data saturation**, which involves sampling to the point at which no new information is obtained and redundancy is achieved.

- Ethnographers make numerous sampling decisions, including not only *whom* to sample but also *what* to sample (e.g., activities, events, documents, artifacts); decision making is often aided by **key informants** who serve as guides and interpreters of the culture.

- Phenomenologists typically work with a small sample of people (usually 15 or fewer) who meet the criterion of having lived the experience under study.

- Grounded theory researchers typically use **theoretical sampling** in which sampling decisions are guided in an ongoing fashion by the emerging theory. Samples of about 20 to 30 people are typical.

- In-depth interviews are the most widely used method of collecting data for qualitative studies. Self-reports in qualitative studies include completely **unstructured interviews**, which are conversational discussions on the topic of interest; **semi-structured** (or *focused*) interviews, using a broad **topic guide; focus group interviews**, which involve discussions with small groups; **diaries**, in which respondents are asked to maintain daily records about some aspects of their lives; and **photo elicitation** interviews, which are guided and stimulated by photographic images, sometimes using photos that participants themselves take (**photovoice**). The **think-aloud method** is a technique for collecting data about cognitive processes, such as thinking, problem-solving, and decision making.

- In qualitative research, self-reports are often supplemented by direct observations in naturalistic settings. One type of unstructured observation is **participant observation**, in which the researcher gains entrée into a social group and participates to varying degrees in its functioning while making in-depth observations of activities and events. **Logs** of daily events and **field notes** of the experiences and interpretations are the major data collection documents.

REFERENCES

Beck, C. T. (2025). Survivors of placenta accreta: What blogs can tell us. *Journal of Perinatal Education*. 34(1), 6–14. https://doi.org/10.1891/JPE-2023-0037

Braun, V., & Clarke, V. (2022). *Thematic analysis: A practical guide*. Sage.

Brown, K. S., & Gale, J. (2022). Dyadic interviews: A chronological review of the literature with research recommendations. *Journal of Ethnography and Qualitative Research*, 16, 196–206.

Dahlberg, K., Dahlberg, H., & Nystrom, M. (2008). *Reflective lifeworld research*. Studentlitteratur.

Daltviet, S., Kleppe, L., Petterteig, M. O., & Moi, A. L. (2024). Photographs in burn patient diaries: A qualitative study of patients' and nurses' experiences. *Intensive & Critical Care Nursing*, 82, 10333619. https://doi.org/10.1016/j.iccn.2023.103619

Fonteyn, M. E., Kuipers, B., & Grobe, S. J. (1993). A description of think aloud method and protocol analysis. *Qualitative Health Research*, 3(4), 430–441. https://doi.org/10.1177/104973239300300403

George, S., Nalini, M., Kumar, S., D'Silva, F., & Shenoy, P. (2024). Physical and psychosocial burden experienced by women on maintenance hemodialysis. *Journal of Education and Health Promotion*, 12, 456. https://doi.org/10.4103/jehp.jehp_1449_22

Hladek, M. D., Wilson, D., Krasnansky, K., McDaniel, K. M., Shanbhag, M., McAdams-DeMarco, M., Crews, D. C., Brennan, D. C., Taylor, J., Segev, D., Walston, J., Xue, Q. L.,

& Szanton, S. L. (2024). Using photovoice to explore the lived environment and experience of older adults with frailty on their kidney transplant journey. *Kidney*, *360*(5), 589–598. https://doi.org/10.34067/kid.0000000000000380

Kaldal, M. H., Voldbjerg, S. L., Gronkjaer, M., Conroy, T., & Feo, R. (2024). Newly graduated nurses' commitment to the nursing profession and their workplace during their first year of employment: A focused ethnography. *Journal of Advanced Nursing*, *80*(3), 1058–1071. https://doi.org/10.1111/jan.15883

Kristiansen, S. (2022). Qualitative online data collection: Towards a framework of ethical decision-making. *The Qualitative Report*, *27*(12), 2686–2700. https://doi.org/10.46743/2160-3715/2022.5048

Kyololo, O. M., Stevens, B. J., & Songok, J. (2023). Photo-elicitation technique: Utility and challenges in clinical research, *International Journal of Qualitative Methods*, *22*, 1–8. https://doi.org/10.46743/2160-3715/2022.5048

Lyons, R., Colbert, A., Browning, M., & Jakub, K. (2024). The relationship between urban greenspace perception and use within the adolescent population: A focused ethnography. *Journal of Advanced Nursing*, *80*, 2869–2879. https://doi.org/10.1111/jan.15905

Mage, S., Benton, D., Gonzalez, A., Zaragoza, G., Wilber, K., Tucker-Seeley, R., & Meyer, K. (2024). "I lay awake at night": Latino family caregivers' experiences covering out-of-pocket costs when caring for someone living with dementia. *The Gerontologist*, *64*, 1–11. https://doi.org/10.1093/geront/gnad011

Malterud, K., Siersma, V. D., & Guassora, A. D. (2016). Sample size in qualitative interview studies: Guided by information power. *Qualitative Health Research*, *26*(13), 1753–1760. https://doi.org/10.1177/1049732315617444

Missel, M., Donsel, P. O., Petersen, R. H., & Beck, M. (2024). Ready to go home? Nurses' perspectives of prolonged admission for patients undergoing video-assisted thoracic surgery for non-small-cell lung cancer in Denmark. *Qualitative Health Research*, *34*(11), 1096–1107. https://doi.org/10.1177/10497323231191709

Morse, J. M. (1991). Strategies for sampling. In J. M. Morse (Ed.), *Qualitative nursing research: A contemporary dialogue* (pp. 127–145). Sage.

Morse, J. M. (2015). "Data were saturated…". *Qualitative Health Research*, *25*(5), 587–588. https://doi.org/10.1177/1049732315576699

Ollivier, R., Aston, M., Price, S., Shepppard-LeMoine, D., & Steenbeek, A. (2024). "Feeling ready": A feminist post-structural analysis of postpartum sexual health. *Qualitative Health Research*, *34*(3), 252–262. https://doi.org/10.1177/10497323231209842

Patriksson, K., Andersson, O., Stierna, F., Haglund, K., & Thies-Lagergren, L. (2024). Midwives' experiences of intact cord resuscitation in nonvigorous neonates after vaginal birth in Sweden. *Journal of Obstetric, Gynecologic, and Neonatal Nursing*, *53*, 255–263. https://doi.org/10.1016/j.jogn.2023.12.003

Patton, M. Q. (2015). *Qualitative research & evaluation methods* (4th ed.). Sage.

Pekyiğit, A., Yildiz, D., Deniz, A. Ö., & Bağriyanik, B. C. (2024). White tears: A phenomenological study of perinatal loss. *OMEGA—Journal of Death and Dying*, 302228241234381. https://doi.org/10.1177/00302228241234381

Ruan, J., Liu, C., Yang, Z., Kuang, Y., Yuan, X., Oiu, J., Tang, L., & Xing, W. (2024). Suffering and adjustment: A grounded theory study of the process of coping with financial toxicity among young women with breast cancer. *Supportive Care in Cancer*, *32*, 96. https://doi.org/10.1007/s00520-024-08305-9

Srichalerm, T., Jacelon, C. S., Sibeko, L., Granger, J., & Briere, C. E. (2024). Thai novice nurses' lived experiences and perspectives of breastfeeding and human milk in the Neonatal Intensive Care Unit. *International Breastfeeding Journal*, *19*, 20. https://doi.org/10.1186/s13006-024-00620-5

Thiengtham, S., Chiang-Hanisko, L., D'Avolio, D., & Sritanyarat, W. (2024). Experience of transitional care among Thai-Isan older stroke survivors and their family caregivers. *Qualitative Health Research*, *34*(12), 1191–1202. https://doi.org/10.1177/10497323241232937

12 Understanding Mixed Methods Research, Quality Improvement, and Other Special Types of Research

Learning Objectives

On completing this chapter, you will be able to:

- Understand the advantages of mixed methods research and describe specific applications
- Describe strategies and designs for conducting mixed methods research
- Distinguish research and quality improvement (QI), and describe QI strategies
- Identify the purposes and some of the distinguishing features of specific types of research (e.g., clinical trials, evaluations, outcomes research, surveys)
- Define new terms in the chapter

Key Terms

- Clinical trial
- Comparative effectiveness research (CER)
- Convergent design
- Delphi survey
- Economic (cost) analyses
- Evaluation research
- Explanatory sequential design
- Exploratory sequential design
- Health services research
- Improvement science
- Intervention research
- Intervention theory
- Methodologic study
- Mixed methods research
- Nursing sensitive outcome
- Outcomes research
- Patient-centered outcomes research
- Plan-Do-Study-Act (PDSA)
- Pragmatism
- Process analyses
- Quality improvement (QI)
- Root cause analysis (RCA)
- Secondary analysis
- Sequential design
- Survey

In this final chapter on research designs, we explain several special types of research. We begin by discussing mixed methods research that combines qualitative and quantitative approaches.

MIXED METHODS RESEARCH

A growing trend in nursing research is the planned collection and integration of qualitative and quantitative data within a single study or coordinated clusters of studies. This section discusses the rationale for such **mixed methods research** and presents a few applications.

Rationale for Mixed Method Research

The dichotomy between quantitative and qualitative data represents a key methodologic distinction. It is now widely believed, however, that many areas of inquiry can be enriched by integrating qualitative and quantitative data. The advantages of a mixed methods (MM) design include the following:

- *Complementarity.* Qualitative and quantitative data are complementary. By using MM, researchers can avoid the limitations of a single approach.
- *Practicality.* Given the complexity of phenomena, it is practical to use whatever methodologic tools are best suited to addressing pressing research questions.
- *Enhanced validity.* When a hypothesis or model is supported by multiple and complementary types of data, researchers can be more confident about their inferences.

Perhaps the strongest argument for MM research, however, is that some questions *require* MM. The paradigm called **pragmatism** is often associated with MM research—a paradigm that some consider offers an "umbrella worldview" for a study (Creswell & Plano Clark, 2018, p. 69). Pragmatist researchers consider that it is the research question that should drive the research design. They reject a forced choice between the traditional positivist and constructivist modes of inquiry.

Purposes and Applications of Mixed Methods Research

In MM research, there are inevitably at least two research questions, each of which requires a different approach. For example, MM researchers may ask both exploratory (qualitative) and confirmatory (quantitative) questions. In an MM study, researchers can examine causal *effects* in a quantitative component but can shed light on causal *mechanisms* in a qualitative component. In addition to mono-method questions, MM studies ideally ask a specific MM question relating to the integration of qualitative and quantitative data and that makes explicit what will be answered through such integration.

Creswell and Plano Clark (2018) identified seven broad types of research situations that are especially well suited to MM research. Here are a few examples:

1. Neither a qualitative nor a quantitative approach, by itself, is adequate in addressing the complexity of the research problem.
2. The findings from one approach can be greatly enhanced with a second source of data that has explanatory power.
3. Quantitative results from an intervention study require qualitative data to help to explain and interpret the results.
4. A program (or formal instrument) needs to be developed and evaluated.

As this list suggests, MM research can be used in various situations. Some major applications include the following:

- *Hypothesis generation.* In-depth qualitative studies are often fertile with insights about constructs and relationships among them. These insights then can be tested with larger samples in quantitative studies.
- *Explication.* Qualitative data are sometimes used to explicate the *meaning* of quantitative relationships. Quantitative methods can demonstrate that variables are systematically related but may fail to explain *why* they are related.
- *Instrument development.* Nurse researchers sometimes gather qualitative data as the basis for generating construct-valid questions for quantitative scales that are then subjected to rigorous testing.
- *Intervention development.* Qualitative research also plays an important role in the development of nursing interventions that are then rigorously tested for efficacy.

> **Example of mixed methods in intervention development research**
> Cuzco et al. (2021) describe a mixed method protocol they will implement to understand patients' lived experiences of being discharged from an intensive care unit in Spain. They will use the data obtained from these interviews to develop an intervention aimed at reducing patients' anxiety and depression levels during the discharge process.

Mixed Method Designs and Strategies

In designing MM studies, researchers make many important decisions. We briefly describe a few.

Design Decisions and Notation

Two decisions in MM design concern sequencing and prioritization. There are three options for sequencing components of an MM study: Qualitative data are collected first, quantitative data are collected first, or both types are collected simultaneously. When the data are collected at the same time, the approach is convergent. The design is sequential when the two types of data are collected in phases. In well-conceived **sequential designs**, the analysis and interpretation in one phase informs the collection of data in the second.

In terms of prioritization, researchers decide which approach—qualitative or quantitative—to emphasize. One option is to give the two components (*strands*) equal, or roughly equal, weight. Usually, however, one approach is given priority. The distinction is sometimes referred to as *equal status* versus *dominant status*.

Morse (1991) proposed a notation system for sequencing and prioritization. In this system, priority is designated by upper- and lowercase letters: QUAL/quan designates an MM study in which the dominant approach is qualitative, whereas QUAN/qual designates the reverse. If neither approach is dominant (i.e., both are equal), the notation is QUAL/QUAN. Sequencing is indicated by the symbols + or →. The arrow designates a sequential approach. For example, QUAN → qual is the notation for a primarily quantitative MM study in which qualitative data are collected in phase 2. When both approaches occur concurrently, a plus sign is used (e.g., QUAL + quan).

Specific Mixed Methods Designs

Numerous design typologies have been proposed by different MM methodologists. We illustrate the three core designs described by Creswell and Plano Clark (2018): convergent, explanatory sequential, and exploratory sequential.

The purpose of the **convergent design** is to obtain different, but complementary, data about the central phenomenon under study. The goal of this design is to converge on "the truth" about a problem or phenomenon by allowing the limitations of one approach to be offset by the strengths of the other. In this design, qualitative and quantitative data are collected simultaneously, with equal priority (QUAL + QUAN).

> **Example of a convergent design**
> Mandal and Seethalakshmi (2023) conducted a mixed method study using a convergent design to explore the link of environmental constraints with missed nursing care. They randomly selected 225 nurses involved in direct patient care across four acute care hospitals in India and had them complete a survey that specifically addressed missed care. They used maximum variation sampling to conduct in-depth interviews with 12 nurses to further explore their experiences with missed care.

Explanatory sequential designs are sequential designs with quantitative data collected in the first phase, followed by qualitative data collected in the second phase. Either the qualitative or the quantitative strand can be given a stronger priority: The design can be either QUAN → qual or quan → QUAL. In explanatory designs, qualitative data from the second phase are used to build on or explain the quantitative data from the initial phase. This design is especially suitable when results are complex and tricky to interpret.

> **Example of an explanatory sequential design**
> Zhang and colleagues (2023) conducted a sequential explanatory mixed method design to explore the multidimensional aspects of caregiver burden among family caregivers of people experiencing advanced cancer in a palliative care context. The research team recruited family caregivers meeting inclusion criteria from a palliative care department in a tertiary hospital in China. After collecting quantitative data from a total of 150 caregivers, the researchers invited a subgroup of 22 caregivers to participate in semi-structured interviews.

Exploratory sequential designs are sequential MM designs, with qualitative data being collected first. The design has as its central premise the need for initial in-depth exploration of a phenomenon, often to better understand contextual or cultural issues relevant to a phenomenon. Its intent is to use rich contextualized information to inform the development of a quantitative feature, such as a new measure, survey, intervention, or digital tool such as a website or app. The overall design of the previously described MM project by Cuzco et al. (2021) would be considered exploratory sequential. The first phase includes collection of qualitative data from critical care units across three tertiary-level hospitals in Spain. The data from these interviews will inform the development and implementation of the empowerment intervention for patients being discharged from critical care units.

Other Mixed Methods Designs

In addition to the three core designs, Creswell (2022) added complex designs as other types of MM designs. In these complex designs, one or more core designs are embedded within a larger framework or another methodology. Examples of complex designs can include embedded core designs into an experimental study or into an evaluation study or a participatory action research study.

Morse (2012, 2017) has argued that a qualitative-qualitative MM study is a legitimate form of inquiry, using either a simultaneous (her term for convergent) or sequential design. One of the qualitative methods is a complete design such as grounded theory or phenomenology, and the other is a supplemental design that is not sufficiently complete to stand on its own.

Sampling and Data Collection in Mixed Methods Research

Sampling and data collection in MM studies are often a blend of approaches described in earlier chapters. A few special issues for an MM study merit brief discussion.

MM researchers can combine sampling designs in various ways. The quantitative component is likely to rely on a sampling strategy that enhances the researcher's ability to generalize from the sample to a population. For the qualitative component, MM researchers usually adopt purposive sampling methods to select people who are good informants about the phenomenon of interest. Sample sizes are also likely to be different in the qualitative and quantitative strands, with larger samples for the quantitative component. A unique sampling issue in MM studies concerns whether the same people will be in both the strands. The best strategy depends on the study purpose and research design, but using overlapping samples can be advantageous. Indeed, a popular strategy is a *nested* approach in which a subset of participants from the quantitative strand is included in the qualitative strand.

> **Example of nested sampling**
> LeBlanc and colleagues (2022) conducted an explanatory sequential MM study to understand how social networks influence therapeutic self-care behaviors and health among older people in the Northeast United States who are living with multiple long-term conditions. They first conducted 89 telephone interviews with adults older than 65 years of age and then used a nested sample of 12 participants to conduct follow-up open-ended interviews.

In terms of data collection, all of the data collection methods discussed previously can be creatively combined and triangulated in an MM study. Thus, possible sources of data include group and individual interviews, psychosocial scales, observations, biophysiologic measures, records, diaries, and so on. MM studies can involve *intramethod mixing* (e.g., structured and unstructured self-reports) and *intermethod mixing* (e.g., biophyisologic measures and unstructured observation). A fundamental issue concerns the methods' complementarity—that is, having the limitations of one method be balanced and offset by the strengths of the other.

TIP One challenge in doing MM research concerns how best to analyze the qualitative and quantitative data. The benefits of MM research require an effort to merge results from the two strands and to develop interpretations and recommendations based on integrated understandings.

QUALITY IMPROVEMENT

Quality improvement (QI) involves assessments of a problem in patient care with the aim of improving clinical care and patient outcomes within a health care organization. A decade ago, there was a lot of discussion in nursing journals about the differences and similarities among QI, research, and evidence-based practice projects. All three have a lot in common, notably the use of systematic methods of solving health problems with an overall aim of fostering improvements in health care.

Shirey and colleagues (2011) created a comparison chart describing the similarities and differences of the three types of efforts on over 20 dimensions. On some dimensions, the differences noted in the chart continue to be relevant. For example, one issue is whether approval from an ethics committee is needed. Most QI efforts are not subject to the regulations protecting human subjects in research, and patient informed consent is typically not obtained.

On other dimensions, however, differences between QI and research are becoming less clear-cut. For example, one dimension on the comparison chart was "expectations for knowledge dissemination." A decade ago, publication in a professional journal was considered by many a criterion for classifying something as "research" rather than QI, but this is no longer the case. Many QI projects are described in professional journals, and several journals are now devoted specifically to improvement activities.

A related dimension on which QI, evidence-based practice, and research were compared by Shirey and colleagues (2011) was the generalizability of the knowledge gained from the project. Their chart stated that knowledge from QI is not generalizable—it is specific to the organization in which the QI is undertaken. However, the growing interest in health care improvement has led to efforts to inspire more systematic, rigorous, theoretical, and replicable improvement activity—in short, to develop improvement science (Marshall et al., 2015). Increasingly, improvement researchers are developing their own base of QI evidence.

Features of Quality Improvement and Improvement Science

QI projects typically have as their primary goal the swift attainment of positive change in a health care service. QI projects are practical and typically focus on a specific problem identified in a local context. QI can also involve an ongoing process in which interprofessional teams collaborate to improve systems and processes, with the goals of reducing waste, increasing efficiency, and improving satisfaction. The ongoing nature of such efforts is integral to a quality management philosophy called *continuous quality improvement* (CQI). CQI encourages members of health care teams to continuously ask such questions as, "How are we doing?" and "Can we do this better?"

Several features characterize many QI projects. For example, the intervention or protocol for an improvement project can change as it is being evaluated to incorporate new ideas and insights—unlike what occurs in a research study. Another feature is that QI projects are designed to achieve an improvement that is sustainable. Typically, QI projects are interprofessional, involving a team with diverse perspectives on a problem.

For the past decade, a growing group of advocates have been promoting improvement science as a distinct discipline. Marshall and colleagues (2015) argued that improvement science "aims to generate local wisdom and generalisable or transferable knowledge with robust, well established research methods applied in highly pragmatic ways" (p. 419). They and other commentators have noted that QI projects are often methodologically weak and called for the adoption of a more scientific approach to health care improvement. Kline and Payne (2020) view improvement science as a partner in basic and clinical research. The field of implementation science continues to expand significantly (Chambers & Emmons, 2024).

 TIP Considering nurses are the largest segment of the health care workforce and spend the most time with patients, they are being encouraged to not only participate in QI efforts, but also to play a lead role (Sherwood, 2021).

Efforts to improve quality and safety in health care organizations have involved a wide variety of strategies to effect positive change. QI interventions include (1) provider education (teaching health care teams how best to manage particular situations), (2) provider reminders (providing decision support materials to prompt health care professionals to undertake some action), (3) patient education (increasing patient's understanding of a prevention or treatment strategy), (4) patient reminders (reminding patients to keep appointments or adhere to regimens), and (5) structural changes (creating care coordination or case management systems).

Example of reminders and education in a quality improvement project ••••
Pfingstag (2024) conducted a QI project aimed at increasing the catch-up HPV vaccination rate for those aged 19 to 26 years at a sexual and reproductive health clinic. To do so, they implemented electronic health record prompts, in-clinic education, and the scheduling of a follow-up visit.

Quality Improvement Planning Tools

During the planning of QI initiatives, a major issue is the identification of a problem on which to focus. This is likely to involve discussions with key stakeholders, brainstorming, a review of institutional trends, a search for relevant evidence, and the creation of flowcharts and process maps.

Once a problem or process has been selected for improvement, the QI team usually tries to investigate the *causes* of the problem. It is difficult to develop solutions to institutional problems without understanding the underlying factors contributing to them. QI teams often undertake what is called a **root cause analysis (RCA)**, which involves efforts to identify underlying process deficiencies (Haxby & Shuldham, 2018).

One tool for identifying the root cause of a problem is a process called the *5 Whys*. The process begins by identifying the specific problem and then asking why the problem happens. If the answer fails to get to the underlying cause, "Why" is asked again. Figure 12.1 shows an example for the problem "Oral mucosal injury related to an endotracheal tube (ETT) holder."

QI teams use such tools to determine the causes of undesirable outcomes and to understand why current practices deviate from best practices. Then, the team can consider specific aspects of a problem that will be addressed.

Quality Improvement Approaches

QI projects typically are based on one of several broad models to guide processes and activities. For example, health care institutions have used the *lean approach* (also called the *Toyota Production System*) in efforts to achieve improved quality and efficiency at lower costs. A major feature of lean is that it strives to eliminate three types of waste: (1) unnecessary actions, (2) unevenness and variability in product or in flow of information, and (3) unreasonableness of a process for a person's capability. The goal of a lean process is to eliminate non–value-added steps, to identify what "value" means to customers (patients), and to serve customers' needs.

The most widely used QI model in health care is **Plan-Do-Study-Act (PDSA)**, which is sometimes called *Plan-Do-Check-Act* (PDCA). The PDSA cycle was originally introduced as a framework for CQI in business and manufacturing. Typically, PDSA relies on multiple *rapid cycles* of investigating and acting on a problem. The idea underpinning

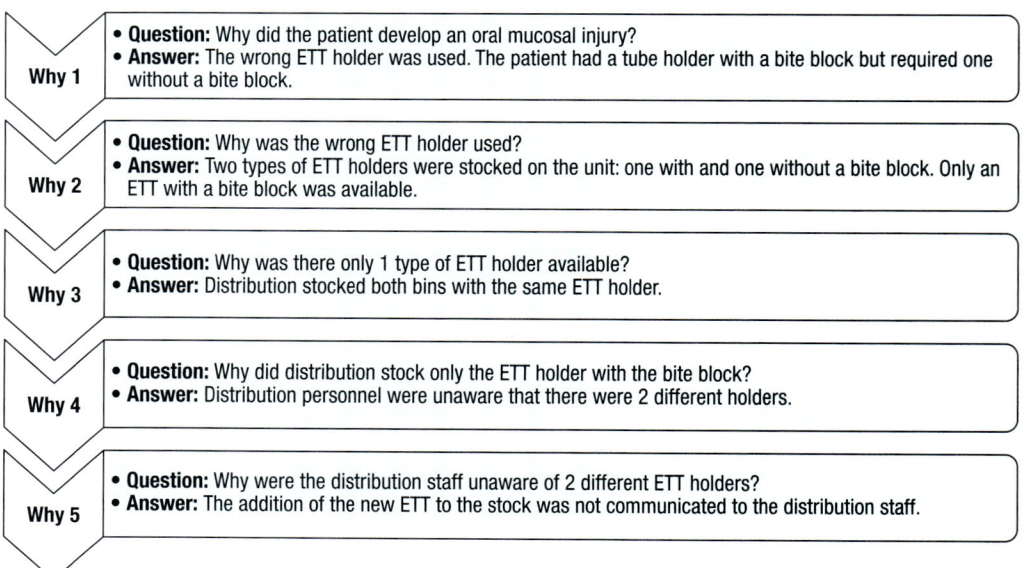

Figure 12.1 The 5 Whys for an oral mucosal injury related to an endotracheal tube (ETT) holder. (Reprinted with permission from Whiteman, K., Yaglowski, J., & Stephens, K. [2021]. Critical thinking tools for quality improvement projects. *Critical Care Nurse*, *41*[2], e1–e9. https://doi.org/10.4037/ccn2021914. Copyright ©2021 by the American Association of Critical-Care Nurses. All rights reserved. Used with permission.)

rapid cycle improvement is to first try an improvement strategy on a small scale to see how well it works and then modify it and try it again until there is confidence in the effectiveness of the change.

PDSA allows the QI team to test improvement strategies in a controlled manner, to measure results of these strategies, and to drive further improvements. The PDSA/PDCA process involves the following:

1. **Plan:** The QI team initially works on developing explicit strategies or interventions to address the problem identified before the project gets underway. During this phase, the team also develops a plan for data collection and identifies measures that will be used to assess improvement. Baseline (pre-QI intervention) data typically are collected during this phase.
2. **Do:** The team then implements the QI intervention and collects data on key outcomes to assess whether improvement occurred. In a PDSA cycle, each improvement is tested on a fairly small scale.
3. **Study/Check:** Data from the trial run are analyzed to see if a positive change occurred.
4. **Act:** If the QI project resulted in improved outcomes, the team considers how best to sustain (and perhaps disseminate) the practice change. If no improvements were observed, or were modest, the team would work through the PDSA/PSCA cycle again, starting with decisions on what changes to make next.

Many QI projects use simple research designs. Conducting projects within real-world health care settings makes it challenging to use powerful designs, but those who promote a more rigorous approach are urging QI teams to consider designs that offer better internal validity. Randomized controlled trials (RCTs) are rare in the field of QI, but they do exist. RCTs are especially suitable when an improvement intervention is being considered for widespread use based on early evidence.

Most QI teams adopt quasi-experimental designs to test the effectiveness of changes to systems or processes of care. Before–after designs, which measure changes to key outcomes after implementing a QI intervention, are especially common, but they are notably weak designs. Time series–type designs are especially useful for sorting out the effects of seasonal or cyclical trends from QI intervention effects.

> **Example of a quality improvement project** •
> Pratt and Howard-Ruben (2024) collaborated with an interdisciplinary team from two hospitals in the midwestern United States to assess and treat postoperative nausea and vomiting (PONV). They used a pre/postimplementation QI design and the Donabedian structure–process–outcomes and quality-of-care model to institute a PONV preoperative assessment checklist and a PONV management protocol. Findings indicated that PONV rates decreased from 56% to 43.6% during the project implementation phase.

 TIP Many QI projects use MM designs that involve collecting both qualitative and quantitative data. Qualitative methods are especially well suited during the planning phase and during the "Act" phase when the QI team must consider what to do next.

OTHER SPECIAL TYPES OF RESEARCH

The remainder of this chapter briefly describes types of research that vary by study purpose rather than by research design or tradition.

Intervention Research

In Chapter 8, we discussed RCTs and other designs for testing the effects of interventions. In actuality, intervention research is often more complex than a simple experimental–control group comparison of outcomes—indeed, intervention research often relies on MM to develop, refine, test, and understand the intervention and its effects.

Different disciplines have developed their own approaches and terminology in connection with intervention efforts. *Clinical trials* are associated with medical research, *evaluation research* is linked to the fields of education and public policy, and nurses are developing their own tradition of intervention research. We briefly describe these three approaches.

Clinical Trials

Clinical trials test clinical interventions. Clinical trials that are undertaken to evaluate an innovative therapy or drug are often designed in a series of phases:

- *Phase I* of the trial is designed to establish safety, tolerance, and dose with a simple design (e.g., one-group pretest–posttest). The focus is on developing the best treatment.
- *Phase II* is a pilot test of treatment effectiveness. Researchers see if the intervention is feasible and holds promise. This phase is designed as a small-scale experiment or quasi-experiment.
- *Phase III* is a full experimental test of the intervention—an RCT with random assignment to treatment conditions. The objective is to develop evidence about the treatment's *efficacy*—that is, whether the intervention is more efficacious than usual care or an alternative. When the term *clinical trial* is used, it often is referring to a phase III trial.
- *Phase IV* of clinical trials involves studies of the *effectiveness* of an intervention in the general population. The emphasis in effectiveness studies is on the external validity of an intervention that has demonstrated efficacy under controlled (but artificial) conditions.

Evaluation Research

Evaluation research focuses on developing useful information about a program or policy—information that decision makers need on whether to adopt, modify, or abandon the program.

Evaluations are undertaken to answer various questions. Questions about program effectiveness rely on experimental or quasi-experimental designs, but other questions do not. Many evaluations are MM studies with distinct components.

For example, a **process analysis** is often undertaken to obtain descriptive information about the process by which a program gets implemented and how it actually functions. A process analysis addresses such questions as the following: What exactly *is* the treatment, and how does it differ from traditional practices? What are the barriers to successful program implementation? How do staff and clients feel about the intervention? Qualitative data play a big role in process analyses.

Evaluations may also include an **economic** (or **cost**) **analysis** to assess whether program benefits outweigh its monetary costs. Administrators make decisions about resource allocation for health services not only on the basis of whether something "works" but also based on economic viability. Cost analyses are often done when researchers are also evaluating program efficacy.

> **Example of an economic analysis**
> Iovino and colleagues (2024) assessed the cost effectiveness of a nurse-delivered heart failure self-care education program compared to usual care. The nurse-led program was aimed at improving the outcomes for people living in Italy with heart failure. They

conducted a cost analysis examining data over a 20-year period and found that nurse-led program resulted in an extra cost of $1.356 million while gaining 247 quality-adjusted life years compared with usual care, and the incremental cost-effectiveness ratio was greater than $5,700 per quality-adjusted life year.

TIP Some nurse researchers have begun to undertake a *realist evaluation*, which is a theory-driven approach to evaluating programs—especially complex programs or interventions. The realist approach acknowledges that interventions are not always effective for everyone because people are diverse and embedded in complicated social and cultural contexts. In a realist evaluation, the focus is on understanding why certain groups benefited from an intervention, whereas others did not benefit.

Nursing Intervention Research

Both clinical trials and evaluations involve *interventions*. However, the term **intervention research** is increasingly being used by nurse researchers to describe an approach characterized by a distinctive *process* of planning, developing, and testing interventions—especially *complex interventions*. Proponents of the process are critical of the simplistic, atheoretical approach that is often used to design and evaluate interventions. The recommended process involves an in-depth understanding of the problem and the target population; careful, collaborative planning with a diverse team; and the development or adoption of a theory to guide the inquiry.

Similar to clinical trials, nursing intervention research that involves the development of a complex intervention typically involves several phases: (1) basic developmental research, (2) pilot research, (3) evaluation of intervention efficacy, and (4) implementation research.

Conceptualization, a major focus of the development phase, is supported through collaborative discussions, consultations with experts, critical literature reviews, and in-depth qualitative research to understand the problem. The construct validity of the intervention is enhanced through efforts to develop an **intervention theory** that clearly articulates what must be done to achieve desired outcomes. The intervention design, which emerges from the intervention theory, specifies what the clinical inputs should be. During the developmental phase, key *stakeholders*—people who have a stake in the intervention—are often identified and "brought on board." Stakeholders include potential beneficiaries of the intervention and their families, advocates and community leaders, and health care staff.

The second phase of nursing intervention research is a pilot test of the intervention. The central activities during the pilot test are to secure preliminary evidence of the intervention's benefits, to assess the feasibility of a rigorous test, and to refine the intervention theory and intervention protocols. The feasibility assessment should involve an analysis of factors that affected implementation during the pilot (e.g., recruitment, retention, and adherence problems). Qualitative research can be used to gain insight into how the intervention should be refined.

As in a classic clinical trial, the third phase involves a full experimental test of the intervention. The final phase focuses on implementation and effectiveness in real-world clinical settings.

Example of nursing intervention research •
D'Avolio and colleagues (2023) conducted a pilot test on an 8-week nurse-coached intervention aimed at improving (1) family caregiver stress and well-being and (2) the nutritional status via increased protein intake for the caregiver and care recipient dyad.

> All family caregivers received information on stress reduction, and each dyad received nutrition education and a protein prescription of 1.2 g/kg body weight/day. In addition, those randomized to the coached group received weekly nutrition and stress-reduction coaching.

Comparative Effectiveness Research

Comparative effectiveness research (CER) involves direct comparisons of two or more health interventions. Like realist approaches, CER seeks insights into which intervention works best for which patients. CER has emerged as a major force in health research. Disappointment with some of the methods favored for evidence-based practice—especially the strong reliance on tightly controlled RCTs with placebo comparators—has led to the development of new ideas, new models, and new methods of research that fall within the umbrella of CER.

The impetus for CER in the United States crystallized when the Institute of Medicine published a report (2009) that proposed priorities for CER. CER was defined as follows: "Comparative effectiveness research (CER) is the generation and synthesis of evidence that compares the benefits and harms of alternative methods to prevent, diagnose, treat, and monitor a clinical condition or to improve the delivery of care. The purpose of CER is to assist consumers, clinicians, purchasers, and policy makers to make informed decisions that will improve health care at both the individual and population level" (p. 41).

Another major stimulus for CER in the United States was the creation in 2010 of the independent nonprofit organization, the *Patient-Centered Outcomes Research Institute* (PCORI). PCORI specifically sponsors CER—in fact, CER is sometimes referred to as **patient-centered outcomes research**. PCORI funds research that is designed to help patients select the health care options that best meet their needs. CER studies often incorporate outcomes that are especially important to patients and their caregivers. The standard outcomes used in medical research (e.g., blood pressure, mortality) are increasingly being supplemented by outcomes in which patients have a strong interest, such as functional limitations, quality of life, and experiences with care.

Designs for CER vary widely. Some studies are RCTs involving a comparison of two or more active (nonplacebo) treatments. Some CER projects, however, are observational studies using data from large databases, such as patient registries. CER is described at greater length in Chapter 18.

> **Example of comparative effectiveness research**
> Chen and colleagues (2023) conducted a randomized clinical trial in China to compare the effectiveness of Tai Chi Chuan versus fitness walking for improving cognitive function in older adults with type 2 diabetes and mild cognitive impairment.

Health Services and Outcomes Research

Health services research is the broad interdisciplinary field that studies how organizational structures and processes, health technologies, social factors, and personal behaviors affect access to health care, the cost and quality of health care, and, ultimately, people's health and well-being. **Outcomes research**, a subset of health services research, comprises efforts to understand the end results of particular health care practices and to assess the effectiveness of health care services. Outcomes research represents a response to the increasing demand from policy makers and the public to justify care practices in terms of improved patient outcomes and costs.

Many nursing studies evaluate patient outcomes, but efforts to appraise the quality and impact of nursing care—as distinct from care provided by the overall health care system—are less common. A major obstacle is attribution—that is, linking patient outcomes to specific nursing actions, distinct from those of other members of the health care team. It is also often difficult to ascertain a causal connection between outcomes and health care interventions because factors outside the health care system (e.g., patient characteristics) affect outcomes in complex ways.

Donabedian (1987), whose pioneering efforts created a framework for outcomes research, emphasized three factors in appraising quality in health care services: structure, process, and outcomes. The *structure* of care refers to broad organizational and administrative features. Nursing skill mix, for example, is a structural variable that has been found to be related to patient outcomes. *Processes* involve aspects of clinical management and decision making. *Outcomes* refer to specific clinical end results of patient care. Much progress has been made in identifying **nursing sensitive outcomes**—patient outcomes that improve if there is greater quantity or quality of nurses' care.

Several modifications to Donabedian's (1987) framework for appraising health care quality have been proposed, the most noteworthy of which is the Quality Health Outcomes Model developed by the American Academy of Nursing (Mitchell et al., 1998). This model is more dynamic than Donabedian's original framework and takes client characteristics (e.g., illness severity) and system characteristics into account.

Outcomes research usually concentrates on studying linkages within such models rather than on testing the overall model. Some studies have examined the effect of health care structures on health care processes or outcomes, for example. Outcomes research in nursing often has focused on the process–patient–outcomes nexus. Examples of nursing process variables include nursing actions, nurses' problem-solving and decision making, clinical competence and leadership, and specific activities or interventions (e.g., communication, touch).

> **Example of outcomes research**
> Labrague et al. (2024) conducted a descriptive, cross-sectional study, enrolling 1,237 nurses in Oman to explore the mediating role of adherence to clinical safety guidelines within the nurse practice environment and missed nursing care. They found that a positive nurse practice environment was associated with outcomes of higher adherence to clinical safety guidelines and less frequency of missed nursing care.

Survey Research

A **survey** obtains quantitative information about the prevalence, distribution, and interrelations of variables within a population. Political opinion polls are examples of surveys. Survey data are used primarily in correlational studies and are often used to gather information from nonclinical populations (e.g., college students, nurses).

Surveys obtain information about people's actions, knowledge, intentions, and opinions by self-report. Surveys may be either cross-sectional or longitudinal. Any information that can reliably be obtained by direct questioning can be gathered in a survey, although surveys include mostly closed-ended questions and thus yield quantitative data primarily.

Survey data can be collected in various ways, but the most respected method is through personal interviews in which interviewers meet in person with respondents to ask them questions. Personal interviews are expensive because they involve a lot of personnel time, but they yield high-quality data and refusal rates tend to be low. Telephone interviews are less costly, but when the interviewer is unknown, respondents may be uncooperative on the phone. Self-administered questionnaires (especially those delivered over the internet) are an economical approach to doing a survey but are not appropriate for surveying certain populations (e.g., the elderly, children) and tend to yield especially low response rates.

The greatest advantage of surveys is their flexibility and broadness of scope. Surveys can be used with many populations and can focus on a wide range of topics. The information obtained in surveys, however, tends to be relatively superficial: Surveys rarely probe deeply into complexities of human behavior and feelings.

> **Example of a survey**
> Lake and colleagues (2023) surveyed 148 clinicians from federally qualified health centers to explore their practice related to recommending HPV vaccination for patients across age groups ranging from 9 to 45 years. They sought to specifically examine factors associated with HPV vaccination recommendation in 9- to 10-year-old patients.

A Few Other Types of Research

Most quantitative nursing studies are the types described thus far in this and earlier chapters. However, nurse researchers have pursued a few other specific types of research, as briefly described here.

- **Secondary analysis**. Secondary analyses involve the use of existing data from a previous or ongoing study to test new hypotheses or answer questions that were not initially envisioned. Secondary analyses are often based on quantitative data from a large data set (e.g., from national surveys), but secondary analyses of data from qualitative studies are also undertaken.
- **Delphi surveys**. Delphi surveys were developed as a tool for short-term forecasting. The technique involves a panel of experts who are asked to complete several rounds of questionnaires focusing on their judgments about a topic of interest. Multiple iterations are used to achieve consensus.
- **Methodologic studies**. Nurse researchers have undertaken many methodologic studies, which focus on the development, validation, and assessment of methodologic tools or strategies (e.g., the psychometric testing of a new scale).

CRITICAL APPRAISAL OF STUDIES DESCRIBED IN THIS CHAPTER

It is difficult to provide guidance on appraising the types of studies described in this chapter because they are so varied and because many fundamental methodologic issues require an appraisal of the overall design. Guidelines for evaluating design-related issues were presented in previous chapters.

You should, however, consider whether researchers took appropriate advantage of the possibilities of an MM design. Collecting both qualitative and quantitative data is not always necessary or practical, but in appraising studies, you can consider whether the study would have been strengthened by integrating different types of data. In studies in which MM were used, you should carefully consider whether the inclusion of both types of data was justified and whether the researcher really made use of both types of data to enhance knowledge on the research topic. Box 12.1 offers a few specific questions for appraising the types of studies included in this chapter.

Box 12.1 Guidelines for Critically Appraising Studies Described in Chapter 12

a. Was the study exclusively qualitative or exclusively quantitative? If so, could the study have been strengthened by incorporating both approaches?
b. If the study used an MM design, did the inclusion of both approaches contribute to enhanced validity? In what other ways (if any) did the inclusion of both types of data strengthen the study and further the aims of the research?
c. If the study used an MM approach, what was the design—how were the components sequenced, and which had priority? Was this approach appropriate?
d. In a QI project, were adequate methods used to identify the root cause of the problem being addressed? Was PDSA (or another QI model) used to guide the process, and was it used appropriately? Was a good research design used to assess the effects of the QI changes?
e. If the study was a clinical trial or intervention study, was adequate attention paid to developing an appropriate intervention? Was there a well-conceived intervention theory that guided the endeavor? Was the intervention adequately pilot tested?
f. If the study was a clinical trial, evaluation, or intervention study, was there an effort to understand how the intervention was implemented (i.e., a process-type analysis)? Were the financial costs and benefits assessed? If not, should they have been?
g. If the study was outcomes research, which segments of the structure–process–outcomes model were examined? Would it have been desirable (and feasible) to expand the study to include other aspects? Do the findings suggest possible improvements to structures or processes that would be beneficial to patient outcomes?
h. If the study was a survey, was the most appropriate method used to collect the data (i.e., in-person interviews, telephone interviews, mail or internet questionnaires)?

RESEARCH EXAMPLES WITH CRITICAL THINKING EXERCISES

The nursing literature abounds with studies of the types described in this chapter. Here, we describe an example. Read the summary, and then answer the critical thinking questions that follow, referring to the full research report if necessary.

EXAMPLE 1: MIXED METHODS STUDY

Study: "Feasibility of a nurse-coached walking intervention for informal dementia caregivers" (Flanagan et al., 2022)

Statement of Purpose: The purpose of this study was to investigate the feasibility of a nurse-coached walking intervention for informal caregivers of people experiencing dementia. The study had two aims: (1) to determine the feasibility of a nurse-coached walking program using wireless pedometers to track steps in informal caregivers of people experiencing dementia and (2) to understand participants' overall experience of participating in a walking program using wireless pedometers.

Method: The study used an explanatory sequential MM (QUANT→ QUAL) design to enroll a total of 32 participants who were provided a wearable tracking device and randomly assigned to either a nurse-coached or control group. The control group received information about the benefits of walking, whereas those in the intervention group received this education plus weekly coaching via telephone or text message. At the end of the intervention phase, all participants were qualitatively interviewed to gain insights into the intervention.

Data Analysis and Integration: Statistical methods were used to answer the first research question. For example, descriptive statistics were used to characterize the demographics of the sample. The outcome measures (e.g., number of steps/miles walked) were examined for the intervention and control group separately before calculating the mean values at the start and at the end of the study. Then, the *t*-test statistic for the two groups and the associated *p*-values were calculated along with Cohen's *d* to determine effect size. The second aim was addressed using a content analysis of the qualitative data concerning the participants' experiences of the walking program intervention. After determining codes and identifying categories, themes were developed. The qualitative data provided insights into aspects of the walking intervention that were impossible to understand based on the quantitative data alone.

Key Findings: A statistical difference was noted in the number of steps walked ($p = .01$ control; $p = .02$ intervention) with a large effect size (0.90). However, there were no statistical differences noted in the other outcome measures and moderate effect size in perceived stress (0.51). The feasibility of the intervention was supported by adherence to pedometer use, self-reported user ease with technology, and a 100% retention rate. However, four themes indicated that there were challenges not captured in the quantitative data, including participants' reports of loneliness and grief and a need to connect with others who understood their experiences.

Critical Thinking Exercises

1. Answer the relevant questions from Box 12.1 regarding this study.
2. What might be an advantage of using a sequential rather than a concurrent design in this study?
3. If the results of this study are valid, what are some of the uses to which the findings might be put in clinical practice?

Summary Points

- **Mixed methods (MM) research** involves the collection, analysis, and integration of both qualitative and quantitative data within a study or series of studies, often with an overarching goal of achieving both discovery and verification.

- MM research has numerous advantages, including the complementarity of qualitative and quantitative data and the practicality of using methods that best address a question. MM research has many applications, including the development and testing of instruments, theories, and interventions.

- The paradigm most often associated with MM research is **pragmatism**, which has as a major tenet "the dictatorship of the research question."

- Key decisions in designing an MM study involve how to sequence the components and which strand (if either) will be given priority. In terms of sequencing, MM designs are either **convergent** (both strands occurring in one simultaneous phase) or **sequential** (one strand occurring prior to and informing the second strand).

- Notation for MM research often designates priority—all capital letters for the dominant strand and all lowercase letters for the nondominant strand—and sequence. An arrow is used for sequential designs, and a "+" is used for concurrent designs. QUAL → quan, for example, is a sequential, qualitative-dominant design.

- Core MM designs include the **convergent design** (e.g., QUAL + QUAN), **explanatory sequential design** (e.g., QUAN → qual), and **exploratory sequential design** (e.g., QUAL → quan).

- Sampling in MM studies can involve the same or different people in the different strands. *Nesting* is a common sampling approach in which a subsample of the participants in the QUAN strand also participates in the QUAL strand.

- **Quality improvement (QI)** projects are designed to improve practices in a specific organization. The growing interest in rigorous QI projects has led to the emergence of **improvement science**, the discipline devoted to the systematic generation of evidence for cultivating positive changes in health care institutions.

- During the planning phase of a QI study, the team can use various strategies to understand the problem, such as a **root cause analysis (RCA)**, which is designed to understand underlying process deficiencies.

- The most widely used QI model in health care is called **Plan-Do-Study-Act (PDSA)** (or *Plan-Do-Check-Act* [PDCA]), which involves multiple *rapid cycles* of improvements and testing. Designs for QI projects are usually quasi-experimental.

- Different disciplines have developed different approaches to (and terms for) efforts to evaluate interventions. **Clinical trials**, which are studies designed to assess clinical interventions, often involve a series of phases. *Phase I* is designed to finalize features of the intervention. In *Phase II*, researchers seek preliminary evidence of efficacy and feasibility. *Phase III* is a full experimental test of treatment *efficacy*. In *Phase IV*, the researcher focuses primarily on generalized *effectiveness*.

- **Evaluation research** focuses on the efficacy of a program, policy, or procedure to assist decision makers in choosing a course of action. Evaluations can answer a variety of questions. **Process analyses** describe the process by which a program gets implemented and how it functions in practice. **Economic (cost) analyses** seek to determine whether the monetary costs of a program are outweighed by benefits. *Realist evaluations* constitute a theory-driven approach to evaluating programs; the focus is on understanding why certain groups benefited from an intervention and others did not.

- **Intervention research** is a term sometimes used to refer to a distinctive *process* of planning, developing, testing, and disseminating interventions—especially *complex interventions*. The construct validity of an emerging intervention is enhanced through efforts to develop an **intervention theory** that conceptualizes what must be done to achieve desired outcomes.

- **Comparative effectiveness research (CER)** involves direct comparisons of health interventions to gain insights into which work best for which patients—as well as which have greater risks of harm. The PCORI is a major funder of CER, which is sometimes referred to as **patient-centered outcomes research**.

- Outcomes research (a subset of **health services research**) is undertaken to document the quality and effectiveness of health care and nursing services. A model of health care quality encompasses several broad concepts: *structure* (e.g., nursing skill mix), *process* (nursing interventions and actions), and *outcomes* (the specific end results of patient care in terms of patient functioning). Efforts have been made to identify **nursing sensitive outcomes**.

- **Survey** research examines people's characteristics, behaviors, intentions, and opinions by asking them to answer questions. Surveys can be administered through personal (face-to-face) interviews, telephone interviews, or self-administered questionnaires.

REFERENCES

Chambers, D. A., & Emmons, K. M. (2024). Navigating the field of implementation science towards maturity: Challenges and opportunities. *Implementation Science*, 19(1), 26. https://doi.org/10.1186/s13012-024-01352-0

Chen, Y., Qin, J., Tao, L., Liu, Z., Huang, J., Liu, W., Xu, Y., Tang, Q., Liu, Y., Chen, Z., Chen, S., Liang, S., Chen, C., Xie, J., Liu, J., Chen, L., & Tao, J. (2023). Effects of Tai Chi Chuan on cognitive function in adults 60 years or older with type 2 diabetes and mild cognitive impairment in China: A randomized clinical trial. *JAMA Network Open*, 6(4), e237004. https://doi.org/10.1001/jamanetworkopen.2023.7004

Creswell, J. W. (2022). *A concise introduction to mixed methods research* (2nd ed.). Sage.

Creswell, J. W., & Plano Clark, V. L. (2018). *Designing and conducting mixed methods research* (3rd ed.). Sage.

Cuzco, C., Castro Rebollo, P., Marín Pérez, R., Núñez Delgado, A. I., Romero García, M., Martínez Momblan, M. A., Estrada Reventós, D., Martínez Estalella, G., & Delgado-Hito, P. (2021). Mixed-method research protocol: Development and evaluation of a nursing intervention in patients discharged from the intensive care unit. *Nursing Open*, 8(6), 3666–3676. https://doi.org/10.1002/nop2.894

D'Avolio, D., Gropper, S. S., Appelbaum, M., Thiengtham, S., Holt, J., & Newman, D. (2023). The impact of a pilot telehealth coaching intervention to improve caregiver stress and well-being and to increase dietary protein intake of caregivers and their family members with dementia—Interrupted by COVID-19. *Dementia*, 22(4), 1241–1258. https://doi.org/10.1177/14713012231177491

Donabedian, A. (1987). Some basic issues in evaluating the quality of health care. In L. T. Rinke (Ed.), *Outcome measures in home care* (Vol. I, pp. 3–28). National League for Nursing.

Flanagan, J., Post, K., Hill, R., & DiPalazzo, J. (2022). Feasibility of a nurse coached walking intervention for informal dementia caregivers. *Western Journal of Nursing Research*, 44(5), 466–476. https://doi.org/10.1177/01939459211001395

Haxby, E., & Shuldham, C. (2018). How to undertake a root cause analysis investigation to improve patient safety. *Nursing Standard*, 32, 41–46. https://doi.org/10.7748/ns.2018.e10859

Institute of Medicine. (2009). *Initial priorities for comparative effectiveness research*. The National Academies Press.

Iovino, P., D'Angelo, D., Vellone, E., & Ruggeri, M. (2024). A cost-effectiveness analysis of community nurse-led self-care education for heart failure patients. *Collegian*, 31(4), 258–266. https://doi.org/10.1016/j.colegn.2024.05.003

Kline, J. N., & Payne, A. S. (2020). Improvement science is a partner in basic and clinical research. *Journal of Investigative Medicine*, 68(3), 724–727. https://doi.org/10.1136/jim-2019-001260

Labrague, L. J., Al Sabei, S., AbuAlRub, R., Burney, I., & Al Rawajfah, O. (2024). The role of nurses' adherence to clinical safety guidelines in linking nurse practice environment to missed nursing care. *Journal of Nursing Scholarship: An Official Publication of Sigma Theta Tau International Honor Society of Nursing*, 57(2), 354–362. https://doi.org/10.1111/jnu.13017

Lake, P., Fuzzell, L., Brownstein, N. C., Fontenot, H. B., Michel, A., McIntyre, M., Whitmer, A., Rossi, S. L., Perkins, R. B., & Vadaparampil, S. T. (2023). HPV vaccine recommendations by age: A survey of providers in federally qualified health centers. *Human Vaccines & Immunotherapeutics*, 19(1), 2181610. https://doi.org/10.1080/21645515.2023.2181610

LeBlanc, R. G., Chiodo, L., & Jacelon, C. S. (2022). Social relationship influence on self-care and health among older people living with long term conditions: A mixed-methods study. *International Journal of Older People Nursing*, 17(4), e12450. https://doi.org/10.1111/opn.12450

Mandal, L., & Seethalakshmi, A. (2023). Experience of missed nursing care: A mixed method study. *Worldviews on Evidence-Based Nursing*, 20(3), 212–219. https://doi.org/10.1111/wvn.12653

Marshall, M., Pronovost, P., & Dixon-Woods, M. (2015). Promotion of improvement as a science. *Lancet*, 381, 419–421. https://doi.org/10.1016/S0140-6736(12)61850-9

Mitchell, P., Ferketich, S., & Jennings, B. (1998). Quality health outcomes model. American Academy of Nursing Expert Panel on Quality Health Care. *Image: The Journal of Nursing Scholarship*, 30, 43–46. https://doi.org/10.1111/j.1547-5069.1998.tb01234.x

Morse, J. M. (1991). Approaches to qualitative-quantitative methodological triangulation. *Nursing Research*, 40, 120–123. https://doi.org/10.1097/00006199-199103000-00014

Morse, J. M. (2012). Simultaneous and sequential qualitative mixed method designs. In P. Munhall (Ed.), *Nursing research: A qualitative perspective* (pp. 553–569). Jones & Bartlett Learning.

Morse, J. M. (2017). *Essentials of qualitatively driven mixed method designs*. Routledge.

Pfingstag, C. S. (2024). Increasing rates of human papillomavirus catch-up vaccination at a sexual and reproductive health clinic: A quality improvement project. *Journal of Midwifery & Women's Health*, 69(2), 294–299. https://doi.org/10.1111/jmwh.13568

Pratt, S., & Howard-Ruben, J. (2024). Implementation of electronic postoperative nausea and vomiting assessment and best practice advisory tools to improve patient care. *Journal of Nursing Care Quality*, 39(2), 136–143. https://doi.org/10.1097/NCQ.0000000000000735

Sherwood, G. (2021). Driving forces for quality and safety: Changing mindsets to improve health care. In G. Sherwood & J. Barnsteiner (Eds.), *Quality and safety in nursing: A competency approach to improving outcomes* (3rd ed.). John Wiley & Sons, 3-22.

Shirey, M. R., Hauck, S. L., Embree, J. L., Kinner, T. J., Schaar, G. L., Phillips, L. A., Ashby, S. R., Swenty, C. F., & McCool, I. A. (2011). Showcasing differences between quality improvement, evidence-based practice, and research. *Journal of Continuing Education in Nursing*, 42(2), 57–70. https://doi.org/10.3928/00220124-20100701-01

Zhang, Y., Zhang, S., Liu, C., Chen, X., Ding, Y., Guan, C., & Hu, X. (2023). Caregiver burden among family caregivers of patients with advanced cancer in a palliative context: A mixed-method study. *Journal of Clinical Nursing*, 32(21–22), 7751–7764. https://doi.org/10.1111/jocn.16872

Part 4: Analysis, Interpretation, and Application of Nursing Research

13 Understanding Statistical Analysis of Quantitative Data

Learning Objectives

On completing this chapter, you will be able to:

- Describe the four levels of measurement and identify which level was used for measuring specific variables
- Describe characteristics of frequency distributions and identify and interpret various descriptive statistics
- Describe the logic and purpose of parameter estimation and interpret confidence intervals
- Describe the logic and purpose of hypothesis testing and interpret p values
- Specify appropriate applications for t-tests, analysis of variance, chi-squared tests, and correlation coefficients and interpret the meaning of the calculated statistics
- Identify several types of multivariate statistics and describe situations in which they could be used
- Identify indices used in assessments of reliability and validity
- Understand the results of simple statistical procedures described in a research report
- Define new terms in the chapter

Key Terms

- Absolute risk (AR)
- Absolute risk reduction (ARR)
- Alpha (α)
- Analysis of covariance (ANCOVA)
- Analysis of variance (ANOVA)
- Central tendency
- Chi-squared test
- Coefficient alpha
- Cohen's kappa
- Confidence interval (CI)
- Continuous variable
- Correlation
- Correlation coefficient
- Crosstabs table
- d statistic
- Descriptive statistics
- Effect size
- F ratio
- Frequency distribution
- Hypothesis testing
- Inferential statistics
- Interval measurement
- Intraclass correlation coefficient
- Level of measurement
- Level of significance
- Logistic regression
- Mean
- Median
- Mode

- Multiple regression
- Multivariate statistics
- N
- Negative relationship
- Nominal measurement
- Nonsignificant result (NS)
- Normal distribution
- Number needed to treat (NNT)
- Odds ratio (OR)
- Ordinal measurement
- p value
- Parameter
- Parameter estimation
- Pearson's r
- Positive relationship
- Predictor variable
- Range
- Ratio measurement
- Repeated measures ANOVA
- Skewed distribution
- Standard deviation
- Statistic
- Statistical test
- Statistically significant
- Symmetric distribution
- Test statistic
- t-Test
- Type I error
- Type II error
- Variability

Statistical analysis is used in quantitative research for four main purposes—to describe the data (e.g., sample characteristics), to estimate population values, to test hypotheses, and to provide evidence regarding measurement properties of quantified variables. This chapter provides a brief overview of statistical procedures for these purposes. We begin, however, by explaining levels of measurement.

TIP Although the thought of learning about statistics may be anxiety-provoking, consider Florence Nightingale's view of statistics: "To understand God's thoughts we must study statistics, for these are the measure of His purpose."

LEVELS OF MEASUREMENT

Statistical operations depend on a variable's **level of measurement**. There are four major levels of measurement.

Nominal measurement, the lowest level, involves using numbers simply to categorize attributes. Sex is an example of a nominally measured variable (e.g., female = 1, male = 2, other = 3). The numbers used in nominal measurement do not have quantitative meaning and cannot be treated mathematically. It makes no sense to compute a sample's average sex.

Ordinal measurement ranks people on an attribute. For example, consider this ordinal scheme to measure the ability to perform activities of daily living (ADL): 1 = completely dependent; 2 = needs another person's assistance; 3 = needs mechanical assistance; and 4 = completely independent. The numbers signify incremental ability to perform ADL independently, but they do not tell us how much greater one level is than another. As with nominal measures, the mathematic operations with ordinal-level data are restricted.

Interval measurement occurs when researchers can rank people on an attribute *and* specify the distance between them. Most psychological scales and tests yield interval-level measures. For example, the Stanford-Binet Intelligence (IQ) test is an interval measure. The difference between a score of 140 and 120 is equivalent to the difference between 120 and 100. Some statistical procedures require interval data.

Ratio measurement is the highest level. Ratio scales, unlike interval scales, have a meaningful zero and provide information about the absolute magnitude of the attribute. Many physical measures, such as a person's weight, are ratio measures. It is meaningful to say that someone who weighs 200 pounds is twice as heavy as someone who weighs 100 pounds. Statistical procedures suitable for interval data are also appropriate for ratio-level data. Variables with interval and ratio measurements often are called **continuous variables**.

> **Example of different measurement levels** ••••••••••••••••••••••••••••
> LaRowe et al. (2024) describe a study protocol for a longitudinal study in which they plan to explore the prevalence and characteristics of chronic pain in older adults. Demographic variables such as ethnicity will be captured as nominal-level variables. Income and educational level will be captured as ordinal measures. Several other variables such as sleep, fatigue, anxiety, and depression will be measured on interval-level scales. Other variables will be measured at the ratio level (e.g., height).

Researchers usually strive to use the highest levels of measurement possible because higher levels yield more information and are amenable to more powerful analyses.

> **HOW-TO-TELL TIP** How can you tell a variable's measurement level? A variable is *nominal* if the values could be interchanged (e.g., 1 = male, 2 = female *OR* 1 = female, 2 = male). A variable is usually *ordinal* if there is a quantitative ordering of values AND if there are a small number of values (e.g., excellent, good, fair, poor). A variable is usually considered *interval* if it is measured with a composite scale or test. A variable is *ratio* level if it makes sense to say that one value is twice as much as another (e.g., 100 mg is twice as much as 50 mg).

DESCRIPTIVE STATISTICS

Statistical analysis enables researchers to make sense of numeric information. **Descriptive statistics** are used to synthesize and describe data. When indices such as averages and percentages are calculated with population data, they are **parameters**. A descriptive index from a sample is a **statistic**. Most research questions are about parameters; researchers calculate statistics to estimate parameters and use *inferential statistics* to make inferences about the population.

Descriptively, data for a continuous variable can be depicted in terms of three characteristics: the shape of the distribution of values, **central tendency**, and variability.

Frequency Distributions

Data that are not organized are overwhelming. Consider the 60 numbers in Table 13.1. Assume that these numbers are the scores of 60 preoperative patients on an anxiety scale. Visual inspection of these numbers provides little insight into patients' anxiety.

A **frequency distribution** is an arrangement of values from lowest to highest and a count or percentage of how many times each value occurred. A frequency distribution for the 60 anxiety scores (Table 13.2) makes it easy to see the highest and lowest scores, where scores clustered, and how many patients were in the sample (total sample size is designated as *N* in research reports).

Frequency data can be displayed graphically in a *frequency polygon* (Fig. 13.1). In such graphs, scores typically are on the horizontal line, and counts or percentages are on the vertical axis. Distributions can be described by their shapes. **Symmetric distribution** occurs if, when folded over, the two halves of a frequency polygon would be superimposed (Fig. 13.2). In an *asymmetric* or **skewed distribution**, the peak is off center and one tail is longer than the other. When the longer tail points to the right, the distribution has a *positive skew*, as in Figure 13.3A. Personal income is positively skewed: Most people have moderate incomes, with relatively few people with high incomes at the distribution's right end. If the longer tail points to the left, the distribution has a *negative skew* (Fig. 13.3B). Age at death is negatively skewed: Most people are at the right end of the distribution, with fewer people dying young.

Another aspect of a distribution's shape concerns how many peaks it has. A *unimodal distribution* has one peak (Fig. 13.2A), whereas a *multimodal distribution* has two or more peaks—two

TABLE 13.1 Patients' Anxiety Scores

22	27	25	19	24	25	23	29	24	20	26	16	20	26	17
22	24	18	26	28	15	24	23	22	21	24	20	25	18	27
24	23	16	25	30	29	27	21	23	24	26	18	30	21	17
25	22	24	29	28	20	25	26	24	23	19	27	28	25	26

TABLE 13.2 Frequency Distribution of Patients' Anxiety Scores

Score	Frequency	Percentage (%)
15	1	1.7
16	2	3.3
17	2	3.3
18	3	5.0
19	2	3.3
20	4	6.7
21	3	5.0
22	4	6.7
23	5	8.3
24	9	15.0
25	7	11.7
26	6	10.0
27	4	6.7
28	3	5.0
29	3	5.0
30	2	3.3
	$N = 60$	100.0%

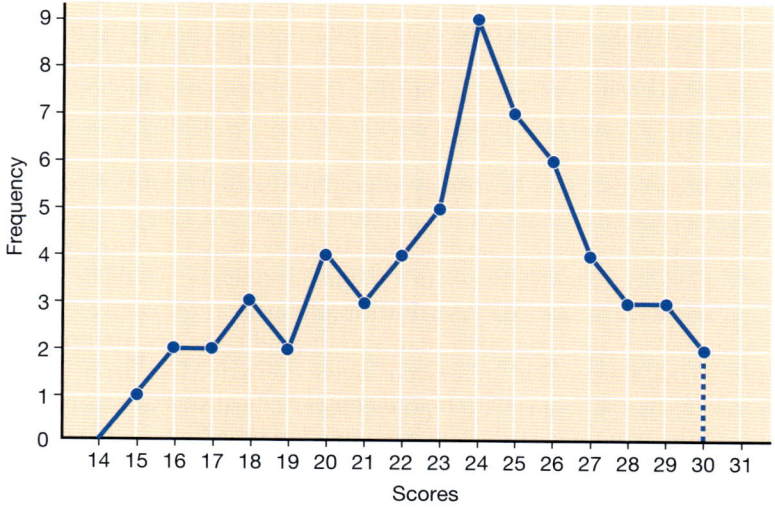

Figure 13.1 Frequency polygon of patients' anxiety scores.

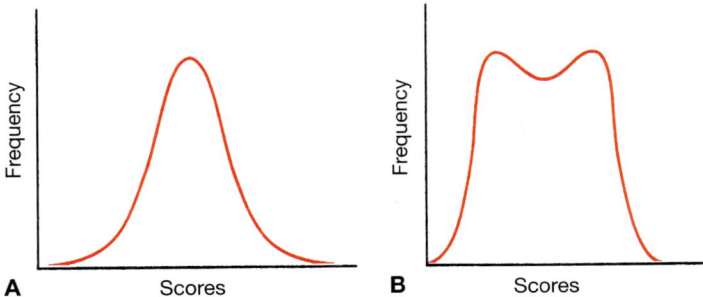

Figure 13.2 Examples of unimodal (**A**) and bimodal (**B**) symmetric distributions.

or more values of high frequency. A distribution with two peaks is *bimodal* (Fig. 13.2B). A special distribution called the **normal distribution** (*a bell-shaped curve*) is symmetric, unimodal, and not very peaked (Fig. 13.2A). Many human attributes (e.g., height, intelligence) approximate a normal distribution.

Central Tendency

Frequency distributions clarify patterns, but an overall summary often is desired. Researchers ask questions such as "What is the *average* daily calorie consumption of nursing home residents?" Such a question seeks a single number to summarize a distribution. Indices of central tendency indicate what is "typical." There are three indices of central tendency: the mode, the median, and the mean.

- **Mode:** The mode is the number that occurs most frequently in a distribution. In the following distribution, the mode is 53:

    50 51 51 52 53 53 53 53 54 55 56

  The value of 53 occurred four times more than any other number. The mode of the patients' anxiety scores in Table 13.2 was 24. The mode identifies the most "popular" value.

- **Median:** The median is the point in a distribution that divides scores in half. Consider the following set of values:

    2 2 3 3 4 5 6 7 8 9

  The value that divides the cases in half is midway between 4 and 5; thus, 4.5 is the median. The median anxiety score is 24, the same as the mode. The median does not take into account individual values and is insensitive to extremes. In the given set of numbers, if the value of 9 were changed to 99, the median would remain 4.5.

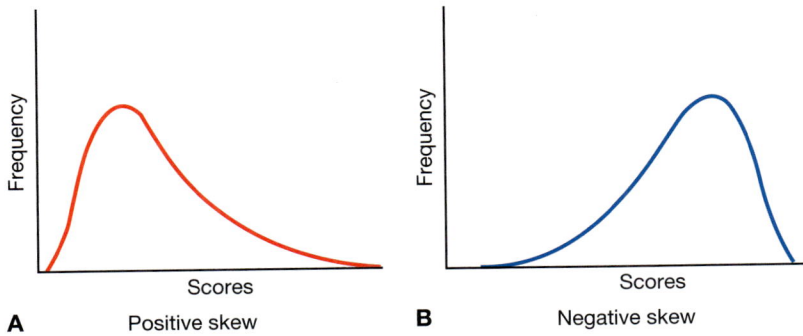

Figure 13.3 Examples of skewed positive skew (**A**) and negative skew (**B**) distributions.

- **Mean:** The mean equals the sum of all values divided by the number of participants—what we usually call the average. The mean of the patients' anxiety scores is 23.4 (1,405/60). As another example, here are the weights of eight people:

  85 109 120 135 158 177 181 195

  In this example, the mean is 145. Unlike the median, the mean is affected by the value of every score. If we exchanged the 195-pound person for a person weighing 275 pounds, the mean would increase from 145 to 155 pounds. In research articles, the mean is often symbolized as M or $\bar{X}$ (e.g., $\bar{X} = 145$).

  For continuous variables, the mean is usually reported. Of the three indices, the mean is most stable: If repeated samples were drawn from a population, the means would fluctuate less than the modes or medians. Because of its stability, the mean usually is the best estimate of a population's central tendency. When a distribution is skewed, however, the median is preferred. For example, the median is a better index for a sample's average (typical) income than the mean because income is usually positively skewed.

Variability

Two distributions with identical means could differ with respect to how spread out the data are—how people are different from one another on the attribute. This section describes the **variability** of distributions.

Consider the two distributions in Figure 13.4, which represent hypothetical scores for students from two schools on an IQ test. Both distributions have a mean of 100, but school A has a wider range of scores, with some below 70 and some above 130. In school B, there are few low or high scores. School A is more *heterogeneous* (i.e., more varied) than school B, and school B is more *homogeneous* than school A. Researchers compute an index of variability to express the extent to which scores in a distribution differ from one another. Two common indices are the range and standard deviation.

- **Range:** The range is the highest minus the lowest score in a distribution. The chief virtue of the range is ease of computation. Because it is based on only two scores, the range is unstable: From sample to sample drawn from a population, the range can fluctuate greatly.
- **Standard deviation:** The most widely used variability index is the standard deviation. Like the mean, the standard deviation is calculated based on every value in a distribution. The standard deviation summarizes the *average* amount of deviation of values from the mean. In the example of patients' anxiety scores (Table 13.2), the standard deviation is 3.725. In research reports, the standard deviation is often abbreviated as *SD*.

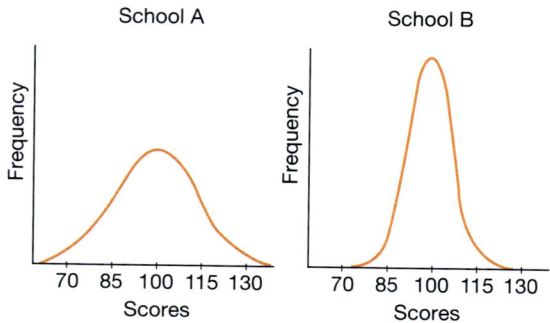

Figure 13.4 Two distributions of different variability.

TIP SDs sometimes are shown in relation to the mean without a label. For example, the anxiety scores might be displayed as M = 23.4 (3.7) or M = 23.4 ± 3.7, where 23.4 is the mean and 3.7 is the standard deviation.

A standard deviation is more difficult to interpret than the range. For the *SD* of anxiety scores, you might ask, 3.725 *what?* What does the number mean? We can answer these questions from several angles. First, the *SD* is an index of how variable the scores in a distribution are. For example, if male and female patients had means of 23.0 on the anxiety scale, but their *SD*s were 7.0 and 3.0, respectively, then females were more homogeneous (i.e., their scores were more similar to one another) than males.

The *SD* represents the *average* of deviations from the mean. The mean tells us the best value for summarizing an entire distribution, and an *SD* tells us how much, on average, the scores deviate from the mean. A standard deviation can be interpreted as our degree of error when we use a mean to describe an entire sample.

In normal and near-normal distributions, there are roughly three *SD*s above and below the mean. For example, for a normal distribution with a mean of 50 and an *SD* of 10 (Fig. 13.5), a fixed percentage of cases fall within certain distances from the mean. Sixty-eight percent of all cases fall within 1 *SD* above and below the mean. Thus, nearly 7 of 10 scores are between 40 and 60. In a normal distribution, 95% of the scores fall within 2 *SD*s of the mean. Only a handful of cases—about 2% at each extreme—lie more than 2 *SD*s from the mean. Using this figure, we can see that a person with a score of 70 achieved a higher score than about 98% of the sample.

Example of descriptive statistics
McCann and colleagues (2024) conducted a cross-sectional study to explore the differences in perceived harms of cigarette and e-cigarette use and perceived birth and health outcomes in a sample of pregnant people in the United States who smoked in the past 30 days. They used descriptive statistics to describe the sample. For example, the authors reported that the sample ranged in age from 18 to 40 years, with a mean age of 29.3 years (*SD* = 5.5). Additionally, in the sample of 267 participants, 53.2% were non-Hispanic White, 18.0% were non-Hispanic Black or African American, and 10.9% were Hispanic.

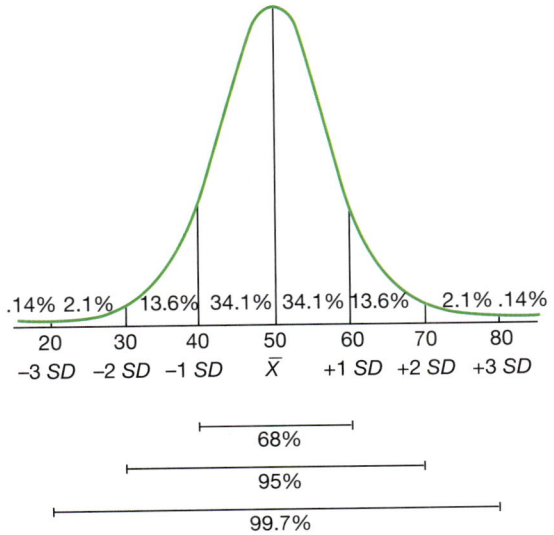

Figure 13.5 Standard deviations in a normal distribution.

TIP Descriptive statistics (percentages, means, *SD*s) are most often used to describe sample characteristics and key research variables and to document methodologic features (e.g., response rates). They are seldom used to answer research questions; inferential statistics usually are used for this purpose.

Bivariate Descriptive Statistics

So far, our discussion has focused on *univariate* (one variable) *descriptive statistics*. Bivariate (two variables) *descriptive statistics* describe relationships between two variables.

Crosstabulations

A **crosstabs table** is a two-dimensional frequency distribution in which the frequencies of two variables are *crosstabulated*. Suppose we had data on patients' gender and whether they did not smoke, smoked less than 1 pack of cigarettes a day, or smoked 1 or more packs a day. The question is whether men smoke more heavily than women, or vice versa (i.e., whether there is a *relationship* between smoking and gender). Fictitious data for this example are shown in Table 13.3. Six *cells* are created by placing one variable (gender) along one dimension and the other variable (smoking status) along the other dimension. After participants' data are allocated to the appropriate cells, percentages are computed. The crosstab shows that women in this sample were more likely than men to not smoke (45.4% vs. 27.3%) and less likely to smoke 1 or more packs a day (18.2% vs. 36.4%). Crosstabs are used with nominal data or ordinal data with few values. In this example, gender is nominal, and smoking, as operationalized, is ordinal.

Correlation

Relationships between two variables can be described by **correlation** methods. The correlation question is, *To what extent are two variables related to each other*? For example, to what degree are anxiety scores and blood pressure values related? This question can be answered by calculating a **correlation coefficient**, which describes *intensity* and *direction* of a relationship.

Two variables that are related are height and weight: Taller people tend to weigh more than shorter people. The relationship between height and weight would be a *perfect relationship* if the tallest person in a population was the heaviest, the second tallest person was the second heaviest, and so on. A correlation coefficient indicates how "perfect" a relationship is. Possible values for a correlation coefficient range from −1.00 through .00 to +1.00. If height and weight were perfectly correlated, the correlation coefficient would be 1.00 (the actual correlation coefficient is in the vicinity of .50 to .60 for a general population). Height and weight have a **positive relationship** because greater height tends to be associated with greater weight.

When two variables are unrelated, the correlation coefficient is zero. One might anticipate that women's shoe size is unrelated to their intelligence. Women with larger feet are

TABLE 13.3 Crosstabs Table for Relationship Between Gender and Smoking Status

Smoking Status	Gender				Total	
	Women		Men			
	n	%	*n*	%	*N*	%
Nonsmoker	10	45.4	6	27.2	16	36.4
Light smoker	8	36.4	8	36.4	16	36.4
Heavy smoker	4	18.2	8	36.4	12	27.2
TOTAL	22	100.0	22	100.0	44	100.0

as likely to perform well on IQ tests as those with smaller feet. The correlation coefficient summarizing such a relationship would be in the vicinity of .00.

Correlation coefficients between .00 and −1.00 express a **negative** (*inverse*) **relationship**. When two variables are inversely related, higher values on one variable are associated with lower values in the second. For example, there is a negative correlation between depression and self-esteem. This means that, on average, people with *high* self-esteem tend to be *low* on depression. If the relationship were perfect (i.e., if the person with the highest self-esteem score had the lowest depression score), then the correlation coefficient would be −1.00. In actuality, the relationship between depression and self-esteem is moderate—usually in the vicinity of −.30 or −.40. Note that the higher the *absolute value* of the coefficient (i.e., the value disregarding the sign), the stronger the relationship. A correlation of −.50, for instance, is stronger than a correlation of +.30.

The most widely used correlation statistic is **Pearson's r**, the *product–moment correlation coefficient*, which is computed with continuous measures. (*Spearman's rho* is a correlation index used for ordinal-level data, or when sample sizes are very small.) There are no guidelines on what should be interpreted as strong or weak correlations because it depends on the variables. If we measured patients' body temperature orally and rectally, an r of .70 between the two measurements would be low. For most psychosocial variables (e.g., stress and depression), however, an r of .70 would be high.

 TIP Correlation coefficients are sometimes reported in tables displaying a two-dimensional *correlation matrix*, in which every variable is displayed in both a row and a column, and coefficients between pairs of variables are displayed at the intersections. An example is presented later in this chapter.

Example of a correlation
Yang et al. (2024) conducted a cross-sectional study to examine the correlation of psychological resilience with social support in patients with Parkinson disease. They found that in patients with Parkinson disease, the level of psychological resilience was significantly and positively correlated with social support ($r = .371$, $p < .01$).

Describing Risk

The evidence-based practice (EBP) movement has made decision making based on research findings an important issue. Several descriptive indices can be used to facilitate such decision making. Many of these indices involve calculating risk differences—for example, differences in risk before and after exposure to a beneficial intervention.

We focus on describing dichotomous outcomes (e.g., had a fall/did not have a fall) in relation to exposure or nonexposure to a beneficial treatment or protective factor. This situation results in a 2 × 2 crosstabs table with four cells. The four cells in the crosstabs table in Table 13.4 are labeled so that various indices can be explained. *Cell a* is the number of cases with an undesirable outcome (e.g., a fall) in an intervention/protected group, *cell b* is the number with a desirable outcome (e.g., no fall) in an intervention/protected group, and *cells c* and *d* are the two outcome possibilities for a nontreated/unprotected group. We can now explain the meaning and calculation of some indices of interest to clinicians.

Absolute Risk

Absolute risk can be computed for those exposed to an intervention/protective factor and for those not exposed. **Absolute risk (AR)** is simply the proportion of people who experienced

TABLE 13.4 Indices of Risk and Association in a 2 × 2 Table

	Outcome		
Exposure	Undesirable Outcome	Desirable Outcome	Total
Yes, exposed (E) to intervention–experimentals (or, NOT exposed to a risk factor)	a	b	a + b
No, not exposed (NE) to intervention–controls (or, exposed to a risk factor)	c	d	c + d
TOTAL	a + c	b + d	a + b + c + d
Absolute risk, exposed group (AR_E)		= a/(a + b)	
Absolute risk, nonexposed group (AR_{NE})		= c/(c + d)	
Absolute risk reduction (ARR)		= $AR_{NE} - AR_E$	
Odds ratio (OR)		= $\dfrac{a/b}{c/d}$	
Number needed to treat (NNT)		= $\dfrac{1}{ARR}$	

an undesirable outcome in each group. Suppose 200 people who smoke were randomly assigned to a smoking cessation intervention or to a control group (Table 13.5). The outcome is smoking status 3 months later. Here, the AR of continued smoking is .50 in the intervention group and .80 in the control group. Without the intervention, 20% of those in the experimental group would presumably have stopped smoking anyway, but the intervention boosted the rate to 50%.

Absolute Risk Reduction

The **absolute risk reduction (ARR)** index, a comparison of the two risks, is computed by subtracting the absolute risk for the exposed group from the absolute risk for the unexposed group. This index is the estimated proportion of people who would be spared the undesirable outcome through exposure to an intervention/protective factor. In our example, the value of ARR is .30: 30% of the control group subjects would presumably have stopped smoking if they had received the intervention, over and above the 20% who stopped without it.

TABLE 13.5 Hypothetical Data for Smoking Cessation Intervention Example, Risk Indices

	Outcome		
Exposure to Smoking Cessation Intervention	Continued Smoking	Stopped Smoking	Total
Yes, exposed: E (experimental group)	50 (a)	50 (b)	100
No, not exposed: NE (control group)	80 (c)	20 (d)	100
TOTAL	130	70	200
Absolute risk, exposed group (AR_E)		= 50/100 = .50	
Absolute risk, nonexposed group (AR_{NE})		= 80/100 = .80	
Absolute risk reduction (ARR)		= .80 − .50 = .30	
Odds ratio (OR)		= $\dfrac{(50/50)}{(80/20)}$ = .25	
Number needed to treat (NNT)		= 1/.30 = 3.33	

Odds Ratio

The odds ratio is a widely reported risk index. The *odds*, in this context, is the proportion of people *with* the adverse outcome relative to those *without* it. In our example, the odds of continued smoking for the intervention group is 1.0: 50 (those who continued smoking) divided by 50 (those who stopped). The odds for the control group is 80 divided by 20, or 4.0. The **odds ratio (OR)** is the ratio of these two odds—here, .25. The estimated odds of continuing to smoke are one fourth as high among intervention group members as for control group members. Turned around, the estimated odds of continued smoking is 4 times higher among people who smoke and do not get the intervention than among those who do.

> **Example of odds ratios** •••
> Fiske and colleagues (2024) examined the nutritional status of older adults receiving home nursing care in Norway considering living alone versus living with others and polypharmacy. They found that the risk for malnutrition was higher in those living with others with an adjusted OR of 2.23 (1.20 to 4.13). Higher odds for malnutrition risk were associated with the use of 0 to 5 drugs as compared to polypharmacy (≥6 drugs) with an adjusted OR of 1.97 (1.04 to 3.75).

Number Needed to Treat

The **number needed to treat (NNT)** index estimates how many people would need to receive an intervention to prevent one undesirable outcome. NNT is computed by dividing 1 by ARR. In our example, ARR = .30, and so NNT is 3.33. About three smokers would need to be exposed to the intervention to avoid one person's continued smoking. The NNT is valuable because it can be integrated with monetary information to show if an intervention is likely to be cost-effective.

> **TIP** Another risk index is known as *relative risk* (RR). The RR is the estimated proportion of the original risk of an adverse outcome (in our example, continued smoking) that persists when people are exposed to the intervention. In our example, RR is .625 (.50/.80): The risk of continued smoking is estimated as 62.5% of what it would have been without the intervention.

INTRODUCTION TO INFERENTIAL STATISTICS

Descriptive statistics are useful for summarizing data, but researchers usually do more than describe. **Inferential statistics**, based on the *laws of probability*, provide a means for drawing inferences about a population, given data from a sample. Inferential statistics are used to test research hypotheses.

Sampling Distributions

Inferential statistics are based on the assumption of random sampling of cases from populations—although this assumption is widely ignored. Even with random sampling, however, sample characteristics are seldom identical to those of the population. Suppose we had a population of 100,000 nursing home residents whose mean score on a physical function (PF) test was 500 with an *SD* of 100. We do not know these parameters—assume we must estimate them based on scores from a random sample of 100 residents. It is unlikely that we would obtain a mean of exactly 500. Our sample mean might be, say, 505. If we drew a new random sample of 100 residents, the mean PF score might be 497. Sample statistics fluctuate and are unequal to the parameter because of *sampling error*. Researchers need a way to assess whether sample statistics are good estimates of population parameters.

To understand the logic of inferential statistics, we must perform a mental exercise. Consider drawing 5,000 consecutive samples of 100 residents from the population of all residents. If we calculated a mean PF score each time, we could plot the distribution of these sample means, as shown in Figure 13.6. This distribution is a *sampling distribution of the mean*. A sampling distribution is theoretical: No one *actually* draws consecutive samples from a population and plots their means. Statisticians have shown that sampling distributions of means are normally distributed, and their mean equals the population mean. In our example, the mean of the sampling distribution is 500, the same as the population mean.

For a normally distributed sampling distribution of means, the probability is 95 out of 100 that a sample mean lies between +2 *SD* and −2 *SD* of the population mean. The *SD* of the sampling distribution—called the *standard error of the mean* (or SEM)—can be estimated using a formula that uses two pieces of information: the *SD* for the sample and sample size. In our example, the SEM is 10 (Fig. 13.6), which is the estimate of how much sampling error there would be from one sample mean to another in an infinite number of samples of 100 residents.

We can now estimate the probability of drawing a sample with a certain mean. With a sample size of 100 and a population mean of 500, the chances are 95 out of 100 that a sample mean would fall between 480 and 520—2 *SD*s above and below the mean. Only 5 times out of 100 would the mean of a random sample of 100 residents be less than 480 or greater than 520.

The SEM is partly a function of sample size, so a larger sample improves the accuracy of the estimate. If we used a sample of 400 residents to estimate the population mean, the SEM would be only 5. The probability would be 95 in 100 that a sample mean would be between 490 and 510. The chance of drawing a sample with a mean very different from that of the population is reduced as sample size increases.

You may wonder why you need to learn about these abstract statistical notions. Consider, though, that we are talking about the accuracy of researchers' results. As an intelligent consumer, you need to evaluate critically how believable research evidence is so that you can decide whether to incorporate it into your nursing practice.

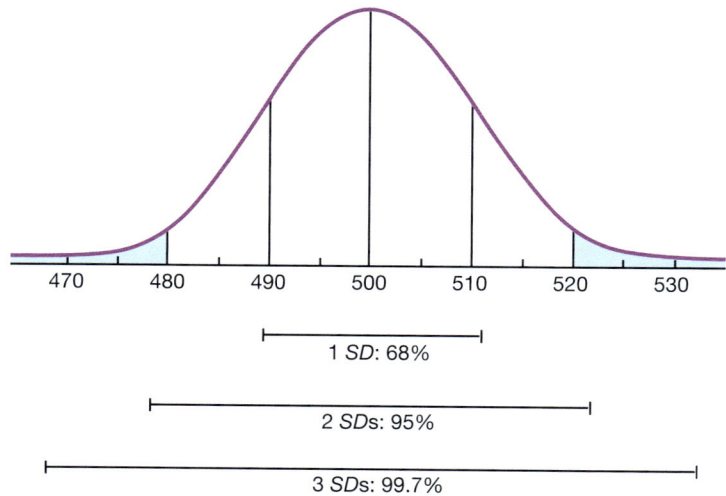

Figure 13.6 Sampling distribution of a mean.

Parameter Estimation

Statistical inference consists of two techniques: parameter estimation and hypothesis testing. **Parameter estimation** is used to estimate a population parameter—for example, a mean, a proportion, or a difference in means between two groups (e.g., people who smoke vs. people who do not smoke). *Point estimation* involves calculating a single statistic to estimate the parameter. In our example, if the mean PF score for a sample of 100 nursing home residents were 510, this would be the point estimate of the population mean.

Point estimates convey no information about the estimate's margin of error. *Interval estimation* of a parameter provides a range of values within which the parameter has a specified probability of lying. With interval estimation, researchers construct a **confidence interval (CI)** around the point estimate. The CI around a sample mean establishes a range of values for the population value and the probability of being right. By convention, researchers use either a 95% or a 99% CI.

As noted previously, 95% of the scores in a normal distribution lie within about 2 *SD*s (more precisely, 1.96 *SD*s) from the mean. In our example, if the point estimate for mean scores is 510 with an $SD = 100$, the SEM for a sample of 100 would be 10. We can build a 95% CI using this formula: $95\% \text{ CI} = (\bar{X} \pm 1.96 \times \text{SEM})$. The confidence is 95% that the population mean lies between the values equal to 1.96 times the SEM, above and below the sample mean. In our example, with an SEM of 10, the 95% CI around the sample mean of 510 is between 490.4 and 529.6.

CIs reflect how much risk of being wrong researchers take. With a 95% CI, researchers risk being wrong 5 times out of 100. A 99% CI sets the risk at only 1% by allowing a wider range of possible values. In our example, the 99% CI around 510 is 484.2 to 535.8. With a lower risk of being wrong, precision is reduced. For a 95% interval, the CI range is about 39 points; for a 99% interval, the range is about 52 points. The acceptable risk of error depends on the nature of the problem, but for most studies, a 95% CI is sufficient.

> **Example of confidence intervals around odds ratio**
> Hoelscher et al. (2024) conducted an exploratory mixed-methods study to identify changes in nursing documentation between February and November 2022 during the COVID-19 pandemic. They assessed documentation patterns from 175 North American nurse leaders and informaticists. Findings indicated significant differences between rural and urban settings ($p = .02$), with urban areas showing higher odds of changes to care plans (OR, 4.889; 95% CI, 1.27 to 18.78).

Hypothesis Testing

With statistical **hypothesis testing**, researchers use objective criteria to decide whether hypotheses should be accepted or rejected. Suppose we hypothesized that maternity patients who received online interactive breastfeeding/chestfeeding support would breastfeed/chestfeed longer than those who did not. The mean number of days of breastfeeding/chestfeeding is 131.5 for 25 intervention group participants and 125.1 for 25 control group participants. Should we conclude that our hypothesis has been supported? Group differences are in the predicted direction, but in another sample, the group means might be more similar. Two explanations for the observed outcome are possible: (1) The intervention was effective in encouraging breastfeeding/chestfeeding or (2) the mean difference in this sample was due to chance (sampling error).

The first explanation is the *research hypothesis*, and the second is the *null hypothesis*, which is that there is no relationship between the independent variable (the intervention) and the dependent variable (breastfeeding/chestfeeding duration). Statistical hypothesis testing is a process of disproof. It cannot be demonstrated directly that the research hypothesis is correct. But it is possible to show that the null hypothesis has a high probability of being incorrect, and such evidence lends support to the research hypothesis. Hypothesis testing helps researchers to make objective decisions about whether results are likely to reflect chance differences or hypothesized effects. Researchers use **statistical tests** in the hope of rejecting the null hypothesis.

Null hypotheses are accepted or rejected based on sample data, but hypotheses are about population values. The interest in testing hypotheses, as in all statistical inference, is to use a sample to make inferences about a population.

Type I and Type II Errors

Researchers decide whether to accept or reject the null hypothesis by estimating how probable it is that observed group differences are due to chance. Without population data, it cannot be asserted that the null hypothesis is or is not true. Researchers must be content to say that hypotheses are either *probably* true or *probably* false.

Researchers can make two types of errors: rejecting a true null hypothesis or accepting a false null hypothesis. Figure 13.7 summarizes possible outcomes of researchers' decisions. Researchers make a **Type I error** by rejecting a null hypothesis that is, in fact, true. For instance, if we decided that online support effectively promoted breastfeeding/chestfeeding when, in fact, group differences were merely due to sampling error, we would be making a Type I error—a false-positive conclusion. If we decided that differences in breastfeeding/chestfeeding were due to sampling fluctuations, when the intervention actually *did* have an effect, we would be making a **Type II error**—a false-negative conclusion.

Level of Significance

Researchers do not know when they have made an error in statistical decision making. However, they control the risk for a Type I error by selecting a **level of significance**, which is the probability of making a Type I error. The two most frequently used levels of significance (referred to as **alpha** or **α**) are .05 and .01. With a .05 significance level, we accept the risk that out of 100 samples from a population, a true null hypothesis would be wrongly rejected 5 times. In 95 out of 100 cases, however, a true null hypothesis would be correctly accepted. With a .01 significance level, the risk of a Type I error is lower: In only 1 sample out of 100 would we wrongly reject the null. By convention, the minimal acceptable alpha level is .05.

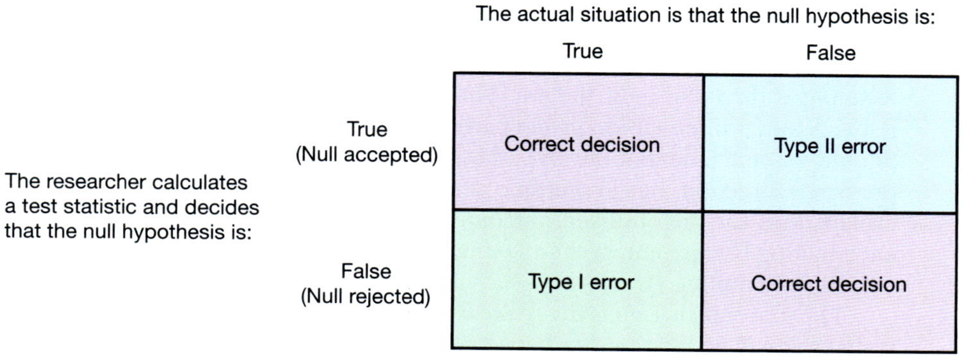

		The actual situation is that the null hypothesis is:	
		True	False
The researcher calculates a test statistic and decides that the null hypothesis is:	True (Null accepted)	Correct decision	Type II error
	False (Null rejected)	Type I error	Correct decision

Figure 13.7 Outcomes of statistical decision making.

TIP Levels of significance are analogous to the CI values described earlier—an alpha of .05 is analogous to the 95% CI, and an alpha of .01 is analogous to the 99% CI.

Researchers would like to reduce the risk of committing both types of error, but unfortunately, lowering the risk of a Type I error increases the risk of a Type II error. Researchers can reduce the risk of a Type II error, however, by increasing the sample size. The probability of committing a Type II error can be estimated through *power analysis*, the procedure we mentioned in Chapter 9 for estimating sample size needs. *Power* is the ability of a statistical test to detect true relationships. Researchers ideally use a sample size that gives them a minimum power of .80, and thus, a risk for a Type II error of no more than .20 (i.e., a 20% risk).

TIP If a report indicates that a research hypothesis was not supported by the data, consider whether a Type II error might have occurred as a result of an inadequate sample size.

Tests of Statistical Significance

In hypothesis testing, researchers use study data to compute a **test statistic**. For every test statistic, there is a theoretical sampling distribution. Hypothesis testing uses theoretical distributions to establish *probable* and *improbable* values for the test statistics, which are used to accept or reject the null hypothesis.

An example can illustrate this process. In our example of a physical functioning test for nursing home residents, suppose that there are population *norms*, which are values derived from large, representative samples. Let us assume that in the sampling distribution for the norming data, the mean is 500 with an SEM of 10, as in Figure 13.6. Now, let us say that we recruited 100 nursing home residents to participate in an intervention to improve physical functioning. The null hypothesis is that those receiving the intervention have mean posttest scores that are not different from those in the overall population—that is, 500—but the research hypothesis is that they will have higher average scores. After the intervention, the mean PF score for the sample is 528. As we can see by examining Figure 13.6, a mean score of 528 is more than 2 standard deviations above the population mean—it is a value that is *improbable* if the null hypothesis is true. Thus, we accept the research hypothesis that the intervention resulted in higher physical functioning scores than those in the population.[1]

We would not be justified in saying that we had *proved* the research hypothesis because the possibility of a Type I error remains—but the possibility is less than 5 in 100. Researchers reporting the results of hypothesis tests state whether their findings are **statistically significant**. The word *significant* does not mean important or meaningful. In statistics, the term *significant* means that results are not likely to have been due to chance, at some specified level of probability. **A nonsignificant result** means that any observed difference or relationship could have been the result of chance.

Overview of Hypothesis Testing Procedures

In the next section, a few statistical tests are discussed. We emphasize applications and interpretations of statistical tests, not computations. Each statistical test can be used with specific kinds of data, but the overall hypothesis testing process is similar for all tests:

1. *Select an appropriate statistical test.* Researchers select a test based on such factors as the variables' level of measurement.

---

[1] The design for our fictitious example is highly flawed, with several serious threats to internal validity. We used this contrived example purely as a simple way to illustrate hypothesis testing.

2. *Specify the level of significance.* An α level of .05 is usually chosen.
3. *Compute a test statistic.* The value for a test statistic is calculated with study data.
4. *Determine degrees of freedom.* The term *degrees of freedom (df)* refers to the number of observations free to vary about a parameter. The concept can be confusing, but computing degrees of freedom is easy.
5. *Compare the test statistic to a theoretical value.* Theoretical distributions exist for all test statistics. The computed value of the test statistics is compared to a theoretical value to establish significance or nonsignificance.

When a computer is used for the analysis, as is almost always the case, researchers follow only the first step. The computer calculates the test statistic, degrees of freedom, and the actual probability that the relationship being tested is due to chance. For example, the printout may indicate that the probability (p) of an intervention group having a higher mean number of days of breastfeeding than a control group on the basis of chance alone is .025. This means that fewer than 3 times out of 100 (only 25 times out of 1,000) would a group difference of the size observed occur by chance. The computed ***p* value** is then compared with the desired alpha. In this example, if we had set the significance level to .05, the results would be significant because .025 is more stringent than .05. Any computed probability greater than .05 (e.g., .15) indicates a nonsignificant relationship (*NS*), that is, one that could have occurred by chance in more than 5 out of 100 samples.

 TIP Most tests discussed in this chapter are *parametric tests*, which are ones that focus on population parameters and involve certain assumptions about variables in the analysis, notably the assumption that they are normally distributed in the population. *Nonparametric tests*, by contrast, do not estimate parameters and involve less restrictive assumptions about the distribution's shape.

BIVARIATE STATISTICAL TESTS

Researchers use a variety of statistical tests to make inferences about their hypotheses. Several frequently used bivariate tests are briefly described and illustrated.

t-Tests

Researchers frequently compare two groups of people on an outcome. A ***t*-test** is a parametric test for testing differences in two group means.

Suppose we wanted to test the effect of early discharge of maternity patients on perceived maternal competence. We administer a scale of perceived maternal competence at discharge to 20 primiparas who had a vaginal delivery: 10 who remained in the hospital 25 to 48 hours (regular discharge group) and 10 who were discharged 24 hours or less after delivery (early discharge group). Data for this example are presented in Table 13.6. Mean scores on the perceived maternal competence measure for these two groups are 25.0 and 19.0, respectively. Are these differences *real* (i.e., Do they exist in the population of early and regular discharge birthing parents?), or do group differences reflect chance fluctuations? The 20 scores vary from one person to another, ranging from a low of 13 to a high of 30. Some variation reflects individual differences in maternal competence; some might result from participants' moods on a particular day, and so forth. The research question is whether a significant amount of the variation is associated with the independent variable—time of hospital discharge. The *t*-test allows us to make inferences about this question objectively.

TABLE 13.6 Fictitious Data for *t*-Test Example: Scores on a Perceived Maternal Competence Scale

Regular Discharge Mothers		Early Discharge Mothers	
30	32	23	26
27	17	17	16
25	18	22	13
20	28	18	21
24	29	20	14
Mean = 25.0		Mean = 19.0	

$t = 2.86$; $df = 18$; $p = .011$

The formula for calculating the t statistic uses group means, variability, and sample size. The computed value of t for the data in Table 13.6 is 2.86. Degrees of freedom here is the total sample size minus 2 ($df = 20 − 2 = 18$). For an α level of .05, the cutoff value for t with 18 degrees of freedom is 2.10. *This value is the upper limit to what is probable if the null hypothesis is true.* Thus, the calculated t of 2.86, which is larger than the theoretical value of t, is improbable (i.e., statistically significant). The primiparas discharged early had significantly lower perceived maternal competence than those who were not discharged early. In fewer than 5 out of 100 samples would a difference in means this large be found by chance. In fact, the actual p value is .011: Only in about 1 sample out of 100 would a mean difference of 6.0 on the dependent variable be found by chance.

The situation we just described requires an *independent groups t-test*: Birthing parents in the two groups were different people, independent of each other. There are situations for which this type of *t*-test is not appropriate. For example, if means for a single group of people measured before and after an intervention were being compared, researchers would compute a *paired t-test* (also called a *dependent groups t-test*), using a different formula.

> **Example of *t*-tests**
> Munroe and colleagues (2022) conducted a quasi-experimental pre-post study to examine if using an emergency nursing framework improved the accuracy of clinical documentation. Two-sample *t*-tests were used to determine differences in the continuous variables between the pre- and postgroups. Findings indicate the pre-post documentation of vital signs increased. For example, heart rate (29 [49.2%] vs. 37 [61.7%], $p = .02$) and blood pressure (17 [28.8%] vs. 25 [41.7%], $p = .029$).

In lieu of *t*-tests, CIs can be constructed around the difference between two means. In the example in Table 13.6, we can construct CIs around the mean difference of 6.0 in maternal competence scores (25.0 − 19.0 = 6.0). For a 95% CI, the confidence limits are 1.6 and 10.4: We can be 95% confident that the difference between population means for early and regular discharge mothers lies between these values. With CI information, we can also see that the mean difference is significant at $p < .05$ *because the range does not include 0*. There is a 95% probability that the mean difference is not lower than 1.6, so this means that there is less than a 5% probability that there is no difference at all—thus, the null hypothesis can be rejected.

Analysis of Variance

Analysis of variance (ANOVA) is used to test mean group differences of three or more groups. ANOVA sorts out the variability of an outcome variable into two components: variability due to the independent variable (e.g., experimental group status) and variability due to all other sources (e.g., individual differences). Variation *between* groups is contrasted with variation *within* groups to yield an **F ratio** statistic.

Suppose we were comparing the effectiveness of interventions to help people stop smoking. Group A people who smoke receive nurse counseling; Group B people who smoke receive a nicotine patch; and a control group (Group C) gets no intervention. The outcome is 1-day cigarette consumption 1 month after the intervention. Thirty people who smoke are randomly assigned to one of the three groups. The null hypothesis is that the population means for posttreatment cigarette smoking are the same for all three groups, and the research hypothesis is inequality of means. Table 13.7 presents fictitious data for the 30 participants. The mean numbers of posttreatment cigarettes consumed are 16.6, 19.2, and 34.0 for groups A, B, and C, respectively. These means are different, but are they significantly different or do differences reflect random fluctuations?

An ANOVA applied to these data yields an F ratio of 4.98. For $\alpha = .05$ and $df = 2$ and 27 (2 df between groups and 27 df within groups), the theoretical F value is 3.35. Because our obtained F value of 4.98 exceeds 3.35, we reject the null hypothesis that the population means are equal. The *actual* probability, as calculated by a computer, is .014. In only 14 samples out of 1,000 would group differences this great be obtained by chance alone.

ANOVA results support the hypothesis that different treatments were associated with different cigarette smoking, but we cannot tell from these results whether treatment A was significantly more effective than treatment B. Statistical analyses known as *post hoc tests* (or *multiple comparison procedures*) are used to isolate the differences between group means that result in the rejection of the overall null hypothesis.

A type of ANOVA known as **repeated measures ANOVA** (RM-ANOVA) can be used when the means being compared are means at different points in time (e.g., mean blood pressure at 2, 4, and 6 hours after surgery). When two or more groups are measured several times, a repeated measures ANOVA provides information about a main effect for time (Do the measures change significantly over time, irrespective of group?), a main effect for groups (Do the group means differ significantly, irrespective of time?), and an *interaction effect* (Do the groups differ more at certain times?).

Example of an ANOVA

In a sample of caregivers of people with schizophrenia, Bagheri and colleagues (2023) explored the effect of a caring science-based health promotion program on the caregivers' sense of coherence and well-being. Participants were allocated to four study groups, and a one-way ANOVA was used to assess the differences among the four groups. Results indicated that in the intervention group, there was a significant difference in change in all the variables ($p < .001$).

TABLE 13.7 Fictitious Data for One-Way ANOVA Example: Number of Cigarettes Smoked in 1-Day Postintervention

Group A Nurse Counseling		Group B Nicotine Patch		Group C Untreated Controls	
28	19	0	27	33	35
0	24	31	0	54	0
17	0	26	3	19	43
20	21	30	24	40	39
35	2	24	27	41	36
Mean$_A$ = 16.6		Mean$_B$ = 19.2		Mean$_C$ = 34.0	

ANOVA, analysis of variance.
$F = 4.98$; $df = 2, 27$; $p = .01$.

Chi-Squared Test

The **chi-squared (χ^2) test** is used to test hypotheses about differences in proportions, as in a crosstabs. For example, suppose we were studying the effect of nursing instruction on patients' compliance with self-medication. Nurses implement a new instructional strategy with 50 patients, whereas 50 control group patients receive usual care. The research hypothesis is that a higher proportion of people in the intervention than in the control condition will be compliant. Some fictitious data for this example are presented in Table 13.8, which shows that 60% of those in the intervention group were compliant, compared to 40% in the control group. But is this 20 percentage point difference statistically significant—that is, likely to be "real"?

The value of the χ^2 statistic for the data in Table 13.8 is 4.00, which we can compare with the value from a theoretical chi-squared distribution. In this example, the theoretical value that must be exceeded to establish significance at the .05 level is 3.84. The obtained value of 4.00 is larger than would be expected by chance (the actual $p = .046$). We can conclude that a significantly larger proportion of experimental than control patients were compliant.

> **Example of chi-squared test**
> Lindsay and Decker (2022) conducted an EBP project to improve the diagnosis and treatment of depression in an adult primary care practice. After instituting the intervention, reminding providers to administer the Patient Health Questionnaire--9 (PHQ-9) instrument, the researchers used the chi-squared test to determine the difference pre-post intervention. They found that the postintervention sample screening rate was significantly higher than preintervention sample rate (90% vs. 23.3%; $\chi^2 = 54.3$, $df = 1$, $p < .000$).

As with means, we can construct CIs around the difference between two proportions. In our example, the group difference in proportion compliant was .20 (.60 − .40 = .20). The 95% CI around .20 is .06 to .34. We can be 95% confident that the true population difference in compliance rates between the groups is between 6% and 34%. This interval does not include 0%, so we can be 95% confident that group differences in the population are "real."

Correlation Coefficients

Pearson's r is both descriptive and inferential. As a descriptive statistic, r summarizes the magnitude and direction of a relationship between two variables. As an inferential statistic, r tests hypotheses about population correlations; the null hypothesis is that there is no relationship between two variables, that is, that the population correlation = .00.

Suppose we were studying the relationship between patients' self-reported level of stress (higher scores indicate more stress) and the pH level of their saliva. With a sample of

TABLE 13.8 Observed Frequencies for Chi-Squared Example: Rates of Compliance With Medications

	Group				Total
	Experimental		Control		
Patient Compliance	n	%	n	%	N
Compliant	30	60.0	20	40.0	50
Noncompliant	20	40.0	30	60.0	50
TOTAL	50	100.0	50	100.0	100

$\chi^2 = 4.0$, $df = 1$, $p = .046$.

50 patients, we find that $r = -.29$. This value indicates a tendency for people with high stress to have lower pH levels than those with low stress. But is the r of $-.29$ a random fluctuation observed only in this sample, or is the relationship significant? Degrees of freedom for correlation coefficients equal N minus 2—48 in this example. The theoretical value for r with $df = 48$ and $\alpha = .05$ is .28. Because the absolute value of the calculated r is .29, the null hypothesis is rejected: The relationship between patients' stress level and the acidity of their saliva is statistically significant.

> **Example of Pearson's r**
> Yu et al. (2025) conducted a cross-sectional analysis of 309 nurse leaders in China. They used Pearson correlations to determine the relationships among ethical climate, moral resilience, and ethical competence. They found that in the nurse leaders, the ethical climate score positively impacted ethical competence ($r = 0.208$, $p < .001$), and ethical climate could affect ethical competence through the mediating role of moral resilience.

Effect Size Indices

Effect size indices are estimates of the magnitude of effects of an "I" component on an "O" component in PICO questions—an important issue in EBP. Effect size information can be crucial because, with large samples, even minuscule effects can be statistically significant. The p values tell you whether results are likely to be *real*, but effect sizes suggest whether they are important. Effect size plays an important role in systematic reviews.

It is beyond our scope to explain effect sizes in detail, but we offer an illustration. A frequently used effect size index is the **d statistic**, which summarizes the magnitude of differences in two means, such as the difference between intervention and control group means on an outcome. Thus, d can be calculated to estimate the effect size when t-tests are used. When d is zero, it means that there is no effect—the means of the two groups being compared are the same. By convention, a d of .20 or less is considered *small*, a d of .50 is considered *moderate*, and a d of .80 or greater is considered *large*.

Different effect size indices and interpretive conventions are associated with different situations. For example, the r statistic can be interpreted directly as an effect size index, as can the OR. The key point is that they encapsulate information about how powerful the effect of an independent variable is on an outcome.

 TIP Researchers who conduct a *power analysis* to estimate how big a sample size they need to adequately test their hypotheses (i.e., to avoid a Type II error) must estimate in advance how large the effect size will be—usually based on prior research or a pilot study.

> **Example of calculated effect size**
> Ramsdale et al. (2024) describe a study protocol in which they aim to conduct a cluster randomized control trial to assess the feasibility and effectiveness of deprescribing interventions in older adults starting chemotherapy who are identified as meeting the criteria for polypharmacy. They estimate that a sample size of 32 participants per group will provide 80% power with a medium effect size (Cohen's *h* value of 0.6).

Guide to Bivariate Statistical Tests

The selection of a statistical test depends on several factors, such as number of groups and the levels of measurement of the research variables. To aid you in evaluating the appropriateness

TABLE 13.9 Guide to Major Bivariate Statistical Tests

Name	Test Statistic	Purpose	Measurement Level	
			Independent Variable	Dependent Variable
t-Test for independent groups	t	To test the difference between the means of two independent groups (e.g., experimental vs. control, men vs. women)	Nominal	Continuous[a]
t-Test for paired groups	t	To test the difference between the means of a paired group (e.g., pretest vs. posttest for the same people)	Nominal	Continuous[a]
Analysis of variance (ANOVA)	F	To test the difference among the means of 3+ independent groups	Nominal	Continuous[a]
Repeated measures ANOVA	F	To test differences among the means for the same group over time or to compare 2+ groups over time	Nominal	Continuous[a]
Pearson's correlation coefficient	r	To test the existence and strength of a relationship between two variables	Continuous[a]	Continuous[a]
Chi-squared test	χ^2	To test the difference in proportions in 2+ independent groups	Nominal (or ordinal, few categories)	Nominal (or ordinal, few categories)

[a]Continuous measures are on an interval- or ratio-level scale.

of statistical tests used by nurse researchers, Table 13.9 summarizes key features of the bivariate tests mentioned in this chapter.

TIP Every time a report presents information about statistical tests such as those described in this section, it means that the researcher was testing hypotheses—whether those hypotheses were formally stated in the introduction or not.

MULTIVARIATE STATISTICAL ANALYSIS

Many quantitative nursing studies today rely on **multivariate statistics** that involve the analysis of three or more variables simultaneously. The increased use of sophisticated analytic methods has resulted in greater rigor in nursing studies, but it can be challenging for those without statistical training to fully understand research reports.

Given the introductory nature of this book and the fact that many of you are not proficient with even basic statistical tests, we present only a brief description of only three widely used types of multivariate statistical analyses: multiple regression, analysis of covariance, and logistic regression.

Multiple Regression

Correlations enable researchers to make predictions. For example, if the correlation between secondary school grades and nursing school grades were .60, nursing school administrators could make predictions—albeit imperfect ones—about applicants' performance in nursing school. Researchers can improve their prediction of an outcome by performing a **multiple regression** in which several independent variables are included in the analysis. As an example, we might predict infant birth weight (the outcome) from such variables as birthing parent's smoking status, amount of prenatal care, and gestational period. In multiple regression, outcome variables are continuous variables. Independent variables (often called **predictor variables** in regression) are either continuous variables or dichotomous nominal-level variables, such as does/does not smoke.

> **Example of multiple regression analysis**
> Flanagan, one of the authors of this book, and colleagues (2023) conducted a secondary analysis of the minimum data set of patients admitted to skilled nursing facilities (SNFs) from acute care hospitals in Massachusetts. They examined the effects of fee-for-service occupational therapy (OT), physical therapy (PT), and a combination of the two on the change in physical function (PF) from admission to quarterly assessment or discharge. For people with dementia ($N = 6,396$), the multiple regression analysis indicated that none of the interventions resulted in a change of PF (OT: β, .01; 95% CI, −0.006 to 0.03; $p = .14$; PT: β, −.01; 95% CI, −0.06 to 0.03; $p = .14$; OT+PT: β, −.01; 95% CI, −0.05 to 0.03; $p = .59$).

Analysis of Covariance

Analysis of covariance (ANCOVA), which combines features of ANOVA and multiple regression, is used to control confounding variables statistically—that is, to attempt to "equalize" groups being compared. This approach is valuable in certain situations, like when a nonequivalent control group design has been used. When control through randomization is lacking, ANCOVA offers the possibility of statistical control.

In ANCOVA, the confounding variables being controlled are called *covariates*. ANCOVA tests the significance of differences between group means on an outcome after removing the effect of covariates. ANCOVA yields F statistics for testing the significance of group differences.

> **Example of ANCOVA**
> Oladokun and colleagues (2025) aimed to validate the defining characteristics of the nursing diagnosis "impaired mood regulation" among individuals experiencing mood problems while under care in Nigeria. They found that after eliminating the covariates of age and gender, the diagnosis was significant when combined with the duration of illness, $F(38, 87) = 2.38$, $p = .036$.

Logistic Regression

Logistic regression analyzes relationships between multiple independent variables and a nominal-level outcome (e.g., compliant vs. noncompliant). It is similar to multiple regression, although it employs a different statistical estimation procedure. Logistic regression transforms the probability of an event occurring (e.g., that a person will practice breast self-examination or not) into its *odds*. After further transformations, the analysis examines the relationship of the predictor variables to the transformed outcome variable. For each predictor, the logistic regression yields an *OR*, which is the factor by which the odds change for a unit change in the predictors after controlling for other predictors. Logistic regression yields ORs for each predictor, as well as CIs around the ORs.

> **Example of logistic regression**
> Kim and colleagues (2023) aimed to determine whether low healthy lifestyle status was associated with alcohol and food addiction risk among college students in South Korea. Logistic regression analysis revealed that when gender and healthy lifestyle status were combined, women had a higher risk of food addiction than men (OR = 2.34, 95% CI [1.09, 5.04]). When considering healthy lifestyle and alcohol consumption, the problematic drinking group risk was 3.06 times higher (OR = 3.06, 95% CI [1.97, 4.90]) than in the low-risk group.

MEASUREMENT STATISTICS

In Chapter 9, we described two measurement properties that are key aspects of measurement quality—reliability and validity. When a new measure is developed, researchers undertake a psychometric assessment to estimate its reliability and validity. Such psychometric assessments rely on statistical analyses, using indices that we briefly describe here. Researchers often report measurement statistics when they describe the measures they opted to use to provide evidence that their data can be trusted.

Reliability Assessment

Reliability, it may be recalled, is the extent to which scores on a measure are consistent across repeated measurements if the trait itself has not changed. In Chapter 9, we mentioned three major types of reliability, each of which relies on different statistical indices: test–retest reliability, interrater reliability, and internal consistency reliability.

- *Test–retest reliability*, which concerns the stability of a measure, is assessed by making two separate measurements of the same people, often 1 to 2 weeks apart, and then testing the extent to which the two sets of scores are consistent. Some researchers use Pearson's r to correlate the scores at Time 1 with those at Time 2, but the preferred index for test–retest reliability is the **intraclass correlation coefficient (ICC)**, which can range in value from .00 to 1.00.
- *Interrater reliability* is used to assess the extent to which two independent raters or observers assign the same score in measuring an attribute. When the ratings are dichotomous classifications (e.g., presence vs. absence of infusion phlebitis), the preferred index is **Cohen's kappa**, whose values also range from .00 to 1.00. If the ratings are continuous scores, the ICC is usually used.
- *Internal consistency reliability* concerns the extent to which the various components of a multicomponent measure (e.g., items on a psychosocial scale) are consistently measuring the same attribute. Internal consistency is estimated by an index called **coefficient alpha** (or *Cronbach's alpha*). If a psychosocial scale includes several subscales, coefficient alpha is usually computed for each subscale separately.

For all of these reliability indices, the closer the value is to 1.00, the stronger is the evidence of good reliability. Although opinions about minimally acceptable values vary, values of .80 or higher are usually considered good. Researchers try to select measures with previously demonstrated high levels of reliability, but if they are using a multi-item scale, they usually compute coefficient alpha with their own data as well.

Validity Assessment

Validity is the measurement property that concerns the degree to which an instrument is measuring what it purports to measure. Like reliability, validity has several aspects. Unlike reliability, however, it is challenging to establish a measure's validity. Validation is a process of evidence building, and typically, multiple forms of evidence are sought.

Content Validity

Content validity is relevant for composite measures, such as multi-item scales. The issue is whether the content of the items adequately reflects the construct of interest. Content validation usually relies on expert ratings of each item, and the ratings are used to compute an index called the *content validity index (CVI)*. A value of .90 or higher has been suggested as providing evidence of good content validity.

Criterion Validity

Criterion validity concerns the extent to which scores on a measure are consistent with a "gold standard" criterion. The methods used to assess criterion validity depend on the level of measurement of the focal measure and the criterion.

When both the focal measure and the criterion are continuous, researchers administer the two measures to a sample and then compute a Pearson's *r* between the two scores. Larger coefficients are desirable, but there is no threshold value that is considered a minimum. Usually, statistical significance is the standard for concluding that criterion validity is adequate.

If both the measure and the gold standard are dichotomous variables, researchers often use methods of assessing *diagnostic accuracy*. **Sensitivity** is the ability of a measure to correctly identify a "case," that is, to correctly screen in or diagnose a condition. A measure's sensitivity is its rate of yielding *true positives*. **Specificity** is the measure's ability to correctly identify noncases, that is, to screen *out* those without the condition. Specificity is an instrument's rate of yielding *true negatives*.

To assess an instrument's sensitivity and specificity, researchers need a highly reliable and valid criterion of "caseness" against which scores on the instrument can be assessed. For example, if we wanted to test the validity of adolescents' self-reports about smoking (yes/no in past 24 hours), we could use urinary cotinine level, using a cutoff value for a positive test of ≥200 ng/mL as the gold standard. Sensitivity would be calculated as the proportion of teenagers who said they smoked *and* who had high concentrations of cotinine, divided by all real smokers as indicated by the urine test. Specificity would be the proportion of teenagers who accurately reported they did not smoke, or the true negatives, divided by all *real* negatives. Both sensitivity and specificity can range from .00 to 1.00. It is difficult to set standards of acceptability for sensitivity and specificity, but both should be as high as possible.

When the focal measure is continuous and the gold standard is dichotomous, researchers often use a statistical tool called a *receiver operating characteristic (ROC) curve*. An ROC curve involves plotting each score on the focal measure against its sensitivity and specificity for correct classification based on a dichotomous criterion. A discussion of ROC curves is beyond the scope of this book, but interested readers can consult Polit and Yang (2016).

Construct Validity

Construct validity concerns the extent to which a measure is truly measuring the target construct and is often assessed using hypothesis testing procedures like those described earlier in this chapter. For example, a researcher might hypothesize that scores on a new measure (e.g., a scale of fear of hospitalization) would correlate with scores on another established measure (e.g., an anxiety scale). Pearson's *r* would be used to test this hypothesis, and a significant correlation would provide some evidence of construct validity. For known-groups validity, which involves testing hypotheses about expected group differences on a new measure, an independent groups *t*-test could be used. Both bivariate and multivariate statistical tests are appropriate in assessments of a new measure's construct validity.

READING AND UNDERSTANDING STATISTICAL INFORMATION

Unless researchers are reporting a psychometric assessment, measurement statistics are most likely to be presented in the methods section of a report, in their descriptions of the measures they used. Statistical *findings* for a substantive study, however, are communicated in the results section, both in the text and in tables (or, less frequently, in figures). This section offers assistance in reading and interpreting statistical information.

Tips on Reading Text With Statistical Information

Both descriptive and inferential statistics are presented in research reports. Descriptive statistics typically summarize sample characteristics. Information about the participants' background helps readers to draw conclusions about the people to whom the findings can be applied. Researchers may provide statistical information for evaluating biases. For example, when a quasi-experimental or case-control design has been used, researchers may test the equivalence of the groups being compared on baseline or background variables, using tests such as t-tests.

For hypothesis testing, the text of research articles usually provides the following information about statistical tests: (1) the test used, (2) the value of the calculated statistic, and (3) the level of statistical significance. Examples of how the results of various statistical tests might be reported in the text are shown below.

1. t-Test: $t = 1.68, p = .09$
2. Chi-squared: $\chi^2 = 16.65, p < .001$
3. Pearson's r: $r = .36, p < .01$
4. ANOVA: $F = 0.18$, *NS*

The preferred approach is to report significance as the computed probability that the null hypothesis is correct, as in Example 1. In this case, the observed group mean differences could be found by chance in 9 out of 100 samples. This result is not statistically significant because the mean difference had an unacceptably high chance of being spurious. The probability level is sometimes reported simply as falling below or above certain thresholds (Examples 2 and 3). Both these results are significant because the probability of obtaining such results by chance is less than 1 in 100. You must be careful to read the symbol following the p value correctly: The symbol < means *less than*. The symbol > means *greater than*—that is, the results are not significant if the p value is .05 or greater. When results do not achieve statistical significance at the desired level, researchers may simply indicate that the results were not significant (*NS*), as in Example 4.

Statistical information often is noted parenthetically in a sentence describing the findings, as in "Patients in the intervention group had a significantly lower rate of infection than those in the control group ($\chi^2 = 5.41, p = .02$)." In reading research reports, the values of the test statistics (e.g., $\chi^2 = 5.41$) are of no inherent interest. What is important is whether the statistical tests indicate that the research hypotheses were accepted as probably true (as demonstrated by significant results) or rejected as probably false (as demonstrated by nonsignificant results).

Tips on Reading Statistical Tables

Tables allow researchers to condense a lot of statistical information. Consider, for example, putting information about dozens of correlation coefficients in the text. Tables are efficient, but they may be daunting for novice readers, partly because of the absence of standardization. There is no universally accepted format for presenting t-test results, for example. Thus, each table may present a new deciphering challenge.

We have a few suggestions for helping you to comprehend statistical tables. First, read the text and the tables simultaneously—the text may help you figure out what the table is communicating. Second, before trying to understand the numbers in a table, try to glean information from the accompanying words. Table titles and footnotes often present critical information. Table headings should be carefully scrutinized because they indicate what the variables in the analysis are (often listed as row labels in the first column, as in Table 13.10) and what statistical information is included (often specified as column headings). Third, you may find it helpful to consult the glossary of symbols on the inside back cover of this book to check the meaning of a statistical symbol. Not all symbols in this glossary were described in this chapter, so it may be necessary to refer to a statistics textbook for further information.

TABLE 13.10 Selected Demographic and Clinical Characteristics of Participants in Study on Social Jetlag and Body Mass Index (BMI) Among Shift-Working Nurses in Korea

Sample Characteristic	(N)	Percentage	Median	SD	Range
Gender					
Male	34	18.6			
Female	149	81.4			
Marital status					
Married	36	19.7			
Not married	147	80.3			
Years in nursing career			3.83		(2.00–7.00)
Age			27		25.00–30.00
Exercise time (per week)			1 hour:50 minutes		1:00–3:00 hours
Smoking					
No	167	91.3			
Yes	16	8.7			
Drinking					
No	29	15.8			
Yes	154	84.2			
BMI				21.5	19.53–23.23
Underweight	9	4.9			
Normal	122	66.7			
Overweight	37	20.2			
Obese	15	8.2			
Eating habits					
Regular	79	43.2			
Irregular	104	56.9			
Sleep duration (hours/minutes)			6:45		5:18–7:37
Social jetlag (hours/minutes)			3:31	1:19	

Adapted from Table 1 of Hwang, K. R., Lee, M., & Jang, S. J. (2024). Social jetlag and body mass index among shift-working nurses in Korea: A cross-sectional study. *International Journal of Nursing Knowledge, 35*(2), 195–202. https://doi.org/10.1111/2047-3095.12410. Copyright © 2023 NANDA International, Inc. Reprinted by permission of John Wiley & Sons, Inc.

TIP In tables, probability levels associated with significance tests are sometimes presented directly in the table, in a column labeled "*p*" (e.g., *p* = .03). However, researchers sometimes indicate significance levels in tables with asterisks placed next to the value of the test statistic. One asterisk usually signifies $p < .05$, two asterisks signify $p < .01$, and three asterisks signify $p < .001$. (There should be a key at the bottom of the table indicating what the asterisks mean.) Thus, a table might show $t = 3.00$ in one column and $p < .01$ in another. Alternatively, the table might show $t = 3.00**$. The absence of an asterisk would signify a nonsignificant result.

CRITICAL APPRAISAL OF QUANTITATIVE ANALYSES

It is often difficult to critically appraise statistical analyses. We hope this chapter has helped to demystify statistics, but we recognize the limited scope of our coverage. It would be unreasonable to expect you to be adept at evaluating statistical analyses, but you can be on the lookout for certain things in reviewing research articles. Some guidance is presented in Box 13.1.

One aspect of the appraisal should focus on which analyses were reported. You should assess whether the statistical information adequately describes the sample and reports the results of statistical tests for all hypotheses. Another presentational issue concerns the researcher's judicious use of tables to summarize statistical information.

A thorough critical appraisal also addresses whether researchers used the appropriate statistics. See Table 13.9 for guidelines for some frequently used bivariate statistical tests. The major issues to consider are the number of independent and dependent variables, the levels of measurement of the research variables, and the number of groups (if any) being compared.

If researchers did not use multivariate statistics, you should consider whether the bivariate analysis adequately tests the relationship between the independent and dependent variables. For example, if a *t*-test or ANOVA was used, could the internal validity of the study have been enhanced through the statistical control of confounding variables, using ANCOVA? The answer will often be "yes."

Finally, you can be alert to possible exaggerations or subjectivity in the reported results. Researchers should never claim that the data proved, verified, confirmed, or demonstrated

---

Box 13.1 Guidelines for Critically Appraising Statistical Analyses

a. Did the descriptive statistics in the report sufficiently describe the major variables and demographic characteristics of the sample?
b. Was a power analysis conducted to determine sample size?
c. Did the researchers report any inferential statistics?
d. Was information provided about hypothesis testing?
e. Was an effect size reported?
f. Overall, did the reported statistics provide readers with sufficient information about the study results?
g. Were any multivariate procedures used?
h. Were the results of any statistical tests significant?
i. What factors might have undermined the study's statistical conclusion validity?
j. Was information about the reliability and validity of measures reported?
k. Was there an appropriate amount of statistical information?
l. Are the tables clear, with good titles and row/column labels?

that the hypotheses were correct or incorrect. Hypotheses should be described as *supported* or *not supported*, *accepted* or *rejected*.

The main task for beginning consumers in reading the results section of a research report is to understand the meaning of the statistical tests. What do the quantitative results indicate about the researcher's hypothesis? How believable are the findings? The answer to such questions forms the basis for interpreting the research results, a topic discussed in Chapter 14.

RESEARCH EXAMPLES WITH CRITICAL THINKING EXERCISES

In this section, we provide details about the analysis in a nursing study, followed by some questions to guide critical thinking. Read the summary for Example 1, and then answer the critical thinking questions that follow. The critical thinking questions for Example 2 are based on the study that appears in its entirety in Appendix A of this book.

EXAMPLE 1: DESCRIPTIVE AND INFERENTIAL STATISTICS

Study: "Social jetlag and body mass index among shift-working nurses in Korea: A cross-sectional study" (Hwang et al., 2024)

Statement of Purpose: Hwang and colleagues aimed to explore the association between social jetlag and obesity among shift-working nurses.

Methods: The authors used a cross-sectional approach. The sample included nurses with at least 1 year of experience who worked all three rotating shifts (days, evenings, and nights).

Analysis: Through a power analysis, the minimal sample size was set at 166, assuming a significance level (p *value*) of .05. Descriptive statistics were used to describe the sample characteristics such as sex, age, marital status, and living status. While this study reports the use of several inferential statistics, the chi-squared analysis, used to explore the relationships of those in the sample with obesity versus those without obesity, and the multiple logistic regression analysis, used to identify the association between social jetlag and obesity, are the two inferential statistics we will focus on in the results section and for the critical thinking questions.

Results: Demographic information about the sample of the 183 participants is provided in Table 13.10. The sample was mostly female (81.4%) and single (80.3%) with a mean age of 27 years. The chi-square analysis (Table 13.11) shows that nurses with obesity had irregular eating habits 86.7% ($n = 13$) and a social jetlag of 3 hours and 31 min or higher 86.7% ($n = 13$). The multiple linear regression analysis indicated that among shift-working nurses with a social jetlag score over 3 hours and 31 minutes, the odds for obesity were 8.44 times higher (95% CI: 1.66–42.99).

Multivariate Analyses:

Critical Thinking Exercises

1. Answer the relevant questions in Box 13.1 regarding this study.
2. Referring to Table 13.10, what is the median amount of time this sample exercised per week?
3. Referring to Table 13.10, what was the median time for social jet lag?
4. What was the standard deviation for social jet lag?

5. What percentage of the participants with obesity also had high social jetlag (Table 13.11)? Was this statistically significant?
6. In this sample, was drinking a significant factor in those with obesity (Table 13.11)? Was irregular eating a significant factor in those with obesity?

TABLE 13.11 **Differences in Select Characteristics of Participants With and Without Obesity**

Categories	Obesity No N/%	Obesity Yes N/%	χ^2	p Value
Social jetlag			9.19	.003
Low (<3:31)	91 (54.2)	2 (13.3)		
High (≥3:31)	77 (45.8)	13 (86.7)		
Eating habits			5.73	.026
Regular eating	76 (45.2)	2 (13.3)		
Irregular	92 (54.8)	13 (86.7)		
Drinking			0.08	>.99
No	27 (16.1)	2 (13.3)		
Yes	141 (83.9)	13 (86.7)		

Adapted from Table 2 of Hwang, K. R., Lee, M., & Jang, S. J. (2024). Social jetlag and body mass index among shift-working nurses in Korea: A cross-sectional study. *International Journal of Nursing Knowledge, 35*(2), 195–202. https://doi.org/10.1111/2047-3095.12410. Copyright © 2023 NANDA International, Inc. Reprinted by permission of John Wiley & Sons, Inc.

EXAMPLE 2: STATISTICAL ANALYSIS IN THE STUDY IN APPENDIX A

Read the Results section of Cheng and colleagues' (2024) study "Advance care planning affects end-of-life treatment preferences among patients with heart failure: A randomized controlled trial" in Appendix A of this book.

Critical Thinking Exercises

1. Answer the relevant questions in Box 13.1 regarding this study.
2. Referring to Table 1, what was the most frequently reported religion in both the control group and the intervention group?
3. Referring to Table 1, what is the median age of the control group?
4. What was the standard deviation for the age of the control group?
5. Was there a pre-post difference in the total Life Support Preference Questionnaire (LSPQ) for the intervention group (Table 2)?
6. Was there a statistically significant difference in mean score changes between the intervention and control groups for antibiotics?

Summary Points

- There are four **levels of measurement:** (1) **nominal measurement**—the classification of attributes into mutually exclusive categories, (2) **ordinal measurement**—the ranking of people based on their relative standing on an attribute, (3) **interval measurement**—indicating not only people's rank order but also the distance between them, and (4) **ratio measurement**—distinguished from interval measurement by having a rational zero point. Interval- and ratio-level measures are often called **continuous**.

- **Descriptive statistics** are used to summarize and describe quantitative data.

- In **frequency distributions**, numeric values are ordered from lowest to highest, together with a count of the number (or percentage) of times each value was obtained.

- Data for a continuous variable can be described in terms of the shape of the distribution, central tendency, and variability.

- A distribution's shape can be **symmetric** or **skewed**, with one tail longer than the other; it can also be unimodal with one peak (i.e., one value of high frequency) or multimodal with more than one peak. A **normal distribution** (bell-shaped curve) is symmetric, unimodal, and not too peaked.

- Indices of **central tendency** represent the average or typical value of a set of scores. The **mode** is the value that occurs most frequently, the **median** is the point above which and below which 50% of the cases fall, and the **mean** is the arithmetic average of all scores. The mean is the most stable index of central tendency.

- Indices of **variability**—how spread out the data are—include the range and standard deviation. The **range** is the distance between the highest and lowest scores. The **standard deviation** (*SD*) indicates how much, on average, scores deviate from the mean.

- In a normal distribution, 95% of values lie within 2 *SD*s above and below the mean.

- A **crosstabs table** is a two-dimensional frequency distribution in which the frequencies of two nominal- or ordinal-level variables are crosstabulated.

- **Correlation coefficients** describe the direction and magnitude of a relationship between two variables; they range from –1.00 (perfect **negative correlation**) through .00 to +1.00 (perfect **positive correlation**). The most frequently used correlation coefficient is **Pearson's *r***, used with continuous variables.

- Statistical indices that describe the effects of exposure to risk factors or interventions provide useful information for clinical decisions. A widely reported risk index is the **odds ratio (OR)**, which is the ratio of the odds for an exposed versus unexposed group, with the *odds* reflecting the proportion of people with an adverse outcome relative to those without it.

- **Inferential statistics**, based on laws of probability, allow researchers to make inferences about population **parameters** based on data from a sample.

- The *sampling distribution of the mean* is a theoretical distribution of the means of an infinite number of same-sized samples drawn from a population. Sampling distributions are the basis for inferential statistics.

- The *standard error of the mean (SEM)*—the *SD* of this theoretical distribution—indicates the degree of average error of a sample mean; the smaller the SEM, the more accurate are estimates of the population value.

- Statistical inference consists of two approaches: hypothesis testing and **parameter estimation** (estimating a population value).

- *Point estimation* is a single value of a population estimate (e.g., a mean). *Interval estimation* provides a range of values—a **confidence interval (CI)**—within which the population value is expected to fall, at a specified probability. Most often, the 95% CI is reported, which indicates that there is a 95% probability that the true population value lies between the lower and upper confidence limits.

- **Hypothesis testing** through statistical tests enables researchers to make objective decisions about relationships between variables.

- The *null hypothesis* is that no relationship exists between variables; rejection of the null hypothesis lends support to the research hypothesis. In testing hypotheses, researchers compute a **test statistic** and then see if the statistic falls beyond a critical region on the theoretical distribution. The value of the test statistic indicates whether the null hypothesis is "improbable."

- A **Type I error** occurs if a null hypothesis is wrongly rejected (false positives). **A Type II error** occurs when a null hypothesis is wrongly accepted (false negatives).

- Researchers control the risk of making a Type I error by selecting a **level of significance** (or **alpha** level), which is the probability that such an error will occur. The .05 level (the conventional standard) means that in only 5 out of 100 samples would the null hypothesis be rejected when it should have been accepted.

- The probability of committing a Type II error is related to *power*, the ability of a statistical test to detect true relationships. The standard criterion for an acceptable level of power is .80. Power increases as sample size increases.

- Results from hypothesis tests are either significant or nonsignificant; **statistically significant** means that the obtained results are not likely to be due to chance fluctuations at a given probability (*p* value).

- Both the ***t*-test** and **analysis of variance (ANOVA)** can be used to test the significance of the difference between group means; ANOVA is used when there are three or more groups. **Repeated measures ANOVA** (RM-ANOVA) is used when data are collected at multiple time points.

- The **chi-squared test** is used to test hypotheses about group differences in proportions.

- Pearson's *r* can be used to test whether a correlation is significantly different from zero.

- **Effect size** indices (such as the *d* **statistic**) summarize the strength of the effect of an independent variable (e.g., an intervention) on an outcome variable.

- **Multivariate statistics** are used in nursing research to untangle complex relationships among three or more variables.

- **Multiple regression analysis** is a method for understanding the effect of two or more **predictor** (independent) **variables** on a continuous dependent variable.

- **Analysis of covariance (ANCOVA)** controls confounding variables (called *covariates*) before testing whether differences in group means are statistically significant.

- **Logistic regression** is used to predict an outcome that is dichotomous on the basis of two or more predictor variables.

- Statistical methods are also used in psychometric assessments to quantify a measure's reliability and validity.

- For test–retest reliability, the preferred index is the **intraclass correlation coefficient (ICC)**. **Cohen's kappa** is used to estimate interrater reliability when the ratings of two independent raters are dichotomous. The index used to estimate internal consistency reliability is **coefficient alpha (α)**. Reliability coefficients of .80 or higher are desirable.

- In terms of content validity, expert ratings of items on a scale are used to compute a *CVI*.

- Criterion validity is assessed with different statistical methods depending on the measurement level of the focal measure and the criterion. When both are dichotomous, sensitivity and specificity are usually calculated. **Sensitivity** is the instrument's ability to identify a case correctly (i.e., its rate of yielding true positives). **Specificity** is the instrument's ability to identify noncases correctly (i.e., its rate of yielding true negatives).

- Construct validity is evaluated using hypothesis testing procedures, so statistical tests such as those described in this chapter (e.g., Pearson's *r*, *t*-tests) are appropriate.

REFERENCES

Bagheri, S., Zarshenas, L., Rakhshan, M., Sharif, F., Sarani, E. M., Shirazi, Z. H., & Sitzman, K. (2023). Impact of Watson's human caring-based health promotion program on caregivers of individuals with schizophrenia. *BMC Health Services Research*, *23*(1), 711. https://doi.org/10.1186/s12913-023-09725-9

Fiske, M., Moen, A., Mdala, I., & Straand, J. (2024). Malnutrition and polypharmacy in older adult patients receiving home care nursing services: A cross-sectional Study. *Journal of the American Medical Directors Association*, *25*(3), 526–531. https://doi.org/10.1016/j.jamda.2023.11.016

Flanagan, J., Boltz, M. & Ji, M. (2023). Post-acute rehabilitation in persons with and without dementia. *Annals of Long-Term Care*. https://www.hmpgloballearningnetwork.com/site/altc/practical-research/postacute-rehabilitation-patients-and-without-dementia

Hoelscher, S. H., McBride, S., Bumpus, S., Gilder, R. E., & Elkind, E. (2024). A study to determine consensus for nursing documentation reduction in times of crisis. *Computers, Informatics, Nursing*, *42*(10), 712–721. https://doi.org/10.1097/CIN.0000000000001180

Hwang, K. R., Lee, M., & Jang, S. J. (2024). Social jetlag and body mass index among shift-working nurses in Korea: A cross-sectional study. *International Journal of Nursing Knowledge*, *35*(2), 195–202. https://doi.org/10.1111/2047-3095.12410

Kim, C. H., Kang, K. A., & Shin, S. (2023). Healthy lifestyle status related to alcohol and food addiction risk among college students: A logistic regression analysis. *Journal of American College Health*, *71*(3), 775–781. https://doi.org/10.1080/07448481.2021.1908302

LaRowe, L. R., Miaskowski, C., Miller, A., Mayfield, A., Keefe, F. J., Smith, A. K., Cooper, B. A., Wei, L.-J., & Ritchie, C. S. (2024). Chronic pain and pain management in older adults: Protocol and pilot results. *Nursing Research*, *73*(1), 81–88. https://doi.org/10.1097/NNR.0000000000000683

Lindsay, M., & Decker, V. B. (2022). Improving depression screening in primary care. *Journal of Doctoral Nursing Practice*, *15*(2), 84–90. https://doi.org/10.1891/JDNP-2021-0005

McCann, R., Richardson, E., Schisler, E. D., Sudduth, A., & Dobbs, P. D. (2024). Cigarette and E-cigarette harm perceptions during pregnancy. *Nursing Research*, *73*(4), 286–293. https://doi.org/10.1097/NNR.0000000000000742

Munroe, B., Curtis, K., Fry, M., Shaban, R. Z., Moules, P., Elphick, T. L., Ruperto, K., Couttie, T., & Considine, J. (2022). Increasing accuracy in documentation through the application of a structured emergency nursing framework: A multisite quasi-experimental study. *Journal of Clinical Nursing*, *31*(19–20), 2874–85. https://doi.org/10.1111/jocn.16115

Oladokun, M. O., Olaogun, A. A., & Mosaku, S. K. (2025). Clinical validation of the nursing diagnosis of impaired mood regulation among individuals with experience of mood disorders. *International Journal of Nursing Knowledge*, *36*(1), 39–47. https://doi.org/10.1111/2047-3095.12460

Polit, D. F., & Yang, F. (2016). *Measurement and the measurement of change: A primer for health professionals*. Wolters Kluwer.

Ramsdale, E., Mohamed, M., Holmes, H. M., Zubkoff, L., Bauer, J., Norton, S. A., & Mohile, S. (2024). Decreasing polypharmacy in older adults with cancer: A pilot cluster-randomized trial protocol. *Journal of Geriatric Oncology*, *15*(2), 101687. https://doi.org/10.1016/j.jgo.2023.101687

Yang, M., Xue, J., Kong, X., Liu, W., Wang, Y., Zou, Y., Wang, L., & Dong, C. (2024). Correlation of psychological resilience with social support and coping style in Parkinson's disease: A cross-sectional study. *Journal of Advanced Nursing*. https://doi.org/10.1111/jan.16408

Yu, Q., Huang, C., Yan, J., Yue, L., Tian, Y., Yang, J., Li, X., Li, Y., & Qin, Y. (2025). Ethical climate, moral resilience, and ethical competence of head nurses. *Nursing Ethics*, *32*(1), 56–70. https://doi.org/10.1177/09697330241230526

14 Interpreting Quantitative Findings and Evaluating Clinical Significance

Learning Objectives

On completing this chapter, you will be able to:

- Describe dimensions for interpreting quantitative research results
- Describe the mindset conducive to a critical interpretation of research results
- Identify approaches to an assessment of the credibility of quantitative results and undertake such an assessment
- Distinguish statistical and clinical significance
- Identify some methods of drawing conclusions about clinical significance at the group and individual levels
- Critically appraise researchers' interpretation of their results in discussion sections of research reports
- Define new terms in the chapter

Key Terms

- Benchmark
- Change score
- Clinical significance
- CONSORT guidelines
- Minimal important change (MIC)
- Responder analysis
- Results

In this chapter, we consider approaches to interpreting researchers' statistical results, which require consideration of the various theoretical, methodologic, and practical decisions that researchers make in undertaking a study. We also discuss an important but seldom discussed topic: **clinical significance**.

INTERPRETATION OF QUANTITATIVE RESULTS

Statistical **results** are summarized in the results section of a research article. Researchers present their interpretations of the results in the discussion section. It is difficult for the researchers to be totally objective, though, so you should develop your own interpretations.

Aspects of Interpretation

Interpreting study results involves attending to different but overlapping considerations.

- The credibility and accuracy of the results
- The precision of the estimate of effects
- The magnitude of effects and importance of the results

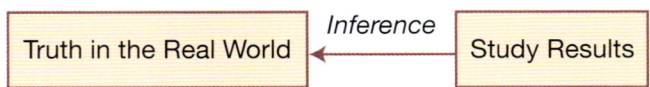

Figure 14.1 Inferences in interpreting research results.

- The meaning of the results, especially with regard to causality
- The generalizability and applicability of the results
- The implications of the results for nursing practice, theory development, or further research

Before discussing these considerations, we want to remind you about the role of inference in research thinking and interpretation.

Inference and Interpretation

An *inference* involves drawing conclusions based on limited information, using logical reasoning. Interpreting research findings entails making multiple inferences. In research, virtually everything is a "stand-in" for something else: a sample is a stand-in for a population, a scale score is a proxy for the magnitude of an abstract attribute, and so on.

Research findings are meant to reflect "truth in the real world"—the findings are proxies for the true state of affairs (Fig. 14.1). Inferences about the real world are valid to the extent that researchers make good decisions in selecting proxies. This chapter offers several vantage points for assessing whether study findings really reflect "truth in the real world."

The Interpretive Mindset

Evidence-based practice (EBP) involves integrating research evidence into clinical decision making. EBP encourages clinicians to think critically about clinical practice and to challenge the status quo when it conflicts with "best evidence." Thinking critically and demanding evidence are also part of a research interpreter's job. Just as clinicians should ask, "What *evidence* is there that this intervention will be beneficial?" so must interpreters ask, "What *evidence* is there that the results are real and true?"

To be a good interpreter of research results, you can profit by starting with a skeptical ("show me") attitude and a null hypothesis. The "null hypothesis" in interpretation is that the results are wrong and the evidence is flawed. The "research hypothesis" is that the evidence reflects the truth. Interpreters decide whether the null hypothesis has merit by critically examining methodologic evidence. The greater the evidence that the researcher's design and methods were sound, the less plausible is the null hypothesis that the evidence is inaccurate.

CREDIBILITY OF QUANTITATIVE RESULTS

A critical interpretive task is to assess whether the results are *right*. If the results are not judged to be credible, the remaining interpretive issues (the meaning, magnitude, precision, generalizability, and implications of results) are unlikely to be relevant.

A credibility assessment requires a careful analysis of the study's methodologic and conceptual limitations and strengths. To come to a conclusion about whether the results closely approximate "truth in the real world," each aspect of the study—its design, sampling plan, data collection, and analyses—must be subjected to critical scrutiny.

There are various ways to approach the issue of credibility, including the use of the critical appraisal guidelines we have offered throughout this book and the overall appraisal protocol presented in Table 3.1 in Chapter 3. We share some additional perspectives in this section.

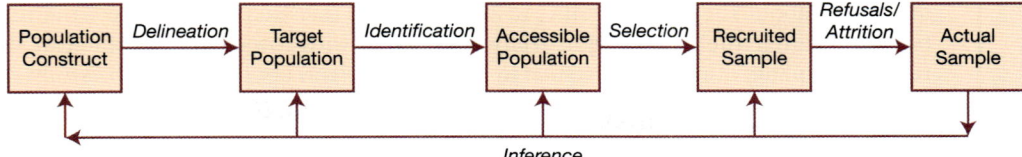

Figure 14.2 Inferences about populations: from final sample to the population.

Proxies and Interpretation

Researchers begin with constructs and then devise ways to operationalize them. The constructs are linked to actual research tactics in a series of approximations; the better the proxies, the more credible the results are likely to be. In this section, we illustrate successive proxies using sampling concepts to highlight the potential for inferential challenges.

When researchers formulate research questions, the population of interest is often abstract. For example, suppose we wanted to test the effectiveness of an intervention to increase physical activity in low-income women. Figure 14.2 shows the series of steps between the abstract population construct (low-income women) and actual study participants. Using data from the actual sample on the far right, the researcher would like to make inferences about the effectiveness of the intervention for a broader group, but each proxy along the way represents a potential problem for achieving the desired inference. In interpreting a study, readers must consider how *plausible* it is that the actual sample reflects the recruited sample, the accessible population, the target population, and the population construct.

Table 14.1 presents a description of a hypothetical scenario in which the researchers moved from the population construct (low-income women) to a sample of 163 participants (recent public assistance recipients from two neighborhoods in Los Angeles) who provided postintervention data. The table identifies questions that could be asked in drawing

TABLE 14.1 Example of Successive Series of Proxies in Sampling

Element	Description	Possible Inferential Challenges
Population construct	Low-income women	
Target population	All women who receive public assistance (cash welfare) in California	• Why only welfare recipients? Why not low-income women who are not eligible for public assistance? • Why California?
Accessible population	All women who receive public assistance in Los Angeles and who speak English or Spanish	• Why Los Angeles? • What about non-English/non-Spanish speakers?
Recruited sample	A consecutive sample of 282 female public assistance recipients (English or Spanish speaking) who applied for benefits in January 2022 at two welfare offices in Los Angeles; 267 were deemed eligible	• Why only new applicants? What about women with long-term receipt? • Why only two offices? Are these representative? • Is January a typical month?
Randomized sample	200 women from the recruited sample who agreed to participate in the study	• How did the 200 participants differ from the 67 who declined to participate?
Final actual sample	163 women who were included in the analysis sample	• How did dropouts differ from those in the final sample?

inferences about the study results. Answers to these questions would affect the interpretation of whether the intervention *really* is effective with low-income women or only with recent recipients of public assistance in Los Angeles who cooperated in the study.

Researchers make methodologic decisions that affect inferences, but prospective participants' behavior also needs to be considered. In our example, only 200 of the 267 eligible women agreed to participate in the study, and only 163 provided data for the analysis. The sample of 163 women almost surely would differ in important ways from the 104 who either declined to participate in the study or who dropped out.

Fortunately, researchers are increasingly documenting participant flow in their studies—especially in intervention studies. Guidelines called the Consolidated Standards of Reporting Trials or **CONSORT guidelines** have been adopted by major health care journals to help readers track study participants. CONSORT flow charts, when available in a report, should be scrutinized in interpreting study results. Figure 14.3 provides an example of such a flowchart for the intervention study just described. The chart shows that 282 people were assessed for eligibility, but 82 either did not meet eligibility criteria or refused to be in the study. Of the 200 people who agreed to participate, half were randomized to the intervention group and the other half to the control group ($N = 100$ per group). However, only 80 in the experimental group received the full intervention. At the 3-month

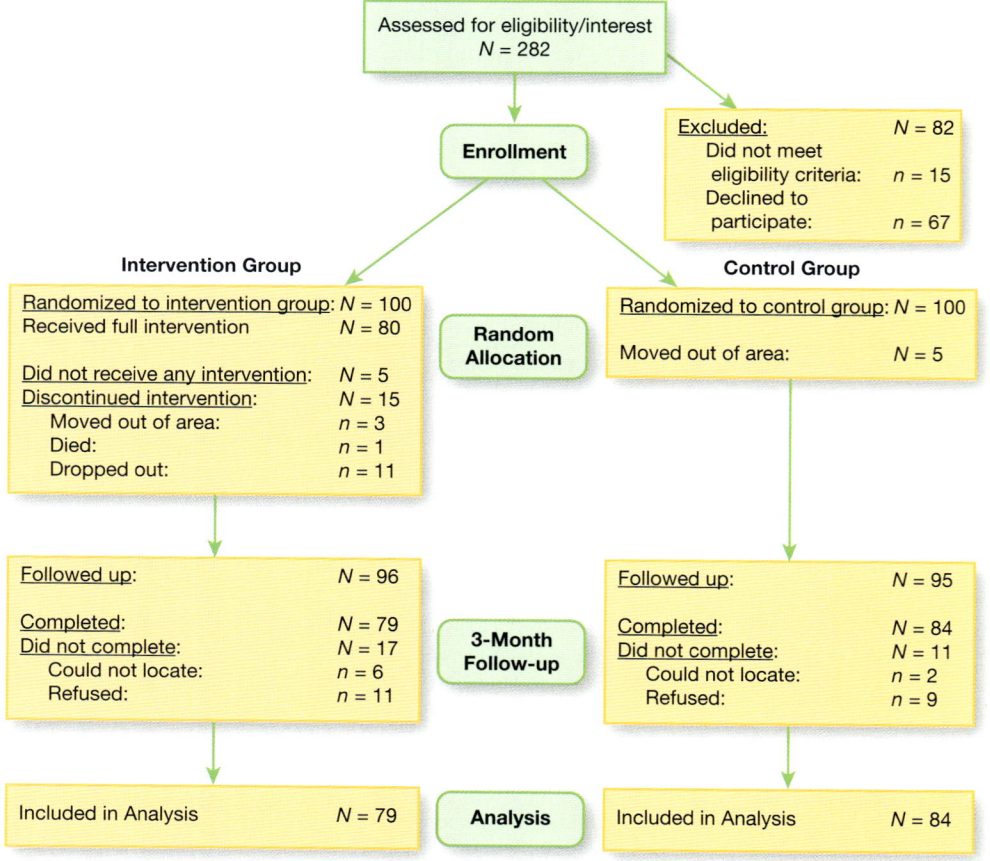

Figure 14.3 Example of CONSORT guidelines flowchart: progression of participants in an intervention study.

follow-up, researchers attempted to obtain data from 96 people in the intervention group and 95 in the control group (everyone who did not move or die). They obtained follow-up data from 79 in the intervention group and 84 in the control group, and these 163 comprised the analysis sample.

Credibility and Validity

Inference and validity are inextricably linked. To be careful interpreters, readers must search for evidence that the desired inferences are, in fact, valid. Part of this process involves considering alternative competing hypotheses about the credibility and meaning of the results.

In Chapter 8, we discussed four types of validity that relate to the credibility of study results: statistical conclusion validity, internal validity, external validity, and construct validity. We use our sampling example (Fig. 14.2; Table 14.1) to demonstrate the relevance of methodologic decisions to all four types of validity—and hence to inferences about study results.

In our example, the population construct is *low-income women*, which was translated into population eligibility criteria stipulating California public assistance recipients. Yet, there are alternative operationalizations of the population construct (e.g., women living below the official poverty level). Construct validity, it may be recalled, involves inferences from the particulars of the study to higher order constructs. So it is fair to ask: Do the eligibility criteria adequately capture the population construct, low-income women?

Statistical conclusion validity—the extent to which correct inferences can be made about the existence of "real" group differences—is also affected by sampling decisions. Ideally, researchers would do a power analysis at the outset to estimate how large a sample they needed. In our example, let us assume (based on previous research) that the effect size for the exercise intervention would be small to moderate, with $d = .40$. For a power of .80, with risk of a Type I error set at .05, we would need a sample of about 200 participants. The actual sample of 163 yields a nearly 30% risk of a Type II error, that is, wrongly concluding that the intervention was not successful.

External validity—the generalizability of the results—is affected by sampling. To whom would it be safe to generalize the results in this example—to the population construct of low-income women? To all recipients of public assistance in California? To all new recipients in Los Angeles who speak English or Spanish? Inferences about the extent to which the study results correspond to "truth in the real world" must take sampling decisions and sampling problems (e.g., recruitment and attrition difficulties) into account.

Finally, the study's internal validity (the extent to which a causal inference can be made) is also affected by sample composition. In this example, attrition would be a concern. Were those in the intervention group more likely (or less likely) than those in the control group to drop out of the study? If so, any observed differences in outcomes could be caused by individual differences in the groups (e.g., differences in motivation to stay in the study), rather than by the intervention itself.

Methodologic decisions and the careful implementation of those decisions—whether they be about sampling, intervention design, measurement, research design, or analysis—inevitably affect the rigor of a study. All of them can affect the four types of validity, and hence the interpretation of the results.

Credibility and Bias

A researcher's job is to translate abstract constructs into appropriate proxies. Another major job concerns efforts to eliminate, reduce, or control biases—or, as a last resort, to detect and understand them. As a reader of research reports, your job is to be on the lookout for biases and to factor them into your assessment about the credibility of the results.

TABLE 14.2 Selected List of Major Biases or Errors in Quantitative Studies in Four Research Domains

Research Design	Sampling	Measurement	Analysis
Expectation bias	Sampling error	Social desirability bias	Type I error
Hawthorne effect	Volunteer bias	Acquiescence bias	Type II error
Contamination of treatments	Nonresponse bias	Naysayers bias	
Carryover effects		Extreme response bias	
Noncompliance bias		Recall/memory bias	
Selection bias		Reactivity	
Attrition bias		Observer biases	
History bias			

Biases create distortions and undermine researchers' efforts to reveal "truth in the real world." Biases are pervasive and virtually inevitable. It is important to consider what types of bias might be present and how extensive, sizable, and systematic they are. We have discussed many types of bias in this book—some reflect design inadequacies (e.g., selection bias), others reflect recruitment problems (nonresponse bias), and others relate to measurement (social desirability bias). Table 14.2 presents biases and errors mentioned in this book. This table is meant to serve as a reminder of some of the problems to consider in interpreting study results.

Credibility and Corroboration

Earlier, we noted that research interpreters should seek evidence to disconfirm the "null hypothesis" that research results are wrong. Some evidence to discredit this null hypothesis comes from the quality of the proxies that stand in for abstractions. Ruling out biases also undermines the null hypothesis. Another strategy is to seek corroboration for the results.

Corroboration can come from internal and external sources, and the concept of *replication* is an important one in both cases. Interpretations are aided by considering prior research on the topic, for example. Interpreters can examine whether the study results are congruent with those of other studies. Consistency across studies tends to discredit the "null hypothesis" of erroneous results.

Researchers may have opportunities for replication themselves. For example, in multi-site studies, if the results are similar across sites, this suggests that something "real" is occurring. Triangulation can be another form of replication. We are strong advocates of mixed methods studies (see Chapter 12). When findings from the analysis of qualitative data are consistent with the results of statistical analyses, internal corroboration can be especially powerful and persuasive.

OTHER ASPECTS OF INTERPRETATION

If an assessment leads you to accept that the results of a study are probably "real," you have made important progress in interpreting the study findings. Other interpretive tasks depend on a conclusion that the results are likely credible.

Precision of the Results

Results from statistical hypothesis tests indicate whether a relationship or group difference is probably "real." A p value in hypothesis testing offers information that is important (whether the null hypothesis is probably false) but incomplete. Confidence intervals (CIs), by contrast, communicate information about how precise the study results are. It is widely recognized that *p* values on their own are not informative and that CIs strengthen the evidence about the outcomes of interest such as treatment benefit. Therefore, CIs are important to report because they allow for the interpretation of study results and their relevance to practice.

Magnitude of Effects and Importance

In quantitative studies, results that support the researcher's hypotheses are described as *significant*. A careful analysis of study results involves evaluating whether, in addition to being statistically significant, the effects are large and clinically important.

Attaining statistical significance does not necessarily mean that the results are meaningful to nurses and clients. Statistical significance indicates that the results are unlikely to be due to chance—not that they are important. With large samples, even modest relationships are statistically significant. For instance, with a sample of 500, a correlation coefficient of .10 is significant at the .05 level, but a relationship this weak may have little practical relevance. Estimating the magnitude and importance of effects is relevant to the issue of clinical significance, a topic we discuss later in this chapter.

The Meaning of Quantitative Results

In quantitative studies, statistical results are in the form of *p* values, effect sizes, and CIs, to which researchers and consumers must attach meaning. Questions about the meaning of statistical results often reflect a desire to interpret causal connections. Interpreting what descriptive results mean is not typically a challenge. For example, suppose we found that, among patients undergoing electroconvulsive therapy, the percentage who experience an electroconvulsive therapy–induced headache is 59.4% (95% CI = 56.3, 63.1). This result is directly interpretable. But if we found that headache prevalence is significantly lower in a cryotherapy intervention group than among patients given acetaminophen, we would need to interpret what the results mean. In particular, we need to interpret whether it is plausible that cryotherapy *caused* the reduced prevalence of headaches. In this section, we discuss the interpretation of research outcomes within a hypothesis testing context, with an emphasis on causal interpretations.

Interpreting Hypothesized Results

Interpreting statistical results is easiest when hypotheses are supported—that is, when there are *positive results*—because existing evidence and theory presumably laid the foundation for the hypotheses. Nevertheless, a few caveats should be kept in mind.

It is important to avoid the temptation of going beyond the data to explain what results mean. For example, suppose we hypothesized that pregnant women's anxiety level about childbearing is correlated with the number of children they have. The data reveal a significant negative relationship between anxiety levels and parity ($r = -.40$). We interpret this to mean that increased experience with childbirth results in decreased anxiety. Is this conclusion supported by the data? The conclusion appears logical, but in fact, there is nothing in the results that leads to this interpretation. An important, indeed critical, research precept is *correlation does not prove causation*. The finding that two variables are related offers no evidence suggesting which of the two variables—if either—caused the other. In our example, perhaps causality runs in the opposite direction, that is, a person's anxiety level influences how many children they bear. Or maybe a third variable, such as the person's relationship with their partner, influences both anxiety and number of children. Inferring causality is especially difficult in studies that have not used an experimental design.

Empirical evidence supporting research hypotheses never constitutes *proof* of their veracity. Hypothesis testing is probabilistic. It is important to note that not all studies state the hypotheses. It is often implied, while other research reports may instead propose a research question and discuss the findings accordingly. There is always a possibility that observed relationships resulted from chance—that is, that a Type I error has occurred. Researchers (and consumers) should be tentative about interpreting results—even when the results are in line with expectations.

> **Example of reporting probabilistic results**
> Underwood and colleagues (2024) posed the question as to whether older adults with diabetes who maintained target ranges of hemoglobin A_{1c} levels (HbA_{1c}) over time were at a lower risk of Alzheimer disease and related dementias (ADRD). They conducted a retrospective cohort study examining data from the Veterans Health Administration and Medicare to examine 374,021 veterans over the age of 65 years with a diagnosis of diabetes. Findings indicated that stable HbA_{1c} levels over time, as opposed to out of range (higher or lower levels), were associated with a lower risk of ADRD.

This study's findings support work that suggests glucose level variability is associated with an increased risk of ADRD incidence. The authors are careful to point out several limitations to the study and appropriately indicate the findings support—but do not prove—the association of HbA_{1c} control with the diagnosis of ADRD. The report highlights the limitations of the findings, such as the sample included primarily older males and did not examine other factors such as social determinants of health or the presence of the *APOE4* genetic mutation associated with AD. Therefore, it is important to keep in mind that while these findings are plausible, as the authors suggest, there could be confounding variables that impacted the results.

Interpreting Nonsignificant Results

Nonsignificant results pose interpretative challenges. Statistical tests are geared toward disconfirmation of the null hypothesis. Failure to reject a null hypothesis can occur for many reasons, and the real reason may be hard to figure out.

The null hypothesis *could* actually be true, accurately reflecting the absence of a relationship among research variables. On the other hand, the null hypothesis could be false. Retention of a false null hypothesis (a Type II error) can result from such methodologic problems as poor internal validity, an anomalous sample, a weak statistical procedure, or unreliable measures. In particular, failure to reject null hypotheses is often a consequence of insufficient power, reflecting too small a sample. It is important to recognize that a null hypothesis that is not rejected does not confirm the *absence* of relationships among variables. Nonsignificant results provide no evidence of the truth or the falsity of the hypothesis.

Because statistical procedures are designed to test support for rejecting null hypotheses, they are not well suited for testing *actual* research hypotheses about the absence of relationships or about equivalence between groups. Yet sometimes, this is exactly what researchers want to do, especially in clinical situations in which the goal is to test whether one's practice is as effective as another—but perhaps less painful or costly.

In feasibility and acceptability trials, the efficacy of the intervention is not being tested, but researchers may be testing what they think may be appropriate measures. If the study's approach also includes a mixed method approach known as an explanatory sequential approach, qualitative interviews may provide insight into what may be more appropriate measures for an efficacy trial.

When the actual research hypothesis is null (e.g., a prediction of *no* group difference), stringent additional strategies must be used to provide supporting evidence. It is useful for the researchers to compute effect sizes or CIs to illustrate that the risk of a Type II error was small.

> **Example of nonsignificant results**
> Flanagan, one of the authors of this book, and colleagues (2022) conducted a feasibility trial with informal caregivers of people experiencing dementia. The authors aimed to explore if a nurse-coached walking intervention for informal caregivers was a feasible intervention to address caregiver health. Thirty-two participants were enrolled in an 8-week walking program and were assigned either to the intervention (nurse coaching) or control group (no nurse coaching). They used validated, reliable measures of steps walked, well-being, and perceived stress. While they found that in terms of steps walked, each group experienced a statistical difference ($p = .01$ control; $p = .02$ intervention) and large effect size (0.90), neither group experienced a change in well-being ($p = .38$ control; $p = .08$ intervention) nor perceived stress ($p = .56$ control; $p = .18$ intervention). However, the intervention group achieved a large effect size in well-being (1.38) but only a moderate effect size for perceived stress (0.51). The large effect sizes (steps walked, well-being) reduce the possibility of a Type II error, but the moderate effect size for perceived stress might indicate that they needed a larger sample size, a longer intervention period, or other interventions that addressed stress. The qualitative findings indicated that participants described loneliness and grief. However, they also reported that the walking intervention helped them to feel socially connected, suggesting that social connection may be an appropriate measure for future work. As you can see from this study, nonsignificant results in preliminary work may help design future studies.

Interpreting Unhypothesized Significant Results

Unhypothesized significant results can occur in two situations. The first involves results from analyses that were not considered when the study was designed. For example, in examining correlations among research variables, a researcher might notice that two variables that were not central to the research questions were nevertheless significantly correlated and interesting.

> **Example of significant findings not hypothesized**
> Keels et al. (2025) conducted a systematic review and meta-analysis to examine the relationship between antidiabetic agents and the clinical outcomes of patients with T2DM who were admitted with COVID-19. The findings from this work found that those on metformin and DPP-4 inhibitors had a decreased rate of mortality compared to those who were on insulin. Although the authors note the need for more research, these findings indicate patients admitted with COVID-19 on metformin and DPP-4 may have better outcomes than those who were converted to insulin, as is typically done.

The second situation is more perplexing: obtaining results *opposite* to those hypothesized. For instance, a researcher might hypothesize that individualized teaching about AIDS risks is more effective than group instruction, but the results might indicate that the group method was better. Although this might seem disconcerting, research should not be undertaken to corroborate predictions but to arrive at truth. When significant findings are opposite to what was hypothesized, the interpretation should involve comparisons with other research, a consideration of alternate theories, and a critical scrutiny of the research methods.

> **Example of significant results contrary to hypotheses**
> Hedley and colleagues (2024) conducted a longitudinal study to explore the potential role of psychological well-being as a moderator between depressive symptoms and thoughts of self-harm in autism. After controlling for the effects of depression on thoughts of self-harm, they found their primary hypothesis that psychological well-being would not moderate the relationship between depression and thoughts of self-harm was not supported. Further, autistic traits and depression were the only statistically significant predictors of thoughts of self-harm.

In summary, interpreting the meaning of research results is a demanding task, but it offers the possibility of intellectual rewards. Interpreters must play the role of scientific detectives, trying to make pieces of the puzzle fit together so that a coherent picture of the truth emerges.

Generalizability and Applicability of the Results

Researchers typically seek evidence that can be used by others. If a new nursing intervention is found to be successful, others might want to adopt it. Therefore, another interpretive question is whether the intervention will "work" or whether the relationships will "hold" in other settings, with other people. Part of the interpretive process involves asking the question, "To what groups, environments, and conditions can the results reasonably be applied?" In interpreting a study's generalizability, it is useful to consider our earlier discussion about proxies. For which higher order constructs, which populations, which settings, or which versions of an intervention were the study operations good "stand-ins"? This issue is discussed at greater length in Chapter 18.

Implications of the Results

Once you have reached conclusions about the credibility, precision, importance, meaning, and generalizability of the results, you are ready to think about their implications. You might consider the implications of the findings with respect to future research: What should other researchers in this area do—what is the right "next step"? You are most likely to consider the implications for nursing practice: How should the results be used by nurses in their practice?

All of the interpretive dimensions we have discussed are critical in evidence-based nursing practice. With regard to generalizability, it may not be enough to ask a broad question about to whom the results could apply—you need to ask, "Are these results relevant to *my* clinical situation?"

CLINICAL SIGNIFICANCE

It has long been recognized that statistical hypothesis testing provides limited information for interpretation purposes. In particular, attaining statistical significance does not address the question of whether a finding is clinically meaningful or relevant. With a large enough sample, a trivial relationship can be statistically significant. Broadly speaking, we define **clinical significance** as the practical importance of research results in terms of whether they have genuine, palpable effects on the daily lives of patients or on the health care decisions made on their behalf.

In fields other than nursing, notably in medicine and psychotherapy, attention has been paid to defining clinical significance and developing ways to operationalize it. There has been no consensus on either front, but a few conceptual and statistical solutions are being used with some regularity. Here, we provide a brief overview of recent advances in defining and operationalizing clinical significance; further information is available in Polit and Yang (2016).

In statistical hypothesis testing, consensus was reached decades ago—for better or worse—that a p value of .05 would be the standard criterion for statistical significance. It is unlikely that a uniform standard will ever be adopted for clinical significance, however, because of its complexity. For example, in some cases, *no change* over time could be clinically significant if it means that a group with a progressive disease has not deteriorated. In other cases, clinical significance is associated with improvements. Another issue concerns whose *perspective* on clinical significance is relevant. Sometimes, clinician perspective is key because of implications for health management. For other outcomes, the patient's view is what matters (e.g., improved quality of life). Two other issues concern whether clinical significance is for group-level findings or about individual patients, and whether clinical significance is attached to point-in-time outcomes or to **change scores**. Most recent work is about the clinical significance of change scores for individual patients (e.g., a change from a baseline measurement to a follow-up measurement). We begin, however, with a brief discussion of group-level clinical significance.

Clinical Significance at the Group Level

Many studies concern group-level comparisons. For example, one-group pretest–posttest designs involve comparing a group at two or more points in time to examine whether or not a change in outcomes has, on average, occurred. In randomized controlled trials and case-control studies, the central comparison is about average differences for different groups of people. Group-level clinical significance typically involves using statistical information other than p values to draw conclusions about the meaningfulness. The most widely used statistics for this purpose are effect size indexes, CIs, and number needed to treat (NNT).

Effect size indexes summarize the magnitude of a change or a relationship and thus provide insights into how a group, *on average*, might benefit from a treatment. In most cases, a clinically significant finding at the group level means that the effect size is sufficiently large to have relevance for patients. CIs are espoused by several writers as useful tools for understanding clinical significance; CIs provide the most plausible range of values, at a given level of confidence, for the unknown population parameter. NNTs are sometimes promoted as good indicators of clinical significance because the information is relatively easy to understand. For example, if the NNT for an important outcome is found to be 2.0, only two patients have to receive a particular treatment in order for one patient to benefit. If the NNT is 10.0, however, 9 patients out of 10 receiving the treatment would get no benefit.

With any of these group-level indexes, researchers should designate in advance what would constitute clinical significance—just as they would establish an alpha value for statistical significance. For example, would an effect size of .20 (for the d index described in Chapter 13) be considered clinically significant? A d of .20 has been described as a "small" effect, but sometimes, small improvements can have clinical relevance. Claims about attainment of clinical significance for groups should be based on defensible criteria.

> **Example of clinical significance at the group level** • • • • • • • • • • • • • • • • • •
> Moore et al. (2024) conducted a meta-analysis to explore the relationship between obesity severity, body composition, and explicit and implicit food reward in 133 adolescents with obesity. In this population, they found degree of obesity significantly predicted the implicit desire for sweet foods independent of metabolic state.

Clinical Significance at the Individual Level

Clinicians usually are not interested in what happens in a *group* of people—they are concerned with individual patients. A key goal in EBP is to personalize "best evidence" into decisions for a specific patient's needs within a particular clinical context.

Dozens of approaches to defining and operationalizing clinical significance at the individual level have been developed, but they share one thing in common: They involve establishing a **benchmark** (or *threshold*) that designates the score value on a measure (or the value of a change score) that would be considered clinically important. With an established benchmark for clinical significance, each person in a study can be classified as having or not having a score or change score that is clinically significant.

> **Example of a benchmark for clinical significance**
> Perelman et al. (2023) conducted a study to understand the psychopathology in people experiencing binge eating disorders. They found that 60.2% (n = 230) reported fear of loss of control, and 27.5% of the sample reported resignation to loss of control (n = 105). They also found that participants with a fear of loss of control reported significantly higher depression scores than those with no fear/resignation ($p < .001$). Although further research is needed and not explicitly stated by the authors, the feeling of loss of control and depression could be important benchmarks in people experiencing binge eating disorders.

Conceptual Definitions of Clinical Significance

Numerous definitions of clinical significance can be found in the health literature, most of which concern change scores on measures of patient outcomes (e.g., a score at Time 1 subtracted from a score at Time 2). One approach to conceptualizing clinical significance dominates medical research. In the classic paper by Jaeschke and colleagues (1989), they offered the following definition: "The minimal clinically important difference (MCID) can be defined as the smallest difference in score in the domain of interest which patients perceive as beneficial and which would mandate, in the absence of troublesome side effects and excessive cost, a change in the patient's management" (p. 408). Although these researchers referred to the conceptual threshold for clinical significance as a minimal clinically important *difference*, we follow an influential group of measurement experts in using the term **minimal important change (MIC)** because the focus is on individual change scores, not differences between groups.

Operationalizing Clinical Significance: Establishing the Minimal Important Change Benchmark

Jaeschke and colleagues' (1989) definition of change score benchmarks has inspired researchers to go in different directions to quantify it. The MIC benchmark is usually operationalized as a value for the amount of change in score points on a measure that an individual patient must achieve to be considered as having a clinically important change.

A traditional approach to setting a benchmark for health outcomes is to obtain input from a panel of health care experts—sometimes called a *consensus panel*. For example, a consensus panel that was convened to establish the clinical significance of changes in self-reported pain intensity (e.g., on a visual analog scale) established the benchmark as a 30% reduction in pain.

Another approach is to undertake a study to determine what patients themselves think is a minimally important change on a focal measure. The developers of some new multi-item scales now use this approach to estimate the MIC as part of the psychometric assessment of their instrument. Calculating an MIC using patient ratings of important change requires a careful research design with a large sample of people whose change over time is expected to vary.

A third approach to defining the MIC is based on the distributional characteristics of a measure. Most often, the MIC using this approach is set to a threshold of 0.5 *SDs*—that is, one half a standard deviation (*SD*) on a distribution of baseline scores. For example, if the baseline *SD* for a scale were 6.0, then the MIC using the 0.5 *SD* criterion would be 3.0. This value, like any MIC, can be used as the benchmark to classify individual patients as having or not having experienced clinically meaningful change.

Many researchers have used the MIC to interpret group-level findings. The MIC is, however, an index of *individual* change, not group differences. Experts have warned that it is inappropriate to interpret mean differences in relation to the MIC. For example, if the MIC on an important outcome has been established as 4.0, this value should not be used to interpret the clinical significance of the mean difference between two groups. If the mean group difference were found to be 3.0, for instance, it would be wrong to conclude that the results were not clinically significant. A mean difference of 3.0 suggests that a sizable percentage of participants *did* achieve a clinically meaningful benefit—that is, an improvement of 4 points or more.

MIC thresholds can be used to calculate rates of clinical significance for individual study participants. Once the MIC is known, researchers can classify all people in a study in terms of their having attained or not attained the threshold. Then, researchers can compare the percentage of people who "responded" at clinically important levels in the study groups (e.g., those in the intervention and those in the control group). Such a **responder analysis** is easy to understand and has strong implications for EBP.

> **Example of a responder analysis**
> Thanarajasingam et al. (2022) conducted an exploratory study with 65 men who had undergone treatment for metastatic prostate cancer to understand patients' perspectives as to whether their treatment was worthwhile. They used the Was It Worth It (WIWI) questionnaire as a metric to explore the patients' perspectives about factors related to the disease treatment and outcomes, such as adverse events, quality of life, bone scan response, and overall survival. They found that those who responded "no" or "uncertain" to the question of whether the treatment was worth it discontinued treatment due to adverse events more frequently than those responding "yes" (36% vs. 7.5%, *p* = .004) and experienced a decline in quality of life from baseline (−2.5 vs. −0.2 mean change, *p* < .001).

CRITICAL APPRAISAL OF INTERPRETATIONS

Researchers interpret their findings and discuss what the findings might imply for nursing in the discussion section of research articles. When critically appraising a study, your own interpretation can be contrasted against those of the researchers.

A good discussion section should point out study limitations. Researchers are in the best position to detect and assess sampling deficiencies, data quality problems, and so on, and it is a professional responsibility to alert readers to these difficulties. Of course, researchers are unlikely to note all relevant limitations. Your task as reviewer is to develop your own interpretation and assessment of methodologic problems and to challenge conclusions that do not appear to be warranted.

You should also carefully scrutinize causal interpretations, especially in nonexperimental studies. Sometimes, even the titles of reports suggest potential problems. If the title of a nonexperimental study includes terms like "the effect of …," or "the impact of …," this may signal the need for critical scrutiny of the researcher's inferences.

In addition to comparing your interpretation with that of the researchers, your appraisal should also draw conclusions about the stated implications of the study. Some researchers make grandiose claims or offer unfounded recommendations based on modest results.

> **Box 14.1 Guidelines for Critically Appraising Interpretations/Discussions in Quantitative Research Reports**
>
> **Interpretation of the Findings**
> a. Were all the important results discussed?
> b. Did the researchers discuss any study limitations and their possible effects on the credibility of the findings? In discussing limitations, were key threats to the study's validity and possible biases reviewed? Did the interpretations take limitations into account?
> c. What types of evidence were offered in support of the interpretation, and was that evidence persuasive? Were results interpreted in light of findings from other studies?
> d. Did the researchers make any unjustifiable causal inferences? Were alternative explanations for the findings considered? Were the rationales for rejecting these alternatives convincing?
> e. Did the interpretation take into account the precision of the results and/or the magnitude of effects?
> f. Did the researchers draw any unwarranted conclusions about the generalizability of the results?
>
> **Implications of the Findings and Recommendations**
> g. Did the researchers discuss the study's implications for clinical practice or future nursing research? Did they make specific recommendations?
> h. If yes, are the stated implications appropriate, given the study's limitations and the magnitude of the effects as well as evidence from other studies? Are there important implications that the report neglected to include?
>
> **Clinical Significance**
> i. Did the researchers mention or assess clinical significance? Did they make a distinction between statistical and clinical significance?
> j. If clinical significance was examined, was it assessed in terms of group-level information (e.g., effect sizes) or individual-level results? How was clinical significance operationalized?

The conceptualization and operationalization of clinical significance have not received much attention in nursing, so studies that do not mention clinical significance should not be faulted for this omission—but researchers who do address clinical significance should be lauded. We hope that nurse researchers will pay more attention to this issue in the years ahead.

Some guidelines for evaluating researchers' interpretation are offered in Box 14.1.

RESEARCH EXAMPLES WITH CRITICAL THINKING EXERCISES

In this section, we discuss the critical appraisal of interpretations. The critical thinking questions for Example 1 are based on the study that appears in its entirety in Appendix A.

EXAMPLE 1: DISCUSSION SECTION IN THE STUDY IN APPENDIX A

Read the "Discussion" section of Cheng and colleagues' 2024 study, "Advance care planning affects end-of-life treatment preferences among patients with heart failure: A randomized controlled trial" in Appendix A of this book.

Critical Thinking Exercises

1. Answer the relevant questions in Box 14.1 regarding this study.
2. Was a CONSORT-type flow chart used in this study?
3. Can you think of any limitations that the researchers did not mention?

Summary Points

- The interpretation of quantitative **results** (the outcomes of the statistical analyses) typically involves consideration of (1) the credibility of the results, (2) precision of estimates of effects, (3) magnitude of effects, (4) underlying meaning, (5) generalizability, and (6) implications for nursing practice and future research.
- The particulars of the study—especially the methodologic decisions made by researchers—affect the inferences that can be made about the correspondence between study results and "truth in the real world."
- A cautious outlook is appropriate in drawing conclusions about the credibility and meaning of study results.
- An assessment of a study's credibility can involve various approaches, one of which involves an evaluation of the degree of congruence between abstract constructs or idealized methods on the one hand and the proxies actually used on the other.
- Credibility assessments also involve an assessment of study rigor through an analysis of validity threats and biases that could undermine the accuracy of the results.
- Corroboration (replication) of results, through either internal or external sources, is another approach in a credibility assessment.
- Researchers can facilitate interpretations by carefully documenting methodologic decisions and the outcomes of those decisions (e.g., by using the **CONSORT guidelines** to document participant flow).
- Broadly speaking, **clinical significance** refers to the practical importance of research results—that is, whether the effects are genuine and palpable in the daily lives of patients or in the management of their health.
- Clinical significance for group-level results is often evaluated based on such statistics as effect size indexes, CIs, and NNT. However, clinical significance is most often discussed in terms of effects for individual patients—especially, whether they have achieved a clinically meaningful change.
- Definitions and operationalizations of clinical significance for individuals typically involve a **benchmark** or threshold to designate a meaningful amount of change. This benchmark is often called a **minimal important change (MIC)**, which is a value for the amount of **change score** points on a measure that an individual patient must achieve to be classified as having clinically meaningful change.
- MIC benchmarks can be used to ascertain whether each person in a sample has or has not achieved a change greater than the MIC, and then a **responder analysis** can be undertaken to compare the percentage of people meeting the threshold in different study groups.
- In their discussions of study results, researchers should themselves point out known study limitations, but readers should draw their own conclusions about the rigor of the study and about the plausibility of alternative explanations for the results.

REFERENCES

Flanagan, J., Post, K., Hill, R., & DiPalazzo, J. (2022). Feasibility of a nurse coached walking intervention for informal dementia caregivers. *Western Journal of Nursing Research*, *44*(5), 466–476. https://doi.org/10.1177/01939459211001395

Hedley, D., Uljarevic´, M., Bury, S. M., Haschek, A., Richdale, A. L., Trollor, J. N., & Stokes, M. A. (2024). Examination of the potential moderating role of psychological wellbeing in the relationship between depression and thoughts of self-harm in autistic adolescents and adults: A two-year longitudinal study. *Journal of Autism and Developmental Disorders*. https://doi.org/10.1007/s10803-024-06489-x

Jaeschke, R., Singer, J., & Guyatt, G. H. (1989). Measurement of health status. Ascertaining the minimal clinically important difference. *Controlled Clinical Trials*, *10*(4), 407–415. https://doi.org/10.1016/0197-2456(89)90005-6

Keels, J. N., McDonald, I. R., Lee, C. S., & Dwyer, A. A. (2025). Antidiabetic agent use and clinical outcomes in patients with diabetes hospitalized for COVID-19: A systematic review and meta-analysis. *Frontiers in Endocrinology*, 15, 1482853. https://doi.org/10.3389/fendo.2024.1482853

Moore, H., Pereira, B., Fillon, A., Miguet, M., Masurier, J., Beaulieu, K., Finlayson, G., & Thivel, D. (2024). The association between obesity severity and food reward in adolescents with obesity: A one-stage individual participant data meta-analysis. *European Journal of Nutrition*, 63(4), 1241–1255. https://doi.org/10.1007/s00394-024-03348-4

Perelman, H., Gilbert, K., Grilo, C. M., & Lydecker, J. A. (2023). Loss of control in binge-eating disorder: Fear and resignation. *The International Journal of Eating Disorders*, 56(6), 1199–1206. https://doi.org/10.1002/eat.23929

Polit, D. F., & Yang, F. M. (2016). *Measurement and the measurement of change: A primer for health professionals*. Lippincott Williams & Wilkins.

Thanarajasingam, G., Basch, E., Mead-Harvey, C., Bennett, A. V., Mazza, G. L., Schwab, G., Roydhouse, J., Rogak, L. J., & Dueck, A. C. (2022). An exploratory analysis of the "Was It Worth It?" Questionnaire as a novel metric to capture patient perceptions of cancer treatment. *Value in Health: The Journal of the International Society for Pharmacoeconomics and Outcomes Research*, 25(7), 1081–1086. https://doi.org/10.1016/j.jval.2021.11.1368

Underwood, P. C., Zhang, L., Mohr, D. C., Prentice, J. C., Nelson, R. E., Budson, A. E., & Conlin, P. R. (2024). Glycated hemoglobin A1c time in range and dementia in older adults with diabetes. *JAMA Network Open*, 7(8), e2425354. https://doi.org/10.1001/jamanetworkopen.2024.25354

15 Understanding the Analysis of Qualitative Data

Learning Objectives

On completing this chapter, you will be able to:

- Describe activities that qualitative researchers perform to manage and organize their data
- Discuss the procedures used to analyze qualitative data, including both general procedures and those used in ethnographic, phenomenologic, and grounded theory, and qualitative descriptive research
- Assess the adequacy of researchers' descriptions of their analytic procedures and evaluate the suitability of those procedures
- Define new terms in the chapter

Key Terms

- Axial coding
- Basic social process (BSP)
- Central category
- Coding scheme
- Constant comparison
- Core category
- Domain
- Emergent fit
- Hermeneutic circle
- Metaphor
- Open coding
- Paradigm case
- Qualitative content analysis
- Selective coding
- Substantive codes
- Taxonomy
- Thematic analysis
- Theme
- Theoretical codes

Qualitative research data are derived from such narrative materials as transcripts of audiotaped interviews or participant observers' field notes. This chapter describes methods for analyzing such qualitative data.

INTRODUCTION TO QUALITATIVE ANALYSIS

Qualitative data analysis is challenging, for several reasons. First, there are no universal rules for analyzing qualitative data. Second, an enormous amount of work is required. Qualitative analysts must organize and make sense of hundreds of pages of narrative materials. Qualitative researchers typically scrutinize their data carefully, often reading the data over and over in a search for understanding. Also, doing qualitative analysis proficiently requires creativity and strong inductive skills (generating universals from particulars). A qualitative analyst must be adept at discerning patterns and weaving them together into an integrated whole.

Another challenge comes in reducing data for reporting purposes. Quantitative results can often be summarized in a few tables. Qualitative researchers, by contrast, must balance the need to be concise with the need to maintain the richness of their data.

 TIP Qualitative analyses are more difficult to *do* than quantitative ones, but qualitative findings are easier to understand than quantitative ones because the stories are told in everyday language. Qualitative analyses are often hard to critically appraise, however, because readers cannot know if researchers adequately captured thematic patterns in the data.

QUALITATIVE DATA MANAGEMENT AND ORGANIZATION

Qualitative analysis is supported by several tasks that help to organize and manage the mass of narrative data.

Developing a Coding Scheme

Qualitative researchers usually begin their analysis by developing a method to classify and index their data. Researchers must be able to access parts of the data without having repeatedly to reread the data set in its entirety. The usual procedure is to create a **coding scheme**, based on actual data, and then code data according to the categories in the coding scheme. Developing a good coding scheme involves a careful reading of the data, with an eye to identifying underlying concepts.

Saldaña defined a code in qualitative analysis as "most often a word or short phase that symbolically assigns a summative, salient, essence-capturing, and/or evocative attribute for a portion of language-based or visual data" (2021, p. 5). Saldaña identified 33 different types of coding approaches that vary along several dimensions, such as amount of detail and level of abstraction.

The same excerpt can be coded in various ways—there is no single "right" way to code data, and two people are unlikely to develop identical codes for the same data. The nature of the research question and the desired end product influence the type of codes that get created.

> **Example of a descriptive coding scheme**
> Hoffman and Fredkove (2024) conducted in-depth interviews with 33 war-affected Korean mothers and 26 of their children who resettled in the Midwestern United States. The purpose of the study was to explore the maternal caregivers' decision making and disclosure of torture and war trauma experiences to their children. The researchers used the following three main categories of communication codes to analyze the data: direct, indirect, and silencing.

Coding Qualitative Data

After a coding scheme has been developed, the data are read in their entirety and coded for correspondence to the categories. This can be a difficult task—it sometimes takes several readings of the material to grasp its nuances. Researchers often discover during coding that the initial coding scheme needs to be modified. Ideas may emerge for new codes, for example. In such a case, it would be necessary to reread all previously coded material to check if the new code should be applied.

Data Extract	Codes
"While I was lying down, they were making sure I was feeling well and began to move me to confirm that the emergency transfer blanket was under me. As they sat me up, **I immediately started to feel like I couldn't breathe**, and **my chest felt like a ton of bricks were on it**. I felt **nauseous**. I was **screaming that I couldn't breathe**. I was **begging them to save my life** and not to let me die. This all happened **within 30 minutes** of my water breaking."	sudden inability to breathe ton of bricks on chest nauseous screaming can't breathe begging to save her life short period of time

Figure 15.1 Example of a coded excerpt. (From the author's records for the study reported in the following paper: Beck, C. T. [2025]. In a flash: A qualitative descriptive study of amniotic fluid embolism survivors. *MCN: The American Journal of Maternal Child Nursing, 50*[2], 107–113. https://doi.org/10.1097/NMC.0000000000001081)

Paragraphs from transcribed interviews often contain elements relating to three or four different codes. Figure 15.1 shows an example of a paragraph with multiple codes—this is an excerpt from Beck's, one of the authors of this textbook, study of the experiences of amniotic fluid embolism survivors (2025).

Methods of Organizing Qualitative Data

Computer-assisted qualitative data analysis software (CAQDAS) has advanced extensively, changing how researchers manage and analyze qualitative data. Current CAQDAS removes the labor-intensive project of cutting up pages of narrative material by digitizing the complete workflow. Researchers can now store and easily access entire datasets—uploading text, audio, and video—on a computer, engage in coding relevant portions of the data, and organize text segments tagged with identifiable codes for deep analysis and reflection. Many platforms now offer integrated transcription services enhanced by artificial intelligence (AI), utilizing speech recognition and machine learning algorithms to convert audio or video files into precise text transcription. A popular option is sophisticated theory-building software, which permits researchers to examine relationships between concepts, develop hierarchies of codes, construct diagrams, and generate hyperlinks to create nonhierarchical networks. Examples of theory-building packages include NVivo, ATLAS.ti, HyperRESEARCH, MAXQDA, Quirkos, and QDA Miner, most of which are available in Mac and PC versions.

Advanced AI coding offers both automated and semi-automated coding designed to enrich and streamline the coding process. For example, ATLAS.ti offers AI coding (open and descriptive coding), intentional AI coding (results tailored to specific research questions or goals), AI summaries (condensed data to allow the researcher to gain critical insights), and conversational AI (responds to the researcher's queries augmenting engagement with the data).

Researchers must consider the ethical, legal, and logistical implications of using AI. It is important for researchers to have deep knowledge of the AI system they are using, establishing whether it operates on an Open AI (open source), proprietary AI (closed source), or combination of both. Misuse or disclosure of human subjects' data violates ethical principles of research. Developing and training AI models requires a systematic process that may result in inherent bias in the output. Therefore, AI models hold the potential to reflect bias in their training, possibly skewing the interpretation of qualitative data analysis. AI can enhance data analysis, but ultimately researchers need to remember these are merely tools. Researchers must continue to act as the critical thinkers and analysts who shape the interpretation and comprehension of the data.

van Manen asked "What do the capabilities of ChatGPT [Chat Generative Pre-training Transformer] say about distinctions between humanity and technology? What aspects of writing and interpretation of texts are uniquely human?" (2023, p. 1135). Proponents of AI use in qualitative data analysis stress that it can rapidly generate codes and sort text into categories. A warning, however, for qualitative researchers is that the coding ChatGPT does is accomplished without understanding the meaningfulness or significance of the text. What ChatGPT generates is based on probabilistic modeling instead of on meaningfulness. van Manen worries that qualitative researchers may simply rely on AI to analyze their data and bypass the essential hard work of meaningful reading and interpreting data.

Although computer programs offer many advantages for managing qualitative data, some researchers prefer manual data analysis (paper–pencil method) to engage intensely with the data, cultivating a deep-rooted connection with the transcripts. This approach evades technologic challenges such as software incompatibility, data loss, or technology crashes. Some researchers have raised objections to having a process that is basically cognitive turned into an activity that is mechanical.

ANALYTIC PROCEDURES

Data *management* in qualitative research is reductionist in nature: It involves converting masses of data into smaller, more manageable segments. By contrast, qualitative data *analysis* is constructionist: It involves putting segments together into meaningful conceptual patterns. Various approaches to qualitative data analysis exist, but some elements are common to several of them.

A General Analytic Overview

The analysis of qualitative materials often begins with the identification of broad *categories*, which are clusters of codes that are connected conceptually. Figure 15.1 shows a coded excerpt from Beck's 2025 study of amniotic fluid embolism survivors where two of the codes ("sudden inability to breathe" and "ton of bricks on chest") were clustered with other codes to form the theme "in a flash." Ideas for categories or themes usually begin to emerge during coding and would likely be documented in analytic memos.

In many qualitative studies, the next phase involves the identification of themes. In their review of how the term *theme* is used among qualitative researchers, DeSantis and Ugarriza offer this definition: "A **theme** is an abstract entity that brings meaning and identity to a current experience and its variant manifestations. As such, a theme captures and unifies the nature or basis of the experience into a meaningful whole" (2000, p. 362).

The search for themes involves not only discovering commonalities across participants but also seeking variation. Themes are never universal. Researchers must attend not only to what themes arise but also to how they are patterned. Does the theme apply only to certain types of people or in certain contexts? Thus, qualitative analysts must be sensitive to patterns and relationships within the data.

 TIP Qualitative researchers often use major themes and subthemes as subheadings in the Results section of their reports. For example, in their analysis of interview data for a study of the understanding of resilience among Generation Z baccalaureate nursing students, Boyden and colleagues (2024) identified the major theme of "Maneuvering the murky water" with four subthemes that were used to organize their qualitative results: "Not a crushing train," "Choosing the hard push," "Building more confidence," and "Adopting a positive mindset."

Researchers' search for themes and patterns in the data can sometimes be facilitated by devices that enable them to chart the evolution of behaviors and processes. For example, for qualitative studies that focus on dynamic experiences (e.g., decision making), flow charts or timelines can be used to highlight time sequences or major decision points.

Some qualitative researchers use metaphors as an analytic strategy. A **metaphor** is a symbolic comparison, using figurative language to evoke a visual analogy. Metaphors can be expressive tools for qualitative analysts, but they can run the risk of "supplanting creative insight with hackneyed cliché masquerading as profundity" (Thorne & Darbyshire, 2005, p. 1111).

Example of a metaphor
Hulse and coresearchers (2024) examined the use of language in the context of meaning-making among women with metastatic breast cancer. Semi-structured interviews were conducted to consider the war metaphor's impact on 22 women's illness experiences.

In the final analysis stage, researchers strive to weave the thematic pieces into an integrated whole. The various themes are integrated to provide an overall structure (such as a theory or a taxonomy) to the data. Successful integration demands creativity and intellectual rigor.

 TIP Although relatively few qualitative researchers make formal efforts to quantify features of their data, be alert to quantitative implications when you read a qualitative report. Qualitative researchers routinely use words like "some," "most," or "many" in characterizing participants' experiences and actions, which implies some level of quantification.

Qualitative Content Analysis and Thematic Analysis

In the remainder of this section, we discuss analytic procedures used by ethnographers, phenomenologists, and grounded theory researchers. Qualitative researchers who conduct descriptive qualitative studies may, however, simply say that they performed a content analysis or a thematic analysis.

Qualitative content analysis involves analyzing the content of narrative data to identify prominent themes and patterns among the themes. Qualitative content analysis involves breaking down data into smaller units, coding and naming the units according to the content they represent, and grouping coded material based on shared concepts.

Content analysts often make the distinction between manifest and latent content. *Manifest content* is what the text actually says. In purely descriptive studies, qualitative researchers may focus mainly on summarizing the manifest content communicated in the text. Often, however, content analysts also analyze what the text talks *about*, which involves interpretation of the meaning of its *latent content*. Interpretations vary in depth and level of abstraction and are usually the basis for themes.

Krippendorff (2019) and Kyngäs et al. (2020) are two of the most frequently cited content analysis methods. Both address inductive and deductive content analysis. Krippendorff's inductive content analysis uses dendrograms to help cluster codes and categories. A dendrogram is a tree diagram that illustrates the arrangement of clusters in a hierarchically ordered system. Figure 15.2 is an example of a dendrogram created by Beck (2023) for her study on women's experiences of hyperemesis gravidarum.

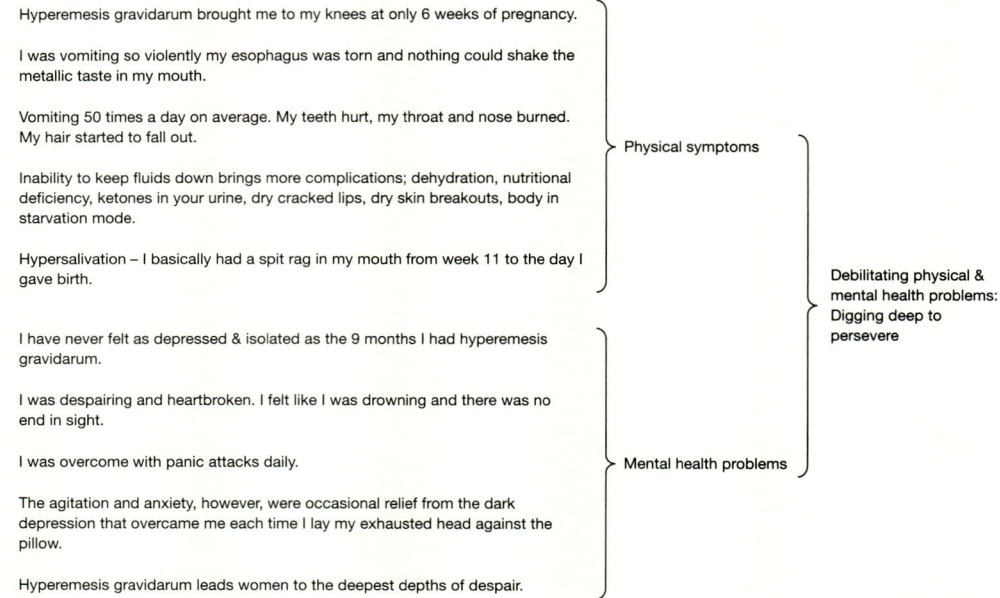

Figure 15.2 Example of a dendrogram for theme 1: Debilitating physical and mental health problems: Digging deep to persevere. (Reprinted with permission from Beck, C. T. [2023]. Survivors' experiences of hyperemesis gravidarum. *Journal of Infusion Nursing*, *46*[6], 338–346. https://doi.org/10.1097/NAN.0000000000000520. Copyright © 2023 Infusion Nurses Society)

Kyngäs et al.'s approach uses inductive content analysis when the purpose is to create categories and themes from the qualitative data. In deductive content analysis, on the other hand, the researcher would apply either a structured or semi-structured matrix of analysis to the data. Researchers would choose deductive content analysis when the starting point of their study is prior theoretical knowledge.

> **Example of a qualitative content analysis**
> Anyiam and colleagues (2024) used inductive content analysis to analyze data from semi-structured interviews with 10 pregnant and postpartum Black women on their perspectives of birth centers and midwifery care. All the women shared experiences of discrimination and bias they received during obstetric care. Participants expressed a desire to receive care in birth centers and midwifery care, but financial and institutional barriers hindered access to this care.

Many qualitative nurse researchers use the **thematic analysis** methods suggested by Braun and Clarke (2022). Their reflexive thematic analysis is differentiated from other thematic analyses by an emphasis on the reflexivity of the researcher. It involves a six-phase process: familiarizing oneself with the data set; coding; generating initial themes; developing and reviewing themes; refining, defining, and naming themes; and writing up.

> **Example of a thematic analysis**
> In China, Song and colleagues (2024) studied the experiences of returning to work in 24 patients with schizophrenia after treatment. Interviews were conducted at three different times: first when patients were close to discharge from the hospital, then within one month, and again at 6 months post discharge. Using thematic analysis, the researchers identified themes for each phase.

Ethnographic Analysis

In an ethnography, analysis typically begins the moment ethnographers set foot in the field. Ethnographers are continually looking for *patterns* in the behavior and thoughts of participants, comparing one pattern against another. As they analyze patterns of everyday life, ethnographers acquire a deeper understanding of the culture being studied. Maps, flowcharts, and organizational charts are also useful tools that help to crystallize and illustrate the data being collected. Matrices (two-dimensional displays) can also help to highlight a comparison graphically and to discover emerging patterns.

Spradley's (1979) classic approach is sometimes used for ethnographic data analyses. His 12-step sequence included strategies for both data collection and data analysis. In Spradley's method, there are four levels of data analysis: *domain analysis*, *taxonomic analysis*, *componential analysis*, and *theme analysis*. **Domains** are broad categories that represent units of cultural knowledge. During this first level of analysis, ethnographers identify relational patterns among terms in the domains that are used by members of the culture. The ethnographer focuses on the cultural meaning of terms and symbols (objects and events) used in a culture and their interrelationships.

In *taxonomic analysis*, the second level in Spradley's data analytic method, ethnographers decide how many domains the analysis will encompass. After making this decision, a **taxonomy**—a system of classifying and organizing terms—is developed to illustrate the internal organization of a domain.

In *componential analysis*, multiple relationships among terms in the domains are examined. The ethnographer analyzes data for similarities and differences among cultural terms in a domain. Finally, in *theme analysis*, cultural themes are uncovered. Domains are connected in cultural themes, which help to provide a holistic view of the culture being studied. The discovery of cultural meaning is the outcome.

> **Example using Spradley's method**
> Hwang and coresearchers (2024) studied the sociocultural context of nursing research in a clinical setting at a Korean tertiary hospital. The researchers conducted ethnographic interviews with six registered nurses working in a medical-surgical unit; participant observation also occurred. They used Spradley's ethnographic method to analyze the data, which included domain analysis, taxonomic analysis, componential analysis, and theme analysis. The overarching theme identified for nursing research culture in clinical practice was the development of a driving force for growth within the clinical environment.

Other approaches to ethnography have been developed. For example, in Leininger's ethnonursing method, as described in McFarland and Wehbe-Alamah (2015), ethnographers follow a four-phase data analysis guide. In the first phase, ethnographers collect, describe, and record data. The second phase involves identifying and categorizing descriptors. In phase 3, data are analyzed to discover repetitive patterns in their context. The fourth and final phase involves abstracting major themes and presenting findings.

> **Example using Leininger's method**
> Nwozichi and coresearchers (2024) used Leininger's ethnonursing method to study the worldview, institutional, and contextual factors affecting cancer care in Nigeria. Researchers conducted participant observation for 6 months in a cancer care setting and interviewed seven nurses and six patients with cancer. Results revealed that unfavorable institutional factors, such as lack of equipment and staff and intensified workload, constrained cancer care.

Phenomenologic Analysis

Schools of phenomenology have developed different approaches to data analysis. Three frequently used methods for descriptive phenomenology are the methods of Colaizzi (1978), Giorgi (1985), and van Kaam (1966), all of whom are from the *Duquesne School* of phenomenology, based on Husserl's philosophy.

The basic outcome of all three methods is the description of the essential nature of an experience, often through the identification of essential themes. Some important differences among these three approaches exist. Colaizzi's (1978) method, for example, is the only one that calls for a validation of results by querying study participants. Giorgi's (1985) view is that it is inappropriate either to return to participants to validate findings or to use external judges to review the analysis. van Kaam's (1966) method requires that intersubjective agreement be reached with other expert judges. Figure 15.3 provides an illustration of the steps involved in Colaizzi's data analysis approach.

> **Example of a study using Colaizzi's method**
> In Italy, Monaco and an interprofessional team (2024) conducted a descriptive phenomenologic study to understand the experiences of motherhood and daily life among women diagnosed with fibromyalgia. In-depth interviews were conducted with 10 mothers, and the data were analyzed using Colaizzi's method. Five themes were identified: "A trauma preceding diagnosis," "Pervasive feelings of misunderstanding," "A struggle to maintain strength among limitations," "Challenges in fulfilling maternal roles," and "Persistent sexual discomfort."

Phenomenologists from the *Utrecht School*, such as van Manen (1997), combine characteristics of descriptive and interpretive phenomenology. According to van Manen, thematic aspects of experience can be uncovered from participants' descriptions of the experience by three methods: the holistic, selective, or detailed approach. In the *holistic approach*, researchers

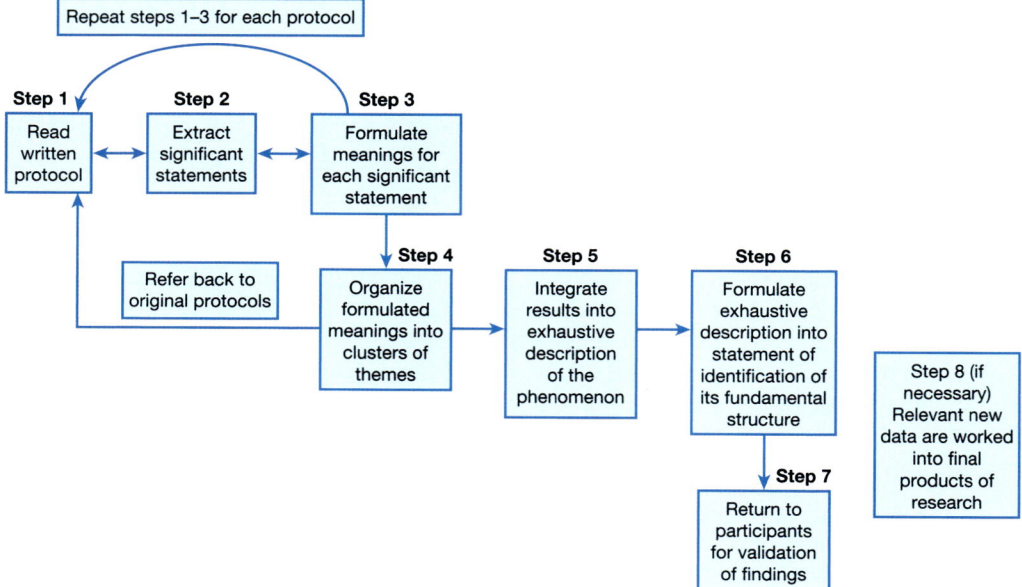

Figure 15.3 Colaizzi's procedural steps in phenomenologic data analysis. (Reprinted with permission from Beck, C.T. [2009]. The arm: There is no escaping the reality for mothers of children with obstetric brachial plexus injuries. *Nursing Research, 58*[4], 237–245. https://doi.org/10.1097/NNR.0b013e3181ac10da)

view the text as a whole and try to capture its meanings. In the *selective* (or highlighting) *approach*, researchers pull out statements that seem essential to the experience under study. In the *detailed* (or line-by-line) *approach*, researchers analyze every sentence. Once themes have been identified, they become the objects of interpretation through follow-up interviews with participants. Through this process, essential themes are discovered.

> **Example of a study using van Manen's method**
> Petreca and colleagues (2024) used van Manen's method to explore the experience of being a sex offender for 14 men who were reintegrating into society. Five major themes were identified: "Exposed secret leads to humiliation," "Being considered a sex offender is living in fear of the unknown," "Stigma and shame consume the identity of the individual charged with a sexual offense," "Reframing and 'leveling' of the crime are coping strategies," and "Path toward healing and forgiveness is complex."

In addition to identifying themes from participants' descriptions, van Manen (1997) also called for gleaning thematic descriptions from artistic sources. van Manen urged qualitative researchers to keep in mind that literature, painting, and other art forms can provide rich experiential data that can increase insights into the essential meaning of the experience being studied.

A third school of phenomenology is an interpretive approach called Heideggerian hermeneutics. Central to analyzing data in a hermeneutic study is the notion of the **hermeneutic circle**. The circle signifies a methodologic process in which, to reach understanding, there is continual movement between the parts and the whole of the text being analyzed.

Benner (1994) offered an analytic approach for hermeneutic analysis that involves three interrelated processes: the search for paradigm cases, thematic analysis, and analysis of exemplars. **Paradigm cases** are "strong instances of concerns or ways of being in the world" (p. 113). Paradigm cases are used early in the analytic process as a strategy for gaining understanding. Thematic analysis is done to compare and contrast similarities across cases. Paradigm cases and thematic analysis can be enhanced by exemplars that illuminate aspects of a paradigm case or theme. Paradigm cases and exemplars presented in research reports allow readers to play a role in consensual validation of the results by deciding whether the cases support the researchers' conclusions.

> **Example using Benner's hermeneutical analysis**
> Watson (2024) explored the meaning behind professional identity in 20 intensive care nurses who cared for patients with COVID-19. The researcher used Benner's interpretive phenomenologic method to analyze semi-structured interview transcripts. Four themes were identified: "Keep them alive," "We are survivors," "I am an intensive care unit nurse," and "I was meant for this."

Grounded Theory Analysis

Grounded theory methods emerged in the 1960s when two sociologists, Glaser and Strauss, were studying dying in hospitals (Glaser & Strauss, 1967). The two co-originators eventually split and developed divergent approaches (Corbin and Strauss, 2015; Glaser, 1978). A third analytic approach by Charmaz (2025), constructivist grounded theory, has also emerged.

Glaser's Grounded Theory Method

Grounded theory in all three analytic methods uses **constant comparison**, a method that involves comparing elements present in one data source (e.g., in one interview) with those in another. The process continues until the content of all sources has been compared so that commonalities are identified.

Coding in the Glaserian (1978) approach is used to conceptualize data into patterns. Coding helps the researcher to discover the basic problem with which participants must contend. The substance of the topic under study is conceptualized through **substantive codes**, of which there are two types: open and selective. **Open coding**, used in the first stage of constant comparison, captures what is going on in the data. Open codes may be the actual words participants used. There are three levels of open coding that vary in degree of abstraction. *Level I codes* (or *in vivo codes*) are derived directly from the language of the substantive area. They have vivid imagery and "grab."

As researchers constantly compare new level I codes with previously identified ones, they condense them into broader *level II codes*. *Level III codes* (or theoretical constructs) are the most abstract. Collapsing level II codes aids in identifying constructs.

Open coding ends when the core category is discovered, and then selective coding begins. The **core category** (or *core variable*) is a pattern of behavior that is relevant and/or problematic for study participants. In **selective coding**, researchers code only those data that are related to the core category. One kind of core category is a **basic social process (BSP)** that evolves over time in two or more phases. All BSPs are core categories, but some core categories are not BSPs.

Glaser (1978) provided criteria to help researchers decide on a core category. Here are a few examples: It must be central, meaning that it is related to many categories; it must reoccur frequently in the data; it relates meaningfully and easily to other categories; and it has clear and grabbing implications for formal theory.

Theoretical codes provide insights into how substantive codes relate to each other. Theoretical codes help grounded theorists to weave the broken pieces of data back together again. Glaser (1978) proposed 18 families of theoretical codes that researchers can use to conceptualize how substantive codes relate to each other (although he subsequently expanded possibilities in 2005). Four examples of his families of theoretical codes include the following:

- Process: stages, phases, passages, transitions
- Strategy: tactics, techniques, maneuverings
- Cutting point: boundaries, critical junctures, turning points
- The six Cs: causes, contexts, contingencies, consequences, covariances, and conditions

Throughout coding and analysis, grounded theory analysts document their ideas about the data and emerging conceptual scheme in *memos*. Memos encourage researchers to reflect on and describe patterns in the data, relationships between categories, and emergent conceptualizations.

The product of a typical Glaserian grounded theory analysis is a theoretical model that endeavors to explain a pattern of behavior that is relevant for study participants. Once the basic problem emerges, the grounded theorist goes on to discover the process these participants experience in coping with or resolving this problem.

> **Example of a Glaserian grounded theory analysis**
> Didier and colleagues (2023) conducted a classic Glaserian grounded theory study of hospitalized patients' perceptions of being cared for by interprofessional health care teams in Switzerland. "Protecting personhood" emerged as the core category, which involved the process hospitalized patients went through to achieve a balance in their sense of self as they pivoted between personhood and patienthood. The process consisted of four phases: introspection, preservation, rupture, and reconciliation.

Glaser cautioned against consulting the literature before a framework is stabilized, but he also saw the benefit of scrutinizing other work. Glaser (1978) discussed the evolution of grounded theories through the process of **emergent fit** to prevent individual substantive theories from being "respected little islands of knowledge" (p. 148). As he noted, generating grounded theory does not necessarily require discovering all new categories or ignoring ones previously identified in the literature. Through constant comparison, researchers can compare concepts emerging from the data with similar concepts from existing theory or research to evaluate which parts have emergent fit with the theory being generated.

Corbin and Strauss' Approach

The Corbin and Strauss' approach to grounded theory analysis, most recently described in 2015, differs from the original Glaser and Strauss' method with regard to method, processes, and outcomes. Table 15.1 summarizes major analytic differences between the Glaser, Corbin and Strauss, and Charmaz grounded theory analysis methods.

Glaser (1978) stressed that to generate a grounded theory, the basic problem must emerge from the data—it must be discovered. The theory is, from the very start, grounded in the data rather than starting with a preconceived problem. Strauss and Corbin, however, argued that research problems can, for example, come from the literature or a researcher's personal and professional experience.

The Corbin and Strauss' (2015) method involves two types of coding: open and axial coding. In *open coding*, data are broken down into parts and concepts identified for interpreted meaning of the raw data. In **axial coding**, the analyst codes for context. Here, the analyst is "locating and linking action-interaction within a framework of subconcepts that give it meaning and enable it to explain what interactions are occurring, and why and what consequences real or anticipated are happening" (Corbin & Strauss, 2015, p. 156). The *paradigm* is used as an analytic strategy to help integrate structure and process. The basic components of the paradigm include conditions, actions–interactions, and consequences or outcomes. Corbin and Strauss suggested the conditional/consequential matrix as an analytic strategy for considering the range of possible conditions and consequences that can enter into the context.

The first step in integrating the findings is to decide on the **central category** (sometimes called the *core category*), which is the main construct in the research. The outcome of the Corbin and Strauss' approach is a full conceptual description. The original grounded theory method, by contrast, generates a theory that explains how a basic social problem that emerged from the data is processed in a social setting.

TABLE 15.1 Comparison of Alternative Grounded Theory Approaches

	Glaser	Corbin and Strauss	Charmaz
Initial data analysis	Breaking down and conceptualizing data, with comparisons so that patterns emerge	Breaking down and conceptualizing data, which includes taking apart a single sentence, observation, or incident	Creating link between collecting data and developing emergent theory; defining what is occurring in data and beginning to analyze what it means
Types of coding	Open, selective, theoretical	Open, axial, and selective	Initial, focused
Connections between categories: strategies	18 coding families plus theoretical codes from different disciplines	Paradigm (conditions, actions–interactions, and consequences or outcomes) and the conditional/consequential matrix	Analytic strategies are emergent rather than procedural application; categories, subcategories, and links
Outcome	Emergent theory (discovery)	Conceptual description (verification)	A theory co-constructed by the researcher with the participants

> **Example of Corbin and Strauss' grounded theory analysis**
> Michaels and Meeker (2024) used Corbin and Strauss' grounded theory method to study family caregiving for older adults who lived at home and required daily assistance in rural areas. The researchers conducted two interviews each with 15 family caregivers for a total of 30 interviews. Results revealed that family caregivers engaged in the process of orchestrating care by growing into their caregiving role, integrating technology, and using networks when providing caregiving.

Constructivist Grounded Theory Approach

The constructivist approach to grounded theory is in some ways similar to Glaserian methods. According to Charmaz, in constructivist grounded theory, the "coding generates the bones of your analysis. Theoretical integration will assemble these bones into a working skeleton" (2025, p. 113). Charmaz offered guidelines for different types of coding: word-by-word coding, line-by-line coding, and incident-to-incident coding. Unlike Glaser's grounded theory approach, in which theory is discovered from data separate from the researcher, Charmaz's position is that researchers construct grounded theories by means of their past and current involvements and interactions with individuals and research practices. A researcher's reflexivity and positionality are central in Charmaz's approach.

Charmaz distinguished *initial coding* and *focused coding*. In initial coding, the pieces of data (e.g., words, lines, segments, incidents) are studied so the researcher can learn what the participants view as problematic. In focused coding, the analysis is directed toward identifying the most significant initial codes, which are then theoretically coded.

> **Example of constructivist grounded theory analysis**
> Lund and colleagues (2024) use constructivist methods to develop a grounded theory of "just pee in the diaper" focusing on moral distress related to neglectful care practices in nursing homes. The researchers conducted 10 individual interviews and 5 focus groups with staff who worked in 17 different nursing homes in Norway. The core category discovered was facilitating staff-centered and self-protective care practices to mitigate their moral distress related to neglectful care practices.

Secondary Qualitative Data Analysis

Like quantitative researchers, qualitative researchers have come to recognize the value of secondary qualitative data analysis of existing data sets (Beck, 2019). In some cases, secondary analysis of a qualitative dataset is undertaken by the same researcher who conducted the original study; in other cases, the data are used by new researchers. Thorne (2013) identified five types of qualitative secondary analyses.

- *Analytic expansion* occurs when a researcher goes back to an original data set to ask new questions that were not envisioned with the primary study.
- *Retrospective interpretation* is a type of analytic expansion that involves a temporal aspect. The analysis occurs long after the results of the primary study were published. The researchers go back to the original data to further examine issues or findings that were only superficially dealt with the first time around.
- *Armchair induction* is undertaken by theoretical scholars who have not conducted any fieldwork themselves. They are removed from the field but analyze existing qualitative data sets to develop different types of results than the primary researcher.
- *Cross-validation* involves the use of multiple datasets from different researchers to confirm or challenge the original interpretations.
- *Amplified sampling* enhances transferability of the original data set by analyzing different qualitative data sets across populations and contexts.

> **Example of a secondary qualitative data analysis**
> Beck (2022) conducted a secondary qualitative analysis combining data from three of her primary studies to examine the metaphors women used to describe their experiences of postpartum depression. Eleven metaphors were identified that women used to help explain what they were experiencing: "being hit by a ton of bricks," "being a tightrope walker," "living in a nightmare," "feeling trapped," "being in the middle of the sea," "feeling like an alien," "being a loner," "being a basket case," "having cobwebs in the brain," "feeling like garbage," and "hitting rock bottom."

CRITICAL APPRAISAL OF QUALITATIVE ANALYSIS

Evaluating a qualitative analysis is not easy to do. Readers do not have access to the information they would need to assess whether researchers exercised good judgment and critical insight in coding and interpreting the narrative materials, developing a thematic analysis, and integrating materials into a meaningful whole. Researchers are seldom able to include more than a handful of examples of actual data in a journal article. Moreover, the process they used to inductively abstract meaning from the data is difficult to describe and illustrate.

In a critical appraisal of qualitative analyses, one focus should be on whether the researchers adequately documented the analytic process and explained their approach. For example, a report for a grounded theory study should indicate whether the researchers used the Glaser, Corbin and Strauss, or constructivist methods.

Another aspect of a qualitative analysis that can be appraised is whether the researchers have documented that they used one approach consistently and were faithful to the integrity of its procedures. Thus, for example, if researchers say they are using the Glaserian approach to grounded theory analysis, they should not also include elements from the Corbin and Strauss' method. An even more serious problem occurs when, as sometimes happens, the researchers "muddle" traditions. For example, researchers who describe their study as a grounded theory study should not present *themes* because grounded theory analysis does not yield themes. Researchers who attempt to blend elements from two traditions may not have a clear grasp of the analytic precepts of either one.

Some further guidelines that may be helpful in evaluating qualitative analyses are presented in Box 15.1.

> **Box 15.1 Guidelines for Critically Appraising Qualitative Analyses**
>
> a. Was the data analysis approach appropriate for the research design or tradition?
> b. Was the coding scheme described? If so, does the scheme appear logical and complete?
> c. Did the report adequately describe the process by which the actual analysis was performed? Did the report indicate whose approach to data analysis was used (e.g., that of Glaser, Corbin and Strauss, or Charmaz in grounded theory studies)?
> d. What major themes or processes emerged? Were relevant excerpts from the data provided, and do the themes or categories appear to capture the meaning of the narratives? Is the analysis parsimonious—could two or more themes be collapsed into a broader and perhaps more useful conceptualization?
> e. Was a conceptual map, model, or diagram effectively displayed to communicate important processes?
> f. Was the context of the phenomenon adequately described? Did the report give you a clear picture of the social or emotional world of study participants?
> g. Did the analysis yield a meaningful and insightful picture of the phenomenon under study? Is the resulting theory or description trivial or obvious?

RESEARCH EXAMPLES WITH CRITICAL THINKING EXERCISES

This section describes the analytic procedures used in a qualitative study. Read the summary for Example 1, and then answer the critical thinking questions that follow, referring to the full research report if necessary. The critical thinking questions for Example 2 are based on the study that appears in its entirety in Appendix B of this book.

EXAMPLE 1: A SECONDARY QUALITATIVE DATA ANALYSIS

Study: "Intersecting substance use disorder and unmet social needs in rural pregnant women" (Allen et al., 2024)

Statement of Purpose: The aim of this study was to describe the unique challenges faced by rural pregnant women with intersecting substance use disorder (SUD) and unmet social needs.

Method: Thorne's (2013) analytic expansion approach was used for this secondary qualitative analysis where the researchers explored an emerging research question that had not been previously explored in the analysis of the primary dataset. In the primary study, 14 pregnant women were interviewed about their experiences of food insecurity in a rural setting. The sample in this secondary qualitative analysis focused on four participants in recovery from SUD who shared unprompted about the relationship between SUD and their unmet social needs while pregnant. The transcribed interviews of these four participants were the data used in this secondary qualitative analysis.

Analysis: The researchers used Braun and Clarke's (2022) reflexive thematic analysis to analyze the four transcripts. Braun and Clarke's six steps included dwelling with the data set, coding, generating initial themes, refining the themes, defining and naming theme, and writing the report.

Key Findings: Three themes described the intersection of SUD treatment, pregnancy, and unmet social needs of pregnant women in a rural setting: (1) "Experiencing social needs during pregnancy complicates SUD recovery and treatment," (2) "Stigma, social isolation, and mental health challenges overlap with unmet social needs to influence recovery," and (3) "The integration of prenatal care, social supports, and SUD treatment is affirming and helpful."

Critical Thinking Exercises

1. Answer the relevant questions from Box 15.1 regarding this study.
2. Did the researchers identify any limitations of their study?
3. What might be some of the uses to which the findings could be put in clinical practice?

EXAMPLE 2: A PHENOMENOLOGIC ANALYSIS IN APPENDIX B

Read the method and results sections from Morrison et al.'s (2024) phenomenologic study, "Lived experience of fathers after infertility," in Appendix B of this book.

1. Answer the relevant questions from Box 15.1 regarding this study.
2. Comment on the amount of data that had to be analyzed in this study. Do you think saturation was achieved?

Summary Points

- Qualitative analysis is a challenging, labor-intensive activity, with few fixed rules.

- Qualitative analysis usually begins with efforts to understand and manage the mass of narrative data by developing a **coding scheme**. Analysts use *codes* to identify an interesting, salient, or essential feature of the data in relation to the central phenomenon. Data segments can be coded in different ways, depending on research goals.

- Traditionally, researchers organized their data by developing *conceptual files*, which are physical files into which coded excerpts of data for specific codes are placed. Now, however, computer software (CAQDAS) is widely used to perform basic indexing functions and to facilitate data analysis.

- The analysis of qualitative data often involves a search for broad **categories**, which are clusters of codes that are connected conceptually. In many qualitative studies, the next phase involves the identification of themes. A **theme**, which often cuts across several categories, is a recurring regularity that captures meaningful patterns in the data. Identifying themes involves the discovery not only of commonalities across participants but also of natural variation and patterns in the data.

- Researchers whose goal is qualitative description often say they used **qualitative content analysis**. Content analysis can vary in terms of an emphasis on *manifest content* or *latent content*. **Thematic analysis** is another broad approach to extracting themes from descriptive qualitative data.

- In ethnographies, analysis begins as the researcher enters the field. One analytic approach is Spradley's method, which involves four levels of analysis: *domain analysis* (identifying **domains** or units of cultural knowledge), *taxonomic analysis* (selecting key domains and constructing **taxonomies**), *componential analysis* (comparing and contrasting terms in a domain), and a *theme analysis* (to uncover cultural themes).

- There are numerous approaches to phenomenologic analysis, including the descriptive methods of Colaizzi, Giorgi, and van Kaam, in which the goal is to find common patterns of experiences shared by particular instances.

- In van Manen's approach, which involves efforts to grasp the essential meaning of the experience being studied, researchers search for themes, using either a *holistic approach* (viewing text as a whole), a *selective approach* (pulling out key statements and phrases), or a *detailed approach* (analyzing every sentence).

- Central to analyzing data in a hermeneutic study is the notion of the **hermeneutic circle**, which signifies a process in which there is continual movement between the parts and the whole of the text under analysis.

- Benner's approach consists of three processes: searching for **paradigm cases**, thematic analysis, and the analysis of *exemplars*.

- Grounded theorists use the **constant comparative** method of data analysis, a method that involves comparing elements present in one data source (e.g., in one interview) with those in another. *Fit* has to do with how closely concepts fit with incidents they represent, which is related to how thoroughly constant comparison was done.

- One grounded theory approach is the Glaser and Strauss' method, in which there are two broad types of codes: **substantive codes** (in which the empirical substance of the topic is conceptualized) and **theoretical codes** (in which the relationships among the substantive codes are conceptualized).

- Substantive coding involves **open coding** to capture what is going on in the data, and then **selective coding**, in which only variables relating to a core category are coded. The **core category**, a behavior pattern that has relevance for participants, is sometimes a **basic social process (BSP)** that involves a process of coping or adaptation.

- In the Glaserian method, open codes begin with *level I (in vivo) codes*, which are collapsed into a higher level of abstraction in *level II codes*. Level II codes are then used to formulate *level III codes*, which are theoretical constructs. Through constant comparison, researchers compare concepts emerging from the data with similar concepts from existing theory or research to see which parts have **emergent fit** with the theory being generated.

- Corbin and Strauss' method is an alternative grounded theory method whose outcome is a full conceptual description. This approach to grounded theory analysis involves two types of coding: open coding (in which categories are generated) and **axial coding** (where categories are linked with subcategories and integrated).

- In Charmaz's constructivist grounded theory, coding can be word-by-word, line-by-line, or incident-by-incident. Initial coding leads to *focused coding*, which is then followed by theoretical coding.

REFERENCES

Allen, S., Dev, A., Canavan, C., & Goodman, D. (2024). Intersecting substance use disorder and unmet social needs in rural pregnant women. *Journal of Obstetric, Gynecologic, and Neonatal Nursing*, 53(5), 485–490. https://doi.org/10.1016/j.jogn.2024.04.006

Anyiam, S., Woo, J., & Spencer, B. (2024). Listening to Black women's perspectives of birth centers and midwifery care: Advocacy, protection, and empowerment. *Journal of Midwifery & Women's Health*, 69(5), 653–662. https://doi.org/10.1111/jmwh.13635

Beck, C. T. (2019). *Secondary qualitative data analysis in the health and social sciences*. Routledge.

Beck, C. T. (2022). Postpartum depression: A metaphorical analysis. *Journal of the American Psychiatric Nurses Association*, 28(5), 382–390. https://doi.org/10.1177/1078390320959448

Beck, C. T. (2023). Survivors' experiences of hyperemesis gravidarum. *Journal of Infusion Nursing*, 46(6), 338–346. https://doi.org/10.1097/NAN.0000000000000520

Beck, C. T. (2025). In a flash: A qualitative descriptive study of amniotic fluid embolism survivors. *MCN: The American Journal of Maternal Child Nursing*, 50(2), 107–113. https://doi.org/10.1097/NMC.0000000000001081

Benner, P. (1994). The tradition and skill of interpretive phenomenology in studying health, illness, and caring practices. In P. Benner (Ed.), *Interpretive phenomenology: Embodiment, caring, and ethics in health and illness* (pp. 99–127). Sage.

Boyden, G. L., Brisbois, M. D., Kellogg, M. B., & Foli, K. J. (2024). Understanding resilience among generation Z baccalaureate nursing students: A hermeneutical phenomenology study. *Journal of Nursing Education*, 63(7), 460–469. https://doi.org/10.3928/01484834-20240505-02

Braun, V., & Clarke, V. (2022). *Thematic analysis: A practical guide*. Sage.

Charmaz, K. (2025). *Constructing grounded theory* (3rd ed.). Sage.

Colaizzi, P. (1978). Psychological research as the phenomenologist views it. In R. Valle & M. King (Eds.), *Existential-phenomenological alternatives for psychology* (pp. 48–71). Oxford University Press.

Corbin, J., & Strauss, A. (2015). *Basics of qualitative research: Techniques and procedures for developing grounded theory* (4th ed.). Sage.

DeSantis, L., & Ugarriza, D. N. (2000). The concept of theme as used in qualitative nursing research. *Western Journal of Nursing Research*, 22, 351–372. https://doi.org/10.1177/019394590002200308

Didier, A., Nathaniel, A., Scott, H., Look, S., Benaroyo, L., & Zumstein-Shaha, M. (2023). Protecting personhood: A classic grounded theory. *Qualitative Health Research*, 33(13), 1177–1188. https://doi.org/10.1177/10497323231190329

Giorgi, A. (1985). *Phenomenology and psychological research*. Duquesne University Press.

Glaser, B. G. (1978). *Theoretical sensitivity: Advances in the methodology of grounded theory*. Sociology Press.

Glaser, B. G. (2005). *The grounded theory perspective III: Theoretical coding*. Sociology Press.

Glaser, B. G., & Strauss, A. (1967). *The discovery of grounded theory: Strategies for qualitative research*. Aldine de Gruyter.

Hoffman, S. J., & Fredkove, W. M. (2024). Using a constructivist-oriented modified grounded theory approach in the study of intrafamily trauma communication process in war-affected families. *Advances in Nursing Science*, 47(4), E138–E157. https://doi.org/10.1097/ans.0000000000000506

Hulse, S. B., Balogun, Z., Rosenzweig, M. Q., Marsland, A. L., & Palmer, V. M. (2024). I'm still me, I'm still a person: War metaphor use and meaning making in women with metastatic breast cancer. *Supportive Care in Cancer*, 32(2), 108. https://doi.org/10.1007/s00520-024-08309-5

Hwang, H., DeGagne, J. C., Yoo, L., Lee, M., Jo, H. K., & Kim, J. E. (2024). Exploring nursing research culture in clinical practice: Qualitative ethnographic study. *Asian and Pacific Island Nursing Journal*, 8, e50703. https://doi.org/10.2196/50703

Krippendorff, K. (2019). *Content analysis: An introduction to its methodology* (4th ed.). Sage.

Kyngäs, H., Mikkonen, K., & Kääriäinen, M. (Eds.). (2020). *The application of content analysis in nursing science research*. Springer.

Lund, S. B., Malmedal, W. K., Mosqueda, L., & Skolbekken, J. A. (2024). "Just pee in the diaper"—A constructivist grounded theory study of moral distress enabling neglect in nursing homes. *BMC Geriatrics*, 24(1), 366. https://doi.org/10.1186/s12877-024-04920-7

McFarland, M. R., & Wehbe-Alamah, H. B. (2015). *Leininger's culture care diversity and universality: A worldwide nursing theory* (3rd ed.). Jones & Bartlett Learning.

Michaels, J. A., & Meeker, M. A. (2024). Orchestrating care: A grounded theory study of family caregiving for older adults in rural areas. *Qualitative Health Research*, 34(12), 1231–1242. https://doi.org/10.1177/10497323241236308

Monaco, M. L., Alblooshi, S., Mocchio, R. M., Natoli, G., Landa, M. L., & Corrao, S. (2024). The lived experience of mothers living with fibromyalgia syndrome: A phenomenological inquiry. *Musculoskeletal Care, 22*(2), e1889. https://doi.org/10.1002/msc.1889

Nwozichi, C. U., Ramos, M. D., Ogunmuyiwa, A. O., & Gigi, M. B. (2024). Dominant worldviews, institutional, and contextual factors affecting cancer care: Evidence from an institutional ethnonursing study in Nigeria. *Journal of Transcultural Nursing, 35*(3), 216–225. https://doi.org/10.1177/10436596241230998

Petreca, V. G., Flanagan, J., Lyons, K. S., & Burgess, A. W. (2024). The reintegration of men into society after a sexual offense: A hermeneutic phenomenology study. *Issues in Mental Health Nursing, 45*(5), 453–467. https://doi.org/10.1080/01612840.2024.2322008

Saldaña, J. (2021). *The coding manual for qualitative researchers* (4th ed.). Sage.

Song, J., Zhang, Y. X., Qin, M. N., Ren, J. X., Jia, Y. N., You, H., & Zhou, Y. Q. (2024). Experiences of returning to work in patients with schizophrenia after treatment: A longitudinal qualitative study. *International Journal of Social Psychology, 70*(3), 588–600. https://doi.org/10.1177/00207640231223423

Spradley, J. P. (1979). *The ethnographic interview*. Holt, Rinehart, and Winston.

Thorne, S. (2013). Secondary qualitative data analysis. In C. T. Beck (Ed.). *Routledge international handbook of qualitative nursing research* (pp. 393–404). Routledge.

Thorne, S., & Darbyshire, P. (2005). Land mines in the field: A modest proposal for improving the craft of qualitative health research. *Qualitative Health Research, 15*, 1105–1113.

van Kaam, A. (1966). *Existential foundations of psychology*. Duquesne University Press.

van Manen, M. (1997). *Researching lived experience* (2nd ed.). The Althouse Press.

van Manen, M. (2023). What does ChatGPT mean for qualitative health research? *Qualitative Health Research, 33*(13), 1135–1139. https://doi.org/10.1177/10497323231210816

Watson, A. L. (2024). The evolution of professional identity in intensive care nurses during COVID-19—An interpretive phenomenological study. *Intensive & Critical Care Nursing, 80*, 103538. https://doi.org/10.1016/j.iccn.2023.103538

16 Appraising Trustworthiness and Integrity in Qualitative Research

Learning Objectives

On completing this chapter, you will be able to:

- Discuss some controversies relating to the issue of quality and integrity in qualitative research
- Identify the criteria proposed in a major framework for evaluating quality in qualitative research
- Discuss strategies for enhancing quality in qualitative research
- Describe different dimensions relating to the interpretation of qualitative results
- Define new terms in the chapter

Key Terms

- Audit trail
- Authenticity
- Confirmability
- Credibility
- Data triangulation
- Dependability
- Disconfirming cases
- Inquiry audit
- Investigator triangulation
- Member check
- Method triangulation
- Negative case analysis
- Peer debriefing
- Persistent observation
- Positionality statement
- Prolonged engagement
- Reflexivity
- Researcher credibility
- Thick description
- Transferability
- Triangulation
- Trustworthiness

Integrity in qualitative research is a critical issue for both those doing the research and those considering the use of qualitative evidence.

PERSPECTIVES ON QUALITY IN QUALITATIVE RESEARCH

Qualitative researchers agree on the importance of doing high-quality research, yet defining "high quality" has been controversial. We offer a brief overview of the arguments of the debate.

Debates About Rigor and Validity

One controversial issue concerns use of the terms *rigor* and *validity*—terms some people avoid because they are associated with the positivist paradigm. For these critics, the concept of rigor is by its nature a term that does not fit into an interpretive paradigm that values insight and creativity.

Others disagree with those opposing these terms. Morse (2015), for example, has argued that qualitative researchers should return to the terminology of the social sciences—that is, rigor, reliability, validity, and generalizability.

This debate has given rise to several positions. At one extreme are those who think that validity is an appropriate quality criterion in both qualitative and quantitative studies, although qualitative researchers use different methods to achieve it. At the opposite extreme are those who berate the "absurdity" of validity. A widely adopted stance is what has been called a *parallel perspective*. This position was proposed by Lincoln and Guba (1985), who created standards for the **trustworthiness** of qualitative research that parallel the quality standards in quantitative research.

Generic Versus Specific Standards

Another controversy concerns whether there should be a generic set of quality standards, or whether specific standards are needed for different qualitative traditions. Some writers believe that research conducted within different disciplinary traditions must attend to different concerns and that techniques for enhancing integrity vary. Thus, different writers have offered standards for specific forms of qualitative inquiry, such as grounded theory, phenomenology, ethnography, and critical research. Some writers believe, however, that some quality criteria are fairly universal within the constructivist paradigm. For example, Whittemore and colleagues (2001) prepared a synthesis of criteria that they viewed as essential to all qualitative inquiry.

Terminology Proliferation and Confusion

The result of these controversies is that there is no common vocabulary for quality criteria in qualitative research. Terms such as *truth value*, *goodness*, *integrity*, and *trustworthiness* abound, but each proposed term has been refuted by some critics. With regard to actual *criteria* for evaluating quality in qualitative research, dozens have been suggested. Establishing a consensus on what the quality criteria should be, and what they should be named, remains elusive.

FRAMEWORKS FOR QUALITATIVE RESEARCH

Given the lack of consensus, and the heated arguments supporting and contesting various frameworks, it is challenging to provide guidance about quality standards. In this section, we present information about qualitative *criteria*. We then describe *strategies* that researchers use to strengthen integrity in qualitative research. These strategies should provide guidance for considering whether a qualitative study is sufficiently rigorous/trustworthy/valid.

Lincoln and Guba's Quality Criteria

Although not without critics, the criteria often viewed as the "gold standard" for qualitative research are those outlined by Lincoln and Guba (1985). These researchers suggested four criteria for enhancing the trustworthiness of a qualitative inquiry: credibility, dependability, confirmability, and transferability. These criteria represent parallels to the positivists' criteria of internal validity, reliability, objectivity, and external validity, respectively. In later writings, responding to critics and to their own evolving views, a fifth criterion more distinctively aligned with the constructivist paradigm was added: authenticity (Guba & Lincoln, 1994).

Credibility

Credibility refers to confidence in the truth value of the data and interpretations of them. Qualitative researchers must strive to establish confidence in the truth of the findings.

Lincoln and Guba (1985) pointed out that credibility involves two aspects: first, carrying out the study in a way that enhances the believability of the findings, and second, taking steps to *demonstrate* credibility to external readers. Credibility is a crucial criterion in qualitative research that has been proposed in several quality frameworks.

Dependability

Dependability refers to the stability (reliability) of data over time and over conditions. The dependability question is, "Would the study findings be repeated if the inquiry were replicated with the same (or similar) participants in the same (or similar) context?" Credibility cannot be attained in the absence of dependability, just as validity in quantitative research cannot be achieved in the absence of reliability.

Confirmability

Confirmability refers to objectivity—the potential for congruence between two or more independent people about the data's accuracy, relevance, or meaning. This criterion is concerned with establishing that the data represent the information participants provided and that the interpretations of those data are not imagined by the inquirer. For this criterion to be achieved, the findings must reflect the participants' voice and the conditions of the inquiry, and not the researcher's biases.

Transferability

Transferability, analogous to generalizability, is the extent to which qualitative findings have applicability in other settings or groups. Lincoln and Guba (1985) noted that the investigator's responsibility is to provide sufficient descriptive data that readers can evaluate the relevance of the data to other contexts: "Thus the naturalist cannot specify the external validity of an inquiry; he or she can provide only the thick description necessary to enable someone interested in making a transfer to reach a conclusion about whether transfer can be contemplated as a possibility" (p. 316).

Authenticity

Authenticity emerges in a report when it conveys the feeling tone of participants' lives as they are lived. A text has authenticity if it invites readers into a vicarious experience of the lives being described and enables readers to develop a heightened sensitivity to the issues being depicted. When a text achieves authenticity, readers are better able to understand the lives being portrayed "in the round," with some sense of the mood, experience, language, and context of those lives.

Primary and Secondary Qualitative Validity

Whittemore et al. (2001) developed a primary and secondary qualitative validity framework. They proposed four primary criteria as essential to all qualitative inquiry and six secondary criteria that are not relevant to every study but provide supplementary benchmarks for some. The primary criteria are credibility, authenticity, criticality, and integrity. The six secondary criteria include explicitness, vividness, creativity, thoroughness, congruence, and sensitivity.

STRATEGIES TO ENHANCE QUALITY IN QUALITATIVE INQUIRY

This section describes some strategies that qualitative researchers use to establish trustworthiness in their studies. We hope this description will prompt you to carefully assess the steps researchers did or did not take to enhance quality.

We have not organized strategies according to the five criteria described in the previous section (e.g., strategies researchers use to enhance *credibility*) because many strategies simultaneously address multiple criteria. Instead, we have organized strategies by phase of the study—data collection, coding and analysis, and report preparation. Table 16.1 indicates how various quality-enhancement strategies map onto Lincoln and Guba's (1985) criteria.

TABLE 16.1 **Quality-Enhancement Strategies in Relation to Lincoln and Guba's Quality Criteria for Qualitative Inquiry**

Strategy	Credibility	Dependability	Confirmability	Transferability	Authenticity
Throughout the Inquiry					
Reflexivity/reflexive journaling	×				×
Careful documentation, audit trail		×	×		
Data Collection					
Prolonged engagement	×				×
Persistent observation	×				×
Comprehensive field notes	×			×	
Audio recording and verbatim transcription	×				×
Triangulation (data, method)	×	×			
Saturation of data	×			×	
Member checking	×	×			
Data Coding/Analysis					
Transcription rigor/data cleaning	×				
Intercoder reliability checks	×		×		
Triangulation (investigator)	×	×	×		
Search for disconfirming cases/negative case analysis	×				
Peer review/debriefing	×		×		
Inquiry audit		×	×		
Presentation of Findings					
Documentation of quality-enhancement efforts	×			×	
Thick, vivid description				×	×
Impactful, evocative writing					×
Documentation of researcher credentials, background	×				
Documentation of reflexivity	×				

Quality-Enhancement Strategies During Data Collection

Some of the strategies that qualitative researchers use are difficult to discern in a report. For example, intensive listening during an interview, careful *probing* to obtain rich and comprehensive data, and taking pains to gain participants' trust are all strategies to enhance data quality that cannot easily be communicated in a report. In this section, we focus on some strategies that can be described to readers to increase their confidence in the integrity of the study results.

Prolonged Engagement and Persistent Observation

An important step in establishing integrity in qualitative studies is **prolonged engagement**—the investment of sufficient time collecting data to have an in-depth understanding of the culture, language, or views of the people or group under study; to test for misinformation; and to ensure saturation of important categories. Prolonged engagement is also important for building trust with informants, which in turn makes it more likely that useful and rich information will be obtained.

> **Example of persistent observation and prolonged engagement**
> In Canada, Balcom and coresearchers (2024) examined how 14 registered nurses (RNs) and practical nurses (PNs) work together to optimize patient care. The first author shadowed each RN or PN for a minimum of one 8-hour shift and then interviewed each of them. The shadow shifts were also conducted for a 2-month period.

High-quality data collection in qualitative studies also involves **persistent observation**, which concerns the salience of the data being gathered. Persistent observation refers to the researchers' focus on the characteristics or aspects of a situation that are relevant to the phenomena being studied. As Lincoln and Guba (1985) noted, "If prolonged engagement provides scope, persistent observation provides depth" (p. 304).

Reflexivity Strategies

Reflexivity involves awareness that the researcher as an individual brings to the inquiry a unique background, set of values, and professional identity that can affect the research process. Reflexivity requires continually attending to the researcher's effect on the collection, analysis, and interpretation of data. Reflexivity goes hand in hand with positionality and is critical for developing positionality. A **positionality statement** offers researchers the opportunity to define themselves in relation to their research studies (Beck, 2024). By being privy to the researcher's positionality, readers can better interpret the research results and any potential bias of the researchers. In these statements, researchers can share their cultural, political, and social contexts that shaped the perspective through which they made research decisions.

The most widely used strategy for maintaining reflexivity is to maintain a reflexive journal or diary. Reflexive writing can be used to record, in an ongoing fashion, thoughts about how previous experiences and readings about the phenomenon are affecting the inquiry. Through self-interrogation and reflection, researchers seek to be well positioned to probe deeply and to grasp the experience, process, or culture under study through the lens of participants.

 TIP Researchers sometimes begin a study by being interviewed themselves regarding the phenomenon under study.

Data and Method Triangulation

Triangulation refers to the use of multiple referents to draw conclusions about what constitutes truth. The aim of triangulation is to "overcome the intrinsic bias that comes from single-method, single-observer, and single-theory studies" (Denzin, 1989, p. 313). Triangulation can also help to capture a more complete, contextualized picture of the phenomenon under study. Denzin identified four types of triangulation (data triangulation, investigator triangulation, method triangulation, and theory triangulation), and other types have been proposed. Two types are relevant to data collection: data triangulation and method triangulation. Morgan (2024) argued that in order to use triangulation to make qualitative studies trustworthy and rigorous, researchers need to specifically identify which types of triangulation they used in their research.

Data triangulation involves the use of multiple data sources for the purpose of validating conclusions. There are three types of data triangulation: time, space, and person. *Time triangulation* involves collecting data on the same phenomenon or about the same people at different points of time (e.g., at different times of the year). This concept is similar to test–retest reliability assessment—the point is not to study a phenomenon longitudinally to assess change but to establish the congruence of the phenomenon across time. *Space triangulation* involves collecting data on the same phenomenon in multiple sites, to test for cross-site consistency. Finally, *person triangulation* involves collecting data from different types or levels of people (e.g., patients, health care staff), with the aim of validating data through multiple perspectives on the phenomenon.

Method triangulation involves using multiple methods of data collection. In qualitative studies, researchers often use a rich blend of unstructured data collection methods (e.g., interviews, observations, documents) to develop a comprehensive understanding of a phenomenon. Diverse data collection methods provide an opportunity to evaluate the extent to which a consistent and coherent picture of the phenomenon emerges.

> **Example of method triangulation**
> Woodgate and colleagues (2024) explored 29 fathers' experiences of caring for a child with complex care needs in Canada. Data were collected through in-depth interviews, photographs, and ecomaps. The researchers used art-based methodologies of ecomaps and photovoice to help facilitate discussions with fathers and provide a creative approach for fathers to share their stories.

Comprehensive and Vivid Recording of Information

In addition to taking steps to record interview data accurately (e.g., via careful transcriptions of recorded interviews), researchers ideally prepare field notes that are rich with descriptions of what transpired in the field—even if interviews are the only source of data.

Some researchers specifically develop an **audit trail**—a systematic collection of materials that would allow an independent auditor to draw conclusions about the data. An audit trail might include the raw data (e.g., interview transcripts), methodologic and reflexive notes, topic guides, and data reconstruction products (e.g., drafts of the final report). Similarly, the maintenance of a *decision trail* that articulates the researcher's decision rules for categorizing data and making analytic inferences is a useful way to enhance the dependability of the study. When researchers share decision trail information in their reports, readers can better evaluate the soundness of the decisions.

> **Example of an audit trail**
> Jones-Patten and colleagues (2024) explored discrimination experiences and readiness to quit cigarette smoking among 17 African American individuals experiencing

> homelessness by means of five focus groups. The researchers maintained an audit trail of the audio recordings of the focus groups, documentation of meetings with the study team members, and their study timelines.

Member Checking

In a **member check**, researchers provide participants with feedback about emerging interpretations and elicit participants' reactions. The argument is that participants should have an opportunity to assess and validate whether the researchers' interpretations are good representations of their realities. Member checking can be carried out as data are being collected (e.g., through probing to ensure that interviewers have properly interpreted participants' meanings) and more formally after data have been analyzed in follow-up interviews.

Despite the potential that member checking has for enhancing credibility, it has potential drawbacks. For example, member checks can lead to erroneous conclusions if participants share a common façade or a desire to "cover up." Also, some participants might agree with researchers' interpretations out of politeness or in the belief that researchers are "smarter" than they are. Thorne and Darbyshire (2005) cautioned against what they called *adulatory validity*, "a mutual stroking ritual that satisfies the agendas of both researcher and researched" (p. 1110). They noted that member checking tends to privilege interpretations that place participants in a charitable light.

Few strategies for enhancing data quality are as controversial as member checking. Nevertheless, it is a strategy that has the potential to enhance credibility if it is done in a manner that encourages candor and reflection by participants.

> **Example of member checking**
> Thomas and an interdisciplinary team (2024) explored the experiences of 15 Black women advocating for their needs and priorities during the perinatal period. The researchers shared preliminary themes with the participants to make sure the themes resonated with their experiences. Ten of the 15 participants responded and indicated approval of the initial themes with some suggestions on how to refine the wording.

Strategies Relating to Coding and Analysis

Excellent qualitative inquiry is likely to involve the simultaneous collection and analysis of data, so several of the strategies described earlier also contribute to analytic integrity. Member checking, for example, can occur in an ongoing fashion during data collection, but typically also involves participants' review of preliminary analytic constructions. In this section, we introduce a few additional quality-enhancement strategies associated with the coding, analysis, and interpretation of qualitative data.

Investigator Triangulation

Investigator triangulation refers to the use of two or more researchers to make data collection, coding, and analysis decisions. The premise is that through collaboration, investigators can reduce the possibility of biased decisions and idiosyncratic interpretations.

Conceptually, investigator triangulation is analogous to interrater reliability in quantitative studies; it is a strategy often used in coding qualitative data. Some researchers take formal steps to compare two or more independent category schemes or independent coding decisions.

> **Example of independent coding**
> Canli and Aquino (2024) investigated the barriers and challenges 17 Latina nurse leaders had experienced in their ascent to leadership roles. The Latina nurses were interviewed using a semi-structured guide. The two researchers independently coded the transcripts from the interviews. They then met to compare and discuss the codes until consensus was reached.

Collaboration can also be used at the analysis stage. If investigators bring to the analysis task a complementary blend of skills and expertise, the analysis and interpretation can potentially benefit from divergent perspectives.

Searching for Disconfirming Evidence and Competing Explanations

A powerful verification procedure involves a systematic search for data that will challenge a categorization or explanation that emerged early in the analysis. The search for **disconfirming cases** occurs through purposive or theoretical sampling methods. This strategy depends on concurrent data collection and data analysis: Researchers cannot look for disconfirming data unless they have a sense of what they need to know.

Lincoln and Guba (1985) discussed the related activity of **negative case analysis**. This strategy (sometimes called *deviant case analysis*) is a process by which researchers search for cases that appear to disconfirm earlier hypotheses and then revise their interpretations as necessary. The goal of this procedure is to continuously refine a conceptualization or theory until it accounts for *all* cases.

> **Example of a negative case analysis**
> In the United Kingdom, Boucher and colleagues (2024) explored the experiences and choices for a colostomy of 12 individuals following spinal cord injury. Of the 12 individuals, five were early colostomates, five later colostomates, and two did not choose a colostomy. All participants experienced loss of control, loss of self-determination, and loss of dignity. Some participants explained that colostomies transformed their lives, and it felt like "being alive again." The researchers intentionally searched for the negative case to help describe puzzling data which contrasted with major patterns in the data.

Peer Review and Debriefing

Peer debriefing involves external validation, often in face-to-face sessions with the researchers' peers to review aspects of the inquiry. Peer debriefing exposes researchers to the searching questions of others who are experienced in either the methods of constructivist inquiry, the phenomenon being studied, or both.

In a peer review or debriefing session, researchers might present written or oral summaries of their data, categories and themes that are emerging, and interpretations of the data. In some cases, recorded interviews might be played. Among the questions that peer reviewers might address are the following:

- Do the gathered data adequately portray the phenomenon?
- If there are important omissions, what strategies might remedy this problem?
- Are there any apparent errors of fact or errors of interpretation?
- Is there evidence of researcher bias?
- Are the themes and interpretations knit together into a cogent, useful, and creative conceptualization of the phenomenon?

> **Example of peer review**
> In Canada, Boakye and colleagues (2025) explored 24 Black women's experiences of anti-Black medical gaslighting and dismissing of their health concerns when accessing care during pregnancy and childbirth. The researchers conducted a peer review of their preliminary findings with two non-Black racialized colleagues who reviewed and assessed their interpretation of the data and presented themes.

Inquiry Audits

A similar, but more formal, approach is to undertake an **inquiry audit**, a procedure that involves a scrutiny of the actual data and relevant supporting documents by an external reviewer. Such an audit requires careful documentation of all aspects of the inquiry. Once the *audit trail* materials are assembled, the inquiry auditor proceeds to audit, in a fashion analogous to a financial audit, the trustworthiness of the data and the meanings attached to them. Such audits are a good tool for persuading others that qualitative data are worthy of confidence. Relatively few comprehensive inquiry audits have been reported in the literature, but some studies report partial audits.

Strategies Relating to Presentation

This section describes some aspects of the qualitative report itself that can help to persuade readers of the high quality of the inquiry.

Thick and Contextualized Description

Thick description refers to a rich, thorough, and vivid description of the research context, study participants, and events and experiences observed during the inquiry. Transferability cannot occur unless investigators provide information for judging contextual similarity. Lucid and textured descriptions, with judicious inclusion of verbatim quotes from study participants, contribute to the authenticity of a qualitative study.

> **TIP** Sandelowski (2004) cautioned that "the phrase *thick description* likely ought not to appear in write-ups of qualitative research at all, as it is among those qualitative research words that should be seen but not written" (p. 215).

In high-quality qualitative studies, descriptions typically go beyond a faithful rendering of information. Powerful description is evocative and has the capacity for emotional impact. Qualitative researchers must be careful, however, not to misrepresent their findings by sharing only the most poignant stories. Thorne and Darbyshire (2005) warned against "lachrymal validity," a criterion for evaluating research by the extent to which the report can bring tears from its readers. At the same time, they noted the opposite problem with reports that are "bloodless." Bloodless findings are characterized by a tendency of some researchers to "play it safe in writing up the research, reporting the obvious … (and) failing to apply any inductive analytic spin to the sequence, structure, or form of the findings" (p. 1109).

Researcher Credibility

Another aspect of credibility is **researcher credibility**. In qualitative studies, researchers are the data-collecting instruments—as well as creators of the analytic process—so their qualifications, experience, and reflexivity are relevant in establishing confidence in the data. Patton (2015) argued that trustworthiness is enhanced if the report contains information about the researchers, including information about credentials and any personal connections the researchers had to the people, topic, or community under study. For example, it is relevant for a reader of a report on the coping mechanisms of patients with AIDS to know that the researcher is living with HIV. Researcher credibility is also enhanced when reports describe the researchers' efforts to be reflexive.

> **Example of researcher credibility**
> In Korea, Byun and Eom (2024) studied the experiences of nine women who were separated from their newborns when they were transported to neonatal intensive care units to receive treatment. Four themes were extracted: "Outsider left alone," "Enduring in a different world," "The lost starting line," and "Running together." The report noted that one of the researchers worked in the NICU for over 20 years and oversaw tasks related to transfers. The other researcher worked at the referral center for 3 years and had qualitative experience.

INTERPRETATION OF QUALITATIVE FINDINGS

It is difficult to describe the interpretive process in qualitative studies, but there is considerable agreement that the ability to "make meaning" from qualitative texts depends on researchers' immersion in and closeness to the data. *Incubation* is the process of *living* the data, a process in which researchers must try to understand their meaning, find essential patterns, and draw insightful conclusions. Another ingredient in interpretation and meaning-making is researchers' self-awareness and the ability to reflect on their own worldview—that is, reflexivity. Creativity also plays an important role in uncovering meaning in the data. Researchers need to devote sufficient time to achieve the *aha* that comes with making meaning beyond the facts.

For *readers* of qualitative reports, interpretation is hampered by having limited access to the data and no opportunity to "live" the data. Researchers are selective in the amount and types of information to include in their reports. Nevertheless, you should strive to consider some of the same interpretive dimensions for qualitative studies as for quantitative ones (see Chapter 14).

The Credibility of Qualitative Results

As with quantitative reports, you should consider whether the results of a qualitative inquiry are believable. It is reasonable to expect authors of qualitative reports to provide *evidence* of the credibility of the findings. Because consumers view only a portion of the data, they must rely on researchers' efforts to corroborate findings through such strategies as peer debriefings, member checks, audits, triangulation, and negative case analysis. They must also rely on researchers' frankness in acknowledging known limitations.

In considering the believability of qualitative results, it makes sense to adopt the posture of a person who needs to be persuaded about the researcher's conceptualization and to expect the researcher to present evidence with which to persuade you. It is also appropriate to consider whether the researcher's conceptualization is consistent with your own clinical insights.

The Meaning of Qualitative Results

The researcher's interpretation and analysis of qualitative data occur virtually simultaneously in an iterative process. Unlike quantitative analyses, the meaning of the data flows directly from qualitative analysis. Efforts to validate the analysis are necessarily efforts to validate interpretations as well. Nevertheless, prudent qualitative researchers hold their interpretations up for closer scrutiny—self-scrutiny as well as review by external reviewers.

The Importance of Qualitative Results

Qualitative research is especially productive when it is used to describe and explain poorly understood phenomena. However, the phenomenon must be one that merits scrutiny.

You should also consider whether the findings themselves are trivial. Perhaps the topic is worthwhile, but you may feel after reading a report that nothing has been learned beyond what is everyday knowledge—this can happen when the data are "thin" or when the conceptualization is shallow. Readers, like researchers, want to have an *aha* experience when they read about participants' lives. Qualitative researchers often attach catchy labels to their themes, but you should ask yourself whether the labels have really portrayed an insightful construct.

The Transferability of Qualitative Results

Qualitative researchers do not strive for generalizability, but the possible application of the results to other settings is important to evidence-based practice. Thus, in interpreting qualitative results, you should consider how transferable the findings are. In what types of settings and contexts would you expect the phenomena under study to be manifested in a similar fashion? Of course, to make such an assessment, the researchers must have described the participants and context in sufficient detail. Because qualitative studies are context bound, it is only through a careful analysis of the key features of the study context that transferability can be assessed.

The Implications of Qualitative Results

If the findings are judged to be believable and important and if you are satisfied with the interpretation of the results, you can begin to consider what the implications of the findings might be. First, you can consider implications for further research: Should a similar study be undertaken in a different setting? Has an important construct been identified that merits the development of a formal measuring instrument? Do the results suggest hypotheses that could be tested through controlled quantitative research? Second, do the findings have implications for nursing practice? For example, could the health care needs of a subculture (e.g., people who are unhoused) be addressed more effectively as a result of the study? Finally, do the findings shed light on fundamental processes that could play a role in nursing theories?

CRITICAL APPRAISAL OF QUALITY AND INTEGRITY IN QUALITATIVE STUDIES

For qualitative research to be judged trustworthy, investigators must earn the trust of their readers. In a world that is conscious about the quality of research evidence, qualitative researchers need to be proactive in doing high-quality research and persuading others that they were successful.

Demonstrating integrity to others involves providing a good description of the quality-enhancement activities that were undertaken—and yet, many qualitative reports fail to do so. Just as clinicians seek *evidence* for clinical decisions, research consumers need evidence that findings are trustworthy. Researchers should include enough information about their quality-enhancement strategies for readers to draw conclusions about study quality.

Part of the difficulty that qualitative researchers face in demonstrating trustworthiness is that page constraints in journals impose conflicting demands. It takes a precious amount of space to present quality-enhancement strategies adequately and convincingly. Using space for such documentation means that there is less space for the thick description of context

Box 16.1 Guidelines for Critically Appraising Quality and Integrity in Qualitative Studies

a. Did the report discuss efforts to enhance or evaluate the quality of the data and the overall inquiry? If so, was the description sufficiently detailed and clear? If not, was there other information that allowed you to draw inferences about the quality of the data, the analysis, and the interpretations?
b. Did the researchers include their positionality statements?
c. Which specific techniques (if any) did the researcher use to enhance the trustworthiness and integrity of the inquiry? What quality-enhancement strategies were *not* used? Would additional strategies have strengthened your confidence in the study and its evidence?
d. Did the researcher adequately represent the multiple realities of those being studied? Do the findings seem *authentic*?
e. Given the efforts to enhance data quality, what can you conclude about the study's validity/integrity/rigor/trustworthiness?
f. Did the report discuss any study limitations and their possible effects on the credibility of the results or on interpretations of the data?
g. Did the researchers discuss the study's implications for clinical practice or future research? Were the implications well grounded in the study evidence and in evidence from earlier research?

and rich verbatim accounts that support authenticity and vividness. It is helpful to keep the need for compromise in mind in appraising qualitative research reports.

An important point in thinking about quality in qualitative inquiry is that attention needs to be paid to both art and science and to interpretation and description. Creativity and insightfulness need to be attained but not at the expense of soundness. And the quest for soundness cannot sacrifice inspiration, or else the results are likely to be "perfectly healthy but dead" (Morse, 2006, p. 6). Good qualitative work is both descriptively accurate and explicit and interpretively rich and innovative. Some guidelines that may be helpful in evaluating qualitative methods and analyses are presented in Box 16.1.

RESEARCH EXAMPLES WITH CRITICAL THINKING EXERCISES

This section describes quality-enhancement efforts in a grounded theory study. Read the summary for Example 1, and then answer the critical thinking questions that follow, referring to the full research report if necessary. The critical thinking questions for Example 2 are based on the study that appears in its entirety in Appendix B of this book.

EXAMPLE 1: TRUSTWORTHINESS IN A CORBIN AND STRAUSS GROUNDED THEORY STUDY

Study: "Orchestrating care: A grounded theory study of family caregiving for older adults in rural areas" (Michaels & Meeker, 2024).

Statement of Purpose: The purpose was to explain the family caregiving process from the perspective of family caregivers for older adults who live at home in rural areas.

Method: The researchers used Corbin and Strauss's (2015) grounded theory method. Fifteen family caregivers who provided care on a daily basis to older adults living in two rural counties in upstate New York participated in the study. Two semi-structured interviews were conducted with each family caregiver. Initial sampling was purposeful, but as the study progressed, snowball and theoretical sampling were used. Interviews were conducted using Zoom.

Quality-Enhancement Strategies: The researchers provided specific detail about efforts to enhance the trustworthiness of their study. Regarding credibility, the researchers shared they used the actual words of the participants in the findings. Also, the primary researcher provided information about her reflexivity of her personal perspectives through field notes and memos. Focusing on auditability, the researchers described how and why participants were selected. Fittingness was addressed by describing the setting, sample, and theory and how the literature was related to the categories in their grounded theory. The researchers also used what they called the "interviewing the researcher technique," which provided insight into what participants may feel or experience being interviewed. The primary researcher who cared for her older adult parents who lived in a rural area was interviewed by the second author. This taped interview provided the researchers an opportunity to decide if any modifications were needed to their interview guide.

Key Findings: Analysis revealed that the process these family caregivers used to provide caregiving activities to older adults in rural areas was explained by "Orchestrating care," which involved (1) growing into caregiving, (2) integrating technology, and (3) utilizing networks when providing and managing caregiving.

Critical Thinking Exercises

1. Answer the relevant questions from Box 16.1 regarding this study.
2. Which quality-enhancement strategy used by Michaels and Meeker gave you the *most* confidence in the integrity and trustworthiness of their study? Why?
3. Think of an additional type of triangulation that the researchers could have used in their study and describe how this could have been implemented.
4. What might be some of the uses to which the findings could be put in clinical practice?

EXAMPLE 2: TRUSTWORTHINESS IN THE PHENOMENOLOGIC STUDY IN APPENDIX B

Read the method and results sections from Morrison et al.'s (2024) phenomenologic study, "Lived experience of fatherhood after infertility," in Appendix B of this book.

1. Answer the relevant questions from Box 16.1 regarding this study.
2. Suggest one or two ways in which triangulation could have been used in this study.
3. Which quality-enhancement strategy used by Morrison and colleagues gave you the *most* confidence in the integrity and trustworthiness of their study? Why?

Summary Points

- One controversy regarding *quality* in qualitative studies involves terminology. Some argue that *rigor* and *validity* are quantitative terms that are not suitable as goals in qualitative inquiry, but others believe these terms are appropriate. Other controversies involve what criteria to use as indicators of integrity and whether there should be generic or tradition-specific criteria.

- Lincoln and Guba (1985) proposed a framework for evaluating **trustworthiness** in qualitative inquiries, using five criteria: credibility, dependability, confirmability, transferability, and authenticity.

- **Credibility**, which refers to confidence in the truth value of the findings, has been viewed as the qualitative equivalent of internal validity. **Dependability**, the stability of data over time and over conditions, is somewhat analogous to reliability in quantitative studies. **Confirmability** refers to the objectivity of the data. **Transferability**, the analog of external validity, is the degree to which findings can be transferred to other settings or groups. **Authenticity** is the extent to which researchers faithfully show a range of different realities and convey the feeling tone of lives as they are lived.

- Strategies for enhancing quality during qualitative data collection include **prolonged engagement**, which strives for adequate scope of data coverage; **persistent observation**, which is aimed at achieving adequate depth; comprehensive recording of information (including maintenance of an **audit trail**); triangulation; and **member checks** (asking study participants to review and react to emerging conceptualizations).

- **Positionality statements** specify for readers the researchers' cultural, political, and social contexts that shaped their perspectives through which their research decisions were made.

- **Triangulation** is the process of using multiple referents to draw conclusions about what constitutes the truth. This includes **data triangulation** (using multiple data sources to validate conclusions) and **method triangulation** (using multiple methods to collect data about the same phenomenon).

- Strategies for enhancing quality during the coding and analysis of qualitative data include **investigator triangulation** (independent coding and analysis of data by two or more researchers), searching for **disconfirming cases**, undertaking a **negative case analysis** (revising interpretations to account for cases that appear to disconfirm early conclusions), external validation through **peer debriefings** (exposing the inquiry to the searching questions of peers), and launching an **inquiry audit** (a formal scrutiny of audit trail documents by an independent auditor).

- Strategies that can be used to convince readers of the high quality of qualitative inquiries include using **thick description** to vividly portray contextualized information about study participants and the focal phenomenon and making efforts to be transparent about researchers' credentials and reflexivity so that **researcher credibility** can be established.

- Interpretation in qualitative research involves "making meaning"—a process that is difficult to describe or appraise. Yet interpretations in qualitative inquiry need to be reviewed in terms of credibility, importance, transferability, and implications.

REFERENCES

Balcom, S., Doucet, S., & Dubé, A. (2024). Registered nurses and practical nurses working together: An institutional ethnography. *Global Qualitative Nursing Research, 11*, 23333936231225201. https://doi.org/10.1177/23333936231225201

Beck, C. T. (2024). Perspectives on positionality statements in scholarly discourse. *Journal of Obstetric, Gynecologic, and Neonatal Nursing, 53*(6), 581–584. https://doi.org/10.1016/j.jogn.2024.09.010

Boakye, P. N., Prendergast, N., Bailey, A., Sharon, M., Bandari, B., Odutayo, A. A., & Brown, E. A. (2025). Anti-Black medical gaslighting in healthcare: Experiences of Black women in Canada.

Canadian Journal of Nursing Research, 57(1), 59–68. https://doi.org/10.1177/08445621241247865

Boucher, M., Gelling, L., & Tait, D. (2024). The choice for colostomy following spinal cord injury: A grounded theory study. *Journal of Clinical Nursing, 33*(3), 1094–1109. https://doi.org/10.1111/jocn.16885

Byun, H. M., & Eom, J. H. (2024). Phenomenological study of women's experiences of neonatal transport after childbirth in Korea. *Journal of Obstetric, Gynecologic, and Neonatal Nursing, 53*, 151–159. https://doi.org/10.1016/j.jogn.2023.11.004

Canli, U., & Aquino, E. (2024). Barriers and challenges experienced by Latina nurse leaders. *Hispanic Health Care International, 22*(2), 92098. https://doi.org/10.1177/15404153231199175

Corbin, J., & Strauss, A. (2015). *Basics of qualitative research: Techniques and procedures for developing grounded theory*. Sage.

Denzin, N. K. (1989). *The research act* (3rd ed.). McGraw-Hill.

Guba, E., & Lincoln, Y. (1994). Competing paradigms in qualitative research. In N. Denzin & Y. Lincoln (Eds.), *Handbook of qualitative research* (pp. 105–117). Sage.

Jones-Patten, A., Shin, S.S., Nyamathi, A., & Bounds, D. (2024). "Cigarettes play the equalizer": Discrimination experiences and readiness to quit cigarette smoking among African Americans experiencing homelessness: A qualitative analysis. *Addiction Science & Clinical Practice, 19*(1), 1. https://doi.org/10.1186/s13722-023-00432-8

Lincoln, Y. S., & Guba, E. G. (1985). *Naturalistic inquiry*. Sage.

Michaels, J. A., & Meeker, M. A. (2024). Orchestrating care: A grounded theory study of family caregiving for older adults in rural areas. *Qualitative Health Research, 34*(12), 1231–1242. https://doi.org/10.1177/10497323241236308

Morgan, H. (2024). Using triangulation and crystallization to make qualitative studies trustworthy and rigorous. *The Qualitative Report, 29*(7), 1844–1856. https://doi.org/10.46743/2160-3715/2024.6071

Morse, J. M. (2006). Insight, inference, evidence, and verification: Creating a legitimate discipline. *International Journal of Qualitative Methods, 5*(1), 1–7. https://doi.org/10.1177/160940690600500108

Morse, J. M. (2015). Critical analysis of strategies for determining rigor in qualitative inquiry. *Qualitative Health Research, 25*, 1212–1222. https://doi.org/10.1177/1049732315588501

Patton, M. Q. (2015). *Qualitative research & evaluation methods* (4th ed.). Sage.

Sandelowski, M. (2004). Counting cats in Zanzibar. *Research in Nursing & Health, 27*(4), 215–216. https://doi.org/10.1002/nur.20027

Thomas, T. H., Vetterly, S., Kaselitz, E. B., Doswell, W., & Baxter, B. (2024). A qualitative exploration of self-advocacy experiences of Black women in the perinatal period: Who is listening? *Journal of Midwifery & Women's Health, 69*(5), 689–696. https://doi.org/10.1111/jmwh.13630

Thorne, S., & Darbyshire, P. (2005). Land mines in the field: A modest proposal for improving the craft of qualitative health research. *Qualitative Health Research, 15*(8), 1105–1113. https://doi.org/10.1177/1049732305278502

Whittemore, R., Chase, S. K., & Mandle, C. L. (2001). Validity in qualitative research. *Qualitative Health Research, 11*(4), 522–537. https://doi.org/10.1177/104973201129119299

Woodgate, R. L., Gonzalez, M., Ripat, J. D., Edwards, M., & Rempel, G. (2024). Exploring fathers' experiences of caring for a child with complex care needs through ethnography and arts-based methodologies. *BMC Pediatrics, 24*(1), 93. https://doi.org/10.1186/s12887-024-04567-8

17 Learning From Systematic Reviews

Learning Objectives

On completing this chapter, you will be able to:

- Discuss alternative approaches to integrating research evidence and advantages to using systematic methods
- Describe key decisions and steps in doing a systematic review of quantitative and qualitative study findings
- Critically appraise key aspects of a written systematic review
- Define new terms in the chapter

Key Terms

- Aggregative
- Effect size (ES)
- Forest plot
- Frequency effect size
- GRADE
- Intensity effect size
- Interpretive
- Manifest effect size
- Meta-aggregation
- Meta-analysis
- Meta-ethnography
- Meta-summary
- Metasynthesis
- Mixed methods research synthesis
- Primary study
- Publication bias
- Qualitative evidence synthesis (QES)
- Rapid review
- Scoping review
- Statistical heterogeneity
- Subgroup analysis
- Systematic review
- Umbrella review

Systematic reviews, a cornerstone of evidence-based practice (EBP), are inquiries that follow many of the same rules as those for **primary studies**, i.e., original research investigations. This chapter provides guidance in helping you to understand and evaluate the systematic integration of research evidence.

RESEARCH INTEGRATION AND SYNTHESIS

In a **systematic review**, researchers carefully and transparently integrate research evidence about a specific research question using methodical procedures that are spelled out in advance. The review process is disciplined and transparent, so that readers of a systematic review can assess the integrity of the conclusions.

Originally, systematic reviews in health care fields were mainly syntheses of evidence from randomized controlled trials (RCTs) that addressed therapy/intervention questions. Systematic reviews of findings from RCTs—which are at the pinnacle of most evidence hierarchies for therapy questions (see Fig. 1.2)—often involve the statistical integration of evidence in a meta-analysis. The Cochrane Collaboration is a premier organization for creating and disseminating reviews of research evidence; most reviews in the Cochrane Collaboration database involve meta-analyses. Systematic reviews of all types of quantitative evidence—including findings from studies addressing etiology, prognosis, or diagnosis questions—have also burgeoned. As a result, the Preferred Reporting Items for Systematic Reviews and Meta-Analyses (PRISMA) Executive provides guidance on how to conduct and report systematic reviews and other types of reviews that are extensions of systematic reviews, such as scoping reviews, which identify the concepts and definitions under study and explore the available evidence but do not assess the quality of the evidence. Qualitative researchers have also created techniques to integrate evidence from multiple studies. Their products are often called *metasyntheses*. Metasyntheses typically involve integrations of studies focused on abstract phenomena and experiences (e.g., grief following a miscarriage). However, there is emerging interest among health care researchers on synthesizing information on the qualitative aspects of interventions, such as patient acceptance, implementation processes and contexts, and barriers to implementation. Such reviews are often called *qualitative evidence syntheses*.

TIP In the evolving field of evidence synthesis, special types of review are emerging. For example, in a **rapid review**, the reviewers follow streamlined procedures designed to produce an evidence synthesis in a timely (but less rigorous) manner than a standard systematic review. **Umbrella reviews** integrate findings from multiple systematic reviews on a topic. **Mixed methods research syntheses** (also called mixed research syntheses or systematic mixed studies) use disciplined procedures to integrate and synthesize findings from qualitative, quantitative, and mixed methods studies (Hayvaert et al., 2017). With so many types of systematic reviews, Munn et al. (2018) developed a proposed typology to help researchers know which type of review they should conduct.

SYSTEMATIC REVIEWS OF QUANTITATIVE EVIDENCE

In systematic reviews, the "data" are the findings from studies that addressed a specific question (e.g., mean pain levels following receipt of a pain-reducing intervention). Data from the included studies can be integrated in a narrative fashion or statistically in a meta-analysis.

Basics of Meta-Analysis

The essence of a meta-analysis is that findings from each study are used to compute a common index, an *effect size* (ES). ESs are averaged across studies, yielding aggregated information about not only the existence of a relationship between variables but also an estimate of its magnitude.

Advantages of Meta-Analysis

Meta-analysis offers a simple advantage as an integration method: objectivity. It is difficult to draw objective conclusions about a body of evidence using narrative methods when results are inconsistent, as they often are. Narrative reviewers make subjective decisions about how much weight to give findings from different studies, so different reviewers may reach different conclusions in reviewing the same set of studies. Meta-analysts make decisions that are explicit and open to scrutiny. The integration itself is objective because it uses statistical formulas. Readers of a meta-analysis can be confident that another analyst using the same data set and analytic decisions would reach the same conclusions.

Another advantage of meta-analysis concerns *power*, i.e., the probability of detecting a true relationship between variables (see Chapter 13). By combining effects across multiple studies, power is increased. In a meta-analysis, it is possible to conclude that a relationship is real (e.g., that an intervention is effective), even when several small studies yielded nonsignificant findings. In a narrative review, 10 nonsignificant findings would almost surely be interpreted as lack of evidence of effectiveness, which could be the wrong conclusion.

Criteria for Undertaking a Meta-Analysis

Despite its advantages, meta-analysis is not always appropriate, so reviewers need to decide whether statistical integration is suitable. A basic criterion is that the research question should be nearly identical across studies. This means that the independent and dependent variables, and the study populations, are sufficiently similar to merit integration.

Another criterion concerns whether there is a sufficient knowledge base for statistical integration. If there are only a few studies, or if all studies are weakly designed, it usually would not make sense to compute an "average" effect.

One other issue concerns the consistency of the evidence. When the same hypothesis has been tested in multiple studies and the results are highly conflicting, meta-analysis is likely not appropriate. As an extreme example, if half the studies testing an intervention found benefits for those in the intervention group, but the other half found benefits for the controls, it would be misleading to compute an average effect. In this situation, it would be better to do an in-depth narrative analysis of *why* the results are conflicting. Campbell et al. (2020) provide guidance on conducting a systematic review without meta-analysis and identify nine items that should be integral to such a review:

1. How studies are grouped
2. Metrics and method used for each outcome
3. Synthesis methods used
4. How the summary of the results was prioritized
5. Heterogeneity of the results and the appropriateness or not of conducting a metasynthesis
6. How the certainty of the findings was assessed
7. The data presentation methods (e.g., tables)
8. Reporting of a synthesis of the results for each outcome variable
9. Limitations of the synthesis

> **Example of a systematic review without meta-analysis** • • • • • • • • • • • • • • • •
> Mellado-García et al. (2024) used the Synthesis without Meta-Analysis (SWiM) guidelines to conduct a systematic review and synthesis of evidence related to water birth, with a specific focus on the second stage of labor. They identified 11 studies that met the inclusion criteria. Due to the heterogeneity of the methods used, they were unable to complete a meta-analysis. They were able to synthesize findings related to the types of delivery, analgesia use, pain perception, and maternal satisfaction with the water birth experience.

Steps in a Quantitative Systematic Review

Unlike literature reviews, systematic reviews require a team. The team usually includes content experts, statisticians (if there is a meta-analysis), and a librarian or information specialist. Putting together a good team is essential. This section describes major steps in a quantitative systematic review so that you can understand the decisions a review team makes—decisions that affect the quality of the review.

Formulation of the Review Question or Aim

A focused systematic review begins with a carefully framed question. Review questions sometimes follow the PICO format described in Chapter 1, with specification of the **p**opulation, the **i**ntervention or influence, the **c**omparison against which the intervention/influence is contrasted, and **o**utcomes. The careful definition of key constructs is critical for deciding whether a primary study qualifies for the synthesis.

> **Example of a question from a meta-analysis**
> Park and colleagues (2024) suggested that studies on addressing risk factors in metabolic syndrome typically report individual changes for each risk factor rather than a comprehensive approach to lifestyle change and its impact on metabolic syndrome. Although they did not specifically ask a question, the authors aimed to understand the impact of comprehensive lifestyle modifications and adherence to recommended health behaviors in individuals with metabolic syndrome.

A strategy that is gaining momentum is to undertake a *scoping review* to refine the specific question for a systematic review. A scoping review is a preliminary investigation that clarifies the range and nature of the evidence base, using flexible procedures. Such scoping reviews can identify strategies for a full systematic review and can also indicate whether a meta-analysis is feasible.

The Design of a Quantitative Systematic Review

Sampling is an important design issue. In a systematic review, the sample consists of the primary studies that have addressed the research question, and eligibility criteria must be stated. Substantively, the criteria specify the population (P) and the variables (I, C, and O). For example, if the reviewer is integrating findings about the effectiveness of an intervention, which outcomes *must* the researchers have studied? With regard to the population, will (for example) certain age groups be excluded? The criteria might also specify that only studies that used a randomized design will be included. On practical grounds, reports not written in English might be excluded. Another decision is whether to include both published and unpublished reports.

> **Example of sampling criteria for a quantitative review**
> Spiga et al. (2024) conducted a systematic review of RCTs to assess the outcomes of interventions aimed at preventing obesity in children aged 5 to 12 years by modifying dietary intake and/or activity levels and its impact on the changes in body mass index (BMI), zBMI score, and serious adverse events. Inclusion criteria included RCTs in children between 5 and 12 years of age that compared diet and/or activity interventions to prevent obesity with no intervention, usual care, or another eligible intervention over a minimum 12-week period post the baseline assessment, and that occurred in any setting.

Researchers sometimes use study quality as a sampling criterion. Screening out studies of lower quality can occur indirectly if the review team excludes studies that did not use a randomized design. More directly, each potential primary study can be rated for quality and excluded if the quality score falls below a threshold. Alternative ways of dealing with study quality are discussed in a later section. Suffice it to say, however, that evaluations of study quality are part of the integration process, so reviewers must decide how to assess quality and what to do with assessments.

In reviews involving a meta-analysis, another design issue concerns the **statistical heterogeneity** of results in the primary studies. For each study, meta-analysts compute an index to summarize the strength of relationship between an independent variable and a dependent variable. Just as there is inevitably variation *within* studies (not all people in a study have identical scores on outcomes), so there is inevitably variation in effects *across* studies. If the results are highly variable (e.g., results across studies are conflicting), a meta-analysis may be inappropriate. If the results are moderately variable, different analytic techniques might be required.

 TIP Review teams are increasingly expected to prepare a *protocol* of a proposed systematic review. Protocols are often registered in an international database called PROSPERO—so if you are searching for evidence for an EBP project, it is a good idea to check in PROSPERO to see if a review is forthcoming.

The Search for Evidence in the Literature

Systematic reviewers typically aim for an exhaustive search of primary studies that meet the eligibility criteria, but they must decide whether their review will include unpublished findings. Although there is not total agreement about the scope of the search, reviewers are increasingly likely to cast as wide a net as possible and include *gray literature*—that is, studies with a more limited distribution, such as dissertations or unpublished reports. Some people restrict their sample to reports in peer-reviewed journals, arguing that the peer review system is a tried-and-true screen for findings worthy of consideration as evidence.

Excluding unpublished findings, however, runs the risk of biased results. **Publication bias** is the tendency for published studies to systematically overrepresent statistically significant findings. This bias is widespread: Authors may refrain from submitting manuscripts for studies with nonsignificant results, reviewers and editors tend to reject such reports when they are submitted, and users of evidence may ignore the findings if they are published. The exclusion of gray literature in a meta-analysis can lead to the overestimation of effects. Meta-analysts can use various search strategies to locate gray literature, in addition to the usual methods for a literature review. These include contacting key researchers in the field to see if they have done studies (or know of studies) that have not been published and reviewing abstracts from conference proceedings.

Example of a search strategy from a systematic review • • • • • • • • • • • • • • • •
Park et al. (2025) conducted a systematic review and narrative analysis to explore telehealth use in people experiencing disabilities in community or primary care settings. They also sought to explore what telehealth interventions were effective in this population. They conducted a literature search of the following databases: PubMed, EMBASE, CINAHL, Cochrane Library, and PsycINFO.

Evaluations of Study Quality

In systematic reviews, the evidence from primary studies needs to be evaluated to assess how much confidence to place in the findings. Evaluations of study quality sometimes involve overall ratings of study features on a multi-item scale. Dozens of quality assessment rating scales exist, but their use is not universally endorsed. Quality criteria vary from scale to scale, so study quality can be rated differently with different assessment scales or by different raters using the same scale.

The Cochrane Collaboration takes an approach that emphasizes risk of bias, using a "domain" approach (Higgins et al., 2024). *Risk of bias* in intervention studies refers to a potential bias in conclusions about a causal effect. In Cochrane reviews, reviewers rate each study for such internal validity threats as selection bias and attrition bias; each is rated low risk, high risk, or unclear risk of bias. Quality assessments of primary studies, regardless of approach, should be done by two or more qualified individuals. If there are disagreements between the raters, there should be a discussion until a consensus has been reached or until another rater helps to resolve the difference.

> **Example of quality assessments in a systematic review**
> Dickins and colleagues (2021), including one of the authors of this book, conducted an integrative review to assess published research addressing the physical and behavioral health characteristics of women age 50 years and older experiencing homelessness in the United States. After searching six databases and screening for eligibility, 10 studies met the inclusion criteria. Two members of the team graded the quality of the studies using the Johns Hopkins Nursing Evidence-Based Practice Model. Per the Johns Hopkins criteria, all were level III or nonexperimental. Nine studies were graded B or of "good quality," and one was graded C or "lower quality." It is important to note that Johns Hopkins now requires those using its tools to seek permission through their web page at https://www.hopkinsmedicine.org/evidence-based-practice/model-tools.

Extraction and Encoding of Data for Analysis

The next step is to extract and record relevant information about the findings, methods, and study characteristics. If a meta-analysis is being undertaken, the goal is to create a data set amenable to statistical analysis. Basic source information must be recorded (e.g., journal, year of publication). Important methodologic features include sample size, whether participants were randomized to treatments, whether blinding was used, rates of attrition, and length of follow-up. Characteristics of participants must be encoded as well (e.g., their mean age). Finally, information about findings must be extracted. For a meta-analysis, reviewers must either calculate ESs (discussed in the next section) or record sufficient statistical information that computer software can compute them.

As with other decisions, extraction and coding of information should be completed by two or more people, at least for a portion of the studies in the sample. This allows for an assessment of interrater agreement, which should be sufficiently high to persuade readers of the review that the data are accurate.

> **Example of data extraction and intercoder agreement**
> Karimi et al. (2024) conducted a systematic review of studies that examined the association between vaginal bleeding during the first trimester of pregnancy and adverse clinical outcomes. Two members of the team assessed the full text of the articles to extract and code data in terms of the study type, years conducted, sample size, setting, the clinical variable of vaginal bleeding during pregnancy, outcomes associated with vaginal bleeding during the first trimester, and the odds ratios and corresponding 95% confidence interval (CI). Discrepancies were brought to a third member of the team for discussion and resolution.

Calculation of Effects in Meta-Analyses

Meta-analyses depend on the calculation of an **effect size (ES)** index that encapsulates in a single number the relationship between the independent and outcome variables in each study. Effects are captured differently depending on the measurement level of variables. The three most common scenarios for meta-analysis involve comparisons of two groups, such as an intervention versus a control group on a continuous outcome (e.g., body fat percentage), comparisons of two groups on a dichotomous outcome (e.g., stopped smoking vs. continued smoking), or correlations between two continuous variables (e.g., blood pressure levels and anxiety scores).

The first scenario, comparison of two group means, is especially common. When the outcomes across studies are on identical scales (e.g., all outcomes are measures of weight in pounds), the effect is captured by simply subtracting the mean for one group from the mean for the other. For example, if the mean postintervention weight in an intervention group were 182.0 pounds and that for a control group were 194.0 pounds, the ES would be −12.0. Typically, however, outcomes are measured on different scales (e.g., a scale of 0 to 10 vs. 0 to 100 to measure pain). Mean differences across studies cannot in such situations be combined and averaged; researchers need an index that is neutral to the original metric. Cohen's d, the ES index most often used, transforms all effects into standard deviation units. If d were computed to be 0.50, it would mean that the group mean for one group was one half a standard deviation higher than the mean for the other group—regardless of the original measurement scale.

 TIP The term *effect size* (ES) is widely used for d in the nursing literature, but the term usually used for Cochrane reviews is *standardized mean difference* (SMD).

When the outcomes in the primary studies are dichotomies, meta-analysts usually use the odds ratio (OR) or the relative risk (RR) index as the ES statistic. In nonexperimental studies, a common ES statistic is Pearson's r, which indicates the magnitude and direction of effect.

Analysis of Data in a Meta-Analysis

After an ES is computed for each study, as just described, a pooled effect estimate is computed as a *weighted average* of the individual effects. The bigger the weight given to any study, the more that study will contribute to the weighted average. A widely used approach is to give more weight to studies with larger samples.

An important decision concerns how to deal with the heterogeneity of findings—i.e., differences from one study to another in the magnitude and direction of effects. Statistical heterogeneity should be formally tested, and meta-analysts should report their results.

Visual inspection of heterogeneity usually relies on the construction of forest plots, which are often included in meta-analytic reports. A forest plot graphs the ES for each study, together with the 95% CI around each estimate. Figure 17.1 illustrates forest plots for situations in which there is low heterogeneity (panel A) and high heterogeneity (panel B) for five studies. In panel A, all five ES estimates (here, odds ratios) favor the intervention group. The CI information indicates the intervention effect is statistically significant (does not encompass 1.0) for studies 2, 4, and 5. In panel B, by contrast, the results are "all over the map." Two studies favor the control group at significant levels (studies 1 and 5), and two favor the treatment group (studies 2 and 4). Meta-analysis is not appropriate for the situation in panel B.

 TIP Heterogeneity affects not only whether a meta-analysis is appropriate but also which statistical model should be used in the analysis. When findings are similar, the researchers may use a *fixed effects model*. When results are more varied, it is better to use a *random effects model*.

Some meta-analysts seek to understand *why* ES estimates vary across studies. Differences could be the result of clinical characteristics. For example, in intervention studies, variation in effects across studies could be related to whether the intervention agents were nurses or

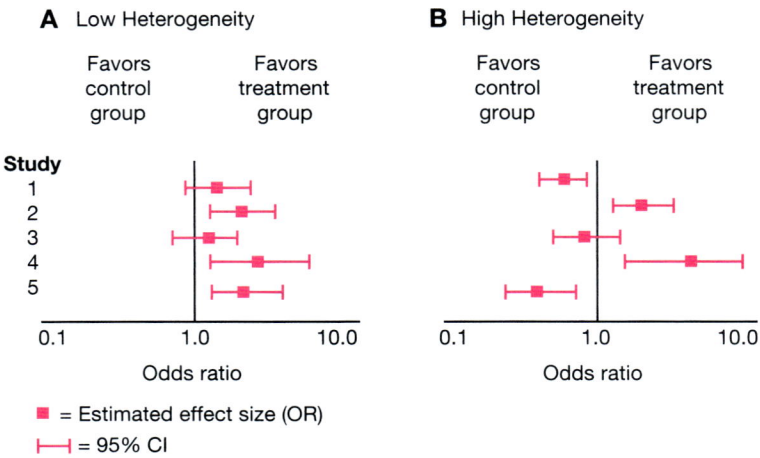

Figure 17.1 Two forest plots.

other health care professionals. Or, variation in results could be explained by differences in participant characteristics (e.g., patients in different age groups). One strategy for exploring systematic differences in ES is to do **subgroup analyses**. Such analyses (sometimes called *moderator* analyses) involve splitting the sample into distinct categorical groups—for example, based on sex. Effects for studies with all-male (or predominantly male) samples could be compared to those for studies with all or predominantly female samples.

> **Example of an investigation of heterogeneity**
> Price and colleagues (2024) conducted a systematic review to explore the effect of age and sex on peak volume of oxygen (VO_2) obtained during arm crank and cycle ergometry exercises with the same participants. Their findings indicated no studies included reported absolute peak VO_2 for the 40 to 49, 60 to 69, or 70 to 79 years age groups for females, limiting the ability to determine the impact of age in females. There was a large amount of heterogeneity in both absolute and relative peak VO_2 in the different types of ergometry. Heterogeneity values for absolute peak VO_2 for males and females were 87%.

Another analytic issue concerns study quality. There are several strategies for dealing with study quality in a meta-analysis. One is to establish a quality threshold for sampling studies (e.g., omitting studies with a poor quality score). A second strategy is to undertake analyses to evaluate whether excluding lower quality studies changes the results (this is called a *sensitivity analysis*). Another approach is to use quality as the basis for a subgroup analysis. For example, do randomized designs yield different average ES estimates than quasi-experimental designs? A mix of strategies is probably a prudent approach to dealing with differences in study quality.

Assessment of Degree of Confidence: GRADE

Until a few years ago, reviewers typically moved from analyzing their data to writing a report. Now, many reviewers undertake a systematic procedure to draw conclusions about how much *confidence* can be placed in the results of the review. Internationally, numerous organizations, including the Cochrane Collaboration, have adopted the Grades of Recommendation, Assessment, Development, and Evaluation **(GRADE)** approach to grading the quality of evidence (Higgins et al., 2024).

GRADE involves a two-part process that was designed to guide the development of clinical guidelines for interventions. In the first step, the quality of evidence about an intervention's effect on specific outcomes is graded. In the second part, a recommendation is made about using or not using the intervention. For those conducting systematic reviews, only the first part is completed—that is, reviewers do not make clinical recommendations.

GRADE ratings are done on an outcome-by-outcome basis and usually are applied to only a subset of outcomes included in a review—the outcomes judged to be critical to those making decisions about adopting an intervention. The GRADE system involves using ratings to make a categorical determination of the *confidence* one can place in the systematic review results—that is, whether confidence in the evidence for a specified outcome (regardless of ES) is high, moderate, low, or very low. A rating of high, for example, corresponds to high confidence that the *true* effect is close to the effect estimated in the review.

TIP There are explicit reporting guidelines for systematic reviews. As mentioned earlier in this chapter, one is *PRISMA*, which is used primarily for reporting systematic reviews of RCTs. The PRISMA guidelines call for the inclusion of a flowchart that documents the identification, screening, and inclusion of studies in a systematic review.

SYSTEMATIC REVIEWS OF QUALITATIVE EVIDENCE

Integration of qualitative findings is a burgeoning and evolving field for which there are no standard procedures—dozens of approaches have been proposed. This section provides a brief overview of some major issues.

Aggregative and Interpretive Qualitative Reviews

Systematic reviews have been characterized as being either *aggregative* or *interpretive/configurative* (Booth et al., 2018). Most qualitative reviews have elements of both aggregation and interpretation. The decision on which broad (and specific) qualitative synthesis approach to use depends on several factors, including the nature of the question and the reviewers' philosophical leanings.

Aggregative Qualitative Reviews

Qualitative reviews that are predominantly aggregative are similar in many respects to quantitative systematic reviews. Aggregative reviews involve the *pooling* of findings (i.e., themes, categories, or processes) across the qualitative studies in the review. Aggregative qualitative reviews tend to be fairly structured, the questions addressed are fairly focused, and exhaustive searching for primary studies is expected. The goal of most aggregative reviews is to provide direct, usable guidance for action.

Research questions that are especially well suited to an aggregative approach often concern how best to address a specific health care problem or how to design or improve an intervention. Examples of such questions include the following: What strategies do people use in efforts to quit smoking? What are patients' barriers to participating in a smoking cessation intervention? What features of a smoking intervention lead to nonparticipation?

Both the Joanna Briggs Institute (JBI) and the Cochrane Collaboration, which typically use the umbrella term **qualitative evidence synthesis (QES),** provide guidance for reviews that would best be characterized as aggregative. At JBI, qualitative reviews use an approach to evidence synthesis called *meta-aggregation* (Aromataris et al., 2024; Lockwood et al., 2015).

Interpretive Qualitative Reviews

Qualitative reviews that are predominantly interpretive emphasize the creation of theories and integrated conceptualizations by interpreting and reconfiguring findings from qualitative primary studies. Interpretive syntheses tend to be loosely structured and may not involve comprehensive searching or quality assessments.

Interpretive syntheses most often focus on questions about meanings, feelings, experiences, and processes—questions typically addressed through phenomenologic, ethnographic, or grounded theory research. Examples of such questions include the following: What is it like for people who smoke to lose a loved one to lung cancer? What is the process by which previous people who smoked succeeded in quitting? In nursing, the term **metasynthesis** has predominated as the term for qualitative evidence synthesis, usually referring to syntheses that are interpretive.

Metasynthesis

Over two decades ago, five leading thinkers on qualitative integration used the term *metasynthesis* as an umbrella term that broadly represented "a family of methodologic approaches to developing new knowledge based on rigorous analysis of existing qualitative research findings" (Thorne et al., 2004, p. 1343). Just as there are many different approaches to doing qualitative research, there are diverse approaches to doing a metasynthesis and to defining what it is.

There is more agreement on what a metasynthesis is *not* than on what it *is*. Metasynthesis is not a literature review—a summary of research findings—nor is it a concept analysis. Schreiber and colleagues (1997) offered a definition of what metasynthesis *is*: "… the bringing together and breaking down of findings, examining them, discovering the essential features and, in some way, combining phenomena into a transformed whole" (p. 314). Most metasynthesis methods involve a transformational process.

Preliminary Steps in a Metasynthesis

Formulation of the Problem

In a metasynthesis, researchers begin with a broad research question or an investigative focus. Booth and colleagues (2018) have described the research question in an aggregative review as an "anchor," but it is more like a "compass" in interpretive reviews. The research question may evolve during the course of the review—it may not be evident at first whether the initial question can be answered, or whether the scope of the review should be expanded or contracted. It is sometimes useful to involve relevant stakeholders in the problem-framing stage of a review. In their reports, metasynthesists sometimes state an overall study purpose rather than a research question.

> **Example of a research question in a metasynthesis** • • • • • • • • • • • • • • • • • •
> Rabben and colleagues (2024) stated that their metasynthesis focuses "specifically on qualitative research relevant to the research question: How do patients, informal carers and healthcare professionals experience and perceive shared decision-making in palliative cancer care?" (p. 407).

 TIP Having a team of at least two researchers to design and implement a metasynthesis is often advantageous because of the subjective nature of interpretive efforts. Investigator triangulation is one strategy for enhancing the integrity of metasyntheses.

Development of Sampling and Search Strategies

Metasynthesists must make sampling decisions. One issue is whether the sample of studies will be exhaustive (i.e., including all relevant studies) or purposive. Some approaches to metasynthesis, notably meta-ethnography, may involve purposive strategies in which studies are selected for conceptual purposes. Another issue is whether to include findings from only peer-reviewed journals. An advantage of including alternative sources is that journal articles have page constraints. Some researchers have included dissertations even when a peer-reviewed journal article is available on the topic because the dissertations often contain richer information. Metasynthesists must also decide whether to search for studies about a phenomenon in a single versus multiple qualitative traditions.

It is generally more difficult to find qualitative than quantitative studies using mainstream approaches such as searching electronic databases. For example, "qualitative" became a medical subject heading (MeSH) term in MEDLINE in 2003, but it is risky for reviewers to assume that all qualitative studies (e.g., ethnographies) are coded as qualitative.

TIP Sample sizes in nursing metasyntheses are highly variable, ranging from five or fewer studies to over 100. Sample size varies as a function of the scope of the inquiry, the extent of prior research, and the type of metasynthesis undertaken. One guideline for sampling adequacy is whether categories in the metasynthesis are saturated.

Evaluations of Study Quality

In general, there is less emphasis on assessing the quality of primary studies in interpretive syntheses than in aggregative ones. Nevertheless, critical appraisal is often used in metasyntheses, sometimes simply to describe the sample of studies in the review but in other cases to make sampling decisions.

Not everyone agrees that study quality should be a criterion for study inclusion. Some have argued that a flawed study does not necessarily invalidate the rich data from those studies. Noblit and Hare (1988), whose meta-ethnographic approach is widely used by nurse researchers, advocated including all relevant studies but suggested giving more weight to higher quality studies. Many nurse researchers use the 10-question assessment tool from the Critical Appraisal Skills Programme (CASP) of the Centre for Evidence-Based Medicine in the United Kingdom. However, Thorne (2022) cautions against such quality appraisals in metasyntheses because they diminish the value of qualitative inquiries, and the decisions to eliminate studies can be arbitrary. Thorne further suggests that in a "discipline such as nursing, in which recognition of multiple knowledge sources is an accepted means by which to enhance and deepen our interpretation of the phenomena of concern to practice, screening out atypical sources seems far less reasonable than does examining them with a critically reflective lens to explore and extract any potential value" (Thorne, 2022, p. 16).

Example of evaluations and sampling decisions in a metasynthesis ●●●●●●●
Jarden and colleague (2025) aimed to search and synthesize findings from qualitative studies exploring patients' experiences and perceptions of their fall in the hospital setting. The authors initially identified 5,542 through searches of seven databases. Of those, 32 were moved to full-text eligibility screening, 22 were found to be ineligible, and 10 publications were included in their metasynthesis.

Extraction of Data

Information about various features of the study needs to be abstracted and coded, such as data source information (e.g., year of publication), sample characteristics, and methodologic features (e.g., research tradition). Most important, the study findings must be extracted and recorded—typically the key themes, metaphors, or categories from each study.

However, *finding* the findings is not always easy. Qualitative researchers intermingle data with interpretation and findings from other studies with their own. Noblit and Hare (1988) advised that, just as primary study researchers must read and reread their data before they can proceed with their analysis, metasynthesists must read the primary studies multiple times to fully grasp the categories or metaphors being described.

Data Analysis and Interpretation in Metasynthesis

Strategies for metasynthesis diverge most markedly at the analysis stage. We briefly describe two approaches. Regardless of approach, metasynthesis is a complex interpretive task that involves "carefully peeling away the surface layers of studies to find their hearts and souls in a way that does the least damage to them" (Sandelowski et al., 1997, p. 370).

The Noblit and Hare Approach

Noblit and Hare (1988), whose approach is called **meta-ethnography**, argued that integration should be interpretive and not aggregative—i.e., that the synthesis should focus on constructing interpretations rather than descriptions. Their approach includes seven phases that overlap and repeat as the metasynthesis progresses:

- The first three phases occur before the analysis:
  - *Phase 1: Deciding on the phenomenon*
  - *Phase 2: Deciding which studies are relevant for the synthesis*
  - *Phase 3: Reading and rereading each study*
- Phases 4 through 6 concern the analysis:
  - *Phase 4: Deciding how the studies are related*. In this phase, the researcher lists the key metaphors (or themes/concepts) in each study and their relation to each other. Studies can be related in three ways: *reciprocal* (directly comparable), *refutational* (in opposition to each other), or in a *line of argument* rather than reciprocal or refutational.
  - *Phase 5: Translating the qualitative studies into one another*. Noblit and Hare (1988) noted that "translations are especially unique syntheses because they protect the particular, respect holism, and enable comparison. An adequate translation maintains the central metaphors and/or concepts of each account in their relation to other key metaphors or concepts in that account" (p. 28).
  - *Phase 6: Synthesizing translations*. Here, the challenge for the researcher is to make a whole into more than the individual parts imply.
- *Phase 7: Writing up the synthesis*. Frances et al. (2019) developed eMERGe criteria to provide guidance on reporting meta-ethnographies to ensure their completeness, clarity, and quality.

> **Example of Noblit and Hare's approach**
> Thoen and colleagues (2024) used Noblit and Hare's approach to conduct a meta-ethnography to explore and synthesize findings from 12 qualitative studies on adults' day surgery and recovery experiences. They found four themes captured the essence of the experience: "Requests for tailored information," "Challenges of recognizing and understanding postoperative symptoms," "Being dependent on continuous professional and personal support," and "Calling for individual adaptation." They concluded that there was a need for more tailored information and support aimed at promoting self-care abilities.

The Sandelowski and Barroso Approach

Sandelowski and Barroso (2007) dichotomized integration efforts based on the degree of synthesis and interpretation in the primary studies. Primary studies are called *summaries* if they yield descriptive synopses of the qualitative data, usually with lists and frequencies of themes. *Syntheses*, by contrast, are more interpretive and involve conceptual or metaphorical reframing. Sandelowski and Barroso have argued that only syntheses should be used in a metasynthesis.

Both summaries and syntheses can, however, be used in a **meta-summary**, which can lay a foundation for a metasynthesis. Sandelowski and Barroso (2007) provided an example of a meta-summary, using studies of mothering within the context of HIV infection. The first step, extracting findings, resulted in almost 800 sentences from 45 reports and represented a comprehensive inventory of findings. The 800 sentences were then reduced to 93 thematic statements or abstracted findings.

The next step involved calculating **manifest effect sizes**, i.e., ESs calculated from the manifest content pertaining to mothering in the context of HIV, as represented in the 93 abstracted findings. (Qualitative ESs should not be confused with effects in a meta-analysis.) Two types of ES can be created. A **frequency effect size**, indicating the *magnitude* of the findings, is the number of reports that contain a given finding, divided by all reports (excluding those with duplicated findings from the same data). For example, Sandelowski and Barroso (2007) calculated an overall frequency ES of 60% for the finding of mothers' struggle about disclosing their HIV status to their children. In other words, 60% of the 45 primary studies had a finding of this nature.

An **intensity effect size** indicates the concentration of findings *within* each study. It is calculated by computing the number of different findings in a given report, divided by the total number of findings in all reports. As an example, one primary study in Sandelowski and Barroso's (2007) meta-summary had 29 out of the 93 total findings, for an intensity ES of 31%.

Metasyntheses can build upon meta-summaries but require findings that are more interpretive, i.e., from studies characterized as syntheses. The purpose of a metasynthesis is not to summarize but to offer novel interpretations of qualitative findings. Such interpretive integrations require metasynthesists to piece the individual syntheses together to craft a new coherent explanation of a target event or experience.

> **Example of Sandelowski and Barroso's approach**
> Baltes and colleagues (2023) conducted a meta-summary using Sandelowski and Barroso's method on the fear of falling from the perspective of older adults. They searched the databases of CINAHL, Medline, PsycINFO, and SSCI for relevant studies as well as gray literature. Out of 2,978 identified studies, 15 met the inclusion criteria. Baltes et al. extracted 578 findings, and then the abstraction process resulted in 183 meta-findings. The frequency ESs were calculated by dividing the number of studies that included a meta-finding by the total number of included studies. Three main topics were identified: "Triggers and reasons for fear of falling," "Consequences attributed to fear of falling," and "Strategies to manage fear of falling in their daily lives."

Meta-Aggregation

JBI uses an aggregative approach to the synthesis of qualitative evidence that is highly structured. Although controversial, JBI maintains that regardless of whether the evidence is quantitative or qualitative, the same review process should be used, with certain steps tailored to accommodate the special nature of the findings. The JBI **meta-aggregation** method is aimed at delivering synthesized findings to inform clinical decision making or policy development.

The JBI reviewer's manual (Aromataris et al., 2024) offers guidance on preparing a *qualitative evidence synthesis* using meta-aggregation. Researchers at JBI also prepared a series of articles describing their approach that appeared in *The American Journal of Nursing* in 2014 (e.g., Munn et al., 2014; Stern et al., 2014). In this section, we briefly mention a few issues relating to the JBI approach.

Preliminary Steps in a Joanna Briggs Institute Qualitative Evidence Synthesis

In a meta-aggregation, an explicit review question is formulated upfront. JBI recommends using the PICO format (**p**opulation, phenomenon of **i**nterest, **co**ntext) for articulating the question (Stern et al., 2014). Reviewers are expected to do comprehensive searching for relevant evidence, including a search of the gray literature. Data are extracted by two independent reviewers using a JBI extraction form, in which findings and a supporting quote from the study's raw data are recorded.

Quality appraisals of the studies are undertaken using the 10-item JBI Critical Appraisal Checklist for Qualitative Research. In addition to appraising each study for its overall methodologic quality, the JBI approach calls for ratings of the *credibility* of each finding in a study. Reviewers assign a rating of *unequivocal* (a finding is beyond a reasonable doubt), *credible* (finding is open to challenge), and *unsupported* (finding is not supported by the data).

Analysis Through Meta-Aggregation

Data synthesis using meta-aggregation is a three-step process that begins with the extraction of findings and illustrations from all included studies. In the second step, findings that are sufficiently similar or related conceptually are collapsed into categories. Each category must have two or more findings. In the final step, the reviewers develop one or more synthesized findings that encompass at least two categories. Reviewers are expected to explain what data they considered as a "finding," the process by which findings were identified, and how findings were grouped to create categories.

> **Example of meta-aggregation**
> Barratt and colleagues (2025) conducted a meta-aggregation systematic review to understand parents' perceptions of quality of life when caring for young and adult children who are experiencing intellectual disability. From the 17 studies included in the analysis, 125 findings were synthesized into 25 categories, which were then synthesized into three findings: "Challenges and rewards of being a parent carer," "The real cost of caregiver burden," and "Surrendering self for duty—the mother's role."

Assessment of Confidence

Inspired by the GRADE rating system for quantitative reviews, a working group at JBI developed a system to rate confidence in the synthesized findings of a QES. The *ConQual* approach, as it is called, requires a score—on a scale from 4 (high) to 1 (very low)—summarizing the reviewers' confidence in each finding. A synthesized qualitative finding is given an initial score of "high" that can be downgraded because of low credibility (e.g., a mix of unequivocal and credible findings results in the loss of a point) or low dependability. The dependability score is based on answers to five specific questions from the JBI critical appraisal tool.

TIP A separate effort was undertaken by a group working with GRADE to develop a means of rating confidence in the findings from a qualitative evidence synthesis—*GRADE-CERQual* (Lewin et al., 2018). Although ConQual and CERQual develop similar rankings, the criteria for scoring in the two systems differ.

CRITICAL APPRAISAL OF SYSTEMATIC REVIEWS

Like all studies, systematic reviews should be thoroughly appraised before the findings are deemed trustworthy and useful in clinical practice. Box 17.1 offers some guidelines for evaluating systematic reviews. We have distinguished questions about analysis separately for quantitative and qualitative reviews. The list of questions is not necessarily comprehensive—supplementary questions might be needed for particular types of review.

Box 17.1 Guidelines for Critically Appraising Systematic Reviews

The Problem
a. Did the report state the research problem and/or research questions? Is the scope of the project appropriate? Was the approach to integration described, and was the approach appropriate?

Search Strategy
b. Did the report describe criteria for selecting primary studies, and are the criteria reasonable?
c. Were the bibliographic databases used by the reviewers identified, and are they appropriate and comprehensive? Were search terms identified?
d. Did the reviewers use adequate supplementary efforts to identify relevant studies?

The Sample
e. Were inclusion and exclusion criteria clearly articulated?
f. Did the search strategy yield a good sample of studies?

Quality Appraisal
g. Did the reviewers appraise the quality of the primary studies? Did they use a well-defined set of criteria or a validated quality appraisal scale?
h. Did two or more people do the appraisals, and was interrater agreement reported?
i. Was quality information used effectively in selecting studies or analyzing results?

Data Extraction
j. Was adequate information extracted about the study design, sample characteristics, and study findings?
k. Were two or more people used to extract and record information for analysis?

Data Analysis—General
l. Did the reviewers explain their method of pooling and integrating the data?
m. Were tables, figures, and text used effectively to summarize findings?

Data Analysis—Quantitative
n. If a meta-analysis was not performed, was there adequate justification for using narrative integration? If a meta-analysis *was* performed, was this justifiable?
o. For meta-analyses, did the report describe how ESs were computed?
p. Was heterogeneity of effects assessed? Was the decision to use a random effects model versus a fixed effects model sound? Were subgroup analyses undertaken, or was the absence of subgroup analyses justified?

(continued)

Box 17.1 Guidelines for Critically Appraising Systematic Reviews (*continued*)

Data Analysis—Qualitative
q. Was the analytic approach mainly aggregative or interpretive?
r. In a metasynthesis, did the reviewers describe the techniques they used to compare the findings of each study, and did they explain their method of interpreting their data?
s. In a metasynthesis, did the synthesis achieve a fuller understanding of the phenomenon to advance knowledge? Do the interpretations seem well grounded?
t. In a meta-aggregation, does the integration of findings into categories and categories into synthesized findings appear insightful and justifiable?

Conclusions
u. Did the reviewers draw reasonable conclusions about their results and the quality of evidence relating to the research question?
v. Did the reviewers use GRADE or another system to rate confidence in the review findings?
w. Were limitations of the review/synthesis noted?
x. Were implications for nursing and health care practice and further research clearly stated?

All systematic reviews | Systematic reviews of quantitative studies | Metasyntheses

In drawing conclusions about a research synthesis, a major issue concerns the nature of the decisions the reviewers made. Sampling decisions, approaches to handling the quality of the primary studies, and analytic approaches should be carefully evaluated. In quantitative reviews, the review team should provide a good rationale if a meta-analysis was not undertaken. Reviewers of qualitative studies should explain why they chose to use a primarily interpretive or aggregative approach.

A thorough discussion section is important in systematic reviews. The discussion should include the reviewers' assessment about the strengths and limitations of the body of evidence, suggestions on further research needed to improve the evidence base, and the implications of the review. Critical appraisals should result in envisioning whether and how clinicians could use the evidence in their practice.

RESEARCH EXAMPLES WITH CRITICAL THINKING EXERCISES

We conclude this chapter with a description of two systematic reviews, one with a meta-analysis and one with a metasynthesis. Read the summaries, and then answer the critical thinking questions that follow, referring to the full research report if necessary.

EXAMPLE 1: A META-ANALYSIS

Study: Antidiabetic agent use and clinical outcomes in patients with diabetes hospitalized for COVID-19: A systematic review and meta-analysis (Keels et al., 2025)

Purpose: The purpose of this study was to examine the relationship between the antidiabetic agent usage and the clinical outcomes of patients with a diagnosis of diabetes mellitus who were admitted with a diagnosis of COVID-19.

Eligibility Criteria: The inclusion criteria for studies for the analysis included English language research papers published in peer-reviewed journals that evaluated the clinical outcomes of adult patients (18+ years) with diabetes mellitus who were hospitalized with a diagnosis of COVID-19 and were receiving antidiabetic agents.

Search Strategy: Five databases were searched: PubMed, Embase, CINAHL, Web of Science, and Cochrane Library. The Boolean search included numerous keywords/MeSH terms, such as "COVID-19" or "SARS-CoV-2" AND "diabetes" or "diabetes type 1" or "diabetes type 2" AND "antidiabetic agents" or "metformin" or "insulin."

Sample: Initially, 6,639 studies were identified, 1,741 of which were duplicates and removed, so 4,898 studies were screened, and of those, 4,780 did not meet eligibility criteria. Of the 118 studies that did meet eligibility, 83 were excluded for reasons such as nonadult population or not having a diagnosis of diabetes present. The final analysis was conducted on 35 studies that met all eligibility criteria.

Quality Appraisal: The Joanna Briggs Institute Critical Appraisal tool was used to appraise the quality of the studies. One study was a prospective design, three were RCTs, and 31 were retrospective designs. Fourteen different countries were represented, with China accounting for the most studies at 42.8% of the reports.

Data Extraction: Two reviewers independently extracted data, and the interrater reliability between the reviewers was 0.68, indicating substantial agreement per the Cohen's κ coefficient. The extracted data included publication information, sample size, country and setting, study design, study aims, participant demographics (age, gender, nationality), reported outcomes, and limitations. All data were uploaded into a table.

Statistical Analyses: To understand the relative risk and prevalence of mortality, the authors conducted random-effects meta-analyses based on the reported incidence of mortality in the studies. To assess the precision of aggregate estimates, 95% CIs, Z-scores, and p-values were used as metrics of evidence against the null hypothesis that there was no difference among antidiabetic agents on mortality in those admitted with COVID-19. The team also quantified heterogeneity for the overall estimate and calculated the total dispersion in ESs across studies and the associated p-values.

Key Findings: After examining each antidiabetic agent's impact on outcomes, the authors conducted a quantitative synthesis across all drug classes. They found a 57% risk reduction among individuals using either metformin or DPP-4 inhibitors compared with control treatment, with an overall risk ratio of 0.432 (95% CI = 0.268 to 0.695, z = 3.45, p < .001). Mortality outcomes across studies were variable (Q = 123.83, df = 11, p < .001, I^2 = 91.1%). Lastly, they found that ESs varied between metformin and DPP-4 inhibitors (Q = 8.80, df = 1, p = .003), suggesting there is not equal effectiveness in preventing mortality.

Discussion: The findings from this systematic review and meta-analyses indicate that metformin and DPP-4 inhibitors were associated with decreased mortality in patients with diabetes mellitus hospitalized with COVID-19. From a practice perspective, this suggests that patients on these agents upon admission should not be converted to insulin if hospitalized for COVID-19. While the authors acknowledge there may be other patient factors that contribute to the higher mortality rate, insulin treatment was found to be associated with an increased mortality rate.

Critical Thinking Exercises

1. Answer the relevant questions from Box 17.1 regarding this study.
2. Were the potential limitations of the meta-analysis reported?

EXAMPLE 2: A META-ETHNOGRAPHY

Study: Meta-ethnography on the experience of women from around the world who exclusively breastfed their full-term infants (Aderibigbe et al., 2024)

Purpose: The purpose of this meta-ethnography was to synthesize evidence from qualitative studies on the experiences of women from around the world who exclusively breastfed their full-term infants.

Eligibility Criteria: A study was included if it (1) focused on women's experience of exclusive breastfeeding of full-term infants for at least 1 month, (2) used qualitative methodology, and (3) was published in English between January 1, 2001, and February 28, 2022, from high-, middle-, and/or low-income countries.

Search Strategy: A search of the following five electronic databases from March 3, 2021, to October 14, 2021, was undertaken by two reviewers, with the assistance of an academic librarian: CINAHL Plus, PubMed, PsycInfo, Scopus, and ProQuest Dissertations and Theses Global. Search terms included "exclusive breastfeeding," "experience," and "women." The researchers included a supplementary appendix detailing their search terms and combinations.

Sample: The report included a PRISMA diagram showing the researchers' sampling progression. There were 1,325 citations initially identified through the database search. After removing 516 duplicates, 809 records remained. Two researchers independently screened titles and/or abstracts and removed 770 records because they were not related to exclusive breastfeeding. They then retrieved the remaining 39 reports and assessed them for eligibility. Nineteen articles were excluded due to not meeting inclusion criteria and three articles due to their CASP score being less than eight. This left 17 studies with CASP scores of 8 or greater in the final sample for the review.

Quality Appraisal: The two researchers used the CASP tool for appraisal of the included studies. They independently critically appraised all the studies; in case of disagreements, they met and reached consensus.

Data Analysis: The analysis was based on Noblit and Hare's (1988) meta-ethnographic approach. Two researchers read and reviewed all 17 studies. These reviewers extracted the demographic and methodologic characteristics of the data from the included studies. Key metaphors and themes were extracted from women's experiences of exclusive breastfeeding. The reviewers determined the studies were reciprocally related. Using reciprocal translations of key metaphors, five overarching themes were identified.

Key Findings: Five overarching themes were identified: "Favorable conditions," "Not a smooth journey," "Support," "Determination and perseverance," and "Reflections on benefits."

Discussion: The reviewers noted that women from around the world shared similar experiences of exclusively breastfeeding their full-term infants. Similarities spanned low-, middle-, and high-income countries.

Critical Thinking Exercises

1. Answer the relevant questions from Box 17.1 regarding this study.
2. Do you think the researchers should have included non-peer-reviewed studies in their review? Why or why not?
3. What might be some of the uses to which the findings could be put in clinical practice?

Summary Points

- EBP relies on rigorous integration of research evidence through systematic reviews. A **systematic review** involves the methodical and transparent integration of findings from multiple **primary studies** about a specific research question using careful sampling and data collection procedures that are spelled out in advance in a *protocol*.

- Systematic reviews are undertaken to synthesize quantitative, qualitative, or mixed-method evidence. Reviews of quantitative studies often involve statistical integration of findings through **meta-analysis**, a procedure whose advantages include objectivity and enhanced power; meta-analysis is not appropriate, however, for broad questions or when there is substantial inconsistency of findings.

- Other types of reviews include **scoping reviews**, which identify the concepts and definitions under study and explore the available evidence; **rapid reviews**, where the reviewers follow streamlined procedures designed to produce an evidence synthesis in a timely (but less rigorous) manner than a standard systematic review; and **umbrella reviews** that integrate findings from multiple systematic reviews on a topic. Another newer type of review is **mixed methods research syntheses** in which disciplined procedures are used to integrate and synthesize findings from qualitative, quantitative, and mixed methods studies.

- Major steps in a systematic review typically involve formulating a question, defining eligibility criteria, searching for and selecting primary studies, evaluating study quality, extracting data, analyzing the data, interpreting and evaluating confidence in the findings, and reporting the findings.

- Reviewers are increasingly likely to search for *gray literature*—i.e., unpublished reports. The concern is the risk of **publication bias** that stems from the underrepresentation of nonsignificant findings in published literature.

- In meta-analyses, findings from primary studies are represented by an **effect size (ES)** index that quantifies the relationship between the independent and dependent variables. The most common ES indexes in nursing are d (the *SMD*), the odds ratio, and correlation coefficients.

- Effects from individual studies are pooled in a meta-analysis to yield an estimate of the population ES by calculating a weighted average of effects, usually giving greater weight to studies with larger samples.

- **Statistical heterogeneity** (diversity in effects across studies) is a major issue in meta-analysis; it affects decisions about which statistical model to use and whether a meta-analysis is justified. Heterogeneity can be examined visually using a **forest plot**.

- Heterogeneity can be explored through **subgroup analyses**, the purpose of which is to see whether effects systematically vary based on clinical, demographic, or methodologic attributes.

- Quality assessments (which may involve formal ratings or risk-of-bias assessments) are sometimes used to exclude weak studies from reviews, but they can also be used to differentially weight studies or to evaluate whether including or excluding weaker studies changes conclusions in a *sensitivity analysis*.

- Systematic reviewers are increasingly likely to use the **GRADE** (Grades of Recommendation, Assessment, Development, and Evaluation) approach to assess the degree of *confidence* that the reviewers have in the estimated effect for specific outcomes in a review.

- Qualitative systematic reviews have been described as either **aggregative** (in which findings from multiple studies are pooled) or **interpretive** (in which the goal is to discover new or enriched ways of understanding phenomena). Aggregative reviews are often called **qualitative evidence syntheses (QES)**. The umbrella term most often used for interpretive reviews is **metasynthesis**. Many qualitative reviews in nursing have elements of both aggregation and interpretation.

- Metasyntheses are more than just summaries of prior qualitative findings; they involve a discovery of essential features of a body of findings and a transformation that yields new interpretations.

- One approach to metasynthesis is called **meta-ethnography**, which was proposed by Noblit and Hare (1988); this approach involves listing key themes or metaphors across studies and then translating them into each other.

- In the approach of Sandelowski and Barroso (2007), a **meta-summary** involves listing abstracted findings from the primary studies and calculating **manifest effect sizes**. A **frequency effect size** is the percentage of reports that contain a given finding. An **intensity effect size** indicates the percentage of all findings that are contained in any given report. A meta-summary can lay the foundation for a metasynthesis.

- The approach to qualitative evidence synthesis used at the Joanna Briggs Institute (JBI) is **meta-aggregation**, which is more structured than a metasynthesis and relies on comprehensive searching and systematic quality appraisals. In a meta-aggregation, similar findings across studies are grouped into *categories*, which in turn are grouped into *synthesized findings*. In JBI qualitative reviews, confidence in the findings is assessed using a rating system called *ConQual*.

REFERENCES

Aderibigbe, T., Srisopa, P., Henderson, W. A., & Lucas, R. (2024). Meta-ethnography on the experiences of women from around the world who exclusively breastfed their full-term infants. *Journal of Obstetric, Gynecologic, and Neonatal Nursing*, 53, 120–131. https://doi.org/10.1016/j.jogn.2023.11.008

Aromataris, E., Lockwood, C., Porritt, K., Pilla, B., & Jordan, Z. (Eds.). (2024). *JBI manual for evidence synthesis*. JBI. https://synthesismanual.jbi.global

Baltes, M., Herber, O. R., Meyer, G., & Stephan, A. (2023). Fear of falling from the perspective of affected persons: A systematic review and qualitative meta-summary using Sandelowski and Barroso's method. *International Journal of Older People Nursing*, 18, e12520. https://doi.org/10.1111/opn.12520

Barratt, M., Lewis, P., Duckworth, N., Jojo, N., Malecka, V., Tomsone, S., Rituma, D., & Wilson, N. J. (2025). Parental experiences of quality of life when caring for their children with intellectual disability: A meta-aggregation systematic review. *Journal of Applied Research in Intellectual Disabilities: JARID*, 38(1), e70005. https://doi.org/10.1111/jar.70005

Booth, A., Noyes, J., Flemming, K., Gerhardus, A., Wahlster, P., van der Wilt, G., Mozygemba, K., Refolo, P., Sacchini, D., Tummers, M., & Rehfuess, E. (2018). Structured methodology review identified seven (RETREAT) criteria for selecting qualitative evidence synthesis approaches. *Journal of Clinical Epidemiology*, 99, 41–52. https://doi.org/10.1016/j.jclinepi.2018.03.003

Campbell, M., McKenzie, J. E., Sowden, A., Katikireddi, S. V., Brennan, S. E., Ellis, S., Hartmann-Boyce, J., Ryan, R., Shepperd, S., Thomas, J., Welch, V., & Thomson, H. (2020). Synthesis Without Meta-analysis (SWiM) in systematic reviews: Reporting guideline. *British Medical Journal (Clinical Research Ed.)*, 368, l6890. https://doi.org/10.1136/bmj.l6890

Dickins, K. A., Philpotts, L. L., Flanagan, J., Bartels, S. J., Baggett, T. P., & Looby, S. E. (2021). Physical and behavioral health characteristics of aging homeless women in the United States: An integrative review. *Journal of Women's Health*, *30*(10), 1493–1507. https://doi.org/10.1089/jwh.2020.8557

France, E. F., Uny, I., Ring, N., Turley, R. L., Maxwell, M., Duncan, E. A. S., Jepson, R. G., Roberts, R. J., & Noyes, J. (2019). A methodological systematic review of meta-ethnography conduct to articulate the complex analytical phases. *BMC Medical Research Methodology*, *19*, 35. https://doi.org/10.1186/s12874-019-0670-7

Hayvaert, M., Hannes, K., & Onghena, P. (2017). *Using mixed methods research synthesis for literature reviews*. Sage.

Higgins, J. P. T., Thomas, J., Chandler, J., Cumpston, M., Li, T., Page, M. J., & Welch, V. A. (Eds.). (2024, August). *Cochrane handbook for systematic reviews of interventions version 6.5*. Cochrane. www.training.cochrane.org/handbook

Jarden, R. J., Cherry, K., Sparham, E., Brockenshire, N., Nichols-Boyd, M., Burgess, S., Grieve, K., Twomey, B., Walters, J., & Rickard, N. (2025). Inpatients' experiences of falls: A qualitative meta-synthesis. *Journal of Advanced Nursing*, *81*(1), 4–19. https://doi.org/10.1111/jan.16244

Karimi, A., Sayehmiri, K., Vaismoradi, M., Dianatinasab, M., & Daliri, S. (2024). Vaginal bleeding in pregnancy and adverse clinical outcomes: A systematic review and meta-analysis. *Journal of Obstetrics and Gynaecology: The Journal of the Institute of Obstetrics and Gynaecology*, *44*(1), 2288224. https://doi.org/10.1080/01443615.2023.2288224

Keels, J. N., McDonald, I. R., Lee, C. S., & Dwyer, A. A. (2025). Antidiabetic agent use and clinical outcomes in patients with diabetes hospitalized for COVID-19: A systematic review and meta-analysis. *Frontiers in Endocrinology*, *15*, 1482853. https://doi.org/10.3389/fendo.2024.1482853

Lewin, S., Booth, A., Glenton, C., Munthe-Kaas, H., Rashidian, A., Wainwright, M., Bohren, M. A., Tunçalp, Ö., Colvin, C. J., Garside, R., Carlsen, B., Langlois, E. V., & Noyes, J. (2018). Applying GRADE-CERQual to qualitative evidence synthesis findings: Introduction to the series. *Implementation Science*, *13*(Suppl 1), 2. https://doi.org/10.1186/s13012-017-0688-3

Lockwood, C., Munn, Z., & Porritt, K. (2015). Qualitative research synthesis: Methodological guidance for systematic reviewers utilizing meta-aggregation. *International Journal of Evidence-Based Healthcare*, *13*(3), 179–187. https://doi.org/10.1097/XEB.0000000000000062

Mellado-García, E., Díaz-Rodríguez, L., Cortés-Martín, J., Sánchez-García, J. C., Piqueras-Sola, B., Higuero Macías, J. C., & Rodríguez-Blanque, R. (2024). Systematic reviews and synthesis without meta-analysis on hydrotherapy for pain control in labor. *Healthcare (Basel, Switzerland)*, *12*(3), 373. https://doi.org/10.3390/healthcare12030373

Munn, Z., Stern, C., Aromataris, E., Lockwood, C., & Jordan, Z. (2018). What kind of systematic review should I conduct? A proposed typology and guidance for systematic reviewers in the medical and health sciences. *BMC Medical Research Methodology*, *18*, 5. https://doi.org/10.1186/s12874-017-0468-4

Munn, Z., Tufanaru, C., & Aromataris, E. (2014). JBI's systematic reviews: Data extraction and synthesis. *The American Journal of Nursing*, *114*(7), 49–54. https://doi.org/10.1097/01.NAJ.0000451683.66447.89

Noblit, G., & Hare, R. D. (1988). *Meta-ethnography: Synthesizing qualitative studies*. Sage.

Park, H. N., Kang, G., Nam, H. J., Lee, S., Kim, B., Lee, H., & Yoon, J. Y. (2025). The use of telehealth for people with disabilities: A systematic literature review and narrative synthesis. *Journal of Advanced Nursing*, *81*(3), 1241–1258. https://doi.org/10.1111/jan.16470

Park, S., Lee, J., Seok, J. W., Park, C. G., & Jun, J. (2024). Comprehensive lifestyle modification interventions for metabolic syndrome: A systematic review and meta-analysis. *Journal of Nursing Scholarship: An Official Publication of Sigma Theta Tau International Honor Society of Nursing*, *56*(2), 249–259. https://doi.org/10.1111/jnu.12946

Price, M. J., Smith, P. M., Bottoms, L. M., & Hill, M. W. (2024). The effect of age and sex on peak oxygen uptake during upper and lower body exercise: A systematic review. *Experimental Gerontology*, *190*, 112427. https://doi.org/10.1016/j.exger.2024.112427

Rabben, J., Vivat, B., Fossum, M., & Rohde, G. E. (2024). Shared decision-making in palliative cancer care: A systematic review and metasynthesis. *Palliative Medicine*, *38*(4), 406–422. https://doi.org/10.1177/02692163241238384

Sandelowski, M., & Barroso, J. (2007). *Handbook for synthesizing qualitative research*. Springer.

Sandelowski, M., Docherty, S., & Emden, C. (1997). Qualitative metasynthesis: Issues and techniques. *Research in Nursing & Health*, *20*, 365–371. https://doi.org/10.1002/(SICI)1098-240X(199708)20:4<365::AID-NUR9>3.0.CO;2-E

Schreiber, R., Crooks, D., & Stern, P. N. (1997). Qualitative meta-analysis. In J. M. Morse (Ed.), *Completing a qualitative project* (pp. 311–326). Sage.

Spiga, F., Davies, A. L., Tomlinson, E., Moore, T. H., Dawson, S., Breheny, K., Savović, J., Gao, Y., Phillips, S. M., Hillier-Brown, F., Hodder, R. K., Wolfenden, L., Higgins, J. P., & Summerbell, C. D. (2024). Interventions to prevent obesity in children aged 5 to 11 years old. *The Cochrane Database of Systematic Reviews*, *5*(5), CD015328. https://doi.org/10.1002/14651858.CD015328.pub2

Stern, C., Jordan, Z., & McArthur, A. (2014). JBI's systematic reviews: Developing the review question and inclusion criteria. *The American Journal of Nursing*, *114*(4), 53–56. https://doi.org/10.1097/01.NAJ.0000445689.67800.86

Thoen, C. W., Saele, M., Strandberg, R. B., Eide, P. H., & Kinn, L. G. (2024). Patients' experiences of day surgery and recovery: A meta-ethnography. *Nursing Open*, *11*(1), e2055. https://doi.org/10.1002/nop2.2055

Thorne, S. (2022). Qualitative meta-synthesis. *Nurse Author Editor*, *32*(1), 15–18. https://doi.org/10.1111/nae2.12036

Thorne, S., Jensen, L., Kearney, M., Noblit, G., & Sandelowski, M. (2004). Qualitative metasynthesis: Reflections on methodological orientation and ideological agenda. *Qualitative Health Research*, *14*, 1342–1365. https://doi.org/10.1177/1049732304269888

18 Putting Research Evidence Into Practice: Evidence-Based Practice and Practice-Based Evidence

Learning Objectives

On completing this chapter, you will be able to:

- Distinguish research utilization and evidence-based practice (EBP)
- Identify several resources available to facilitate EBP in nursing practice
- Identify several models for implementing EBP
- Discuss the five major steps in undertaking an EBP effort
- Describe some limitations of the current EBP model and discuss the concept of practice-based evidence
- Distinguish generalizability and applicability
- Identify some strategies for enhancing applicability
- Define new terms in the chapter

Key Terms

- AGREE II
- Applicability
- Clinical practice guidelines
- Cochrane Collaboration
- Iowa Model
- Knowledge translation
- Patient-centered research
- Practice-based evidence
- Pragmatic clinical trial
- Precision health care
- Research utilization
- Subgroup analysis
- The 5As

Evidence-based practice (EBP) has been a major force in the health professions for the past few decades. In Chapter 1, we offered some preliminary information about EBP—for example, we described EBP-related research purposes, evidence hierarchies, and the PICO (population or patients [P], intervention or influence [I], comparison [C], and outcome [O]) framework for asking well-worded clinical questions. This chapter expands the coverage of EBP and introduces some emerging ideas about how to enhance the production and use of **practice-based evidence**. We begin with some background on EBP.

EVIDENCE-BASED PRACTICE AND RELATED CONCEPTS

As we described in Chapter 1, EBP is usually defined as a decision-making process that incorporates three elements: *best evidence*, *clinical expertise*, and *patient preferences and values*. This definition is fairly well established—and yet, several decades ago, there was little discussion of EBP—and perspectives on EBP are still evolving.

During the 1980s, concern about research utilization began to emerge. **Research utilization (RU)** is the use of findings from a study in a practical application. In RU, the emphasis is on translating new knowledge into real-world applications. EBP is a broader concept than RU because it integrates research findings with other factors, as just noted. Also, whereas RU begins with the research itself (How can I put this new knowledge to use in my clinical setting?), the starting point in EBP typically is a clinical question (What does the evidence suggest is the best approach to solving this clinical problem?).

During the 1980s and 1990s, RU projects were undertaken by numerous hospitals and nursing organizations. These projects were institutional attempts to implement changes in nursing practice based on research findings. During the 1990s, however, the call for RU was superseded by the push for EBP.

The EBP movement originated in the fields of medicine and epidemiology during the 1990s. British epidemiologist Archie Cochrane criticized health care practitioners for failing to incorporate research evidence into their decision making. His work led to the establishment of the **Cochrane Collaboration**, an international partnership with centers established in 43 countries. The Collaboration prepares and disseminates reviews of research evidence and has a goal of making Cochrane "the home of evidence" relating to health care decision making.

Also during the 1990s, a group from McMaster University Medical School in Canada (led by Dr. David Sackett) developed a clinical learning strategy they called *evidence-based medicine*. The evidence-based medicine movement has shifted to a broader conception of using the best evidence by all health care practitioners (not just physicians) in multidisciplinary teams. EBP is considered a major shift for health care education and practice. In the EBP environment, a skillful clinician can no longer rely on a repository of memorized information but rather must be a lifelong learner who is adept at accessing, evaluating, and using new evidence.

RU and EBP involve activities that can be undertaken at the level of individual nurses or at a higher organizational level. A related movement mainly concerns system-level efforts to bridge the gap between knowledge generation and use. **Knowledge translation** (KT) is a term that is often associated with efforts to enhance systematic change in clinical practice. The World Health Organization (WHO) (2005) has defined KT as "the synthesis, exchange, and application of knowledge by relevant stakeholders to accelerate the benefits of global and local innovation in strengthening health systems and improving people's health" (p. 2).

 TIP *Translational science* has emerged as a discipline devoted to developing methods to promote KT. Translational science involves the study of interventions, implementation processes, and contextual factors that affect the uptake of new evidence in health care practice.

In nursing, the need for translational research was an impetus for the development of the Doctor of Nursing Practice degree.

RESOURCES FOR EVIDENCE-BASED PRACTICE IN NURSING

Resources to support EBP are increasingly available. We offer some guidance in this section and urge you to explore other ideas with your mentors and health information experts.

Preprocessed and Pre-Appraised Evidence

Searching for the best evidence requires skill, especially because of the accelerating pace of evidence production. Thousands of primary studies of relevance to nurses are published each month in professional journals, but they are not pre-appraised for quality or clinical utility.

Fortunately, finding evidence useful for practice is often facilitated by the availability of evidence sources that are preprocessed (synthesized) and sometimes pre-appraised. DiCenso and colleagues (2009) have created a "6S" hierarchy of evidence *sources*, which is intended as a guide to evidence retrieval. On the first rung above primary studies are synopses of single studies, followed by systematic reviews, and then synopses of systematic reviews. Clinical practice guidelines are near the top of the hierarchy. At each successive step in the hierarchy, there is greater ease in applying the evidence to clinical practice. We described various types of systematic reviews in the previous chapter, so here we focus on clinical practice guidelines.

Evidence-based **clinical practice guidelines** distill a body of evidence into a usable form. Unlike systematic reviews, clinical practice guidelines (which often are *based* on systematic reviews) give specific recommendations for evidence-based decision making. Guideline development typically involves the consensus of a group of researchers, experts, and clinicians. The use or adaptation of a clinical practice guideline is often a good focus for an EBP project.

Finding clinical practice guidelines can be challenging, however, because there is no single guideline repository. A standard search in bibliographic databases such as MEDLINE will yield many references—including a mixture of citations not only to the actual guidelines but also to commentaries and implementation studies.

A recommended approach is to search in guideline databases or through specialty organizations that have sponsored guideline development. An important nursing guideline resource comes from the Registered Nurses' Association of Ontario (RNAO) (https://rnao.ca/bpg/guidelines).

There are many topics for which practice guidelines have not yet been developed, but the opposite problem is also true: Sometimes, there are multiple guidelines on the same topic. Worse yet, because of differences in the rigor of guideline development and interpretation of evidence, different guidelines may offer different or even conflicting recommendations. Thus, those who wish to adopt clinical practice guidelines should appraise them to identify ones that are based on the strongest evidence, have been meticulously developed, are user-friendly, and are appropriate for local use or adaptation.

Several appraisal instruments are available to evaluate clinical practice guidelines. One with broad support is the Appraisal of Guidelines Research and Evaluation (AGREE) instrument, now in its second version and updated in 2017 (AGREE, 2017; Brouwers et al., 2010). The **AGREE II** instrument has ratings for 23 dimensions within six domains (e.g., scope and purpose, rigor of development, and presentation). As examples, a dimension in the scope and purpose domain is "The population (patients, public, etc.) to whom the guideline is meant to apply is specifically described," and one in the rigor of development domain is "The guideline has been externally reviewed by experts prior to its publication." The AGREE tool should be applied to a guideline by a team of two to four appraisers.

Example of using AGREE II

Zhang and colleagues (2023) conducted a systematic review to assess the quality of clinical guidelines for postpartum hemorrhage. Four reviewers independently assessed seven guidelines using the AGREE II instrument. Three guidelines scored high in all domains of the AGREE II and were determined to be recommended for clinical practice. The four remaining guidelines were categorized as recommended with modifications.

TIP The GRADE system for appraising the confidence in systematic review findings, as described in Chapter 17, is increasingly used in the development of clinical practice guidelines.

Models of the Evidence-Based Practice Process

EBP models offer frameworks for designing and implementing EBP projects in practice settings. Some models focus on the use of research by individual clinicians (e.g., the *Stetler Model*, one of the oldest models that originated as an RU model), but most focus on institutional EBP efforts (e.g., the Iowa Model). The many worthy EBP models are too numerous to list comprehensively, but include the following:

- Advancing Research and Clinical Practice Through Close Collaboration (ARCC) Model (Melnyk & Fineout-Overholt, 2023)
- Diffusion of Innovations Model (Rogers, 1995)
- Iowa Model of Evidence-Based Practice to Promote Quality Care (Buckwalter et al., 2017; Titler et al., 2001)
- Johns Hopkins Nursing Evidence-Based Practice Model (Bissett et al., 2025)
- Promoting Action on Research Implementation in Health Services (PARIHS) Model (Harvey & Kitson, 2016; Rycroft-Malone et al., 2013)
- Stetler Model of Research Utilization (Stetler, 2010)
- Joanna Briggs Institute (JBI) Model for Evidence-Based Healthcare (Jordan et al., 2016)

For those considering undertaking an EBP effort who wish to follow a formal EBP model, the cited references should be consulted. Several models are also nicely synthesized by Melnyk and Fineout-Overholt (2019), and Schaffer and colleagues (2013) identify features to consider in selecting a model to plan an EBP project. Each model offers different perspectives on how to translate research findings into practice, but several steps and procedures are similar across the models. Figure 18.1 shows a diagram of one prominent EBP model, the revised Johns Hopkins Evidence-Based Practice Model (Bissett et al., 2025).

> **Example of using an evidence-based practice model**
> Farr and Palokas (2024) used the JBI Model in their EBP implementation project designed to improve adolescent school-based mental health screening. The evidence summary resulted in four best practices to improve mental health services for school-based health screening.

 TIP Several models of EBP distinguish two broad types of stimuli (triggers) for undertaking an EBP endeavor: (1) *problem-focused triggers*, which are clinical practice problems identified as needing a solution and (2) *knowledge-focused triggers*, which come from readings in the research literature and are thus more akin to RU.

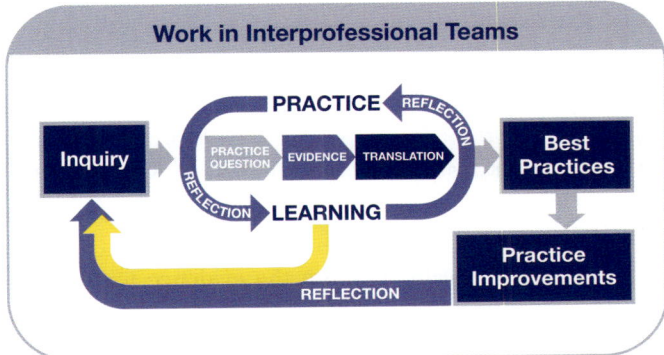

Figure 18.1 Revised Johns Hopkins evidence-based practice model. (Used/reprinted with permission from Bissett, K., Ascenzi, J., & Whalen, M. [2025]. *Johns Hopkins evidence-based practice for nurses and healthcare professionals: Model and guidelines* [5th ed.]. Sigma Theta Tau International.)

INDIVIDUAL AND ORGANIZATIONAL EVIDENCE-BASED PRACTICE

Individual nurses make many decisions and convey important health care information and advice to patients, so they have ample opportunity to put research into practice. Here are three clinical scenarios that provide examples of such opportunities:

- *Clinical Scenario 1.* You work in an allergy clinic and notice how difficult it is for many children to undergo allergy scratch tests. You wonder if an interactive distraction intervention would help reduce children's anxiety when they are being tested.
- *Clinical Scenario 2.* You work in a rehabilitation hospital, and one of your older adult patients, who had a total hip replacement, tells you she is planning a long airplane trip to visit her daughter after rehabilitation treatments are completed. You know that a long plane ride will increase her risk of deep vein thrombosis and wonder if compression stockings are an effective in-flight treatment for her. You decide to look for the best evidence to answer this question.
- *Clinical Scenario 3.* You are caring for a hospitalized cardiac patient who tells you that he has sleep apnea. He confides in you that he is reluctant to undergo continuous positive airway pressure (CPAP) treatment because he worries it will hinder intimacy with his wife. To enable yourself to better address your patient's concerns, you wonder if there is any evidence you could review about what it is like to experience CPAP treatment.

In these and thousands of other clinical situations, research evidence can be put to good use to improve the quality of nursing care. Thus, individual nurses need to have the skills to personally search for, appraise, and apply evidence in their practice.

For some clinical scenarios that trigger an EBP effort, individual nurses have sufficient autonomy to implement research-informed actions on their own (e.g., answering patients' questions about experiences with CPAP). In other situations, however, decisions are best made by a team of nurses (or an interprofessional team) working together to solve a common clinical problem. Institutional EBP efforts typically result in a formal policy or protocol affecting the practice of many nurses and other staff.

Many of the steps in institutional EBP projects are the same as those we describe in the next section, but additional issues are of relevance at the organizational level. For example, some additional activities include assessing whether the question is an organizational priority, forming a team, and conducting a formal evaluation.

 TIP Organizational EBP projects share features with quality improvement efforts, as described in Chapter 12.

MAJOR STEPS IN EVIDENCE-BASED PRACTICE

In this section, we provide an overview of how research evidence can be put to use in clinical settings. In describing the basic steps in the EBP process, we use a mnemonic device (the 5As) that we have adapted from several sources (e.g., Guyatt et al., 2015).

1. *Step 1*: **Ask**: Ask a well-worded clinical question that can be answered with research evidence.
2. *Step 2*: **Acquire**: Search for and retrieve the best evidence to answer the clinical question.
3. *Step 3*: **Appraise**: Critically appraise the evidence for validity and applicability to the problem and situation.
4. *Step 4*: **Apply**: After integrating the evidence with clinical expertise, patient preferences, and local context, apply it to clinical practice.
5. *Step 5*: **Assess**: Evaluate the outcome of the practice change.

The EBP process cannot be undertaken in a vacuum, however. A precondition for the entire undertaking is to have an openness to change and a desire to provide the best possible care, based on evidence showing benefits to patient outcomes. Melnyk and Fineout-Overholt (2023) call this *Step 0*: cultivating a spirit of inquiry. Johnston and Fineout-Overholt (2005) noted that "getting from zero to one" involves having nurses be reflective about their clinical practice. An additional step after Step 5 might be to disseminate information about the EBP project.

Step 1, asking a well-worded question, was described in Chapter 1. We noted that the PICO framework is a widely used system for the wording of clinical questions: (P) **p**opulation, (I) **i**ntervention or influence, (C) **c**omparator to the intervention or influence, and (O) **o**utcome. We describe features of the other four steps in this section.

Step 2: Acquire Research Evidence

By asking clinical questions in a well-worded form, you should be able to more effectively search the research literature for the information you need. Using the templates we provided in Table 1.3, the information inserted into the blanks constitutes *keywords* for undertaking an electronic search of important bibliographic databases.

We noted earlier in this chapter that pre-appraised sources can be used to facilitate an efficient search for evidence. Starting with pre-appraised evidence might lead you to a quick answer—and potentially to a better answer than would be possible if you had to start with individual studies. Researchers who prepare systematic reviews and synopses usually have excellent research skills and use established standards to evaluate the evidence. Thus, when preprocessed evidence is available to answer a clinical question, you may not need to look any further, unless the review is not recent or is of poor quality. When high-quality preprocessed evidence cannot be located or is old, you will need to look for the best evidence in primary studies, using strategies we described in Chapter 6.

 TIP The free Internet resource PubMed offers a special tool for those seeking evidence for clinical decisions. An important database, CINAHL, allows users to restrict a search with an "evidence-based practice" limiter.

Step 3: Appraise the Evidence

The evidence acquired in Step 2 of the EBP process should be appraised before taking clinical action. Critical appraisal for EBP may involve several types of assessments. Various criteria have been proposed for EBP appraisals, including the following:

- *Quality*: To what extent is the evidence valid—how serious is the risk of biases?
- *Magnitude*: How large is the effect of the intervention or influence (I) on the outcome (O) in the population of interest (P)? Are the effects clinically significant?
- *Quantity*: How much evidence is there? How many studies have been conducted, and did those studies involve a large number of participants?
- *Consistency*: How consistent are the findings across various studies?
- *Applicability*: To what extent is the evidence relevant to my clinical situation and patients?

Evidence Quality

The first appraisal issue is the extent to which the findings in a research report are valid. That is, were the study methods sufficiently rigorous that the evidence has a low risk of bias? Melnyk and Fineout-Overholt (2023) propose the following formula: level of evidence (LOE) from an evidence hierarchy (e.g., Fig. 1.2) + quality of evidence = strength of evidence.

Thus, in coming to a conclusion about the quality of the evidence, it is insufficient to simply "level" the evidence using an LOE scale—it must also be appraised. Systematic reviews with a GRADE score of "high confidence" yield evidence of especially high quality. If there are several primary studies and no existing systematic review, you yourself would need to draw conclusions about the body of evidence taken as a whole.

Magnitude of Effects

The appraisal criterion relating to magnitude considers how powerful the effects of an intervention or influence are. Estimating the magnitude of the effect for quantitative findings is especially important when an intervention is costly or when there are potentially negative side effects. If, for example, there is good evidence that an intervention is only modestly effective in improving a health problem, it is important to consider other factors (e.g., evidence regarding its effects on quality of life [QOL]). There are various ways to quantify the magnitude of effects, such as an *effect size index*, discussed in Chapter 13. The magnitude of effects also has a bearing on *clinical significance*, as we discussed in Chapter 14.

Quantity and Consistency of Evidence

A rigorously conducted primary study of a randomized controlled trial (RCT) offers especially strong evidence about the effect of an intervention on an outcome of interest. But *multiple* RCTs are better than a single study. Large-scale studies (such as multisite studies) with a large number of study participants are especially desirable.

If there are multiple studies that address your clinical query, however, the strength of the evidence is likely to be diminished if there are inconsistent results across studies. In the GRADE system, inconsistency of results leads to a lower quality-of-evidence grade. When the results of different studies do not corroborate each other, it is likely that further research will have an impact on confidence about an intervention's effect.

Applicability

It is also important to appraise the evidence in terms of its relevance for the clinical situation at hand—that is, for *your* patient in a specific clinical setting. Best practice evidence can most readily be applied to an individual patient in your care if they are similar to people in the study or studies under review. Would your patient have qualified for participation in the study—or is there some factor, such as age, illness severity, or comorbidity, that would have excluded them? Practitioners must reach conclusions about the applicability of research evidence, but researchers also bear some responsibility for enhancing the applicability of their work. We discuss applicability at greater length later in this chapter.

 TIP An appraisal of evidence for use in your practice may involve additional factors. In particular, costs are likely to be an important consideration. Some interventions are expensive, so the amount of resources needed to put the best evidence into practice would need to be factored into any decision. Of course, the cost of *not* taking action is also important.

Actions Based on Evidence Appraisals

Appraisals of the evidence may lead you to different courses of action. You may reach this point and conclude that the evidence is not sufficiently sound, or that the likely effect is too small, or that the cost of applying the evidence is too high. The evidence may suggest that "usual care" is the best strategy. If, however, the initial appraisal of evidence suggests a promising clinical action, then you can proceed to the next step.

Step 4: Apply the Evidence

As the definition for EBP implies, research evidence needs to be integrated with your own clinical expertise and knowledge of your clinical setting. You may be aware of factors that would make implementation of the evidence, no matter how sound or promising, inadvisable. Patient preferences and values are also important. A discussion with the patient may reveal negative attitudes toward a potentially beneficial course of action, contraindications (e.g., comorbidities), or possible impediments (e.g., lack of health insurance).

Armed with rigorous evidence, your own clinical know-how, and knowledge about your patient's circumstances, you can use the resulting information to make an evidence-based decision or provide research-informed advice. Although the steps in the process, as just described, may seem complicated, in reality, the process can be efficient—*if* there is an adequate evidence base and especially if it has been skillfully preprocessed. EBP is most challenging when findings from research are contradictory, inconclusive, or "thin"—that is to say, when better quality evidence is needed.

One final issue is the importance of integrating evidence from qualitative research, which can provide rich insights about how patients experience a problem or about barriers to complying with a treatment. A new intervention with strong potential benefits may fail to achieve desired outcomes if it is not implemented with sensitivity and understanding of the patients' perspectives. As Morse (2005) so aptly noted, evidence from an RCT may tell you whether a pill is effective, but qualitative research can help you understand why patients may not swallow the pill.

Step 5: Assess the Outcomes of the Practice Change

One last step in many EBP efforts concerns evaluating the outcomes of the practice change. Did you achieve the desired outcomes? Were patients satisfied with the results?

Straus and colleagues (2011) remind us that part of the ongoing evaluation involves how well you are performing EBP. They offer self-evaluation questions that relate to the EBP steps, such as asking answerable questions (Am I asking any clinical questions at all? Am I asking well-formulated questions?) and acquiring external evidence (Do I know the best sources of current evidence? Am I becoming more efficient in my searching?).

EVIDENCE-BASED PRACTICE AND PRACTICE-BASED EVIDENCE

The EBP movement has made enduring contributions to the well-being of human beings. Clinicians no longer rely exclusively on a repository of knowledge acquired during their training—they are expected to be relentless learners who seek and use evidence from rigorous studies about how best to address pressing health problems.

Yet, EBP has limitations that are not always acknowledged. In particular, concerns have been expressed that EBP fails to provide the individualized care patients need (Comer, 2025; Tomkins & Bristow, 2023). Several commentators have noted that high-quality, ethical patient care requires practice-based evidence—evidence that is developed in real-world settings and is responsive to the needs and circumstances of specific patients and contexts (Comer, 2025; Tomkins & Bristow, 2023). In this section, we briefly point out some limitations of the current model of EBP with respect to the applicability of research findings for clinical decision making.

Evidence-Based Practice and Population Models of Evidence

EBP is based on evidence about *populations* of people. Systematic reviews of RCTs, at the pinnacle of evidence hierarchies, are the cornerstone of EBP. Yet, systematic reviews of RCTs cannot affirm that *all* patients receiving an effective intervention will benefit from it—only that the "average" patient in a specified population probably would. Clinicians, however, do not treat "average" patients—they care for people with varying and distinctive traits, preferences, cultures, and health risks. The WHO has described the social determinants of health that influence health outcomes as "the conditions in which people are born, grow, live, work and age, and people's access to power, money and resources that influence health" (WHO, 2024, p. xii) as critical to conducting research and translating evidence into practice.

Subramanian and colleagues (2018) were especially eloquent about this issue, noting that inferences about *average treatment effects* can be misleading or even harmful when responses to an intervention diverge—a situation called *heterogeneity of treatment effects* (HTE). They noted that the "average patient" is a construct, not a reality, and provided some evidence for their claim that "most people taking RCT-validated, effective treatments derive no benefit from them" (p. 78). Universal treatment effects should seldom be assumed. It is not that trial information about average effects is unimportant, but it is often insufficient. For an individual patient, the average effect is of little interest—an intervention either is or is not beneficial for that patient.

Average treatment effects, such as the ones estimated in systematic reviews, are problematic from another perspective: Averages strip away *context*. Context shapes how interventions get implemented and influences their effectiveness. However, population models of EBP provide context-free conclusions about the delivery of effective care.

Evidence-Based Practice and External Validity

In Chapter 8, we noted the tensions between efforts to enhance a study's internal validity (inferences that an intervention *caused* an effect) and external validity (inferences that causal claims generalize across persons, settings, and time). Strategies to reduce threats to internal validity tend to negatively impact external validity, and vice versa.

Researchers who seek to generate evidence for practice have traditionally resolved the tension between internal and external validity in favor of internal validity. Evidence hierarchies, for example, rank study designs based on their ability to eliminate threats to internal validity; external validity is ignored. In systematic reviews, evaluations of study quality and confidence in the findings (GRADE) focus on internal rather than external validity.

Traditional RCTs undermine the generalizability of the results in diverse ways. RCTs have typically been conducted under ideal conditions rather than in normal, real-world situations. All aspects of the study are tightly controlled, including what the exact intervention is, who the interventionists are, where the study takes place, and who participates in the study.

Sampling in RCTs is particularly troublesome for generalizing the results. To reduce confounding, trialists tend to impose exclusion criteria that eliminate key groups of people—often, older people and those with comorbidities, who might especially benefit from, or be harmed by, the intervention under study. This problem is compounded by low rates of participation in RCTs, with refusal rates sometimes approaching 90%. The bottom line is that patients in general usually are very different from ones included in RCTs.

The combined effect of relying on a population model of average effects and using data from highly select study participants is that EBP is often based on evidence of whether an intervention works for a hypothetical "average" patient under ideal, context-neutral conditions. Although the RCT results may be unbiased from an internal validity standpoint, they may be less useful than one would hope in making decisions about individual patients who are neither "ideal" nor "average."

Generalizability, Applicability, and Relevance

The terms *generalizability* and *applicability* have often been used interchangeably, but there is a growing view that they are distinct (Sacristán & Dilla, 2018). *Generalizability* is a term associated with populations—researchers identify characteristics of a population to which their findings might reasonably be generalized.

We define **applicability** as the degree to which research evidence can be applied to individuals, small groups of individuals, or local contexts. Applicability is relevant to clinical decision making because of human heterogeneity—averages are not of much value as decision guides if there is wide diversity in whether an intervention works or how it is viewed, experienced, adhered to, or incorporated into normal life. Sacristán and Dilla (2018) noted, "As health care decisions are becoming more patient centric, the term 'applicability' should evoke 'individual patient' rather than 'average patient'" (p. 165).

New ideas are emerging about how to enhance applicability, generalizability, and relevance. In the context of practice-based evidence, we define *relevance* as evidence that is important to key stakeholders and has the potential to be actionable. **Patient-centered research**, which focuses on developing evidence that is meaningful and valuable to patients, involves efforts to attain relevance.

New Directions in Health Care Research

Concern about the limitations of current models of EBP for guiding decisions about individuals in real-world contexts has led to the emergence of new ideas and innovative methods for *optimizing* evidence. Efforts at optimization have taken shape under various formulations, such as *precision health care*, *personalized health care*, and *patient-centered health care*. Research in these domains has gone in broadly similar directions but with different emphases. Such research typically strives for evidence that is practice-based.

In this section, we describe a few strategies that researchers are using to enhance the applicability of their research findings. We encourage you to think about the benefits of such strategies when you are critically appraising research evidence.

Comparative Effectiveness Research

Comparative effectiveness research (CER), described briefly in Chapter 12, is an important manifestation of emerging directions in health care research. CER emphasizes patient-centeredness and involves direct comparisons of clinical interventions to facilitate decision making. As noted by Greenfield and Kaplan (2012), "CER calls for substantial changes in the way clinical research is conducted, interpreted, and practically applied … the evolving CER paradigm requires … innovations that address three basic questions: what works? for whom? and in whose hands?" (p. 263).

The Institute of Medicine's (2009) report on priorities for CER offered six defining characteristics of CER:

1. *CER's objective is to directly inform clinical decisions.* CER places a high value on the ability to generalize results to real-world decision making. A broad range of relevant stakeholders and decision makers (including patients) should be included in setting priorities, designing studies, and implementing results.
2. *CER involves comparisons of two or more alternative treatments, each of which has potential to be "best practice."* CER avoids the use of placebos, attention controls, or no intervention as comparators in testing an intervention.
3. *CER seeks evidence at both the population and the subgroup level.* A goal of CER is to help providers and patients in individualizing decisions—going beyond "average effects" to effects for people with similar characteristics.

4. *CER uses outcomes that are important to patients*. CER strives to include and give weight to patient-reported outcomes and to attend to benefits, harms, and unintended consequences of health care interventions.
5. *CER uses diverse research designs and methods*. Some comparative effectiveness studies involve experimental designs, but CER also uses other designs, including nonexperimental (observational) approaches.
6. *CER is conducted in real-world settings*. CER studies the effectiveness of interventions in settings similar to those where an intervention would actually be used.

These characteristics of CER diverge in important respects from the research model that has come to be established under EBP, which focuses on internal validity and adheres firmly to evidence from RCTs. Note that these characteristics of CER embody concerns about generalizability (no. 1), applicability (no. 3), and relevance (no. 4).

Pragmatic Clinical Trials

As we noted, features of traditional RCT designs are so tightly controlled that the relevance of the findings to real-life situations can be questioned. Concern about this problem has led to interest in **pragmatic clinical trials (PCTs)**, which have features designed to maximize external validity with minimal negative effect on internal validity (Omerovic et al., 2024). Tunis and colleagues (2003), in a seminal paper, defined pragmatic (practical) clinical trials as "trials for which the hypotheses and study design are formulated based on information needed to make a decision" (p. 1626). Thus, pragmatic trials are consistent with the goals of CER.

 TIP *Pragmatism* as a construct can be applied in most studies. As noted by Sacristán and Dilla (2018), pragmatism is not so much a design type but a "mindset"—pragmatic attitudes can be used in all types of research.

Compared to more traditional *explanatory trials* conducted under optimal conditions with carefully selected participants, PCTs address practical questions about the benefits and risks of an intervention—as well as its costs—as they would unfold in routine clinical practice. Tunis and coauthors (2003) made these recommendations for PCTs: enrollment of diverse populations with fewer exclusions of high-risk patients, recruitment of participants from a variety of practice settings, follow-up over a longer period, inclusion of economic outcomes, and comparisons of clinically viable alternatives.

Trials cannot readily be categorized as *pragmatic* or *explanatory* because they do not represent a dichotomy—pragmatism can be conceptualized as being on a continuum. A tool called *PRECIS-2* (**PR**eferred **E**xplanatory **C**ontinuum **I**ndicator **S**ummary) has been developed to help researchers evaluate how pragmatic their trial is and to help ensure that their designs are congruent with their intended aims (Loudon et al., 2015). The tool covers nine domains (e.g., patient eligibility, patient recruitment), each of which is rated from 1 (very explanatory) to 5 (very pragmatic). For example, the question for the eligibility domain is, "To what extent are the participants in the trial similar to those who would receive this intervention if it was part of usual care?"

> **Example of the use of PRECIS-2**
> Darker and colleagues (2022) described the application of the PRECIS-2 tool to retrospectively evaluate a pilot study focused on a smoking cessation intervention for women living in underresourced areas in Ireland. The goal was to inform the decision-making process for a future study. The team scored the nine domains of the PRECIS-2 tool as either pragmatic or explanatory and found that the trial design was more explanatory than pragmatic.

The most promising (and widely used) designs for PCTs include *cluster randomization* (randomization of groups rather than individuals) and delayed treatment designs (everyone gets the intervention eventually). When a delay-of-treatment strategy is combined with cluster randomization, the result is a *stepped wedge design*, which involves having clusters randomized to receive the intervention at different points (Battaglia & Glasgow, 2018).

PCTs protect internal validity by using familiar bias-reducing strategies such as randomization, allocation concealment, and blinding. Moreover, cluster randomized pragmatic trials can promote internal validity by guarding against contamination of treatments. However, pragmatic trials can suffer from certain problems that are not present in traditional explanatory trials. One issue, for example, is that the interventions are usually less standardized in different real-world settings, perhaps resulting in differential "dosing" of the intervention and different degrees of intervention fidelity.

TIP Nurse researchers have demonstrated growing interest in PCTs. A methods conference at the 2017 meeting of the Council for the Advancement of Nursing Science was devoted to pragmatic trials; a special issue of *Nursing Outlook* included several papers based on conference presentations. In that issue, Battaglia and Glasgow (2018) asserted that pragmatic research "is an area of tremendous opportunity for the nursing science community" (p. 430).

Subgroup Analyses

Some researchers try to develop evidence that is applicable to well-defined groups of people (rather than to entire populations) by conducting subgroup analyses. A **subgroup analysis** involves efforts to disentangle HTEs for subpopulations of people. For example, a subgroup analysis might suggest that an intervention is effective for men but not for women, or more effective for people with comorbidities than for those without them.

Subgroup analyses, which are intuitively appealing to those interested in individualizing care, are often undertaken in the context of RCTs. Evidence suggests that the rate of subgroup analysis is increasing, perhaps because of its prominence in CER. Subgroup analyses are, however, controversial, in part because they are frequently not undertaken properly (Schandelmaier & Guyatt, 2024). The struggle between wanting to go beyond population averages on the one hand and the statistical challenges of subgroup analysis on the other was described by renowned clinical epidemiologist Alvan Feinstein (1998, p. 297) as a "clinicostatistical tragedy."

The statistical challenge in subgroup analyses involves addressing the strong risk of both Type I and Type II errors. False positives (Type I errors) are common because researchers often test multiple subgroups without making adjustments to probabilities. The probability of a false positive might be 5% for one test, but for three independent tests, the risk is 14%. This problem has resulted in many reported subgroup effects that could not be replicated. Potential subgroup effects are also at high risk of being missed because of a Type II error. If a study is adequately powered for the entire sample, it will often be underpowered when the sample is divided into subgroups.

Because of increased interest in personalized health care, the number of scholarly papers devoted to subgroup analyses and HTE has burgeoned in recent years. Advice for those who conduct subgroup analyses includes adopting strategies such as the following:

- *Specifying hypotheses in advance.* Subgroup analysis should be a hypothesis-testing effort, not a fishing expedition. Hypotheses about differential effects should be based on sound theoretical reasoning, biologic plausibility, or previous empirical evidence.

- *Restricting the number of subgroup analyses.* Burke and colleagues (2015) argued that only rarely should more than one or two primary subgroup analyses be performed—the risk of a false positive increases as the number of tests goes up.
- *Avoiding severely underpowered subgroup analyses.* When subgroup analyses are planned, greater power for the overall analyses should likely be used to estimate sample size needs (e.g., 90% rather than the standard 80%).
- *Basing the analyses on variables defined at baseline.* Subgroup analyses should be based on baseline characteristics, not on ones that emerge during the study (e.g., length of intensive care unit [ICU] stay). Frequently used variables for subgroup analyses in medical RCTs include risk factors for the outcome (e.g., smoking status, disease severity, comorbidity), sex, and age (Gabler et al., 2016).
- *Analyzing for subgroup differences using tests for interactions.* Most analyses for subgroup effects are done incorrectly (e.g., Gabler et al., 2016). The typical approach is to test for intervention effects *within* each subgroup—for example, testing intervention–control group differences separately for men and women—and then comparing the results. However, such analyses could lead to erroneous conclusions—for example, the differences might simply be the result of differential subgroup sample sizes. The question that should be addressed is: *Are subgroup treatment effects significantly different from each other?* The appropriate analysis (too complex to explain here) is to test for an *interaction* between the treatment variable and the subgroup variable.

Because the risk of statistical errors is high, it is wise to be cautious in interpreting subgroup results. The most convincing evidence for a subgroup effect comes from replicated results—especially if the effect is supported by a persuasive biologic or theoretic rationale. Corroboration can occur in the context of a systematic review.

> **Example of a subgroup analysis**
> Fukushima and colleagues (2024) conducted a systematic review and meta-analysis to examine the impact of QOL on mortality risk in patients with cancer. In their analysis examining QOL, they considered cancer type and treatment phases. The primary finding was that QOL was significantly associated with mortality risk (hazard ratio: 1.06, 95% confidence interval: 1.05 to 1.07; $p < .00001$). Their subgroup analysis of cancer types suggested many cancers were significantly associated with mortality risk, but not melanoma or pancreatic cancer. Further, all time points of treatment (pre, post, and palliative) were associated with mortality risk, with the pretreatment phase having the greatest impact on QOL.

Precision/Personalized Health Care

A fundamental tenet of **precision health care** (a term sometimes used interchangeably with *personalized health care* or *stratified health care*) is that interventions can be individually tailored to people based on their unique genetic, physiologic, behavioral, lifestyle, and environmental profiles. The goal is not necessarily to develop a unique treatment for every individual but rather to tailor interventions for those with tightly grouped biologic and other features—moving beyond what is possible with subgroup analyses. Personalized health care is being driven by advances in molecular genomics and is heavily dependent on data linkages and integration, data analytics, and machine learning for the identification of patterns in large datasets (big data).

The term *precision health care* has been strongly connected with advances in genomics, but a wide range of biomarkers, data from electronic health records, and data from wearable

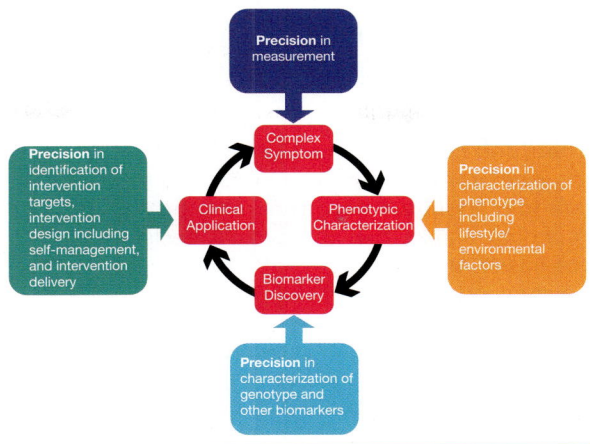

Figure 18.2 The Nursing Science Precision Health Model. (Used/reprinted with permission from Hickey, K. T., Bakken, S., Byrne, M. W., Bailey, D. C. E., Demiris, G., Docherty, S. L., Dorsey, S. G., Guthrie, B. J., Heitkemper, M. M., Jacelon, C. S., Kelechi, T. J., Moore, S. M., Redeker, N. S., Renn, C. L., Resnick, B., Starkweather, A., Thompson, H., Ward, T. M., McCloskey, D. J., … Grady, P. [2019]. Precision health: Advancing symptom and self-management science. *Nursing Outlook, 67*, 462–475. https://doi.org/10.1016/j.outlook.2019.01.003)

sensors are examples of data with relevance to precision health care. This suggests the inevitability of complex statistical models that will be needed for mapping dynamic factors that affect individual health.

Precision health care continues to be an emerging area rather than a broad reality (Kurnat-Thoma et al. 2021), and many challenges remain. However, precision science is advancing rapidly, which bodes well for improving targeted and efficient health care with high levels of applicability. Hickey and colleagues (2019) provide a description of the Nursing Science Precision Health Model that includes "measurement; characterization of phenotype including lifestyle and environment; characterization of genotype and other biomarkers; and intervention target discovery, design, and delivery" (p. 464) (Fig. 18.2).

Concluding Thoughts on Practice-Based Evidence

The push for EBP has led to impressive improvements in health care in all health disciplines, and an ongoing commitment to EBP is warranted. However, for maximum benefit, efforts to generate evidence based on population models will have to be integrated with evidence for individualized care.

Several forces in health research are converging to encourage greater demand for and interest in evidence that is patient-centered, practice-based, and personalized. These include frustration about the limitations of the traditional EBP model on the part of many clinicians, the growth of interest in and funding for CER, and the emerging excitement over opportunities that will become available through precision health care research.

New challenges and new rewards are in store for those who wish to facilitate patient-centered care based on patient-centered evidence. Thus, the overall message in this concluding chapter is to think about the applicability and relevance of research findings when coming to conclusions about "best evidence" in your context.

TIP Every nurse can play a role in using research evidence. Here are some strategies:
- *Read widely and critically.* Professionally accountable nurses keep abreast of research developments relating to their specialty by reading professional journals.
- *Attend professional conferences.* Conference attendees have opportunities to meet researchers and to explore practice implications of new research.
- *Insist on evidence that a procedure is effective.* Every time nurses or nursing students are told about a standard nursing procedure, they have a right to ask: Why? Nurses should expect that the clinical decisions they make are based on sound, evidence-based rationales.
- *Become involved in a journal club.* Many organizations that employ nurses sponsor journal clubs that review studies with potential relevance to practice.
- *Pursue and participate in EBP projects.* Several studies have found that nurses who are involved in research activities (e.g., an EBP project or data collection activities) develop more positive attitudes toward research and better research skills.

CRITICAL APPRAISAL OF APPLICABILITY, RELEVANCE, AND GENERALIZABILITY

Box 18.1 provides a few suggestions for those who wish to consider whether researchers have provided sufficient information for coming to conclusions about a study's relevance, applicability, and generalizability.

In many cases, the researchers' lack of attention to the issues discussed in the section on practice-based evidence might be disappointing. The absence of information on applicability may reflect page constraints in the journal. It may also reflect the fact that most researchers use conventional standards in preparing their articles—standards that have not taken applicability into account. Moreover, the peer review of most articles is undertaken by researchers who may not yet be attuned to changes taking place in health care research. We hope that in the future, researchers will do more to help clinicians answer questions about relevance, applicability, and generalizability.

Box 18.1 Guidelines for Critically Appraising a Study's Generalizability, Applicability, and Relevance[a]

a. Were patients or other stakeholders involved in codesigning the study? In what way were they involved (e.g., identifying the research question, designing the study, disseminating or using the results)?
b. Did the researchers mention that the study was comparative effectiveness research? If the study was a clinical trial, what was the comparator?
c. If the study was a clinical trial, where on the pragmatic-to-explanatory continuum did the trial lie? To what extent was the study conducted in "real-world" circumstances with a broad range of study participants? Did the researchers claim that the trial was pragmatic?
d. What are some of the constraints on the generalizability of the results?
e. Were subgroup effects examined?
f. Did the discussion section of the report adequately address the issues of generalizability, applicability, and relevance?

[a]These questions are primarily relevant for quantitative or mixed methods studies, especially for trials of an intervention.

RESEARCH EXAMPLES WITH CRITICAL THINKING EXERCISES

This section presents brief summaries of two studies completed by nurse researchers relevant to the content of this chapter. Example 1 describes an EBP project. Example 2 describes a PCT. Read the research summaries for these two examples, and then answer the critical thinking questions that follow, referring to the full research reports if necessary.

EXAMPLE 1: AN EVIDENCE-BASED PRACTICE PROJECT

Study: Mindfulness and self-regulation in a summer camp setting: An EBP project (Opalinski & Martinez, 2021)

Purpose: This EBP aimed to implement a mindfulness program for children attending a summer day camp and evaluate the self-regulation skills and behavior of children who partook in the program.

Framework: The project does not describe an EBP framework that guided the project, but the authors do describe the questions guiding the project, a synthesis of the literature that guided the intervention, and the use of a quality assessment guideline in reporting the project to evaluate it.

Approach: There were two questions that guided the project: one around how the mindfulness program could be implemented and the other on the impact of the program on the participants' self-regulation in a camp setting. The program they developed, based on the literature and adapted to the urban day camp setting, included a 40-minute mindfulness program for one session per week over 8 weeks.

Evaluation: Between eight and 19 children attended the sessions. Only 4.4% of children attended all eight sessions, but 56% attended one to two sessions. Outcome measures included a scale measuring distress, the choice of the mindfulness experimental activities, and the counselors' perceptions of what they thought were the most impactful aspects of the mindfulness program on the children's behavior. The authors used descriptive statistics to report the change in distress. Seven campers responded to the questionnaire on distress, and all of them reported some reduction in distress. The most popular experiential activity identified by 57.4% of the attendees was a calm-down jar. Counselors reported several strategies, such as peace corners and mindful anchor words, helped children with self-regulation.

Conclusions: While acknowledging limitations, the authors concluded that the use of the evidence-based mindfulness program in the camp setting extends the reach of mental health promotion for the pediatric population.

Critical Thinking Exercises

1. What would you say was the clinical question on which the EBP team focused? (Use the PICO framework.)
2. What type of trigger was the impetus for the project?
3. What are the merits and limitations of the EBP project?

EXAMPLE 2: PRAGMATIC CLINICAL TRIAL

Study: Transforming nursing assessment in acute hospitals: A cluster randomised controlled trial of an evidence-based nursing core assessment (The ENCORE Trial) (Douglas et al., 2024)

Background: Rapid response teams (RRTs) are widely used in many hospitals globally. The goal of RRTs is to recognize in a timely way patients who are deteriorating and at risk for a medical emergency such as a cardiac arrest. Problems with RRTs include optimal implementation of such teams as well as a focus on the rescue, focusing on the whole issue, for example, what led to the deterioration and interventions that could have prevented it. Improving nurses' ability to assess and intervene early in response to changes in the patient may prevent the need for rescues. The evidence-based nursing core assessment (ENCORE) was developed as a result of a nursing and academic staff collaboration into missed care or delayed recognition of clinical deterioration in general care units at a major hospital in Brisbane, Australia. Through surveys and focus group interviews of staff, the team found issues such as *patient assessment* that was task oriented rather than based on clinical reasoning, reactive, and solely focused on late signs of deterioration. Using this evidence, the team developed the ENCORE to detect and intervene on early changes to prevent patient deterioration.

Program Objectives: The objective of the cluster randomized trial was to examine the impact of strengthening nursing physical assessment (ENCORE) on the rate of RRT activation and serious *adverse events*. The team hypothesized the ENCORE intervention would reduce the rate of RRT activations and serious adverse events.

Trial Description: The practice change related to implementing the ENCORE intervention was grounded in a participatory and action-oriented approach involving the nurses on the care units. A parallel-group cluster-RCT using unequal allocation was used to evaluate the ENCORE intervention in seven acute hospitals in Australia. Hospital units/clusters were randomized to either intervention or control groups. Patient outcome data were collected 6 months after implementation of the intervention. Patients ≥18 years old admitted to the care units under study during the 6 months were prospectively recruited using an opt-out approach for the team to access health records. Patients were blinded to whether they were in the intervention or control group.

Methods: An analysis of intervention effect estimates for patient outcomes (medical team activation, unplanned ICU admission, resuscitation, and mortality) was conducted. Additionally, generalized linear mixed models with care unit/cluster random effects were adjusted for patient age, comorbidities, hospital admission from emergency department, study month, hospital, and care unit type.

Critical Thinking Exercises

1. Answer the relevant questions in Box 18.1 regarding this study.

Summary Points

- Two underpinnings of the EBP movement are the **Cochrane Collaboration** (which is based on the work of British epidemiologist Archie Cochrane) and the clinical learning strategy called *evidence-based medicine* developed at McMaster University Medical School.

- **Research utilization (RU)** and EBP are overlapping concepts that concern efforts to use research as a basis for clinical decisions, but RU *starts* with a research-based innovation that gets evaluated for possible use in practice.

- **Knowledge translation (KT)** is a term used primarily about system-wide efforts to enhance systematic change in clinical practice

- or policies. *Translational science* is a discipline devoted to developing methods to promote KT and the use of evidence.

- Resources to support EBP are growing at a phenomenal pace. Preprocessed (synthesized) and pre-appraised evidence is especially useful for addressing clinical queries. Evidence-based **clinical practice guidelines** are a major example of pre-appraised evidence. Clinical practice guidelines should be carefully and systematically appraised; for example, using the **AGREE II** instrument.

- Many models of EBP have been developed, including models that provide a framework for individual clinicians (e.g., the *Stetler model*) and others for organizations or teams of clinicians (e.g., the **Iowa Model** of Evidence-Based Practice to Promote Quality Care).

- Although organizational projects include additional steps, the most basic steps in EBP for both individuals and teams are as follows (**the 5As**): *Ask* a well-worded clinical question; *Acquire* the best evidence to answer the question; *appraise* and synthesize the evidence; *apply* the evidence after integrating it with patient preferences and clinical expertise; and *assess* the effects of the practice change.

- The EBP movement has made significant contributions to health care worldwide. However, a variety of forces are combining to demand greater attention to **practice-based evidence**—*patient-centered evidence* from real-world settings that is responsive to the needs of specific patients and local contexts.

- The standard EBP model is based on evidence about populations of people; it relies heavily on results from RCTs—which, when integrated in systematic reviews, yield *average treatment effects* within the population of interest.

- *Generalizability* concerns the ability to extrapolate evidence from samples to a specified population. **Applicability** is the degree to which research evidence can be applied to individuals, small groups of individuals, or local contexts.

- *Relevance*, in the context of this discussion, is the degree to which research evidence is important to key stakeholders and has the potential to be actionable. A key strategy for developing practice-based evidence is to involve stakeholders as co-creators of the research process.

- RCTs are seldom designed with the goals of generalizability or applicability in mind. In traditional *explanatory trials*, researchers value internal validity at the expense of external validity and typically focus on average effects at the expense of understanding HTE—individual variation in response to interventions.

- Researchers have begun to address these issues with innovative methodologic strategies. In particular, there is growing interest in *CER*, whose defining characteristics are in line with person-centered research and practice-based evidence.

- Concerns about features of explanatory RCTs (e.g., restrictive eligibility criteria, tight controls) have led to interest in **pragmatic clinical trials** that enroll diverse people from real-world settings and are designed to enhance external validity. The degree to which a trial is "pragmatic" can be evaluated using a tool called *PRECIS-2*.

- **Subgroup analyses** are efforts to disentangle HTEs for subpopulations. Subgroup analyses have been controversial because of risks of both Type I and Type II errors, but guidance for rigorously conducting them has emerged (e.g., prespecification of hypotheses, limiting analyses to a small number of subgroups, testing for interactions).

- Advances in technology and research methods, coupled with increased interest in personalized and **precision health care**, will likely advance the promise of practice-based and patient-centered evidence and contribute to its applicability.

REFERENCES

AGREE Next Steps Consortium. (2017). *The AGREE II instrument* [Electronic version]. http://www.agreetrust.org

Battaglia, C., & Glasgow, R. (2018). Pragmatic dissemination and implementation research models, methods and measures and their relevance for nursing research. *Nursing Outlook*, 66, 430–445. https://doi.org/10.1016/j.outlook.2018.06.007

Bissett, K., Ascenzi, J., & Whalen, M. (2025). *Johns Hopkins evidence-based practice for nurses and healthcare professionals: Model and guidelines* (5th ed.). Sigma Theta Tau International.

Brouwers, M., Kho, M., Browman, G., Burgers, J., Cluzeau, F., Feder, G., Fervers, B., Graham, I. D., Grimshaw, J., Hanna, S. E., Littlejohns, P., Makarski, J., & Zitzelsberger, L.; AGREE Next Steps Consortium. (2010). AGREE II: Advancing guideline development, reporting and evaluation in health care. *Canadian Medical Association Journal*, 182, E839–E842. https://doi.org/10.1503/cmaj.090449

Buckwalter, K., Cullen, L., Hanrahan, K., Kleiber, C., McCarthy, A., Rakel, B., Steelman, V., Tripp-Reimer, T., & Tucker, S.; Authored on behalf of the Iowa Model Collaborative. (2017). Iowa Model of evidence-based practice: Revisions and validation. *Worldviews on Evidence-Based Nursing*, 14, 175–182. https://doi.org/10.1111/wvn.12223

Burke, J., Sussman, J., Kent, D., & Hayward, R. (2015). Three simple rules to ensure reasonably credible subgroup analyses. *BMJ*, 351, h5651. https://doi.org/10.1136/bmj.h5651

Comer, A. (2025). Which values should guide evidence-based practice? *AMA Journal of Ethics*, 27(1), 21–26. https://doi.org/10.1001/amajethics.2025.21

Darker, C., Loudon, K., O'Connell, N., Castello, S., Burke, E., Vance, J., Reynolds, C., Buggy, A., Dougall, N., Williams, P., Dobbie, F., Bauld, L., & Hayes, C. B. (2022). An application of PRECIS-2 to evaluate trial design in a pilot cluster randomized controlled trial of a community-based smoking cessation intervention for women living in disadvantaged areas of Ireland. *Pilot and Feasibility Studies*, 8(1), 19. https://doi.org/10.1186/s40814-022-00969-6

Dicenso, A., Bayley, L., & Haynes, B. (2009). Accessing pre-appraised evidence: Fine-tuning the 5S model into a 6S model. *Evidence-Based Nursing*, 12, 99–101. https://doi.org/10.1136/ebn.12.4.99-b

Douglas, C., Alexeev, S., Middleton, S., Gardner, G., Kelly, P., McInnes, E., Rihari-Thomas, J., Windsor, C., & Morton, R. L. (2024). Transforming nursing assessment in acute hospitals: A cluster randomised controlled trial of an evidence-based nursing core assessment (the ENCORE trial). *International Journal of Nursing Studies*, 151, 104690. https://doi.org/10.1016/j.ijnurstu.2024.104690

Farr, J., & Palokas, M. (2024). Adolescent school-based mental health screening: A best practice implementation project. *JBI Evidence Implementation*, 22(2), 186–194. https://doi.org/10.1097/XEB.0000000000000422

Feinstein, A. R. (1998). The problem of cogent subgroups: A clinicostatistical tragedy. *Journal of Clinical Epidemiology*, 51, 297–299. https://doi.org/10.1016/s0895-4356(98)00004-3

Fukushima, T., Suzuki, K., Tanaka, T., Okayama, T., Inoue, J., Morishita, S., & Nakano, J. (2024). Global quality of life and mortality risk in patients with cancer: A systematic review and meta-analysis. *Quality of Life Research: An International Journal of Quality of Life Aspects of Treatment, Care and Rehabilitation*, 33(10), 2631–2643. https://doi.org/10.1007/s11136-024-03691-3

Gabler, N., Duan, N., Raneses, E., Suttner, L., Ciarametaro, M., Cooney, E., Dubois, R. W., Halpern, S. D., & Kravitz, R. (2016). No improvement in the reporting of clinical trial subgroup effects in high-impact general medical journals. *Trials*, 17, 320. https://doi.org/10.1186/s13063-016-1447-5

Greenfield, S., & Kaplan, S. (2012). Building useful evidence: Changing the clinical research paradigm to account for comparative effectiveness research. *Journal of Comparative Effectiveness Research*, 1, 263–270. https://doi.org/10.2217/CER.12.23

Guyatt, G., Rennie, D., Meade, M., & Cook, D. (2015). *Users' guides to the medical literature: A manual for evidence-based clinical practice* (3rd ed.). McGraw-Hill Education.

Harvey, G., & Kitson, A. (2016). PARIHS revisited: From heuristic to integrated framework for the successful implementation of knowledge into practice. *Implementation Science*, 11, 33. https://doi.org/10.1186/s13012-016-0398-2

Hickey, K. T., Bakken, S., Byrne, M. W., Bailey, D. C. E., Demiris, G., Docherty, S. L., Dorsey, S. G., Guthrie, B. J., Heitkemper, M. M., Jacelon, C. S., Kelechi, T. J., Moore, S. M., Redeker, N. S., Renn, C. L., Resnick, B., Starkweather, A., Thompson, H., Ward, T. M., McCloskey, D. J., ... Grady, P. A. (2019). Precision health: Advancing symptom and self-management science. *Nursing Outlook*, 67, 462–475. https://doi.org/10.1016/j.outlook.2019.01.003

Institute of Medicine. (2009). *Initial national priorities for comparative effectiveness research*. National Academies Press.

Johnston, L., & Fineout-Overholt, E. (2005). Teaching EBP: "Getting from zero to one." Moving from recognizing and admitting uncertainties to asking searchable, answerable questions. *Worldviews on Evidence-Based Nursing*, 2, 98–102. https://doi.org/10.1111/j.1741-6787.2005.05006.x

Jordan, Z., Lockwood, C., Aromataris, E., & Munn, Z. (2016). *The updated JBI model for evidence-based healthcare*. The Joanna Briggs Institute. https://jbi.global/jbi-model-of-EBHC

Kurnat-Thoma, E., Fu, M. R., Henderson, W. A., Voss, J. G., Hammer, M. J., Williams, J. K., Calzone, K., Conley, Y. P., Starkweather, A., Weaver, M. T., Shiao, S. P. K., & Coleman, B. (2021). Current status and future directions of U.S. genomic nursing health care policy. *Nursing Outlook*, 69(3), 471–488. https://doi.org/10.1016/j.outlook.2020.12.006

Loudon, K., Treweek, S., Sullivan, F., Donnan, P., Thorpe, K., & Zwarenstein, M. (2015). The PRECIS-2 tool: Designing trials that are fit for purpose. *BMJ*, 350, h2147. https://doi.org/10.1136/bmj.h2147

Melnyk, B. M., & Fineout-Overholt, E. (2023). *Evidence-based practice in nursing and healthcare* (5th ed.). Lippincott Williams & Wilkins.

Morse, J. M. (2005). Beyond the clinical trial: Expanding criteria for evidence. *Qualitative Health Research*, 15, 3–4. https://doi.org/10.1177/1049732304270826

Omerovic, E., Petrie, M., Redfors, B., Fremes, S., Murphy, G., Marquis-Gravel, G., Lansky, A., Velazquez, E., Perera, D., Reid, C., Smith, J., van der Meer, P., Lipsic, E., Juni, P., McMurray, J., Bauersachs, J., Køber, L., Rouleau, J. L., & Doenst, T. (2024). Pragmatic randomized controlled trials: Strengthening the concept through a robust international collaborative network: PRIME-9—Pragmatic Research and Innovation through Multinational Experimentation. *Trials*, 25(1), 80. https://doi.org/10.1186/s13063-024-07935-y

Opalinski, A. S., & Martinez, L. A. (2021). Mindfulness and self-regulation in a summer camp setting: An EBP project. *Journal of Pediatric Nursing*, 57, 73–78. https://doi.org/10.1016/j.pedn.2020.10.023

Rogers, E. M. (1995). *Diffusion of innovations* (4th ed.). Free Press.

Rycroft-Malone, J., Seers, K., Chandler, J., Hawkes, C., Crichton, N., Allen, C., Bullock, I., & Strunin, L. (2013). The role of evidence, context, and facilitation in an implementation trial: Implications for the development of the PARIHS framework. *Implementation Science*, 8, 28. https://doi.org/10.1186/1748-5908-8-28

Sacristán, J., & Dilla, T. (2018). Pragmatic trials revisited: Applicability is about individualization. *Journal of Clinical Epidemiology, 99*, 164–166. https://doi.org/10.1016/j.jclinepi.2018.02.003

Schaffer, M. A., Sandau, K., & Diedrick, L. (2013). Evidence-based practice models for organizational change: Overview and practical applications. *Journal of Advanced Nursing, 69*, 1197–1209. https://doi.org/10.1111/j.1365-2648.2012.06122.x

Schandelmaier, S., & Guyatt, G. (2024). Same old challenges in subgroup analysis—Should we do more about methods implementation? *JAMA Network Open, 7*(3), e243339. https://doi.org/10.1001/jamanetworkopen.2024.3339

Stetler, C. B. (2010). Stetler model. In J. Rycroft-Malone & T. Bucknall (Eds.), *Models and frameworks for implementing evidence-based practice: Linking evidence to action* (pp. 51–77). Wiley-Blackwell.

Straus, S. E., Glasziou, P., Richardson, W., & Haynes, R. (2011). *Evidence-based medicine: How to practice and teach it* (4th ed.). Churchill Livingstone.

Subramanian, S., Kim, N., & Christakis, N. (2018). The "average" treatment effect: A construct ripe for retirement. A commentary on Deaton and Cartwright. *Social Science & Medicine, 210*, 77–82. https://doi.org/10.1016/j.socscimed.2018.04.027

Titler, M. G., Kleiber, C., Steelman, V., Rakel, B., Budreau, G., Everett, L., Buckwalter, K. C., Tripp-Reimer, T., & Goode, C. (2001). The Iowa Model of evidence-based practice to promote quality care. *Critical Care Nursing Clinics of North America, 13*, 497–509. https://doi.org/10.1016/S0899-5885(18)30017-0

Tomkins, L., & Bristow, A. (2023). Evidence-based practice and the ethics of care: 'What works' or 'what matters'? *Human Relations, 76*(1), 118–143. https://doi.org/10.1177/00187267211044143

Tunis, S. R., Stryer, D., & Clancy, C. (2003). Practical clinical trials: Increasing the value of clinical research for decision making in clinical and health policy. *JAMA, 290*, 1624–1632. https://doi.org/10.1001/jama.290.12.1624

World Health Organization. (2005). *Bridging the "know-do" gap: Meeting on knowledge translation in global health*. https://www.measureevaluation.org/resources/training/capacity-building-resources/high-impact-research-training-curricula/bridging-the-know-do-gap.pdf

World Health Organization. (2024). *Operational framework for monitoring social determinants of health equity*. https://www.who.int/publications/i/item/9789240088320

Zhang, R., Cao, X., Feng, H., Liu, Y., Cui, P., & Jiang, H. (2023). Review of clinical practice guidelines for postpartum hemorrhage according to AGREE II. *Midwifery, 121*, 103659. https://doi.org/10.1016/j.midw.2023.103659

APPENDIX A

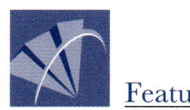 Feature Article

Advance Care Planning Affects End-of-Life Treatment Preferences Among Patients With Heart Failure

A Randomized Controlled Trial

Hui-Chuan Cheng, MSN, RN ○ Shu-Fang Vivienne Wu, PhD, RN ○
Yi-Hui Chen, MSN, RN ○ Ya-Hui Tsan, MSN, RN ○ Shih-Hsien Sung, PhD, MD ○
Li-Shan Ke, PhD, RN

This study explored the effects of advance care planning interventions on end-of-life treatment decisions among patients with heart failure. The study design was a randomized controlled trial. An intervention involving a motivational video, a cartoon version educational brochure, and a guided discussion was implemented. A total of 82 hospitalized patients with heart failure were recruited. Half of the participants received the intervention, and the other half received routine care. The Life Support Preferences Questionnaire was the primary measurement instrument. Before the advance care planning intervention, a significant difference between the experimental and control groups was observed in the cardiopulmonary resuscitation score but not the total, antibiotics, surgery, and artificial nutrition and hydration scores. In the experimental group but not in the control group, significant differences were observed between pretest and posttest total, antibiotics, cardiopulmonary resuscitation, surgery, and artificial nutrition and hydration scores. Significant differences in mean score changes were observed in total and each treatment score between the experimental and control groups. The advance care planning intervention led participants to select fewer medical treatments. This intervention may be suitable for societies where people are unfamiliar with advance care planning and may feel uncomfortable discussing death.

KEY WORDS

advance care planning, end-of-life treatment, heart failure

Hui-Chuan Cheng, MSN, RN, is supervisor, Department of Nursing, Taipei Veterans General Hospital; and PhD candidate, School of Nursing, National Taipei University of Nursing and Health Sciences, Taipei, Taiwan.
Shu-Fang Vivienne Wu, PhD, RN, is president, National Taipei University of Nursing and Health Sciences, Taipei, Taiwan.
Yi-Hui Chen, MSN, RN, is associate head nurse, Department of Nursing, Taipei Veterans General Hospital, Taipei, Taiwan.
Ya-Hui Tsan, MSN, RN, is associate head nurse, Department of Nursing, Taipei Veterans General Hospital, Taipei, Taiwan.
Shih-Hsien Sung, PhD, MD, is attending physician, Department of Internal Medicine, Division of Cardiology, Taipei Veterans General Hospital, Taipei, Taiwan.
Li-Shan Ke, PhD, RN, is assistant professor, School of Nursing, National Taipei University of Nursing and Health Sciences, Taipei, Taiwan.
Address correspondence to Li-Shan Ke, PhD, RN, School of Nursing, National Taipei University of Nursing and Health Sciences, S314, No. 365, Mingde Rd, Beitou District, Taipei City 112303, Taiwan (lske333@gmail.com).
The authors have no conflicts of interest to disclose.
This research was supported by the Taipei Veterans General Hospital (V109A-021).
Copyright © 2023 by The Hospice and Palliative Nurses Association. All rights reserved.
DOI: 10.1097/NJH.0000000000000988

Heart failure is a complex and life-threatening condition that can lead to low cardiac output and pulmonary and systemic congestion.[1] Patients with heart failure often experience psychiatric symptoms that are disabling, painful, and highly stressful.[2] Morbidity and mortality associated with heart failure are substantial, with an estimated 38 million individuals affected worldwide.[3] In a study involving 311 patients with heart failure and 946 patients with cancer, the patients with heart failure were twice as likely as those with cancer to use emergency medical services.[4] A study in South Korea involving 36 patients with heart failure and 107 patients with cancer discovered that patients with heart failure were 3 times more likely than patients with cancer to prefer cardiopulmonary resuscitation (CPR).[5] The disease trajectory of heart failure is highly variable, and time to death cannot be accurately predicted. Treatments intended to alleviate the symptoms of heart failure can also prolong life, which may cause confusion among patients and health care professionals about the actual treatment objectives. It can also lead to unrealistic expectations regarding other treatment modalities, such as mechanical device therapies and CPR.[6]

The American College of Cardiology Foundation/the American Heart Association proposed guidelines for managing heart failure. These guidelines recommend palliative

Appendix A

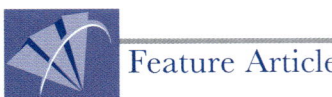
Feature Article

and supportive care for patients with advanced heart failure to improve quality of life.[7,8] The American Heart Association emphasizes the importance of advance care planning (ACP) to prepare for medical care and ensure that treatments are selected that align with the patient's values and preferences.[7] Advance care planning involves a voluntary discussion between a patient and health care professionals, family members, or significant others to identify a patient's preferences before they become unable to make decisions.[9] Patients with heart failure rarely participate in ACP, and the need for palliative care is rarely identified. Only 7% of patients with heart failure receive palliative care, and only 8% to 10% participate in ACP.[10] By contrast, 50% of patients with cancer receive palliative care. Therefore, implementing ACP among patients with heart failure is a challenging task.

Few studies have explored how ACP interventions influence end-of-life (EOL) treatment decisions among patients with heart failure. Unlike cancer or other chronic diseases, heart failure can cause rapid and unexpected clinical deterioration or sudden death throughout the disease trajectory.[7] The ACP outcomes in patients with heart failure often track whether EOL treatments and place of death match what the patient had intended or the effect of ACP on quality of life, satisfaction, EOL communication, and readmission.[11-14] Therefore, the present study investigated the effect of ACP on EOL treatment decisions in patients with heart failure.

METHODS

Study Design

This is a randomized controlled study. The study was conducted between January and December 2020. Study participants were recruited from the cardiology wards of a large medical center (more than 2900 beds) in northern Taiwan.

Participants

Hospitalized patients with heart failure were recruited if they were older than 20 years and if their diagnosis included *International Classification of Diseases, 10th Revision* codes I50.0, I50.1, or I50.9. In addition, the participants had to be physically able to endure the questionnaire interview or self-administer the questionnaire. Patients were excluded if they could not read because of poor eyesight, had severe hearing loss, or were unable to communicate in Chinese or Taiwanese.

Power Analysis

A 2-tailed Wilcoxon-Mann-Whitney test was performed on the 2 groups using the G*power 3.1.9.2 post hoc test. With 41 participants in each group, the α value was .05, the effect size was 0.66, and its power was 0.82.

Intervention

The intervention involved showing participants a motivational video, providing a cartoon version educational brochure, and facilitating a guided discussion. The motivational video was produced by Taichung Veterans General Hospital. The video was 5 minutes 11 seconds long and called "Advance Care Planning: The First Kilometer of Love" (https://www.youtube.com/watch?v=-rj6kuaxBrg). The content of the video depicting the importance of ACP and health care attorneys was utilized in the study to stimulate the participants' motivations for EOL dialogue. The cartoon-illustrated brochure was called "Advance Care Planning for Seniors." The brochure had sections entitled "Becoming Familiar with ACP and Advance Directives," "Participating in Your Medical Care," and "Discussing ACP." The brochure has satisfactory expert validity and encourages consensus on EOL treatment between older adults and their surrogates.[15]

Data Collection

Data were obtained from 2 questionnaires. The first questionnaire collected demographic data on age, sex, education level, marital status, number of children, living conditions, religion, self-report health status, and have ever heard of ACP. The second questionnaire (the Life Support Preferences Questionnaire) collected information on preferred EOL treatments and consisted of 36 questions about 9 medical scenarios and 4 treatment options.[16] The 9 medical scenarios were (1) currently healthy, (2) severe dementia, (3) continuous dyspnea, (4) coma with no chance of recovery, (5) coma with a slight chance of recovery, (6) severe stroke with no chance of recovery, (7) severe stroke with a slight chance of recovery, (8) terminal cancer without pain, and (9) terminal cancer with pain. The 4 treatments were antibiotics, CPR, surgery, and artificial nutrition and hydration (ANH). Questions were rated on a 5-point Likert-type scale with endpoints of 1 (*definitely do not want*) and 5 (*definitely want*). A higher score indicates that participants are more inclined to use medical measures. The questionnaire has been demonstrated to be reliable in studies in the United States and Taiwan.[16,17] The Cronbach α of the questionnaire was 0.97.

Ethical Considerations

The institutional review board of the study hospital approved this study (2019-07-006CC).

Procedures

The researchers had several meetings to establish consensus on the research plan before the study. The researchers presented the study criteria to health care professionals and asked them to refer suitable patients. Eligible patients were then informed of the study plan and agreed to participate by completing consent forms, thereby becoming study participants. Participants completed the questionnaire within

---

Reprinted with permission from Cheng, H. C., Wu, S. F. V., Chen, Y. H., Tsan, Y. H., Sung, S. H., & Ke, L. S. (2024). Advance care planning affects end-of-life treatment preferences among patients with heart failure: A randomized controlled trial. *Journal of Hospice & Palliative Nursing, 26*(1), E13-E19.

Feature Article

the first week of hospitalization. Opaque sealed envelopes were used to randomly assign participants to the experimental or control groups at a ratio of 1:1. The researcher responsible for allocating participants was not involved in participant recruitment, data collection, or data analysis.

The experimental group watched the video after completing the questionnaire. Participants watched the video either on a large screen in a meeting room or on a 13-inch mobile device. After watching the video, the researchers discussed the brochure with the participants, which included introducing EOL treatments with cartoon illustrations to ensure they understood medical approaches to EOL care. The participants were asked to think about their experiences, current health status, future health status, and their practical needs. The participants then recorded their thoughts in writing on the brochure.[15] The process of reviewing the brochure took approximately 30 minutes. The participants were allowed to keep their brochures and review them later privately. After 2 weeks, the participants completed the Life Support Preferences Questionnaire again. The control group was provided routine care and the educational brochure only after they had completed the Life Support Preferences Questionnaire for the second time. All participant-researcher interactions occurred in private meeting rooms or in patients' rooms if they had their own. Upon completion of the Life Support Preferences Questionnaire for the second time, all participants received compensation of NT$200 (approximately US$7).

Data Analysis

Statistical analysis was performed in SPSS 20.0. Statistical significance was indicated by $P < .05$. Descriptive statistics comprised numbers, percentages, means, and standard deviations. To test 2-group homogeneity, the χ^2 test was used for categorical variables, and the Mann-Whitney U test was used for continuous variables. The study investigated whether the ACP intervention influenced EOL treatment decisions in patients with heart failure. Accordingly, total scores and the sum of the scores for each treatment (antibiotics, CPR, surgery, and ANH) were calculated. Total scores and scores for each treatment were compared within and between groups. The mean score change (posttest minus pretest) was also calculated, and the differences between the experimental and control groups were determined. Because of the small sample size, only nonparametric analyses were performed (ie, the Mann-Whitney U and Wilcoxon signed-rank tests).

RESULTS

In total, 82 participants were recruited, with 41 in each group. No significant differences between the groups were observed in age, sex, education level, marital status, number of children, living conditions, religion, self-report health status, and whether they had ever heard of ACP ($P > .05$; Table 1).

Before the ACP intervention, a significant difference was observed between the experimental and control groups in CPR scores ($z = -2.036$, $P < .042$), but no significant differences were observed in total, antibiotics, surgery, or ANH scores ($P > .05$; Table 2). The CPR score was 23.05 (8.26) in the experimental group and 19.71 (10.78) in the control group. The experimental group was more inclined to use CPR than was the control group.

After the ACP intervention, no significant differences in posttest total, antibiotics, CPR, surgery, or ANH scores were observed between the groups ($P > .05$). However, in the experimental group, significant differences were observed between pretest and posttest total ($z = -5.424$, $P < .001$), antibiotics ($z = -5.186$, $P < .001$), CPR ($z = -5.129$, $P < .001$), surgery ($z = -4.680$, $P < .001$), and ANH ($z = -4.952$, $P < .001$) scores. No significant differences were observed between any of the pretest and posttest scores in the control group ($P > .05$). Significant differences in mean score changes were observed between the experimental and control groups. The differences in mean score changes between the groups were as follows: total ($z = -3.799$, $P < .001$), antibiotics ($z = -3.133$, $P = .002$), CPR ($z = -3.775$, $P < .001$), surgery ($z = -3.229$, $P = .001$), and ANH ($z = -3.430$, $P = .001$; Table 2).

DISCUSSION

In this study, the ACP intervention significantly changed the preferences of patients with heart failure for EOL treatments to tend to palliative care in the experimental group, even though the experimental group was more inclined to CPR than the control group before the intervention. A randomized controlled trial involving 246 patients with heart failure older than 64 years observed that an ACP intervention increased the likelihood of participants selecting palliative care and refusing CPR.[18] In a pilot study, an ACP intervention was conducted with 30 patients with New York Heart Association functional class III or IV heart failure who had experienced at least 1 unexpected hospitalization in the previous year. After the intervention, 21 patients (78%) indicated that they would not want to be readmitted and were thus not readmitted during the follow-up period, and 12 patients (40%) died at home during the follow-up period.[19] A South Korean study noted that the tendency to select hospice care was positively correlated with attitude toward ACP.[5] Therefore, ACP can affect EOL treatment decisions among patients with heart failure.

Understanding EOL treatment options and discussing ACP are essential for patients. According to Malhotra et al, patients with heart failure tended to not understand EOL treatments and hold overly optimistic views about their prognosis. As a result, they tended to prefer aggressive

Appendix A

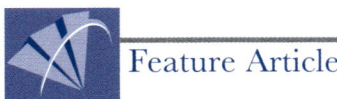

TABLE 1 Demographic Characteristics of Participants (N = 82)

Variables	Control Group (n = 41)	Experimental Group (n = 41)	Statistics	P
Age, mean (SD)	68.07 (17.29)	69.12 (16.86)	$z = -0.167$	.867
Self-reported current health[a]	2.32 (1.04)	2.29 (0.87)	$z = -0.044$	.965
Sex, n (%)				
Male	8 (19.5)	10 (24.4)	$X^2 = 0.285$	.594
Female	33 (80.5)	31 (75.6)		
Educational level, n (%)			$X^2 = 0.813$	.666
Elementary school and below	9 (22.0)	8 (19.5)		
Secondary school	17 (41.5)	21 (51.2)		
College degree and above	15 (36.6)	12 (29.3)		
Marital status, n (%)			$X^2 = 7.131$	.068
Unmarried	5 (12.2)	6 (14.6)		
Married	18 (43.9)	28 (68.3)		
Widowed	11 (26.8)	4 (9.8)		
Others	7 (17.1)	3 (7.3)		
Number of children, n (%)			$X^2 = 0.443$	.801
None	7 (17.1)	8 (19.5)		
1-2 children	11 (26.8)	13 (31.7)		
>3 children	23 (56.1)	20 (48.8)		
Living condition, n (%)			$X^2 = 1.778$	.182
Living with family	27 (67.5)	33 (80.5)		
Living without family	13 (32.5)	8 (19.5)		
Religion, n (%)			$X^2 = 1.906$	.592
None	14 (35.0)	14 (34.1)		
Buddhism	15 (37.5)	16 (39.0)		
Taoism	6 (15.0)	9 (22.0)		
Others	5 (12.5)	2 (4.9)		
Have you ever heard of ACP? n (%)			$X^2 = 0.617$	.432
No	30 (73.2)	33 (80.5)		
Yes	11 (26.8)	8 (19.5)		

Abbreviation: ACP, advance care planning.
[a]The range of self-reported current health was 1 to 5 points, with higher scores indicating healthier.

Reprinted with permission from Cheng, H. C., Wu, S. F. V., Chen, Y. H., Tsan, Y. H., Sung, S. H., & Ke, L. S. (2024). Advance care planning affects end-of-life treatment preferences among patients with heart failure: A randomized controlled trial. *Journal of Hospice & Palliative Nursing, 26*(1), E13-E19.

TABLE 2 LSPQ Scores Before and After the ACP Intervention for Each Group (Experimental Group, n = 41; Control Group, n = 41)

Variables	Pretest Mean (SD)	Pretest z[a]	Pretest P	Posttest Mean (SD)	Posttest z[a]	Posttest P	Within-Group Change (Posttest − Pretest)[b] z	Within-Group Change P	Between-Group Difference (Difference in Change in Mean Scores)[a] Mean (SD)	Between-Group Difference z	Between-Group Difference P
LSPQ total score		−1.252	.210		−0.877	.381				−3.799	<.001
Control group	89.37 (38.40)			84.05 (36.85)			−1.262	.207	−5.32 (25.59)		
Experimental group	95.98 (29.87)			76.44 (29.27)			−5.424	<.001	−19.54 (15.85)		
Antibiotics		−0.599	.549		−1.063	.288				−3.133	.002
Control group	26.27 (10.65)			23.98 (10.34)			−1.738	.082	−2.29 (8.20)		
Experimental group	26.41 (7.66)			21.07 (7.30)			−5.186	<.001	−5.34 (4.56)		
CPR		−2.036	.042		−0.344	.731				−3.775	<.001
Control group	19.71 (10.78)			18.66 (10.06)			−1.050	.294	−1.05 (6.70)		
Experimental group	23.05 (8.26)			17.27 (7.83)			−5.129	<.001	−5.78 (5.07)		
Surgery		−1.393	.164		−0.190	.849				−3.229	.001
Control group	22.78 (10.21)			21.88 (10.43)			−0.925	.355	−0.90 (6.70)		
Experimental group	25.12 (7.78)			20.83 (7.87)			−4.680	<.001	−4.29 (4.48)		
ANH		−0.831	.406		−0.986	.324				−3.430	.001
Control group	20.61 (10.77)			19.54 (9.97)			−0.649	.516	−1.07 (6.70)		
Experimental group	21.39 (9.10)			17.27 (7.97)			−4.952	<.001	−4.12 (4.51)		

Abbreviations: ACP, advance care planning; ANH, artificial nutrition and hydration; CPR, cardiopulmonary resuscitation; LSPQ, Life Support Preferences Questionnaire.
[a]Mann-Whitney test was used.
[b]Wilcoxon signed-rank test was used.

Reprinted with permission from Cheng, H. C., Wu, S. F. V., Chen, Y. H., Tsan, Y. H., Sung, S. H., & Ke, L. S. (2024). Advance care planning affects end-of-life treatment preferences among patients with heart failure: A randomized controlled trial. *Journal of Hospice & Palliative Nursing, 26*(1), E13-E19.

EOL treatments.[20] In the present study, almost 80% of participants had not heard of ACP. The short video and the cartoon illustrations brochure increased participants' understanding of ACP and EOL treatments with less reading burden. Many studies showed that video is useful for educating patients about ACP.[21-24] Although the brochure was developed for older adults, using cartoon illustrations to demonstrate EOL treatments helps patients become less apprehensive about the topic of death, especially among patients with a Chinese cultural background.[15] However, the researchers believe that more than video or educational brochure intervention is needed. As the scholars said, ACP is complex, and individuals' values, diagnosis, prognosis, and family status will affect their EOL choices.[25] Therefore, having an ACP conversation with the patient is crucial. This study adopted the strategy of reviewing the past, discussing the present, and exploring the future to conduct the ACP conversation. Despite many participants needing to become more adept at speaking, in conjunction with writing it down on the brochure, the intervention did change participants' EOL treatment decisions. Such ACP interventions may be particularly appropriate in conservative societies where people are unfamiliar with ACP and may feel uncomfortable talking about death.

Limitations

This study has 2 limitations. First, this study did not collect data on the New York Heart Association functional class of heart failure for any of the participants; whether differences in functional class of heart failure were present between the experimental and control groups is unknown. Such differences might affect the results. Second, the sample was small, which may have caused statistical bias.

CONCLUSION

Guidelines on heart failure account for a large number of clinical factors and have a particular emphasis on palliative care.[7] The ACP intervention significantly changed EOL treatment decisions, causing patients with heart failure to select fewer medical treatments. The ACP intervention consisted of a motivational video, a cartoon version educational brochure, and a guided discussion. This form of intervention may be suitable for societies in which people are not familiar with ACP and may feel uncomfortable talking about death.

References

1. Savarese G, Becher PM, Lund LH, et al. Global burden of heart failure: a comprehensive and updated review of epidemiology. *Cardiovasc Res.* 2023;118(17):3272-3287.
2. Kida K, Doi S, Suzuki N. Palliative care in patients with advanced heart failure. *Heart Fail Clin.* 2020;16(2):243-254.
3. Wang H, Chai K, Du M, et al. Prevalence and incidence of heart failure among urban patients in China: a national population-based analysis. *Circ Heart Fail.* 2021;14(10):e008406.
4. MacKenzie MA, Hanlon A. Health-care utilization after hospice enrollment in patients with heart failure and cancer. *Am J Hosp Palliat Care.* 2018;35(2):229-235.
5. Kim J, Choi J, Shin MS, et al. Do advance directive attitudes and perceived susceptibility and end-of-life life-sustaining treatment preferences between patients with heart failure and cancer differ? *PloS One.* 2020;15(9):e0238567.
6. Howlett J, Morin L, Fortin M, et al. End-of-life planning in heart failure: it should be the end of the beginning. *Can J Cardiol.* 2010;26(3):135-141.
7. Heidenreich PA, Bozkurt B, Aguilar D, et al. 2022 AHA/ACC/HFSA guideline for the management of heart failure: a report of the American College of Cardiology/American Heart Association Joint Committee on Clinical Practice Guidelines. *Circulation.* 2022;145(18):e895-e1032.
8. Yancy CW, Jessup M, Bozkurt B, et al. 2013 ACCF/AHA guideline for the management of heart failure: a report of the American College of Cardiology Foundation/American Heart Association Task Force on Practice Guidelines. *J Am Coll Cardiol.* 2013;62(16):e147-e239.
9. Rietjens JAC, Sudore RL, Connolly M, et al. Definition and recommendations for advance care planning: an international consensus supported by the European Association for Palliative Care. *Lancet Oncol.* 2017;18(9):e543-e551.
10. Schichtel M, MacArtney JI, Wee B, et al. Implementing advance care planning in heart failure: a qualitative study of primary healthcare professionals. *Br J Gen Pract.* 2021;71(708):e550-e560.
11. Malhotra C, Sim D, Jaufeerally FR, et al. Impact of a formal advance care planning program on end-of-life care for patients with heart failure: results from a randomized controlled trial. *J Card Fail.* 2020;26(7):594-598.
12. Kernick LA, Hogg KJ, Millerick Y, et al. Does advance care planning in addition to usual care reduce hospitalisation for patients with advanced heart failure: a systematic review and narrative synthesis. *Palliat Med.* 2018;32(10):1539-1551.
13. Schichtel M, Wee B, Perera R, et al. The effect of advance care planning on heart failure: a systematic review and meta-analysis. *J Gen Intern Med.* 2020;35(3):874-884.
14. Nishikawa Y, Hiroyama N, Fukahori H, et al. Advance care planning for adults with heart failure. *Cochrane Database Syst Rev.* 2020;2(2):Cd013022.
15. Ke LS, Hu WY, Chen CY, et al. A quasi-experimental evaluation of advance care planning improves consistency between elderly individuals and their surrogates regarding end-of-life care preferences: development and application of a decision aid with cartoon pictures. *Patient Educ Couns.* 2021;104(4):815-825.
16. Coppola KM, Bookwala J, Ditto PH, et al. Elderly adults' preferences for life-sustaining treatments: the role of impairment, prognosis, and pain. *Death Stud.* 1999;23(7):617-634.
17. Ke LS, Hu WY, Chen MJ, et al. Advance care planning to improve end-of-life decision-making consistency between older people and their surrogates in Taiwan. *J Palliat Med.* 2020;23(3):325-336.
18. El-Jawahri A, Paasche-Orlow MK, Matlock D, et al. Randomized, controlled trial of an advance care planning video decision support tool for patients with advanced heart failure. *Circulation.* 2016;134(1):52-60.
19. Coster JE, Ter Maat GH, Pentinga ML, et al. A pilot study on the effect of advance care planning implementation on healthcare utilisation and satisfaction in patients with advanced heart failure. *Neth Heart J.* 2022;30(9):436-441.
20. Malhotra C, Hu M, Malhotra R, et al. Instability in end-of-life care preference among heart failure patients: secondary analysis of a randomized controlled trial in Singapore. *J Gen Intern Med.* 2020;35(7):2010-2016.
21. Kang E, Lee J, Choo J, et al. Randomized controlled trial of advance care planning video decision aid for the general population. *J Pain Symptom Manage.* 2020;59(6):1239-1247.

Reprinted with permission from Cheng, H. C., Wu, S. F. V., Chen, Y. H., Tsan, Y. H., Sung, S. H., & Ke, L. S. (2024). Advance care planning affects end-of-life treatment preferences among patients with heart failure: A randomized controlled trial. *Journal of Hospice & Palliative Nursing, 26*(1), E13-E19.

22. Ufere NN, Robinson B, Donlan J, et al. Pilot randomized controlled trial of an advance care planning video decision tool for patients with advanced liver disease. *Clin Gastroenterol Hepatol*. 2022;20(10):2287-2295.e3.
23. Hsieh WT. Virtual reality video promotes effectiveness in advance care planning. *BMC Palliat Care*. 2020;19(1):125.
24. Lai JC-T, Chan HY-L. A video decision aid for advance care planning among community-dwelling older Chinese adults: a cluster randomized controlled trial. *J Palliat Med*. 2023;26(5):637-645.
25. Douglas ML, Simon J, Davison SN, et al. Efficacy of advance care planning videos for patients: a randomized controlled trial in cancer, heart, and kidney failure outpatient settings. *Med Decis Making*. 2021;41(3):292-304.

APPENDIX B

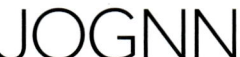

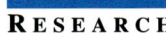

Lived Experiences of Fatherhood After Infertility

Stephanie Morrison, Janet Bryanton, Christina Murray, and Vicki Foley

Correspondence
Stephanie Morrison, RN, MN, Faculty of Nursing, University of Prince Edward Island, 550 University Avenue, Charlottetown, Prince Edward Island, Canada, C1A 4P3.
sawalsh@upei.ca

Keywords
Colaizzi
emotions
family health
fatherhood
infertility
perinatal period
phenomenology
pregnancy
psychological

ABSTRACT

Objective: To explore the lived experiences of fathers in the perinatal period after infertility.
Design: A descriptive, phenomenological study.
Setting: Researcher's private office and participants' homes in an Eastern Canadian province.
Participants: Eight fathers who met the eligibility criteria.
Methods: We recruited a purposive sample of eight participants and held one-on-one interviews in person, by telephone, and via virtual platforms. We analyzed the verbatim transcripts of the audiotaped interviews using Colaizzi's phenomenological data analysis method.
Results: We uncovered seven themes that described the lived experiences of participants: *The Journey: A Long Winding Road, Roles and Responsibilities: Supporter and Protector, Support: The Often-Forgotten Parent, Challenges and Hurdles: Bumps on the Road, So Many Feelings: The Rollercoaster, Coping: Living on the Road,* and *Reflection: An Unforgotten Journey.* Participants shared their experiences of the perinatal period after infertility as long journeys and described how bumps along the road marked these journeys. The journeys were essential parts of their lives that they continued to remember years later.
Conclusion: The perinatal experience after infertility is an important and remembered time for fathers. It is essential to involve and support them in the perinatal process to facilitate positive experiences and overall family health, especially after infertility. There is an ongoing need to conduct research with fathers and to develop evidence-based programming and resources to assist them in the perinatal period after infertility.

JOGNN, 53, 245–254; 2024. https://doi.org/10.1016/j.jogn.2023.12.002

Accepted December 6, 2023; Published online January 16, 2024

Stephanie Morrison, RN, MN, is a clinical nursing instructor, Faculty of Nursing, University of Prince Edward Island, Charlottetown, Prince Edward Island, Canada.

Janet Bryanton, MN, PhD, is a professor emerita, Faculty of Nursing, University of Prince Edward Island, Charlottetown, Prince Edward Island, Canada.

Christina Murray, BA, PhD, RN, is the dean of the Faculty of Nursing and director of Interprofessional Health Education, University of Prince Edward Island, Charlottetown, Prince Edward Island, Canada.

(Continued)

Infertility is a reproductive condition diagnosed when a person is unable to conceive after 1 year of unprotected intercourse (Centers for Disease Control and Prevention, 2023). It is estimated to affect 16% of Canadian couples (Society of Obstetricians and Gynaecologists of Canada, 2023) and one in six people globally (World Health Organization, 2023). The diagnosis and treatment processes are physically and emotionally invasive, and not all people who seek treatment are able to conceive (Mayo Clinic, 2021). Additionally, those who do eventually conceive face potential psychological and emotional distress (Allan et al., 2021).

Proponents of family-centered maternity care maintain that whomever the pregnant person identifies as family must be included and supported during perinatal care (Public Health Agency of Canada, 2022). Fathers endure infertility and are an important part of the family unit. They require support in the perinatal period after infertility just as mothers do (Hanna & Gough, 2017). However, fathers are often forgotten (Vallin et al., 2019). Limited research exists regarding fathers' lived experiences to help us understand their needs from their perspectives.

Literature Review

Men and women can be affected by infertility. Potential causes include lifestyle and biological factors, or the cause can remain unknown (Vander Borght & Wyns, 2018). The often long and invasive diagnosis and treatment process usually begins with a health and sexual history and an extensive assessment (Centers for Disease Control and Prevention, 2023; Mayo Clinic, 2021). Treatment depends on several variables such as cause, age, cost, and the couple's preference. They must

http://jognn.org

© 2023 AWHONN, the Association of Women's Health, Obstetric and Neonatal Nurses.
Published by Elsevier Inc. All rights reserved.

Reprinted from Morrison, S., Bryanton, J., Murray, C., & Foley, V. (2024). Lived experiences of fatherhood after infertility. Journal of Obstetric, Gynecologic & Neonatal Nursing, 53(3), 245-254. https://doi.org/10.1016/j.jogn.2023.12.002. Copyright © 2023 AWHONN, the Association of Women's Health, Obstetric and Neonatal Nurses. With permission.

339

Appendix B

RESEARCH

Fatherhood After Infertility

Fathers' lived experiences during the perinatal period after infertility have not been clearly described, which limits the provision of care that reflects their unique needs.

Vicki Foley, RN, PhD, is an adjunct graduate faculty member, Faculty of Nursing, University of Prince Edward Island, Charlottetown, Prince Edward Island, Canada.

weigh the risks and benefits of treatments that can include addressing lifestyle factors, reproductive anatomy, or diseases; taking medication to facilitate ovulation or sperm production; or undergoing surgery, artificial insemination, or in vitro fertilization (Mayo Clinic, 2021).

Men who experienced infertility described feeling stressed, isolated, and excluded (Arya & Dibb, 2016; Hanna & Gough, 2017). They also reported that they endured and coped with the process differently than women due to social stigma (Hanna & Gough, 2016, 2017). Some men expressed a need to talk about their experience but felt unsupported by health care providers, family, and friends (Arya & Dibb, 2016; Hanna & Gough, 2017). Some preferred to keep the infertility private (Hanna & Gough, 2019) or found it difficult to talk to other men about it (Harlow et al., 2020). In general, all fathers wanted to be involved in the perinatal experience but sometimes lacked information about how to do so (Eggermont et al., 2017; Elmir & Schmied, 2016) and sometimes felt unwelcome (Feenstra et al., 2018; Kowlessar et al., 2015) or overlooked (Hanna & Gough, 2017). This made them feel helpless and left out while trying to protect and support their partners (Feenstra et al., 2018; Hanna & Gough, 2017).

Researchers suggested that fathers who experienced the perinatal period after infertility had similar transitions to fatherhood (Vanska et al., 2017), views of their role as support persons (Herrera, 2013), father–infant attachment (Allan et al., 2021), and quality of life (Orit Taubman et al., 2017) as men whose partners conceived spontaneously. In contrast, in a qualitative study with couples, Allan et al. (2019) found that men's transitions after in vitro fertilization were unique, long, and turbulent compared to those whose partners conceived naturally, and they had ongoing struggles after birth. Some talked about how their transitions to fatherhood began with their infertility experiences, and many said it was stressful and anxiety provoking but rewarding when they became fathers.

Overall, limited current research exists on fathers' experiences during the perinatal period after infertility. We found only two articles written in the past 10 years in which researchers used samples of men. In their quantitative study, Orit Taubman et al. (2017) compared fathers whose partners conceived through artificial reproductive technology to those whose partners conceived spontaneously regarding life satisfaction and found no differences between the groups on any measures of life satisfaction. Using a qualitative approach, Herrera (2013) explored fathers' views of themselves after artificial reproductive technology or adoption. They reported that fathers who experienced artificial reproductive technology viewed themselves as supporters in the process and their partners as the focus. These authors investigated specific aspects of fathers' experiences rather than their lived experiences during the perinatal period after infertility. In systematic reviews, Allan et al. (2021) and Foyston et al. (2023) found that most studies were published more than 10 years ago and that men's experiences were underreported. Furthermore, they did not identify any Canadian studies.

Despite research efforts, fathers' lived experiences during the perinatal period after infertility remain unclear, which limits care that is tailored to their unique needs. Without further exploration of this phenomenon, fathers will continue to endure inequitable care and support and may continue to feel forgotten. By addressing this gap, we will help facilitate more evidence-based, comprehensive, family-centered care. We can potentially enhance nursing practice and allow nurses to fulfill their roles as facilitators and support personnel. Therefore, the purpose of this qualitative, phenomenological study was to explore the lived experiences of fathers in the perinatal period after infertility.

Methods

Design

Phenomenology originated in the disciplines of philosophy and psychology, and phenomenologists explore the "lived experience" and its meaning (Husserl, 1931). They believe that perception cannot be separated from lived experience and that consciousness is not internal; instead, "consciousness is life" (Munhall, 1994, p. 14). People embody the experience of being in the world through touch, taste, smell, sight, and hearing and by how those senses influence their consciousness (Munhall, 1994). To understand the lived experience of a phenomenon, phenomenologists must be open to all aspects of the phenomenon. They must go through the process of phenomenological epoché by intentionally identifying their preexisting thoughts,

Reprinted from Morrison, S., Bryanton, J., Murray, C., & Foley, V. (2024). Lived experiences of fatherhood after infertility. Journal of Obstetric, Gynecologic & Neonatal Nursing, 53(3), 245-254. Copyright © 2023 AWHONN, the Association of Women's Health, Obstetric and Neonatal Nurses. With permission.

attitudes, and assumptions. Phenomenologists must then reduce or not allow their presuppositions to influence the description of the phenomenon. This is known as bracketing (Husserl, 1931).

Descriptive phenomenologists study the essence of a phenomenon and describe its fundamental elements (Husserl, 1931). They return to the original phenomenon, event, or experience (a priori or primordial) to obtain the most faithful description (Colaizzi, 1978). Descriptive phenomenologists bracket their presuppositions and listen intently to what participants say. Then, they analyze the data and organize essential elements into a description of the phenomenon (Husserl, 1931).

Colaizzi's (1978) method is predominantly descriptive but also includes elements of interpretive phenomenology. Like Husserl (1931), Colaizzi believed that to obtain the purest form of a phenomenon, researchers must acknowledge their presuppositions beginning and throughout the study and exclude those thoughts from the description. However, Colaizzi purported that researchers cannot completely bracket their presuppositions but must maintain a close connection with participants' narratives when describing the phenomenon. Because there is little known about fathers' experiences in the perinatal period after infertility, we chose descriptive phenomenology and Colaizzi's method to conduct this study. Colaizzi's descriptive approach had the potential to generate the purest form of the lived experience of this phenomenon.

Before initiating this study, we obtained ethics approval from the University of Prince Edward Island and Health PEI research ethics boards.

Participants

We used purposive sampling to recruit men who had the lived experience of the phenomenon of interest. Men were eligible to participate if they were 18 years of age or older, able to read and speak English, had experienced the perinatal period after infertility, and were in a heterosexual relationship at the time of pregnancy. The time since the perinatal experience did not matter, nor did the time since they experienced infertility.

Setting

We conducted this study in an eastern Canadian province where there is currently no fertility specialist or clinic due to the small size of the population. Access to basic fertility care (e.g., fertility assessment, medications) is available through family doctors and gynecologists; however, individuals must travel out of province for assisted reproductive technology.

Recruitment and Data Collection

We recruited participants through an advertisement placed in obstetricians' offices, two hospitals' obstetric units, and social media. Colaizzi (1978) stated that the phenomenon of interest should guide the sample size; therefore, we reached data saturation when we observed commonalities among eight participants, which helped us gain a comprehensive understanding of the phenomenon (Morse, 2015).

S.M. obtained informed, written consent and advised participants that the study was voluntary and that they could withdraw at any time. Each chose a pseudonym, and S.M. asked for their permission to digitally record the interview and use direct quotes if we protected confidentiality. She collected the data using an in-depth, one-on-one interview with each participant and gave them the choice of how to be interviewed; four were interviewed in person, two by telephone, and two virtually. Some preferred an interview in their own homes; others chose a private office at the university.

We used Colaizzi's (1978) method to guide data collection. S.M. asked participants one question at the beginning of the interview: "Can you please share your thoughts and feelings about your experience before pregnancy, during pregnancy, labor, birth, and after birth following your experience of infertility?" She did not interrupt them while they shared their experiences and used appropriate probes at the end of the interviews to clarify and expand on participants' ideas as needed. Interviews ranged from 30 minutes to 2 hours.

Trustworthiness

Throughout the study, we used various strategies to promote trustworthiness and increase credibility, transferability, dependability, confirmability, and authenticity (Lincoln & Guba, 1985; Polit & Beck, 2021). We were reflexive, maintained careful documentation and a detailed audit trail, and explored our presuppositions at the beginning of and throughout the study as part of our reflexive process. We included the protocols (transcripts), the reflexive journal, notes about the study process, and decisions made in our audit trail. We also detailed when we reached a comprehensive understanding of the phenomenon (data saturation), reviewed each transcript for accuracy, and

Table 1: Steps of Colaizzi's Method of Data Analysis

(1) Review all transcripts (protocols) to gain a clearer understanding of each.
(2) Reread each transcript (protocol). Identify and extract significant statements that address or describe the phenomenon.
(3) Review each significant statement and write a formulated meaning. Refer to the original transcripts to ensure accuracy with the participant's description.
(4) After completing Steps 1, 2, and 3 for each transcript (protocol), cluster the formulated meanings into clusters of themes. Simultaneously, return to original transcripts to ensure you remain true to participants' descriptions.
(5) Organize the results into an exhaustive description of the phenomenon.
(6) Develop the fundamental structure of the phenomenon from the exhaustive description.
(7) Return to the participants seeking reflection and validation of the results. Listen to participants' reflections and adjust results if needed.

Note. From "Psychological Research as the Phenomenologist Views It," by P. F. Colaizzi, 1978, in R. S. Valle & M. King (Eds.), *Existential-phenomenological alternatives for psychology* (pp. 48–71). Oxford University Press.

used investigator triangulation. Finally, we used thick descriptions to explore the phenomenon in the results as well as participant quotes and the descriptions of the themes to share participants' experiences.

Data Analysis

Colaizzi (1978) suggested that before conducting data analysis, researchers must once again reflect on their own presuppositions. He described a series of seven data analysis steps and stressed that they are meant to be flexible and free. See Table 1 for a detailed description of these steps. Before beginning the analysis, we re-examined our presuppositions. Then, after reading and rereading each transcript, we identified and extracted phrases or sentences that addressed or described the phenomenon. Next, we used creative insight to move from what our participants said to what they meant and wrote a formulated meaning for each significant statement. When writing formulated meanings, Colaizzi warned that researchers must remain connected with participants' original descriptions. This is where he suggested slight interpretation rather than exclusive description. See Table 2 for examples of formulated meanings. We then clustered the formulated meanings into seven themes, integrated the results into an exhaustive description of the phenomenon, and developed its fundamental structure. Finally, we e-mailed a copy of the exhaustive description to participants and asked them to reflect on it to determine if, even in part, it represented their experiences. Four participants responded, and no changes were required based on their responses. For example, Sam responded, "I read through the synopsis, and it looks great!! Many of my thoughts and feelings . . . [were] resonating in that synopsis. . . ."

Results

The eight participants ranged in age from 30 to 50 years ($M = 41$ years), and they reported having one to three living children. The couples experienced from one to four pregnancies, and some experienced perinatal loss, including miscarriage ($n = 5$), stillbirth ($n = 1$), and neonatal death ($n = 1$). At the time of the study, participants' experiences of infertility ranged from 2 years to 10 years before the interview. During the perinatal period, participants and their partners accessed various fertility treatments such as medications for ovulation, in vitro fertilization, and surgical procedures. We present additional demographic information in Table 3.

We extracted 843 significant statements and organized them into clusters of subthemes and then seven overarching themes: *The Journey: A Long Winding Road*, *Roles and Responsibilities: Supporter and Protector*, *Support: The Often-Forgotten Parent*, *Challenges and Hurdles: Bumps on the Road*, *So Many Feelings: The Rollercoaster*, *Coping: Living on the Road*, and *Reflection: An Unforgotten Journey*. The first and last themes represented the entire journey, whereas the remaining five described specific points in time during the journey.

The Journey: A Long Winding Road

This initial theme set the stage for how participants envisioned their perinatal experiences that began with infertility and ended in the postpartum period. Although each described a journey, their experiences were not the same, and the distinct roads they took along their travels influenced their experiences. They shared how their knowledge of infertility, process of seeking help from health care providers, infertility treatments, and the desire for

Table 2: Examples of Formulated Meaning From Significant Statements for Theme 2

Significant Statement	Formulated Meaning
"Mostly I think to be strong for both of us because, well because I guess I felt like I had to carry the mental load for both of us and just be that mentally strong person because I didn't feel like it was fair to kind of share that. . . . Just be reassuring even though I wasn't necessarily sure myself." (Rick)	He had to be strong for both of them. He felt like he had to carry the mental load and to be the mentally strong one because he didn't think it was fair to share it. He felt like he should be reassuring even though he wasn't sure himself.
"I got a call saying, from my wife saying that his blood sugar has dropped. So, I was like, I couldn't even believe, like how could that happen. Why is that, like, that shouldn't ever happen. That is bad. I feel so bad." (John)	He got a call from his wife saying that their son's glucose had dropped. He couldn't believe it. He wondered how that could happen. He thought that it should never happen. He felt so bad.

privacy affected their journeys. Sam recalled the process of infertility treatments:

> . . . (doctor) would try . . . [treatment] three times and if that didn't work you would move on . . . when we finally got to the IVF stage . . . you think this is it, right. This is going to work because you are at the end. But . . . we were far closer to the beginning . . . the real challenges lay ahead. . . .

Participants described perinatal losses and infertility as components of the preconception period. Many experienced joy with conception and then sadness with perinatal loss. Billy talked about his desire for privacy and sadness after perinatal loss:

Table 3: Demographic Characteristics of Participants ($N = 8$)

Characteristics	n	%
Marital status		
Married/common law	7	87.5
Single/widowed/divorced	1	12.5
Number of pregnancies conceived		
1	1	12.5
>1	7	87.5
Highest level of education		
Some college/university	2	25
College/university	6	75
Family's gross yearly income (CAD$)		
≤50,000	2	25
51,000–100,000	2	25
>100,000	4	50

"I find it is a lot easier if people don't know; therefore, you can just be more supportive for each other. . . . If a lot of people keep bringing it back . . . makes it a little harder, I find."

Roles and Responsibilities: Supporter and Protector

Participants described a role, responsibility, or sense of duty to support and protect their partners and thought they had a duty to be involved. They also developed a profound respect for their partners and acknowledged their challenges in being the support person. Rick recalled supporting his partner through pregnancy loss, whereas others remembered supporting their partners through infertility. John said, "When she gets depressed, I used to, like, perk her up." Participants also recalled supporting and protecting their partners through the pregnancy and birth. Oscar tried to minimize the stress in the environment during the pregnancy. Max described protecting his wife and son and ensured that they saw one another after the cesarean birth.

A few participants talked about feeling a responsibility to "bear the mental load." They reminisced about how their partners had to endure many additional physical challenges, such as in vitro fertilization and all that it involved and carrying the pregnancy. Rick said, "I felt like I had to carry the mental load for both of us. . . . I didn't feel like it was fair to . . . share that." They also felt profound respect and empathy for their partners and a respect for fatherhood.

Despite being the supporter, protector, and bearer of the mental load, it was sometimes difficult for participants to cope with the experience themselves. Sam described this when he said, "There is unique challenges to being . . . the father . . . because we are not prepared. . . . You want to be supportive. You're doing the best that you can . . . but at the same time you probably need support yourself."

Support: The Often-Forgotten Parent
Our participants talked about how the support they received or did not receive from infertility services, health personnel, family, friends, and employers influenced their journeys positively and negatively. Steve shared his experience of positive support from friends. He noted that it was helpful when his friends were willing to talk about his experience and compared health provider support during the births of his first and subsequent two children: "In the smaller city, it was a lot more inclusive, and in the bigger city, it was a lot more kind of cold . . . it felt like it was conveyor belt . . . in the door, out the door." Limited access to infertility services created a feeling of a lack of support for many participants. Furthermore, a few described how the mother was the focus of care. This was perceived as the status quo for some, whereas others felt forgotten. Rick frequently felt like an "add-on" and a "pest" and that health personnel did not expect him to be as involved as he wanted to be: "I have . . . two babies that nobody apparently expected me to be involved with. . . . But I felt very much like I want to be. . . . It is important to me, and it didn't seem like it was important to anybody else."

Most of the women had cesarean births; our participants described waiting outside the operating room while their partners were inside being prepared. They described how they felt forgotten, scared, worried, unprepared, uninformed, and unimportant in this process. Max stated:

> I had to go out in the hallway by myself for 5 minutes, which was turned into 25 or 30 . . . that was the longest, coldest, loneliest time . . . there should have been a professional . . . come out and say, "How are you doing?" . . . because you are sitting there and your legs are shaking, tears are rolling down, thoughts are going through your mind.

Challenges and Hurdles: Bumps on the Road
Participants described the challenges and hurdles they faced throughout the perinatal experience. They viewed these as bumps on the road rather than dead ends. Challenges included lack of resources, perinatal loss, and an ongoing battle; being left behind; experiencing marital challenges, a tug-of-war between excitement and disbelief, and fear of loss and the unknown; and worrying about the health of their partners and unborn infants.

For some participants, every day of the pregnancy was a challenge, and reaching milestones, such as the age of viability, was an achievement. Sam stated, "Especially in those early stages and you keep wanting . . . to make it to the next day. . . ." Bobby spoke of the progress of the pregnancy: "You look at every trimester and your odds go up." Additional hurdles included encountering birth complications and breastfeeding challenges, caring for sick children, and assisting their partners with healing from cesarean births. Max described his thoughts about potentially losing his son after birth: "These dark thoughts start coming . . . what if something happens. . . . What if we had the pleasure of meeting our son for a week and then he is gone?"

So Many Feelings: The Rollercoaster
The participants' feelings varied and evolved as their journeys progressed through the perinatal period. They experienced a rollercoaster of feelings that fluctuated with the twists, turns, and bumps in the road. Participants shared common feelings: sadness, pain, suffering, frustration, nervousness, fear, excitement, happiness, stress, worry, shock, unpreparedness, helplessness, ease, gratification, joy, fulfillment, reassurance, relief, gratefulness, satisfaction, and disbelief.

In the preconception period, Oscar described his sadness when he realized how devastated his wife was to learn of the infertility. Sam recognized that the infertility was hard for his wife but also hard for him. Participants also talked about having mixed feelings during the prenatal period. Bobby stated, "You kind of go in thinking you are very excited, but you are still leery about how far this is going to go." They discussed negative feelings related to the fear of another pregnancy loss and worry about the health of the mother and child.

Max described labor and birth as a rollercoaster. He shared a mix of positive and negative emotions when he talked about the line between anxiety and excitement. Alternatively, some participants felt relaxed, at ease, and secure during labor. Oscar noted several feelings that he experienced after the birth: "It was kind of surreal . . . waiting so long and the overwhelming joy of my child is here. . . . It was relief and happiness."

Reprinted from Morrison, S., Bryanton, J., Murray, C., & Foley, V. (2024). Lived experiences of fatherhood after infertility. Journal of Obstetric, Gynecologic & Neonatal Nursing, 53(3), 245-254. Copyright © 2023 AWHONN, the Association of Women's Health, Obstetric and Neonatal Nurses. With permission.

Like Oscar, many participants talked about feeling relief at the birth; however, the timing of that joy and relief varied among them. Some felt relief as soon as they heard their newborns cry. For others, it occurred when they held their newborns and looked into their eyes, walked with them to the nursery, or were reunited as a family after cesarean birth.

Participants continued to have a rollercoaster of feelings during the postpartum period. Some shared how they worried about their children dying. Rick had dark thoughts and vivid dreams: "I remember having this reoccurring dream where . . . I would wake . . . and see one of my daughters sitting playing in the middle of the road and having the dream end just before she got hit by a car." Others described positive feelings. Sam noted, "It wasn't that everything that happened . . . didn't matter; it was a feeling of satisfaction that we persevered."

Coping: Living on the Road
Participants coped in various ways depending on their unique journeys. Their coping methods evolved as their journeys progressed; strategies included using caution/self-protection, faith/beliefs, comedy, positivity, distraction, teamwork (with their partners), and knowledge; making a commitment to the journey; being private/insular; gaining perspective; taking control; and monitoring the pregnancy, avoiding risks, and planning for a cesarean birth. Bobby and his wife experienced multiple miscarriages and an unsuccessful in vitro fertilization cycle. When explaining his process of coping throughout the preconception period, he talked about being cautious and remaining prepared that future pregnancies could result in another miscarriage.

Sam remembered how he monitored each of his children during pregnancy, which helped him cope with his fear of another perinatal loss. He said, "Starting at week 7 . . . there might have been 2 weeks . . . where she didn't have an ultrasound." Rick discussed how being involved helped him feel more in control: "That was a way for me to be able to . . . control things. . . . I want something to do because I don't want to be treated like I don't have a part here." He also articulated that he did not realize how he had suppressed his feelings: "I felt like I had to be mentally strong. . . . I suppressed a lot . . . we got home and started living again, that's when a lot of the stuff maybe came back." Steve also mentioned suppressing his feelings.

> **Participants described how their journeys to fatherhood after infertility were long and unique and involved positive and negative experiences.**

Reflection: An Unforgotten Journey
Participants recalled a process of reflection when they described their unique journeys. Although they did not reflect on the same aspects, they all reflected. Most talked about positive and negative memories and how they will never forget their experiences. Some participants envisioned their experiences as normal and believed that they were like fathers who had not endured infertility. Many talked about going home, which was welcomed and exciting for some and fear-provoking for others. Although they were able to move forward, they never forgot their journeys to fatherhood. Sam shared, "We certainly don't forget . . . our experience probably made the postpartum sweeter because . . . having a family was . . . a major accomplishment for us."

Participants also described the stigma surrounding infertility, suggestions for future care, and their desire for more children. For instance, Sam realized how common infertility was and understood how little it was talked about due to stigma. With respect to suggestions for future care, Billy suggested the need for more public awareness about infertility: "When people ask, 'So when is the next one coming?' . . . people don't realize your history and then it just, that brings up all the bad memories." Oscar suggested a video resource to introduce fathers to the operating room: "It would have been nice for someone to say, go look at this and you will know what to expect . . . they told the mother . . . but I had no idea." Other suggestions included helping fathers feel involved throughout the perinatal period and providing coping resources for infertility and perinatal loss. Rick wished that health care providers had acknowledged that perinatal loss would be difficult and recommended that he and his wife see a counselor. He also recommended hard copy resources about perinatal loss.

Discussion
Our participants provided new insights regarding their lived experiences after infertility in their transitions to parenthood. The journey to fatherhood after infertility appears to be unique for each man and cannot be separated from the infertility experience. In a qualitative study with couples,

Allan et al. (2019) concurred that the transition to parenthood began with infertility, was unique, and included "a long, anxious process with many setbacks and losses" (p. 6), which suggested that the experience is not straightforward.

The concept of being the protector and supporter is noteworthy. Like our participants, Herrera (2013) and Foyston et al. (2023) reported that fathers who faced infertility endeavored to protect their partners, which they did by contributing financially, offering emotional support, and attending antenatal appointments (Foyston et al., 2023). Researchers who studied fathers in general also indicated that men tended to focus on their partners rather than themselves (Feenstra et al., 2018; Vallin et al., 2019). This suggests that the responsibility to be a protector and support person may not be unique to the phenomenon under study. Like our participants, researchers reported that all fathers experience helplessness and failure when they cannot protect their partners (Hanna & Gough, 2017; Kowlessar et al., 2015). This underscores the stress that fathers endure during the perinatal period and the uncertainty about how to provide support when they are trying to cope themselves (Eggermont et al., 2017; Feenstra et al., 2018).

Fathers also need support, and whether they receive this support influences their experiences. Poor communication with health care personnel may be perceived as not being supportive. Researchers reported that when providers included fathers with or without infertility (Vallin et al., 2019) or established a healthy level of communication (Elmir & Schmied, 2016), fathers had more positive experiences. Alternatively, when fathers experienced adverse events in their families' care, they developed distrust in health care personnel, and when they believed communication was poor, they perceived the support and experience negatively (Vallin et al., 2019). Employer support also appears to be important. This is consistent with research by Hanna and Gough (2019) who reported that when employers were unsupportive of providing time off for infertility treatment, it caused distress. Researchers also found that fathers who did or did not experience infertility often felt excluded in perinatal care (Feenstra et al., 2018; Hanna & Gough, 2017). This caused distress (Vallin et al., 2019) and feelings of isolation (Feenstra et al., 2018). They recommended a need to be included in care.

Our participants identified many challenges and hurdles throughout the perinatal period; however, they were resilient despite the challenges they faced. Allan et al. (2019) also found that fathers who experienced infertility were resilient. Like our participants, researchers reported a tug-of-war between cautious hopefulness and fear of miscarriage or failure of fertility treatments (Allan et al., 2019; Foyston et al., 2023).

Participants described many feelings throughout their journeys: the highs (positive feelings) and lows (negative feelings) of a rollercoaster and fear, anxiety, and stress. Some appeared to be traumatized by their experiences. The feeling of being on a rollercoaster is consistent with research regarding fathers in general (Kowlessar et al., 2015) and those who experienced infertility (Arya & Dibb, 2016). Given that fathers in general (Feenstra et al., 2018) and those who faced infertility (Allan et al., 2019; Hanna & Gough, 2016) commonly reported fear, anxiety, and stress related to the well-being of their families, it is not clear if our participants' feelings were unique to the phenomenon of the transition to fatherhood after infertility. A lack of clarity remains regarding fathers' mental health experiences and how these are affected by or how they influence the phenomenon under study.

Participants coped in various ways depending on their unique journeys. Like our participants, Allan et al. (2019) and Foyston et al. (2023) noted that fathers who experienced infertility reported a sense of caution and fear of loss. During pregnancy, they coped by taking control, monitoring the pregnancy, and staying positive. Fathers pursued reassurance of fetal well-being through prenatal appointments, ultrasounds, and asking their partners about fetal well-being (Foyston et al., 2023). Additional coping measures shared by our participants and noted by researchers in studies with fathers (with or without infertility) included seeking or having knowledge (Vallin et al., 2019), avoiding risks (Foyston et al., 2023), seeking reassurance from health care personnel (Foyston et al., 2023), talking to people who provide support (Foyston et al., 2023; Vallin et al., 2019), and suppressing their emotions (Vallin et al., 2019).

Our participants reflected on their experiences, and although they moved forward, they never forgot their journeys. Foyston et al. (2023) also reported that families who experienced infertility and then parenthood always remembered the experience. Although fathers who endured infertility have unique journeys, what is less clear is how common their experiences are to fathers in general. Vanska et al. (2017) reported that men

Reprinted from Morrison, S., Bryanton, J., Murray, C., & Foley, V. (2024). Lived experiences of fatherhood after infertility. Journal of Obstetric, Gynecologic & Neonatal Nursing, 53(3), 245-254. Copyright © 2023 AWHONN, the Association of Women's Health, Obstetric and Neonatal Nurses. With permission.

Morrison, S., Bryanton, J., Murray, C., and Foley, V.

RESEARCH

who experienced infertility had similar transitions to those whose partners conceived spontaneously. In contrast, men in the study by Allan et al. (2019) reported that after birth, they struggled with an ongoing identity of being infertile and experienced joys and challenges as they negotiated that transition.

Implications

Nurses and other providers should endeavor to optimize the health and wellness of fathers during the perinatal period after infertility. To limit negative, stressful, and traumatic experiences, they should listen to and advocate for fathers, include them in care, and use a trauma-informed, family-centered approach (Government of Canada, 2018; Public Health Agency of Canada, 2022). Providers need to encourage a shift from a mother–infant focus to an inclusive care plan that includes fathers. They should offer coping resources about perinatal loss, psychosocial support and counseling to cope with the perinatal experience after infertility, education about how to support their partners, and education about the cesarean birth experience. Providers should work with fathers to develop required resources and advocate for local infertility services.

Researchers should use an equity, diversity, and inclusion lens in future research regarding the phenomenon. They should conduct studies about the unique journey, the rollercoaster of emotions and coping strategies, the labor and birth experience, and the experience of being forgotten and fearing loss, which would offer further insight about the phenomenon and could help personnel develop support initiatives for fathers who experience infertility. This may also provide clarity about the similarities and differences between fathers' experiences after infertility and those whose partners conceive naturally. There is an evident lack of consistency about fathers' mental health experiences and how these are affected by or how they influence the phenomenon. Therefore, researchers should conduct additional qualitative studies to explore what all fathers require to feel included and supported during the perinatal period, including those who experience infertility and perinatal loss.

Research with various cultures is needed to enhance our understanding of the potential cultural diversity of this phenomenon. We focused on fathers; however, researchers could focus on the experience for individuals with various sexual and gender identities who most likely have unique experiences and individual support needs.

> **Fathers need to be included, given a voice, and offered support during perinatal care after infertility.**

Limitations

Participants' experiences may have been influenced by the limited access to some infertility services, which potentially reduces transferability. The settings of some interviews created challenges such as distractions, and the variety of methods used to interview may have decreased data quality. Additionally, participants were relatively homogenous with respect to culture, education, and socioeconomic status; this may also limit transferability.

Conclusion

It was evident that the perinatal experience after infertility was significant for our participants. They shared their long, unique journeys that were essential parts of their lives and expressed how important it was to listen to, involve, and support them through the perinatal period. Without this, fathers will continue to endure inequitable care and support and feel forgotten. Nurses and other health care personnel have a responsibility to enhance the experience for all fathers. They must value men's perspectives to facilitate more evidence-based, comprehensive, family-centered care to promote positive experiences and overall family health. Fathers require education regarding how to best support their partners, and there is an ongoing need to conduct research with fathers and to develop evidence-based programming and resources to assist them through the perinatal period after infertility.

CONFLICT OF INTEREST

The authors report no conflict of interest or relevant financial relationships.

FUNDING

None.

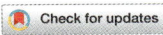

REFERENCES

Allan, H., Mounce, G., Culley, L., van den Akker, O., & Hudson, R. (2019). Transition to parenthood after successful non-donor in vitro fertilization: The effects of infertility and in vitro fertilization on previously infertile couples' experiences of early parenthood. *Health*, *25*(4), 434–453. https://doi.org/10.1177/1363459319891215

Allan, H., van den Akker, O., Culley, L., Mounce, G., Odelius, A., & Symon, A. (2021). An integrative literature review of psychosocial factors in the transition to parenthood following non-donor-assisted reproduction compared with spontaneously conceiving couples. *Human Fertility, 24*(4), 249–266. https://doi.org/10.1080/14647273.2019.1640901

Arya, S. T., & Dibb, B. (2016). The experience of infertility treatment: The male perspective. *Human Fertility, 19*(4), 242–248. https://doi.org/10.1080/14647273.2016.1222083

Centers for Disease Control and Prevention. (2023). *Reproductive health*. https://www.cdc.gov/reproductivehealth/Infertility/

Colaizzi, P. F. (1978). Psychological research as the phenomenologist views it. In R. S. Valle & M. King (Eds.), *Existential-phenomenological alternatives for psychology* (pp. 48–71). Oxford University Press.

Eggermont, K., Beeckman, D., Van Hecke, A., Delbaere, I., & Verhaeghe, S. (2017). Needs of fathers during labour and childbirth: A cross-sectional study. *Women and Birth, 30*(4), e188–e197. https://doi.org/10.1016/j.wombi.2016.12.001

Elmir, R., & Schmied, V. (2016). A meta-ethnographic synthesis of fathers' experiences of complicated births that are potentially traumatic. *Midwifery, 32*, 66–74. https://doi.org/10.1016/j.midw.2015.09.008

Feenstra, M. M., Nilsson, I., & Danbjorg, D. B. (2018). "Dad – A practical guy in the shadow": Fathers' experiences of their paternal role as a father during early discharge after birth and readmission of their newborns. *Sexual & Reproductive Healthcare, 15*, 62–68. https://doi.org/10.1016/j.srhc.2017.11.006

Foyston, Z., Higgins, L., Smith, D. M., & Wittkowski, A. (2023). Parents' experiences of life after medicalized conception: A thematic meta-synthesis of the qualitative literature. *BMC Pregnancy and Childbirth, 23*, Article 520. https://doi.org/10.1186/s12884-023-05727-x

Government of Canada. (2018). *Trauma and violence-informed approaches to policy and practice*. https://www.canada.ca/en/public-health/services/publications/health-risks-safety/trauma-violence-informed-approaches-policy-practice.html#s7

Hanna, E., & Gough, B. (2016). Emoting infertility online: A qualitative analysis of men's forum posts. *Health, 20*(4), 363–382. https://doi.org/10.1177/1363459316649765

Hanna, E., & Gough, B. (2017). Men's accounts of infertility within their intimate partner relationships: An analysis of online forum discussions. *Journal of Reproductive & Infant Psychology, 35*(2), 150–158. https://doi.org/10.1080/02646838.2017.1278749

Hanna, E., & Gough, B. (2019). The impact of infertility on men's work and finances: Findings from a qualitative questionnaire study. *Gender, Work & Organization, 27*(4), 581–591. https://doi.org/10.1111/gwao.12414

Harlow, A. F., Zheng, A., Nordberg, J., Harch, E. E., Ransbotham, S., & Wise, L. A. (2020). A qualitative study of factors influencing male participation in fertility research. *Reproductive Health, 17*, Article 186. https://doi.org/10.1186/s12978-020-01046-y

Herrera, F. (2013). "Men always adopt": Infertility and reproduction from a male perspective. *Journal of Family Issues, 34*(8), 1059–1080. https://doi.org/10.1177/0192513X13484278

Husserl, E. (1931). *Ideas: General introduction to pure phenomenology* (W. R. B. Gibson, Trans.). Macmillan.

Kowlessar, O., Fox, J. R., & Wittkowski, A. (2015). The pregnant male: A metasynthesis of first-time fathers' experiences of pregnancy. *Journal of Reproductive and Infant Psychology, 33*(2), 106–127. https://doi.org/10.1080/02646838.2014.970153

Lincoln, Y. S., & Guba, E. G. (1985). *Naturalistic inquiry*. Sage Publications.

Mayo Clinic. (2021). *Infertility*. https://www.mayoclinic.org/diseases-conditions/infertility/symptoms-causes/syc-20354317

Morse, J. M. (2015). "Data were saturated . . . ". *Qualitative Health Research, 25*(5), 587–588. https://doi.org/10.1177/1049732315576699

Munhall, P. L. (1994). *Revisioning phenomenology: Nursing and health science research*. National League for Nursing Press.

Orit Taubman, B. A., Skvirsky, V., Shua, E. T., & Horowitz, R. (2017). Satisfaction in life among fathers following fertility treatment. *Journal of Reproductive and Infant Psychology, 35*(4), 334–341. https://doi.org/10.1080/02646838.2017.1342787

Polit, D. F., & Beck, C. T. (2021). *Nursing research: Generating and assessing evidence for nursing practice* (11th ed.). Wolters Kluwer.

Public Health Agency of Canada. (2022). *Family-centered maternity and newborn care: National guidelines*. https://www.canada.ca/en/public-health/services/maternity-newborn-care-guidelines.html

Society of Obstetricians and Gynaecologists of Canada. (2023). *Before you conceive: Fertility*. https://www.pregnancyinfo.ca/before-you-conceive/fertility/

Vallin, E., Nestander, H., & Wells, M. B. (2019). A literature review and meta-ethnography of fathers' psychological health and received social support during unpredictable complicated childbirths. *Midwifery, 68*, 48–55. https://doi.org/10.1016/j.midw.2018.10.007

Vander Borght, M., & Wyns, C. (2018). Fertility and infertility: Definition and epidemiology. *Clinical Biochemistry, 62*, 2–10. https://doi.org/10.1016/j.clinbiochem.2018.03.012

Vanska, M., Punamaki, R. L., Tolvanen, A., Lindblom, J., Flykt, M., Unkila-Kallio, L., ... Tiitinen, A. (2017). Paternal mental health trajectory classes and early fathering experiences: Prospective study on a normative and formerly infertile sample. *International Journal of Behavioral Development, 41*(5), 570–580. https://doi.org/10.1177/0165025416654301

World Health Organization. (2023). *Infertility prevalence estimates 1990-2021*.

Reprinted from Morrison, S., Bryanton, J., Murray, C., & Foley, V. (2024). Lived experiences of fatherhood after infertility. Journal of Obstetric, Gynecologic & Neonatal Nursing, 53(3), 245-254. Copyright © 2023 AWHONN, the Association of Women's Health, Obstetric and Neonatal Nurses. With permission.

GLOSSARY

Note: A few entries in this glossary were not explained in this book but are included here because you might come across them in the research literature. These entries are marked with an asterisk (*).

5 As Five steps that are undertaken in an evidence-based practice project: Ask a well-worded question; Acquire best evidence; Appraise the evidence; Apply the evidence to clinical practice; and Assess the outcome.

5 Whys A process involving rounds of successive questioning; used in some quality improvement (QI) projects to gain insight into the root cause of a problem.

Absolute risk (AR) The proportion of people in a group who experienced an undesirable outcome.

Absolute risk reduction (ARR) The difference between the AR in one group (e.g., those exposed to an intervention) and the AR in another group (e.g., those not exposed).

Abstract A brief description of a study, usually located at the beginning of a report.

Accessible population The population available for a study; often a nonrandom subset of the target population.

Acquiescence response set A bias in self-report instruments, especially in psychosocial scales, that occurs when participants characteristically agree with statements ("yea-say"), independent of item content.

Aggregative review A type of review that involves the pooling of findings (i.e., themes, categories, or processes) across qualitative studies in a systematic review.

AGREE II A widely used instrument (Appraisal of Guidelines for Research and Evaluation) for assessing clinical practice guidelines, updated in 2017.

*Allocation concealment The process used to ensure that the people who enroll participants into a clinical trial are unaware of upcoming assignments to treatment conditions.

Alpha (α) (1) In tests of statistical significance, the significance criterion—the risk the researcher is willing to accept of making a Type I error (a false positive); (2) in measurement, an index of internal consistency, that is, Cronbach's alpha.

Analysis The organization and synthesis of data so as to answer research questions or test hypotheses.

Analysis of covariance (ANCOVA) A statistical procedure used to test mean group differences on an outcome variable while controlling for one or more covariates.

Analysis of variance (ANOVA) A statistical procedure for testing mean differences among three or more groups by comparing variability between groups to variability within groups, yielding an F-ratio statistic.

Ancestry approach In literature searches, using citations in relevant studies to track down earlier research on which the studies were based (the "ancestors").

Anonymity Protection of participants' confidentiality such that even the researcher cannot link individuals with the data they provided.

Applicability The degree to which research evidence can be applied to individuals, small groups of individuals, or local contexts (as opposed to broad populations).

*****Applied research** Research conducted to find a solution to an immediate practical problem.

Argument An explanation of what a researcher wants to study, with supportive evidence and background material linked in a manner that provides a rationale.

*****Arm** A particular treatment group to which participants are allocated (e.g., the control *arm* or treatment *arm* of a controlled trial).

*****Ascertainment bias** Systematic differences between groups being compared in how outcome variables are measured, verified, or recorded when data collectors have not been blinded; also called *detection bias*.

Assent The affirmative agreement of a vulnerable person (e.g., a child) to participate in a study, typically to supplement formal consent by a parent or guardian.

Associative relationship An association between two variables that cannot be described as causal.

Assumption A principle that is accepted as being true based on logic or reason, without proof.

Asymmetric distribution A distribution of data values that is skewed, with two halves that are not mirror images of each other.

*****Attention control group** A control group that gets a similar amount of attention as those in the intervention group, without receiving the "active ingredients" of the treatment.

Attrition The loss of participants over the course of a study, which can create bias by changing the composition of the sample initially drawn.

Audit trail In a qualitative study, the systematic documentation of decisions, procedures, and data that allows an independent auditor to draw conclusions about trustworthiness.

Authenticity The extent to which qualitative researchers fairly and faithfully show a range of different realities in the collection, analysis, and interpretation of their data.

Autoethnography An ethnographic study in which researchers study their own culture or group.

Axial coding The second level of coding in a grounded theory study using the Corbin and Strauss approach, involving the process of categorizing, recategorizing, and condensing first-level codes by connecting a category and its subcategories.

Baseline data Data collected at an initial measurement (e.g., prior to an intervention) to enable an assessment of changes.

*****Basic research** Research designed to enhance knowledge in a discipline for the sake of knowledge production rather than for solving an immediate problem.

Basic social process (BSP) The central social process emerging through analysis of grounded theory data; a type of *core variable*.

Belmont Report The 1978 report from the National Commission for the Protection of Human Subjects of Biomedical and Behavioral Research that articulated three primary ethical principles on which standards of ethical research conduct are based: beneficence, respect for human dignity, and justice.

Benchmark In measurement, a threshold value on a measure that corresponds to an important value, such as a threshold for interpreting whether a change in scores is meaningful or clinically significant.

Beneficence An ethical principle that involves maximizing benefits for study participants and preventing harm.

Beta (β) (1) In statistical testing, the probability of a Type II error; (2) in multiple regression, the standardized coefficients indicating the relative weights of the predictor variables in the equation.

Bias Any influence that distorts the results of a study and undermines validity or trustworthiness.

Bibliographic database Data files containing bibliographic (reference) information that can be accessed electronically to conduct a literature search.

Bimodal distribution A distribution of data values with two peaks (high frequencies).

Biomarker An objective, quantifiable characteristic of biologic processes.

Biophysiologic measure A measure that includes both in vivo (e.g., measuring blood pressure) and in vitro measurements (e.g., obtaining and testing blood or tissue samples).

Bivariate statistics Statistical analysis of two variables to assess the empirical relationship between them.

Blind review The review of a manuscript or proposal such that neither the author nor the reviewer is identified to the other party.

Blinding The process of preventing those involved in a study (participants, intervention agents, data collectors, or health care providers) from having information that could lead to a bias, particularly information about which treatment group a participant is in; also called *masking*.

Bracketing In descriptive phenomenologic inquiries, the process of identifying and holding in abeyance any preconceived beliefs and opinions about the phenomena under study; also called *epoché*.

Carryover effect The influence that one treatment (or measurement) can have on subsequent treatments/measurements, notably in crossover designs or test–retest reliability assessments.

*__Case study__ A method involving a thorough, in-depth analysis of an individual, group, or other social unit.

Case–control design A nonexperimental design that compares "cases" (people with a specified condition, such as lung cancer) with matched controls (similar people without the condition), to examine differences that could have contributed to "caseness."

*__Categorical variable__ A variable with discrete categories (e.g., blood type) rather than values along a continuum (e.g., weight).

Category system In studies involving observation, the prespecified plan for recording behaviors and events; in qualitative studies, the system developed from the narrative information to organize the data.

Cause In research cause refers to the phenomenon under study (e.g., lack of sleep) and the potential impact it may have (fatigue).

Cause-and-effect (causal) relationship A relationship between two variables wherein the presence or value of one variable (the "cause") determines the presence or value of the other (the "effect").

Cause-probing research Research designed to illuminate the underlying causes of phenomena.

*__Ceiling effect__ An effect resulting from restricted variation above a certain point on a measurement continuum, which constrains true variability and reduces the amount of upward change that is detectable.

Cell The intersection of a row and column in a table with two dimensions, such as a crosstabs table.

Central category The main category or pattern of behavior in grounded theory analysis; sometimes called the *core category*.

Central tendency A statistical index of what is "typical" in a set of scores, derived from the center of the score distribution; indices of central tendency include the mode, median, and mean.

Certificate of Confidentiality A certificate issued by the National Institutes of Health in the United States to protect researchers against forced disclosure of confidential research information.

Change score A person's score difference between two measurements on the same measure, calculated by subtracting the value at one point in time from the value at the second point.

Checklist An instrument used to record observations, typically with a list of behaviors from a category system in the left column and a space for tallying frequency or duration in the right column.

Chi-squared test A statistical test used in various contexts, most often to assess group differences in proportions; symbolized as χ^2.

CINAHL An electronic database for nurses: **C**umulative **I**ndex to **N**ursing and **A**llied **H**ealth **L**iterature.

Clinical nursing research Research designed to generate knowledge to guide nursing practice and to improve the health and quality of life of nurses' patients.

Clinical practice guidelines Practice guidelines that are evidence-based, combining a synthesis and appraisal of research evidence with specific recommendations for clinical decisions.

Clinical significance The practical importance of research results in terms of whether they have genuine, palpable effects on the daily lives of patients or on the health care decisions made on their behalf.

Clinical trial A study designed to assess the safety, efficacy, and effectiveness of a new clinical intervention, often involving several phases (e.g., Phase III typically is a *randomized controlled trial* [RCT] using an experimental design).

Closed-ended question A question that offers respondents a set of specified response options.

Cluster randomization The random assignment of intact units or organizations (e.g., hospitals), rather than individuals, to treatment conditions.

Cochrane Collaboration An international organization that aims to facilitate well-informed decisions about health care by preparing systematic reviews of the effects of health care interventions.

Code of ethics The fundamental ethical principles established by a discipline or institution to guide researchers' conduct in research with human (or animal) participants.

Coding scheme The process of transforming raw data into standardized form for data processing and analysis; in quantitative research, the process of attaching numbers to categories; in qualitative research, the process of identifying recurring words, themes, or concepts within the data.

Coefficient alpha The most widely used index of internal consistency that indicates the degree to which the items on a multi-item scale are measuring the same underlying construct; also referred to as *Cronbach's alpha*.

Coercion In a research context, the explicit or implicit use of threats (or excessive rewards) to gain people's cooperation in a study.

Cohen's kappa See *kappa*.

Cohort design A nonexperimental design in which a defined group of people (a cohort) is followed over time to study outcomes for subsets of the cohorts; also called a *prospective design*.

Comparative effectiveness research (CER) A patient-centered research approach that focuses on comparisons of alternative treatments to identify which leads to the greatest health improvements.

Comparison group A group of study participants whose scores on outcomes are used to evaluate the outcomes of the group of primary interest (e.g., nonsmokers as a comparison group for smokers); term often used in lieu of *control group* when the study is not a randomized experiment.

Complex hypothesis A hypothesis statement with multiple independent or dependent variables.

Complex intervention An intervention in which complexity exists along one or more dimensions, including number of components, number of targeted outcomes, and the time needed for the full intervention to be delivered.

Composite scale A measure of an attribute, involving the aggregation of responses from multiple items into a single numerical score that places people on a continuum with respect to the attribute.

Concealment A tactic involving the unobtrusive collection of research data without participants' knowledge or consent, used to obtain an accurate view of naturalistic behavior when the behavior would be distorted if participants knew they were being observed.

Concept An abstraction based on observation or self-reporting of behaviors or characteristics (e.g., fatigue, pain).

Concept analysis A systematic process of analyzing a concept or construct, with the aim of identifying the boundaries, definitions, and dimensionality for that concept.

Conceptual definition The abstract or theoretical meaning of a concept of interest.

Conceptual files A manual method of organizing qualitative data, by creating file folders for each category in the coding scheme and inserting relevant excerpts from the data.

Conceptual framework See *framework*.

Conceptual map A schematic representation of a theory or conceptual model that graphically represents key concepts and linkages among them; also called a *schematic model*.

Conceptual model Interrelated concepts assembled in a rational and often explanatory scheme to illuminate relationships but less formally than a theory; sometimes called a *conceptual framework*.

Concurrent design A mixed methods study design in which the qualitative and quantitative strands of data collection occur simultaneously; symbolically designated with a plus sign (e.g., QUAL + QUAN).

*****Concurrent validity** A type of criterion validity that concerns the degree to which scores on a measure are correlated with an external criterion, measured at the same time.

Confidence interval (CI) The range of values within which a population parameter is estimated to lie, at a specified probability (e.g., 95% CI).

Confidentiality Protection of study participants' privacy, such that data they provide are never publicly identified and divulged.

Confirmability A criterion for trustworthiness in a qualitative inquiry, referring to the objectivity or neutrality of the data and interpretations.

Confounding variable A variable that is extraneous to the research question and that confounds the relationship between the independent and dependent variables; confounding variables can be controlled in the research design or through statistical procedures.

Consecutive sampling The recruitment of *all* people from an accessible population who meet the eligibility criteria over a specific time interval or for a specified sample size.

Consent form A written agreement signed by a study participant and a researcher concerning the terms and conditions of voluntary participation in a study.

CONSORT guidelines Widely adopted guidelines (Consolidated Standards of Reporting Trials) for reporting information for an RCT, including a checklist and a flow chart for tracking participants through the trial.

Constant comparison A procedure used in qualitative analysis (especially in grounded theory) wherein newly collected data are compared in an ongoing fashion with data obtained earlier, to refine theoretically relevant categories.

Construct An abstraction or concept that is invented (constructed) by researchers based on inferences from human behavior or human traits (e.g., health locus of control).

Construct validity The degree to which evidence about study particulars supports inferences about the higher order constructs they are intended to represent; in measurement, the degree to which a measure truly captures the focal construct.

Constructivist grounded theory An approach to grounded theory, developed by Charmaz, in which the grounded theory is constructed from shared experiences and relationships between the researcher and study participants and interpretive aspects are emphasized.

Constructivist paradigm An alternative paradigm to the positivist paradigm that holds that there are multiple interpretations of reality, and that the goal of research is to understand how individuals construct reality within their context; associated with qualitative research; also called *naturalistic paradigm*.

Contamination of treatments The inadvertent, biasing influence of one treatment on another treatment condition, for example, when control group members unintentionally receive all or part of the intervention being tested.

Content analysis An approach to extracting, organizing, and synthesizing material from written materials, including transcripts of narrative data from a qualitative study, according to key concepts and themes.

Content validity The degree to which a multi-item measure has an appropriate set of relevant items reflecting the full content of the construct domain being measured.

Content validity index (CVI) An index of the degree to which an instrument is content valid, based on ratings of a panel of experts; content validity for individual items and the overall scale can be assessed.

Continuous quality improvement An approach to health care that involves an environment in which management and staff strive to constantly improve quality.

Continuous variable A variable that can take on an infinite range of values along a specified continuum (e.g., height); less strictly, a variable measured on an interval or ratio scale.

Control group Participants in a clinical trial who do not receive the experimental intervention and whose performance provides a counterfactual against which the effects of an intervention can be measured.

Control, research Procedures used to hold constant confounding influences on the dependent variable (the outcome) under study.

Controlled trial A trial of an intervention that includes a control group, with or without randomization.

Convenience sampling Selection of the most readily available persons as participants in a study.

Convergent design A convergent, equal-priority mixed methods design in which different but complementary data, qualitative and quantitative, are gathered about a central phenomenon under study; symbolized as QUAL + QUAN.

Core category (variable) In a grounded theory study, the central phenomenon that is used to integrate all categories of the data.

Correlation A bond or association between variables, such that variation in one variable is systematically related to variation in another.

Correlation coefficient An index summarizing the degree of relationship between variables, typically ranging from +1.00 (for a perfect positive relationship) through .0 (for no relationship) to −1.00 (for a perfect negative relationship).

Correlation matrix A two-dimensional display showing the correlation coefficients between all pairs of variables in a set of three or more variables.

Correlational research Nonexperimental research that explores the interrelationships among variables of interest, with no researcher intervention.

Correlational studies Studies conducted to examine the relationship between two variables.

Cost (economic) analysis An analysis of the relationship between costs and outcomes of nursing or other health care interventions.

*Counterbalancing The process of systematically varying the order of presentation of stimuli or treatments to control for ordering effects, especially in a crossover design.

Counterfactual The condition or group used as a basis of comparison in a study, embodying what would have happened *to the same people* exposed to a causal factor if they *simultaneously* were *not* exposed to it.

Covariate A variable that is statistically controlled in ANCOVA; typically, a confounding influence on, or a preintervention measure of, the outcome.

Covert data collection The collection of information in a study without participants' knowledge.

Credibility A criterion for evaluating trustworthiness in qualitative studies, referring to confidence in the truth of the data; analogous to internal validity in quantitative research.

Criterion validity The extent to which scores on a measure are an adequate reflection of (or predictor of) a criterion that is considered a "gold standard" measure.

Critical appraisal An objective assessment of a study's strengths, limitations, and relevance, often to reach a conclusion about whether its evidence can be applied to practice.

Critical ethnography An ethnography that focuses on raising consciousness in the group or culture under study in the hope of effecting social change.

Critical theory An approach to viewing the world that involves a critique of society, with the goal of envisioning new possibilities and effecting social change.

Critique A critical appraisal that analyzes both weaknesses and strengths of a research report, often to assess its potential for publication; see also *critical appraisal*.

Cronbach's alpha A widely used index that estimates the internal consistency of a composite measure composed of several subparts (e.g., items); also called *coefficient alpha*.

Crossover design An experimental design in which one group of participants is exposed to more than one condition or treatment, in random order.

Cross-sectional design A study design in which data are collected at one point in time; sometimes used to infer change over time when data are collected from different age or developmental groups.

Crosstabs table A two-dimensional table in which the frequencies of two categorical variables are crosstabulated.

Crosstabulation A calculation of frequencies for two variables considered simultaneously—for example, gender (male/female/other) crosstabulated with smoking status (smoker/nonsmoker).

***d* statistic** An effect size index for comparing two group means, computed by subtracting one mean from the other and dividing by the pooled standard deviation; also called *Cohen's d* or *standardized mean difference*.

Data The pieces of information obtained in a study (singular is *datum*).

Data analysis The systematic organization and synthesis of research data and, in quantitative studies, the testing of hypotheses using those data.

Data collection protocols The formal procedures researchers develop to guide the collection of data in a standardized fashion.

Data saturation The collection of qualitative data to the point where a sense of closure is attained because new data yield redundant information.

Data set The total collection of data on all variables for all study participants.

Data triangulation The use of multiple data sources for the purpose of validating conclusions.

Debriefing Communication with study participants after participation is complete regarding aspects of the study (e.g., explaining the study purpose more fully).

Deception The deliberate withholding of information, or the provision of false information, to study participants, usually to reduce potential biases.

Deductive reasoning The process of developing specific predictions from general principles; see also *inductive reasoning*.

Degrees of freedom (*df*) A statistical concept referring to the number of sample values free to vary (e.g., with a given sample mean, all but one value would be free to vary).

Delayed treatment design A design for an intervention study that involves putting control group members on a waiting list to receive the intervention after follow-up data are collected; also called a *wait-list design*.

Delphi survey A technique for obtaining judgments from an expert panel about an issue of concern; experts are questioned individually in several rounds, with a summary of the panel's views circulated between rounds, to achieve some consensus.

Dependability A criterion for evaluating integrity in qualitative studies, referring to the stability of data over time and over conditions; analogous to reliability in quantitative research.

Dependent variable The variable hypothesized to depend on or be caused by the independent variable; the outcome of interest.

Descendancy approach In literature searches, finding a pivotal early study and searching forward in citation indexes to find more recent studies ("descendants") that cited the key study.

Description question A question aimed at describing a health-related phenomenon.

Descriptive phenomenology An approach to phenomenology that focuses on the careful description of ordinary conscious experiences of everyday life.

Descriptive qualitative study An in-depth study that involves the collection of rich, qualitative data but does not have roots in a particular qualitative tradition; data are often analyzed using content analysis or thematic analysis.

Descriptive research Research that has as a primary objective the accurate portrayal of people's characteristics or circumstances and/or the frequency with which certain phenomena occur.

Descriptive statistics Statistics used to describe and summarize data (e.g., means, percentages).

Descriptive theory A broad characterization that thoroughly accounts for a phenomenon.

Determinism The belief that phenomena are not haphazard or random but rather have antecedent causes; an assumption in the positivist paradigm.

Diagnosis/assessment question A question about the accuracy and validity of instruments to screen, diagnose, or assess patients.

Dichotomous question A question with only two response alternatives (e.g., yes/no).

Directional hypothesis A hypothesis that makes a specific prediction about the direction of the relationship between two variables.

Disconfirming case In qualitative research, a case that challenges the researchers' conceptualizations; sometimes sought as part of a sampling strategy.

Domain In ethnographic analysis, a unit or broad category of cultural knowledge.

*****Dose–response analysis** An analysis to assess whether larger doses of an intervention are associated with greater benefits.

Double-blind study A clinical trial in which two sets of people are blinded with respect to the group that a study participant is in; often a situation in which neither the participants nor those administering the treatment know who is in the intervention or control group.

Economic (cost) analysis An analysis of the relationship between costs and outcomes of alternative health care interventions.

Effect size (ES) A statistical index expressing the magnitude of the relationship between two variables, or the magnitude of the difference between groups on an attribute of interest (e.g., Cohen's *d*); also used in meta-summaries of qualitative research to characterize the salience of a theme or category.

Effectiveness study A clinical trial designed to test the effectiveness of an intervention under ordinary conditions, usually for an intervention already found to be efficacious in an efficacy study.

*****Efficacy study** A tightly controlled trial designed to establish the efficacy of an intervention under ideal conditions, using a design that maximizes internal validity; sometimes called an *explanatory trial*.

Element The most basic unit of a population for sampling purposes, typically a human being.

Eligibility criteria The criteria designating the specific attributes of the target population, by which people are selected for inclusion in a study or excluded from it.

Emergent design A design that unfolds in the course of a qualitative study as the researcher makes ongoing design decisions reflecting what has already been learned.

Emergent fit A concept in grounded theory that involves comparing new data and new categories with previous conceptualizations.

Emic perspective An ethnographic term referring to the way members of a culture view their own world; the "insider's view."

Empirical evidence Evidence rooted in objective reality and gathered using one's senses as the basis for generating knowledge.

Estimation of parameters Statistical procedures that estimate population parameters based on sample statistics.

Ethical dilemma A situation in which there is a conflict between ethical principles and the research methods needed to maximize the quality of study evidence.

Ethics In research, a system of moral values that concerns the degree to which research procedures adhere to professional, legal, and social obligations to study participants.

Ethnography A branch of human inquiry, associated with anthropology, that focuses on the culture of a group of people, with an effort to understand the worldview and customs of those under study.

Ethnonursing research A term coined by Leininger to denote the study of human cultures, with a focus on a group's beliefs and practices relating to nursing care and related health behaviors.

Etic perspective In ethnography, the "outsider's view" of the experiences of a cultural group.

Etiology (causation)/harm question A question about the underlying cause of a health problem, such as an environmental cause or personal behavior (e.g., smoking).

Evaluation research Research aimed at learning how well a program, practice, or policy is working.

Event sampling A type of observational sampling that involves the selection of integral behaviors or events to be observed.

Evidence hierarchy A ranked arrangement of the strength of research evidence based on the rigor of the method that produced it; traditional evidence hierarchies are appropriate primarily for cause-probing research.

Evidence-based practice (EBP) A practice that involves making clinical decisions based on clinical judgment, patient preferences, and on the best available evidence, usually evidence from disciplined research.

Exclusion criteria Criteria specifying characteristics that a target population does *not* have stipulated for the purpose of determining eligibility for a study sample.

Expectation bias The bias that can arise when participants (or research staff) have expectations about treatment effectiveness in intervention research; the expectation can result in altered behavior.

Experiment A true experiment has three elements: an intervention, a control (group), and randomization.

Experimental group The study participants who receive an experimental treatment or intervention.

Experimental research Research using a design in which the researcher controls (manipulates) the independent variable by randomly assigning people to different treatment groups; RCTs use experimental designs.

***Explanatory mixed methods design** A sequential mixed methods design in which quantitative data are collected in the first phase and qualitative data are collected in the second phase to build on or explain quantitative findings.

Explanatory trial A traditional clinical trial, conducted under optimal conditions with carefully selected participants, to enhance internal validity.

Exploratory mixed methods design A sequential mixed methods design in which qualitative data are collected in the first phase and quantitative data are collected in the second phase based on the initial in-depth exploration.

External validity The degree to which study results can be generalized to people or settings other than the one studied.

Extraneous variable A variable that confounds the relationship between the independent and dependent variables and that needs to be controlled either in the research design or through statistical procedures; often called *confounding variable*.

Extreme response set A bias resulting from a respondent's consistent selection of extreme alternatives (e.g., *strongly agree* or *strongly disagree*) to scale items, regardless of item content.

***F* ratio** The statistic obtained in several statistical tests (e.g., ANOVA) in which variation in the outcome that is attributable to different sources (e.g., between groups and within groups) is compared.

Face validity The extent to which an instrument looks as though it is measuring what it purports to measure.

*Factor analysis A statistical procedure for disentangling complex interrelationships among items and identifying the items that "go together" as a unified dimension.

Feminist research Research that seeks to understand how gender and a gendered social order shape women's lives and their consciousness.

Field diary A daily record of events and conversations in the field; also called a *log*.

Field notes The notes recorded by researchers to document the unstructured observations made in the field and the interpretation of those observations.

Field research Research in which the data are collected "in the field," that is, in naturalistic settings.

Fieldwork The activities undertaken by qualitative researchers (especially ethnographers) to collect data out in the field, that is, in natural settings.

Findings The results of the analysis of research data.

Fit An element in Glaserian grounded theory analysis in which the researcher develops categories of a substantive theory that fit the data.

Fixed effects model In meta-analysis, a statistical model in which studies are assumed to be measuring the same overall effect; a pooled effect estimate is calculated under the assumption that observed variation between studies is attributable to chance.

Focus group interview An interview with a small group of individuals assembled to discuss a specific topic, usually guided by a moderator using a semi-structured topic guide.

Focused interview A loosely structured interview in which an interviewer guides the respondent through a set of questions using a topic guide; also called a *semi-structured interview*.

Follow-up study A study undertaken to assess the outcomes of individuals with a specified condition or who have received a specified treatment.

Forest plot A graphic representation of effects across studies in a meta-analysis, permitting a visual assessment of variation in effects across studies (i.e., heterogeneity).

Framework The conceptual underpinnings of a study—e.g., a *theoretical framework* in theory-based studies, or *conceptual framework* in studies based on a conceptual model.

Frequency distribution A systematic array of numeric values from the lowest to the highest, together with a count of the number of times each value was obtained.

Frequency effect size In a meta-summary of qualitative studies, the percentage of reports that contain a given thematic finding.

Full disclosure The communication of complete, accurate information about a study to potential study participants.

Functional relationship A relationship between two variables in which it cannot be assumed that one variable caused the other.

Gaining entrée The process of gaining access to study participants through the cooperation of key gatekeepers in a selected community or site.

Generalizability The degree to which the research methods justify the inference that the findings are true for a broader group than study participants; in particular, the inference that the findings can be generalized from the sample to the population.

GRADE The **G**rades of **R**ecommendation, **A**ssessment, **D**evelopment, and **E**valuation, an approach to grading confidence in findings from a systematic review.

Grand theory A broad theory aimed at describing and explaining large segments of the physical, social, or behavioral world; also called a *macrotheory*.

Grand tour question A broad question asked in an unstructured interview to gain a general overview of a phenomenon, on the basis of which more focused questions are subsequently asked.

Gray literature Unpublished and thus less readily accessible research reports (e.g., dissertations).

Grounded theory An approach to collecting and analyzing qualitative data that aims to develop theories about social psychological processes grounded in real-world observations.

Hawthorne effect The effect on the outcome resulting from people's awareness that they are participants under study.

Health services research The broad interdisciplinary field that studies how organizational structures and processes, health technologies, social factors, and personal behaviors affect access to health care, the cost and quality of health care, and, ultimately, people's health and well-being.

Hermeneutic circle In hermeneutics, the process in which, to reach understanding, there is continual movement between the parts and the whole of the text that is being analyzed.

Hermeneutics A qualitative research tradition, drawing on interpretive phenomenology, that focuses on the lived experiences of humans and on how they interpret those experiences.

Heterogeneity The degree to which objects are dissimilar (characterized by variability) on an attribute.

Heterogeneity of treatment effects (HTE) Variation in the effectiveness of an intervention across a population—that is, the intervention's benefits (or harms) are not universal.

Historical research Systematic studies designed to discover facts and relationships about past events.

History threat The occurrence of events external to an intervention but concurrent with it, which can affect the outcome variable and threaten the study's internal validity.

Homogeneity The degree to which people or objects are similar (i.e., characterized by low variability) on an attribute; sometimes used as a design strategy used to control confounding variables.

Hypothesis A statement of predicted relationships between variables.

Hypothesis testing Statistical procedures for testing whether hypotheses should be accepted or rejected, based on the probability that hypothesized relationships in a sample exist in the population.

Hypothesis-testing validity The extent to which one can corroborate hypotheses regarding how scores on a measure function in relation to scores on measures of other variables; an aspect of construct validity.

*Implementation potential The extent to which an innovation is amenable to implementation in a new setting; implementation potential is sometimes assessed prior to EBP projects.

Implied consent Consent to participate in a study that a researcher assumes has been given based on participants' actions, such as returning a completed questionnaire.

Improvement science An emerging field that focuses on explorations of how to accelerate QI and do it rigorously.

IMRaD format The organization of a research report into four main sections: the **I**ntroduction, **M**ethod, **R**esults, **a**nd **D**iscussion sections.

*Incidence The rate of new cases with a specified condition, determined by dividing the number of new cases over a given period of time by the number at risk for becoming a new case (i.e., free of the condition at the outset of the time period).

Inclusion criteria The criteria specifying characteristics of a population that a prospective participant must have to be considered eligible for a study.

Independent variable The variable that is believed to cause or influence the dependent variable; in experimental research, the manipulated (treatment) variable; the independent variable is both the "I" and the "C" in the PICO framework.

Inductive reasoning The process of reasoning from specific observations to more general rules (see also *deductive reasoning*).

Inference A conclusion drawn from limited information, using logical reasoning; in research, a conclusion drawn from study evidence, taking into account the methods used to generate that evidence.

Inferential statistics Statistics that are used to make inferences about whether results observed in a sample are likely to be reliable, that is, found in the population.

Informant A person who provides information to researchers about a phenomenon under study; a term used mostly in qualitative studies.

Informed consent A process in the ethical conduct of a study that involves obtaining people's voluntary participation in a study, after informing them of possible risks and benefits.

Inquiry audit An independent scrutiny of qualitative data and relevant supporting documents by an external reviewer to determine their dependability and confirmability.

Insider research Research on a group or culture—usually in an ethnography—by a member of that group or culture; in ethnographic research, an *autoethnography*.

Institutional ethnography A type of ethnography that focuses on social organization and institutional processes.

Institutional Review Board (IRB) A term used primarily in the United States to refer to the institutional group that convenes to review proposed and ongoing studies with respect to ethical considerations.

Instrument The device used to collect data (e.g., a questionnaire or observation checklist).

Intensity effect size In a qualitative meta-summary, the percentage of all thematic findings that are contained in any given report.

***Intention to treat** The gold standard strategy for analyzing data in an intervention study that includes participants with the group to which they were assigned, regardless of whether they received or completed the treatment associated with the group.

Interaction effect The effect of two or more independent variables acting in combination (interactively) on an outcome.

Intercoder reliability The degree to which two coders, working independently, agree on coding decisions.

Internal consistency The degree to which items on a composite scale are interrelated and are measuring the same attribute, usually evaluated using coefficient alpha; a measurement property in the reliability domain.

Internal validity The degree to which it can be inferred that an intervention (the independent variable), rather than confounding factors, caused the observed effects on an outcome.

Interpretive A type of qualitative systematic review in which the goal is to discover new or enriched ways of understanding phenomena.

Interpretive phenomenology A type of phenomenology that stresses interpreting and understanding, not just describing, human experience sometimes referred to as *hermeneutics*.

Interrater (interobserver) reliability The degree to which two raters or observers, working independently, assign the same ratings or scores for an attribute being measured.

Interval estimation A statistical estimation approach in which the researcher computes a range of values that are likely, within a given level of confidence (e.g., a 95% CI), to contain the true population parameter.

Interval measurement A measurement level in which an attribute is rank ordered on a scale that has equal distances between points on that scale (e.g., Fahrenheit degrees).

Intervention In experimental research (clinical trials), the treatment being tested; the "I" in the PICO framework.

Intervention fidelity The extent to which the implementation of a treatment is faithful to its plan.

Intervention protocol The specification of what the intervention and alternative (control) treatment conditions are, how they should be administered, and who should administer them.

Intervention research Research involving the development, implementation, and testing of an intervention.

Intervention theory The conceptual underpinning of a health care intervention, which articulates the theoretical basis for the achievement of desired outcomes.

Interview A data collection method in which an interviewer asks questions of a respondent, either face-to-face, by telephone, or over the Internet (e.g., via Skype).

Interview schedule The formal instrument that specifies the wording of all questions to be asked of respondents in studies in which structured self-report data are collected.

Intraclass correlation coefficient (ICC) A statistical index used to estimate the reliability (e.g., test–retest reliability) of a measure.

Inverse relationship A relationship characterized by the tendency of high values on one variable to be associated with low values on the second variable; also called a *negative relationship*.

Investigator triangulation The use of two or more researchers to analyze and interpret data, to enhance trustworthiness.

Iowa Model of evidence-based practice A widely used framework that can be used to guide the development and implementation of a project to promote EBP.

Item A single question on an instrument, such as on a composite scale.

Journal article A report appearing in professional journals such as *Nursing Research* or *International Journal of Nursing Studies*.

Journal club A group that meets in clinical contexts to discuss and critically appraise research articles published in journals.

Kappa A statistical index of chance-corrected agreement or consistency between two nominal (or ordinal) measurements, often used to assess interrater reliability; also called *Cohen's kappa*.

Key informant A person knowledgeable about the phenomenon of research interest and who is willing to share information and insights with the researcher, most often in ethnographies.

Keyword An important term used to search for references on a topic in bibliographic databases, identified by authors or indexers to enhance the likelihood that the report will be found.

Knowledge translation (KT) The exchange, synthesis, and application of knowledge by relevant stakeholders within complex systems to accelerate the beneficial effects of research aimed at improving health care.

Known-groups validity A type of construct validity that concerns the degree to which a measure can discriminate between groups known or expected to differ with regard to the construct of interest.

Lean approach In QI, a model whose aim is to improve quality and efficiency at lower costs; also called the *Toyota Production System*.

Level of evidence (LOE) A scale that rank orders evidence for cause-probing questions in terms of risk of bias, based on evidence hierarchies; Level I evidence is typically systematic reviews of RCTs.

Level of measurement A system of classifying measurements according to the nature of the measurement and the type of permissible mathematical operations; the levels are nominal, ordinal, interval, and ratio.

Level of significance The risk of making a Type I error in a statistical analysis, with the criterion (alpha) established by the researcher beforehand (e.g., $\alpha = .05$).

Likert scale Traditionally, a type of scale to measure attitudes, involving the summation of scores on a set of items that respondents rate for their degree of agreement or disagreement; more loosely, the name often used for summated rating scales.

Literature review A summary of research on a topic, often prepared to put a research problem in context or to summarize existing evidence; typically, less rigorously conducted than a systematic review.

Log In participant observation studies, the observer's daily record of events and conversations.

Logistic regression A multivariate regression procedure that analyzes relationships between one or more independent (predictor) variables and a categorical dependent variable.

Longitudinal design A study design in which data are collected at more than one point in time, in contrast to a cross-sectional design.

Macrotheory A broad theory aimed at describing large segments of the physical, social, or behavioral world; also called a *grand theory*.

Manifest effect size In meta-summaries, an ES index calculated from the manifest content represented in the findings of primary qualitative studies; includes *frequency effect sizes* and *intensity effect sizes*.

*****Manipulation** The introduction of an intervention or treatment in an experimental or quasi-experimental study to assess its impact on outcomes of interest.

*****MANOVA** See *multivariate analysis of variance*.

Masking See *blinding*.

Matching The pairing of participants in one group with those in a comparison group based on their similarity on one or more attributes, to enhance group comparability.

Maturation threat A threat to the internal validity of a study that results when changes to the outcome variable result from the passage of time.

Maximum variation sampling A sampling approach used by qualitative researchers involving the purposeful selection of cases with wide variation on key attributes.

Mean A measure of central tendency, computed by summing all scores and dividing by the total number of cases.

Meaning/process question A question about what health-related phenomena mean to people or about how a process or experience unfolds.

Measure A device whose purpose is to obtain numerical information to quantify an attribute or construct (e.g., a scale).

Measurement The assignment of numbers to objects according to specified rules to characterize quantities of some attribute.

Measurement error The systematic and random error associated with a person's score on a measure, reflecting factors other than the construct being measured and resulting in an observed score that is different from a hypothetical true score.

Measurement property A characteristic reflecting a distinct aspect of a measure's quality (e.g., reliability, validity).

Median A measure of central tendency; the point in a score distribution above and below which 50% of the cases fall.

Mediating variable A variable that mediates or acts like a "go-between" in a causal chain linking two other variables.

MEDLINE The Medical Literature On-Line database.

Member check A method of validating the credibility of qualitative data through debriefings and discussions with study participants.

MeSH Medical Subject Headings, the system used to index articles in MEDLINE.

Meta-aggregation An approach to the synthesis of qualitative evidence in which findings are categorized and summarized rather than transformed, as in a metasynthesis.

Meta-analysis A technique for quantitatively integrating the results of multiple studies addressing the same or highly similar research question.

Meta-ethnography An approach to integrating findings from qualitative studies by translating and interpreting concepts and metaphors across studies; developed by Noblit and Hare.

Metaphor A figurative comparison used by some qualitative analysts to evoke a visual or symbolic analogy.

Meta-summary A type of qualitative research synthesis that involves the development of a list of abstracted findings from primary studies and calculating manifest ESs.

Metasynthesis An interpretive translation of evidence produced by systematically integrating findings from multiple qualitative studies.

Method triangulation The use of multiple methods of data collection about the same phenomenon, to enhance credibility.

Methodologic study A study designed to develop or refine methods of obtaining, organizing, or analyzing data.

Methods, research The steps, procedures, and strategies for designing a study and gathering and analyzing study data.

Middle-range theory A theory that attempts to explain a piece of reality or human experience, focusing on a limited number of concepts (e.g., a theory of stress).

Minimal important change (MIC) A benchmark for interpreting change scores that represents the smallest change that is meaningful to patients or clinicians and thus establishes clinical significance.

Minimal risk Anticipated risks from study participation that are no greater than those ordinarily encountered in daily life or during the performance of routine tests or procedures.

Mixed methods research Research in which both qualitative and quantitative data are collected and analyzed to address different but related questions.

Mixed studies review A systematic review that integrates and synthesizes findings from qualitative, quantitative, and mixed methods studies on a topic.

Mode A measure of central tendency; the value that occurs most frequently in a distribution of scores.

Model A symbolic representation of concepts or variables and interrelationships among them.

Moderator variable A variable that affects (moderates) the strength or direction of a relationship between the independent variable and the outcome variable; can be detected through subgroup analyses.

Mortality threat A threat to the internal validity of a study, referring to differential attrition (loss of participants) from different groups.

Multimodal distribution A distribution of values with more than one peak (high frequency).

Multiple comparison procedures Statistical tests, normally applied after an ANOVA indicates statistically significant group differences, that compare different pairs of groups; also called *post hoc tests*.

Multiple regression A statistical procedure for understanding the effects of two or more independent (predictor) variables on a dependent variable.

Multistage sampling A sampling strategy that proceeds through stages from larger to smaller sampling units (e.g., from states, to census tracts, to households).

Multivariate analysis of variance (MANOVA) A statistical procedure used to test the significance of differences between the means of two or more groups on two or more dependent variables, considered simultaneously.

Multivariate statistics Statistical procedures designed to analyze the relationships among three or more variables (e.g., multiple regression, ANCOVA).

N The symbol designating the total number of participants (e.g., "the total N was 500").

n The symbol designating the number of subjects in a subgroup or cell of a study (e.g., "each of the four groups had an n of 125, for a total N of 500").

Narrative analysis A qualitative approach that focuses on a person's story as the object of the inquiry.

Naturalistic setting A setting for the collection of research data that is natural to those being studied (e.g., homes, places of work).

Naysayer bias A bias in self-report scales created when respondents characteristically disagree with statements ("naysay"), independent of item content.

Negative case analysis The refinement of a theory or description in a qualitative study through the inclusion of cases that appear to disconfirm earlier hypotheses.

Negative relationship A relationship between two variables in which there is a tendency for high values on one variable to be associated with low values on the other (e.g., as stress increases, quality of life decreases); also called an *inverse relationship*.

Negative skew An asymmetric distribution of data values with a disproportionately high number of cases at the upper end; when displayed graphically, the tail points to the left.

Nested sampling An approach to sampling in mixed methods studies in which some, but not all, of the participants from one strand are included in the sample for the other strand.

Netnography Sometimes called *online ethnography*, netnography focuses on cultural experiences of data from social media environments such as Facebook, Instagram, and blogs. In netnography, online traces are studied, which are what people leave behind online when they post text, images, blogs, etc.

Network sampling The sampling of participants based on referrals from others already in the sample; also called *snowball sampling*.

Nominal measurement The lowest level of measurement involving the assignment of numbers to categories (e.g., 1 = married, 2 = not married).

Nondirectional hypothesis A research hypothesis that does not stipulate the expected direction of the relationship between variables.

Nonequivalent control group design A quasi-experimental design involving a comparison group that was not created through random assignment.

Nonexperimental research Studies in which the researcher collects data without introducing an intervention; also called *observational research*.

Nonexperimental study Studies that describe the phenomena and/or do not manipulate the independent variable due to ethics or it being impossible to do so.

Nonparametric tests A class of statistical tests that do not involve stringent assumptions about the distribution of variables in the analysis.

Nonprobability sampling The selection of elements (e.g., participants) from a population using nonrandom methods (e.g., convenience sampling).

Nonresponse bias A bias that can result when a nonrandom subset of people invited to participate in a study decline to participate.

Nonsignificant result The result of a statistical test indicating that group differences or observed relationships could have occurred by chance, at a given probability level; sometimes abbreviated as *NS*.

Normal distribution A theoretical distribution that is bell-shaped, symmetrical, and not too peaked.

Null hypothesis A hypothesis stating the absence of a relationship between the variables under study; used primarily in statistical testing as the hypothesis to be rejected.

Number needed to treat (NNT) An estimate of how many people would need to receive an intervention to prevent one undesirable outcome, computed by dividing 1 by the value of the ARR.

Nursing research Systematic inquiry designed to develop knowledge about issues of importance to the nursing profession.

Nursing-sensitive outcome A patient outcome that improves if there is greater quantity or quality of nursing care.

Objectivity The extent to which two independent researchers would arrive at similar judgments or conclusions (i.e., judgments not biased by personal values or beliefs).

Observation A method of collecting information and/or measuring constructs by directly watching and recording behaviors and characteristics.

Observational study A study that does not involve an intervention—that is, nonexperimental research in which phenomena are merely observed.

Odds An index that summarizes the probability of an event occurring to the probability that it will not occur, calculated by dividing the number of people who experienced an event by the number who did not.

Odds ratio (OR) The ratio of one odds to another odds, e.g., the ratio of the odds of an event in one group to the odds of an event in another group; an OR of 1.0 indicates no difference between groups.

Open coding The first level of coding in a grounded theory study, referring to the basic descriptive coding of the content of narrative materials.

Open-access journal A journal that allows free online access to articles, without user subscription costs; traditional journals may include some articles that are open-access.

Open-ended question A question in an interview or questionnaire that does not restrict respondents' answers to predetermined response options.

Operational definition The definition of a concept or variable in terms of the procedures by which it is to be measured.

Operationalization The process of translating research concepts into measurable phenomena.

Ordinal measurement A measurement level that involves sorting people (or objects) based on their relative ranking on an attribute.

Outcome variable A term often used to refer to the dependent variable, that is, the outcome (endpoint) of interest; the "O" in the PICO framework.

Outcomes research Research designed to document the effectiveness of health care services and the end results of patient care.

p In statistical testing, the probability that the obtained results are due to chance; the probability of a Type I error.

Paradigm A way of looking at natural phenomena—a worldview—that encompasses a set of philosophical assumptions that guides one's approach to inquiry.

Paradigm case In Benner's hermeneutic analysis, a strong exemplar of the phenomenon under study, often used early in the analysis to gain understanding of the phenomenon.

Parameter A characteristic of a population (e.g., the mean age of all registered nurses [RNs]).

Parameter estimation An estimation used to estimate a population parameter—for example, a mean, a proportion, or a difference in means between two groups.

Parametric tests A class of statistical tests that involve assumptions about the distribution of the variables and the estimation of a parameter.

Participant See *study participant*.

Participant observation A method of collecting data through the participation in and observation of a group or culture, most often used in ethnographies.

Participatory action research (PAR) A research approach used with groups or communities that is based on the premise that the use and production of knowledge can be political and used to exert power.

***Path analysis** A regression-based procedure for testing causal models, typically using correlational data.

Patient centeredness A focus, in both health care and research, on individual patients' needs and values, including involving patients in care decisions and research priorities.

Patient-centered research Research that focuses on the development of evidence that is important and relevant to patients, especially about outcomes of special concern to them (e.g., quality of life).

Patient-reported outcomes (PRO) research A health outcome that is measured by directly asking patients for information.

Pearson's *r* A correlation coefficient designating the magnitude of relationship between two interval- or ratio-level variables; also called *the product–moment correlation*.

Peer debriefing A session with peers to review and explore various aspects of a study, often used to enhance trustworthiness in a qualitative study.

Peer reviewer A researcher who reviews and critiques a research report or proposal and makes a recommendation about publishing or funding the research.

***Per protocol analysis** Analysis of data from an RCT that excludes participants who did not obtain the protocol to which they were assigned (or who received an incomplete dose of the intervention).

Perfect relationship A correlation between two variables such that the values of one variable can perfectly predict the values of the other; designated as 1.00 or −1.00.

Persistent observation A qualitative researcher's intense focus on the aspects of a situation that are relevant to the phenomena being studied.

Person triangulation The collection of data from different levels or types of persons, with the aim of validating data through multiple perspectives on the phenomenon.

Phenomenology A qualitative research tradition, with roots in philosophy and psychology, that focuses on the lived experience of humans.

Phenomenon The abstract concept under study; term often used by qualitative researchers in lieu of *variable*.

Photo-elicitation An interview stimulated and guided by photographic images.

Photovoice A technique used in some qualitative studies that involves asking participants to take photographs of their culture or environment and then interpret the photos.

PICO format A framework for asking well-worded questions and for searching for evidence, where P = population, I = intervention or influence, C = comparison, and O = outcome.

Pilot study A small-scale study, or trial run, done in preparation for a major study or to assess feasibility.

Placebo A sham or pseudointervention, sometimes used as a control group condition.

***Placebo effect** Changes in the outcome attributable to a placebo as a result of participants' expectations.

Plan-Do-Study-Act (PDSA) A QI model that involves systematic, rapid cycles of activities; sometimes called *Plan-Do-Check-Act (PDCA)*.

Point estimation A statistical procedure that uses data from a sample (a statistic) to estimate the single value that best represents the population parameter.

Population The entire set of individuals or objects having some common characteristics (e.g., all RNs in California); the "P" in the PICO framework.

Positionality statement Describes how the researchers' identities, experiences, and beliefs are related to their study and to the participants.

Positive relationship A relationship between two variables in which high values on one variable tend to be associated with high values on the other (e.g., as physical activity increases, heart rate increases).

Positive results Research results that are consistent with the researcher's hypotheses.

Positive skew An asymmetric distribution of values with a disproportionately high number of cases at the lower end; when displayed graphically, the tail points to the right.

Positivist paradigm The paradigm underlying the traditional scientific approach, which assumes that there is an orderly reality that can be objectively studied; often associated with quantitative research.

Post hoc test A test for comparing all possible pairs of groups following a significant test of overall group differences (e.g., in an ANOVA).

Poster session A session at a professional conference in which several researchers simultaneously present visual displays summarizing their studies, whereas conference attendees circulate around the room perusing the displays.

Posttest data Data collected after introducing an intervention.

Posttest-only design An experimental design in which outcome data are collected from participants only after the intervention has been introduced.

Power The ability of a design or analysis to detect true relationships that exist among variables.

Power analysis A procedure used to estimate sample size requirements prior to undertaking a study or to estimate the likelihood of committing a Type II error.

Practice-based evidence Research evidence that is developed in real-world settings and is responsive to the needs and circumstances of specific patients and contexts.

Pragmatic clinical trial A trial that addresses practical questions about the benefits, risks, and costs of an intervention as it would unfold in routine clinical practice to enhance clinical decision-making.

Pragmatism A paradigm on which mixed methods research is often said to be based, in that it acknowledges the practical imperative of the "dictatorship of the research question."

Precision The degree to which an estimated population value (a statistic) clusters closely around the estimate, usually expressed in terms of the width of the CI.

Precision health care A model that proposes the customization of health care, with decisions and treatments tailored to individual patients based on their unique genetic, physiologic, behavioral, lifestyle, and environmental profile.

Prediction The use of empirical evidence to make forecasts about how variables will perform in a new setting and with a different sample.

Predictive validity A type of criterion validity concerning the degree to which a measure is correlated with a criterion measured at a future point in time.

Predictor variable A variable (usually the independent variable) used to predict another variable (the outcome); term used primarily in the context of regression analysis.

Pretest (1) Data collected prior to an intervention; often called *baseline data*. (2) The trial administration of a newly developed instrument to identify potential weaknesses.

Pretest–posttest design A design in which data are collected from study participants both before and after introducing an intervention.

Prevalence The proportion of a population having a particular condition (e.g., fibromyalgia) at a given point in time.

Primary source Firsthand reports of facts or findings; in research, the original report prepared by the investigator who conducted the study.

Primary studies In systematic reviews, original studies whose findings are the data in the review.

Priority A feature of mixed methods designs, concerning which strand (qualitative or quantitative) is given more emphasis; in notation, the dominant strand is in all capital letters, as QUAL or QUAN, and the nondominant strand is in lower case, as qual or quan.

Probability sampling The selection of elements (e.g., participants) from a population using random procedures, such that each member has an equal probability of being selected.

Probing Eliciting more useful or detailed information from a respondent in an interview than was volunteered in the initial reply.

Problem statement The articulation of a dilemma or a disturbing situation that needs investigation.

Process analysis A descriptive analysis of the process by which a program or intervention gets implemented and used in practice.

Process consent In a qualitative study, an ongoing, transactional process of negotiating consent with participants, allowing them to collaborate in decision-making about continued participation.

Product–moment correlation coefficient (r) A correlation coefficient designating the magnitude and direction of relationship between two variables measured on at least an interval scale; also called *Pearson's r*.

Prognosis question A question about the consequences or long-term outcomes of a disease or health problem.

Prolonged engagement In qualitative research, the investment of sufficient time during data collection to have an in-depth understanding of the phenomenon under study, thereby enhancing credibility.

Proposal A document communicating a research problem, its significance, proposed methods for addressing the problem, and, when funding is sought, how much the study will cost.

Prospective design A study design that begins with an examination of a presumed cause (e.g., cigarette smoking) and then goes forward in time to measure presumed effects (e.g., lung cancer); also called a *cohort design*.

Psychometric assessment An evaluation of the quality of an instrument, primarily in terms of its reliability and validity.

Psychometrics A field of inquiry concerned with the theory of measurement of abstract psychological constructs and the application of the theory in the development and testing of measures.

Publication bias A bias resulting from the fact that published studies overrepresent statistically significant findings, reflecting the tendency to not publish reports with nonsignificant results.

Purposive (purposeful) sampling A nonprobability sampling method in which the researcher selects participants based on personal judgment about who will be most informative.

Q sort A data collection method in which participants sort statements into piles (usually 9 or 11) according to some bipolar dimension (e.g., most helpful/least helpful).

Qualitative analysis The organization and interpretation of narrative data for the purpose of discovering important underlying themes, categories, and patterns.

Qualitative content analysis An approach to extracting, organizing, and synthesizing material from narrative data from a qualitative study according to key concepts and themes.

Qualitative data Information in narrative (nonnumeric) form, such as the information provided in an unstructured interview.

Qualitative descriptive research Qualitative studies that yield rich descriptions of phenomena but that are not embedded in a qualitative tradition such as phenomenology.

Qualitative evidence synthesis (QES) A systematic review of qualitative evidence, typically using an aggregative approach to evidence synthesis; often focused on qualitative aspects of an intervention (e.g., barriers to participation).

Qualitative research The investigation of phenomena, typically in an in-depth and holistic fashion, through the collection of rich narrative materials using a flexible research design.

Quality improvement (QI) Systematic efforts to improve practices and processes within a specific organization or patient group.

Quantitative analysis The organization of numeric data through statistical procedures for the purpose of describing phenomena or testing the magnitude and reliability of relationships among them.

Quantitative data Information collected in a quantified (numeric) form.

Quantitative research The investigation of phenomena that lend themselves to precise measurement and quantification, often involving a rigorous and controlled design and statistical analysis of data.

Quasi-experiment A type of design for testing an intervention in which participants are not randomly assigned to treatment conditions; also called a *nonrandomized trial*.

Questionnaire A document used to gather self-report data via self-administration of questions.

Quota sampling A nonrandom sampling method in which "quotas" for certain subgroups, based on sample characteristics, are established to increase the representativeness of the sample.

R The symbol for the multiple correlation coefficient, indicating the magnitude (but not direction) of the relationship between a dependent variable and multiple independent (predictor) variables, taken together.

r The symbol for a bivariate correlation coefficient (*Pearson's r*), summarizing the magnitude and direction of a relationship between two variables measured on an interval or ratio scale.

R^2 The squared multiple correlation coefficient, indicating the proportion of variance in the dependent variable explained by a set of independent (predictor) variables.

Random assignment The assignment of participants to treatment conditions in a random manner (i.e., in a manner determined by chance alone); also called *randomization*.

Random effects model In meta-analysis, a model in which studies are not assumed to be measuring the same overall effect but rather reflect a distribution of effects; often preferred to a fixed effect model when variation of effects across studies is extensive.

*Random number table A table displaying hundreds of digits (from 0 to 9) in random order; each number is equally likely to follow any other.

Random sampling The selection of a sample such that each member of a population has an equal probability of being included.

Randomization The assignment of participants to treatment conditions in a random manner (i.e., in a manner determined by chance alone); also called *random assignment*.

Randomized controlled trial (RCT) A full experimental test of an intervention, involving random assignment of participants to different treatment groups.

Randomness An important concept in quantitative research, involving having certain features of the study established by chance rather than by design or personal preference.

Range A measure of variability, computed by subtracting the lowest value from the highest value in a distribution of scores.

Rapid review A type of systematic review in which the team follows streamlined procedures designed to produce an evidence synthesis in a timely (but less rigorous) manner than a standard systematic review.

Rating scale A scale that requires ratings of an object or concept along a continuum.

Ratio measurement A measurement level with equal distances between scores and a true meaningful zero point (e.g., weight).

Raw data Data in the form in which they were collected, without being coded or analyzed.

Reactivity A measurement distortion arising from the study participants' awareness of being observed, or, more generally, from the effect of the measurement procedure itself.

Readability The ease with which written material (e.g., a questionnaire) can be read by people with varying reading skills, often determined through readability formulas.

Realist evaluation A theory-driven approach to evaluating complex programs, designed to examine "What works for whom and under what circumstances?"

Receiver operating characteristic curve (ROC curve) A method used in developing and refining a screening instrument to determine the best cutoff point for "caseness."

Reflective notes Notes that document a qualitative researcher's personal experiences, self-reflections, and progress in the field, especially when collecting observational data.

Reflexive journal A journal where a researcher keeps track of their self-reflections during the research process.

Reflexivity In qualitative studies, the researchers' critical self-reflection about their own biases, preferences, and preconceptions, often recorded in a reflexive journal.

Regression analysis A statistical procedure for predicting values of a dependent variable based on one or more independent (predictor) variables.

Relationship A bond or a connection between two or more variables.

Relative risk (RR) An estimate of the risk of "caseness" in one group compared to another, computed by dividing the AR for one group (e.g., a treated group) by the AR for another (e.g., the untreated group); also called the *risk ratio*.

Relevance In the context of patient-centered research, the degree to which evidence is meaningful and valuable to patients and other stakeholders and has the potential to be actionable.

Reliability The extent to which a measurement is free from measurement error; more broadly, the extent to which scores for people who have not changed are the same for repeated measurements.

Reliability coefficient A quantitative index, usually ranging in value from .00 to 1.00, that provides an estimate of how reliable an instrument is (e.g., the ICC).

Repeated measures ANOVA An ANOVA used when there are multiple measurements of the outcome over time.

Replication The deliberate repetition of research procedures in a second investigation for the purpose of assessing whether earlier results can be confirmed.

Representative sample A sample whose characteristics are comparable to those of the population from which it is drawn.

Representativeness A key criterion for assessing the adequacy of a sample in quantitative studies, indicating the extent to which findings from the study can be generalized to the population.

Research Systematic inquiry that uses orderly, disciplined methods to answer questions or solve problems.

Research control Procedures used to hold constant confounding influences on the outcome under study.

Research design The overall plan for addressing a research question, including strategies for enhancing the study's integrity.

Research hypothesis The actual hypothesis a researcher wishes to test (as opposed to the *null hypothesis*), stating the expected relationship between two or more variables.

Research methods The techniques used to structure a study and to gather and analyze information in a systematic fashion.

Research problem A disturbing or perplexing condition that can be investigated through disciplined inquiry.

Research question A specific query the researcher wants to answer to address a research problem.

Research report A document (often a journal article) summarizing the main features of a study, including the research question, the methods used to address it, the findings, and the interpretation of the findings.

Research utilization The use of some aspect of a study in an application unrelated to the original research.

Researcher credibility The faith that can be put in a researcher, based on their training, qualifications, and experiences.

Respondent In a self-report study, the participant responding to questions posed by the researcher.

Respondents' response The answers a study participant may provide to structured self-reports in quantitative studies.

Responder analysis An analysis that compares people who are *responders* to an intervention, based on their having reached a benchmark on a change score (e.g., the MIC), to people who are nonresponders (have not reached the benchmark).

Response options The prespecified set of answers to a closed-ended question or item.

Response rate The rate of participation in a study, calculated by dividing the number of people participating by the number of people sampled.

Response set bias The measurement error resulting from the tendency of some individuals to respond to items in characteristic ways (e.g., always agreeing), independently of item content.

Results The answers to a researcher's questions or hypothesis tests, obtained through an analysis of the collected data.

Retrospective design A study design that begins with the manifestation of the outcome in the present (e.g., lung cancer), followed by a search for a presumed cause occurring in the past (e.g., cigarette smoking).

Risk/benefit assessment An assessment of the relative costs and benefits, to an individual study participant and to society at large, of participation in a study; also, the relative costs and benefits of implementing an innovation.

ROC curve See *receiver operating characteristic curve*.

Root cause analysis (RCA) In QI, systematic efforts to identify the underlying causes of a problem that needs to be addressed.

Sample A subset of a population comprising those selected to participate in a study.

Sample size The number of people who participate in a study; an important factor in the *power* of statistical analyses and in statistical conclusion validity.

Sampling The process of selecting a portion of the population to represent the population.

Sampling bias Distortions that arise when a sample is not representative of the population from which it was drawn.

Sampling distribution A theoretical distribution of a statistic using the values of the statistic (e.g., the mean) from an infinite number of samples as the data points in the distribution.

Sampling error The fluctuation of the value of a statistic from one sample to another drawn from the same population.

Sampling frame A list of all the elements in the population from which a sample is drawn.

Sampling plan The formal plan specifying a sampling method, a sample size, and procedures for recruiting subjects.

Saturation The collection of qualitative data to the point where a sense of closure is attained because new data yield redundant information.

Scale A composite measure of an attribute or trait involving the aggregation of responses to multiple items into a single numerical score that places people on a continuum with respect to the trait.

Schematic model A graphic representation depicting concepts and linkages between them; also called a *conceptual map*.

Scientific merit The degree to which a study is methodologically and conceptually sound.

Scientific method A set of orderly, systematic, controlled procedures for acquiring dependable, empirical—and typically quantitative—information; the methodologic approach associated with the positivist paradigm.

Scoping review A preliminary review of research findings to clarify the range and nature of the evidence base, often to refine the questions and protocols for a systematic review.

Score A numerical value derived from a measurement that communicates *how much* of an attribute is present in a person or whether the attribute is present or absent.

*Screening instrument An instrument used to assess whether potential subjects for a study meet eligibility criteria, or for determining whether a person tests positive or is at risk for a specified condition.

Secondary analysis A form of research in which the data collected in one study are reanalyzed in another investigation to answer new questions.

Secondary source Secondhand accounts of events or facts; in research, a description of a study written by someone other than the original researcher.

Selection threat A threat to a study's internal validity resulting from preexisting differences between groups under study; the differences affect the outcome in ways extraneous to the effect of the independent variable (e.g., an intervention).

Selective coding A level of coding in a grounded theory study that begins once the core category has been discovered; involves limiting coding to only those categories related to the core category.

Self-determination A person's right to voluntarily decide whether to participate in a study.

Self-report A data collection method that involves direct verbal reporting by a study participant (e.g., in an interview or questionnaire).

Semi-structured interview An open-ended interview in which the researcher is guided by a list of topics to cover rather than specific questions to ask.

Sensitivity The ability of a screening or diagnostic instrument to correctly identify a "case" (true positives).

Sensitivity analysis An effort to test how sensitive the results of a statistical analysis are to changes in assumptions or in the way the analysis was done (e.g., in a meta-analysis, sometimes used to assess whether conclusions are sensitive to the quality of the studies included).

Sequential design A mixed methods design in which one strand of data collection (qualitative or quantitative) occurs prior to the other, informing the second strand; symbolically shown with an arrow (e.g., QUAL → QUAN).

Setting In a research context, the physical location in which data collection takes place in a study (e.g., clinics).

Significance level The probability that an observed relationship could be caused by chance; significance at the .05 level indicates the probability that a relationship of the observed magnitude would be found by chance only 5 times out of 100.

Simple hypothesis A hypothesis statement with a single independent variable and dependent variable.

Simple random sampling Basic probability sampling involving the random selection of sample members from a sampling frame.

Site The overall location where a study is undertaken (e.g., Miami).

Situational analysis A grounded theory approach that focuses on the situation under study as the key unit of analysis and not on discovering one BSP. Several kinds of analytic maps are made to help understand the complexities of a situation.

Skewed distribution An asymmetric distribution of data values around a central point, with two halves that are not mirror images of each other.

Snowball sampling The selection of participants through referrals from earlier participants; also called *network sampling*.

Social desirability response set A bias in self-report instruments created when participants tend to misrepresent their opinions in the direction of views consistent with prevailing social norms.

Space triangulation The collection of data on the same phenomenon in multiple sites to assess cross-site consistency and enhance trustworthiness of the findings.

Spearman's rho A correlation coefficient indicating the magnitude of a relationship between variables measured on the ordinal scale.

Specificity The ability of a screening or diagnostic instrument to correctly identify noncases (true negatives).

Stakeholder In the context of health care, a person or group that has a direct interest in a health care decision, action, or process.

Standard deviation A statistic that describes the "average" amount of variability in a set of scores.

Standard error of the mean The standard deviation of a theoretical sampling distribution, such as the sampling distribution of the mean.

Standardized mean difference (SMD) In meta-analysis, the ES index for comparing two group means, computed by subtracting one mean from the other and dividing by the pooled standard deviation; also called Cohen's *d*.

Statement of purpose A declarative statement of the overall goals of a study.

Statistic An estimate of a population parameter, calculated from sample data.

Statistical analysis The organization and analysis of quantitative data using statistical procedures, including both descriptive and inferential statistics.

Statistical conclusion validity The degree to which inferences about relationships from a statistical analysis of the data are accurate.

Statistical control The use of statistical procedures to control confounding influences on the outcome variable.

Statistical heterogeneity Diversity of effects across primary studies included in a meta-analysis.

Statistical inference An inference about the population based on information from a sample, using laws of probability.

Statistical power The ability of a research design and analytic strategy to detect true relationships among variables.

Statistical significance A term indicating that the results from an analysis of sample data are unlikely to have resulted from chance at a specified level of probability.

Statistical test An analytic tool used to estimate the probability that results from a sample reflect true population values.

Stipend A monetary payment to individuals taking part in a study as an incentive for their participation and/or to compensate for time and expenses.

Strata Subdivisions of the population based on a specified characteristic (e.g., gender); singular is *stratum*.

*Stratification The subdivision of a sample or a population into smaller units (e.g., married and unmarried), typically to enhance representativeness (e.g., in sampling).

Stratified random sampling The random selection of study participants from two or more strata of the population independently.

Study participant An individual who participates and provides information in a study.

Subgroup analysis Analytic efforts to understand whether intervention effects vary for defined groups of people (e.g., men vs. women); undertaken to disentangle HTE.

Subject An individual who participates and provides data in a study; term used primarily in quantitative research.

Subscale A subset of items that measures one aspect or dimension of a multidimensional construct.

Substantive codes Types of codes in grounded theory that consist of two types: open and selective codes.

Summated rating scale A composite scale consisting of multiple items that are added together to yield a total score for an attribute (e.g., a Likert scale).

Survey research Nonexperimental research that involves gathering information about people's activities, beliefs, preferences, and attitudes via direct questioning.

Symmetric distribution A distribution of values with two halves that are mirror images of each other.

Systematic review A rigorous synthesis of research findings on a particular research question, using systematic sampling, data collection, and data analysis procedures specified in a formal protocol.

Systematic sampling The selection of sample members such that every kth (e.g., every 10th) person or element in a sampling frame is chosen.

Tacit knowledge Information about a culture that is so deeply embedded that members do not talk about it or may not be consciously aware of it.

Target population The entire population in which a researcher is interested and to which they would like to generalize study results.

Taxonomy In an ethnographic analysis, a system of classifying and organizing terms and concepts, developed to illuminate a domain's organization and the relationship among the domain's categories.

Test statistic A statistic used to test the reliability of relationships between variables (e.g., t, chi-squared); sampling distributions of test statistics are known for circumstances in which the null hypothesis is true.

Test–retest reliability The type of reliability that concerns the extent to which scores for people who have not changed are the same when a measure is administered twice; an assessment of a measure's stability.

Thematic analysis A flexible approach to analyzing qualitative data from a descriptive qualitative study that follows an established process to identify and define themes.

Theme A recurring regularity emerging from an analysis of qualitative data.

Theoretical codes Codes in grounded theory that focus on how substantive codes are related to each other.

Theoretical framework See *framework*.

Theoretical sampling In qualitative studies, especially in grounded theory studies, the selection of sample members based on emerging findings to ensure adequate saturation of important theoretical categories.

Theory An abstract generalization that presents a systematic explanation about relationships among phenomena or that thoroughly describes a phenomenon.

Therapy/intervention question A question about the effects of a treatment or intervention on patient outcomes.

Thick description A rich and thorough description of the research context, study participants, and the phenomenon of interest in a qualitative study.

Think-aloud method A method used to collect data about cognitive processes in which people's reflections on decisions or problem-solving are captured as they are being made.

Threats to validity In research design, reasons that an inference about the effect of an independent variable (e.g., an intervention) on an outcome could be wrong.

Time sampling In structured observations, the sampling of time periods during which observations will take place.

Time triangulation The collection of data on the same phenomenon or about the same people at different points in time to enhance trustworthiness.

Time-series design A quasi-experimental design involving the collection of data over an extended time period, with multiple data collection points both before and after an intervention.

Topic guide A list of broad question areas to be covered in a semi-structured interview or focus group interview.

Transferability The extent to which qualitative findings can be transferred to other settings or groups; an aspect of trustworthiness.

Translational science A discipline that focuses on how study findings can best be translated into practice.

Treatment An intervention; in experimental research (a clinical trial), the condition being manipulated.

Triangulation The use of multiple methods to collect and interpret data about a phenomenon to converge on an accurate representation of reality.

Trustworthiness The degree of confidence qualitative researchers have in their data and analyses, often assessed using the criteria of credibility, transferability, dependability, confirmability, and authenticity.

***t*-test** A parametric statistical test for testing the difference between two group means.

Type I error An error created by rejecting the null hypothesis when it is true (i.e., the researcher concludes that a relationship exists when, in fact, it does not—a false positive).

Type II error An error created by accepting the null hypothesis when it is false (i.e., the researcher concludes that *no* relationship exists when, in fact, it does—a false negative).

Umbrella review A type of systematic umbrella review in which the team integrates findings from multiple systematic reviews on a topic.

Underpowered A characteristic of a study that lacks sufficient statistical power to minimize the risk of a Type II error (i.e., the risk of concluding that a relationship does not exist when, in fact, it does).

Unimodal distribution A distribution of values with one peak (high frequency).

Unit of analysis The basic unit or focus of a researcher's analysis—typically individual study participants.

Univariate statistics Statistical analysis of a single variable for descriptive purposes (e.g., calculating a mean).

Unstructured interview An interview in which the researcher asks respondents questions without having a predetermined plan regarding the content or flow of information to be gathered.

Unstructured observation The collection of descriptive data through direct observation that is not guided by a formal, prespecified plan for observing, enumerating, or recording the information.

Validity A quality criterion referring to the degree to which inferences made in a study are accurate and well-founded; in measurement, the degree to which an instrument measures what it is intended to measure.

Variability The degree to which values on a set of scores are dispersed, that is, are heterogeneous.

Variable An attribute that varies, that is, takes on different values (e.g., heart rate, anxiety).

***Variance** A measure of variability or dispersion, equal to the standard deviation squared.

Vignette A brief description of an event, person, or situation to which respondents are asked to express their reactions.

Visual analog scale (VAS) A scaling procedure used to measure certain clinical symptoms (e.g., pain, fatigue) by having people indicate on a straight line the intensity of the symptom; usually measured on a 100-mm scale with values from 0 to 100.

Vulnerable groups Special groups of people whose rights in studies need special protection because of their inability to provide meaningful informed consent or because their circumstances place them at higher-than-average risk of adverse effects (e.g., children, unconscious patients).

Wait-list design A design for an intervention study that involves putting control group members on a waiting list for the intervention until follow-up data have been collected; also called a *delayed treatment design*.

Yea-sayers bias A bias in self-report scales created when respondents characteristically agree with statements ("yea-say"), independent of content.

INDEX

A
Absolute risk (AR), 217–218
Absolute risk reduction (ARR), 218
Absolute value, 217, 228
Abstract
  literature search and, 92–96
  in research reports, 43
Accessible population, 142
Acquiescence response set bias, 151
Active reading, 47
Active voice, research reports and, 46
Adaptation Model (Roy), 108
ADRD, 248
Adulatory validity, 280
Advanced AI coding, 259
Aim, research, 77
Ajzen's Theory of Planned Behavior, 110
Alpha (α)
  internal consistency reliability (Cronbach's alpha), 231
  significance level, 222
Alzheimer disease and related dementias (ADRD), 248
American Nurses Association (ANA), 2, 60
American Nurses Credentialing Center, 2
Analysis. *See also* Data analysis; Qualitative analysis; Quantitative analysis
  Clarke's, situational, 169
  concept, 107
  content, 170, 261–262
  cost, 200
  data, 34, 209–236, 257–269 (*See also* Data analysis)
  economic, 200
  narrative, 170
  power, 223, 228
  process, 200
  qualitative, 35, 257–269 (*See also* Qualitative analysis)
  quantitative, 34, 209–236 (*See also* Quantitative analysis)
  responder, 253
  secondary, 204
  sensitivity, 296
  statistical, 33, 44 (*See also* Quantitative analysis; Statistic[s])
Analysis of covariance (ANCOVA), 230
  research design and, 133
Analysis of variance (ANOVA), 225–226
Ancestry approach, literature search, 91
ANCOVA. *See* Analysis of covariance
Animal subjects, ethics and, 68
Anonymity, 65–66, 149
ANOVA. *See* Analysis of variance
Anthropomorphic measure, 154

Applicability, 4, 250, 316
  generalizability and relevance and, 319
Appraisal of evidence, 315–317
Appraisal of Guidelines Research and Evaluation (AGREE) instrument, 312
The Archives of Nursing Leadership, 170
Argument, problem statement and, 74, 76
Artificial intelligence (AI), 96–97, 259
Artistic expressions, phenomenology and, 167, 181
Assent, ethics and, 67
Assessment
  psychometric, 154, 204, 231–232
  research purpose, 11
Associative relationship, 29
Assumption(s)
  paradigms and, 6–7
  parametric tests and, 224
Asymmetric distribution, 211
Attention control group, 123
Attrition, 131, 245
Attrition bias, 135
Audit, inquiry, 282
Audit trail, 279
Authenticity, trustworthiness and, 276, 282, 284–285
Author search, literature search and, 91
Authorities, as knowledge source, 5
Autoethnography, 165
Average, 211, 213
Average treatment effects, 4, 318
Axial coding, 267

B
Bandura's Social Cognitive Theory, 109
Baseline data, 121, 125
Basic social process (BSP), 168, 266
Becker's Health Belief Model (HBM), 110
Being-in-the-world, 167
Bell-shaped curve, 213. *See also* Normal distribution
Belmont Report, 60, 62–63
Benchmark, clinical significance and, 252–253
Beneficence, 61
Best evidence, 14
Bias, 6, 245–246
  attrition and, 135
  "best" evidence and, 14
  blinding and, 53, 118
  credibility and, 245–246
  ethics and, 67
  evidence hierarchies and, 15
  expectation, 118
  full disclosure and, 63
  insider research and, 165

379

Bias (*continued*)
  internal validity and, 134
  measurement error and, 154
  nonresponse, 147
  observational, 153
  publication, 293
  qualitative research and, 276, 278, 281
  randomness and, 53
  reflexivity and, 54 (*See also* Reflexivity)
  research control and, 52
  response, 147
  response set, 151
  sampling, 142, 145
  selection, 134
  social desirability, 151
  statement of purpose and, 78
  systematic, 52
  threats to internal validity, 134–135
  triangulation and, 52, 279
  types of, 246
Bibliographic database, 91–96
Bimodal distribution, 213
Biologic plausibility, causality and, 119
Biomarker, 33, 148, 153–154
Biophysiologic measures, 33, 148, 154
Bivariate statistics
  descriptive, 216–217 (*See also* Descriptive statistics)
  inferential, 224–229 (*See also* Inferential statistics)
Blind review, 43
Blinding, 53, 118, 124, 131, 136
  qualitative research and, 53, 163
Boolean operator, 92
Bracketing, 166–167
Breach of confidentiality, 66
BSP (basic social process), 168, 266

C

Canadian Nurses Association, 60
CAQDAS, 259
Carryover effect, 121, 133
Case
  confirming and disconfirming, 179, 281
  diagnostic accuracy and, 232
Case-control design, 127, 132
Case study, 169
CASP (Critical Appraisal Skills Programme), 299
Categories, qualitative data and, 258
Category system, observational, 152
Causal (cause-and-effect) relationship, 25, 28–29, 119, 120. *See also* Causality
  correlation and, 124, 127, 248
  criteria for, 119
  evidence hierarchy and, 15, 120, 124
  experimental research and, 30, 120–121
  hypotheses and, 81, 124
  internal validity and, 134–135
  nonexperimental research and, 30, 126–127
  quasi-experimental research and, 125–126, 135
Causality, 28, 119. *See also* Causal (cause-and-effect) relationship
  correlation and, 128, 247
  determinism and, 6, 119
  interpretation of, 246–250
  longitudinal design and, 130–131
  mixed methods research and, 193
  in qualitative research, 29, 164

  study purpose and, 12–13
Cause-and-effect relationship. *See* Causal (cause-and-effect) relationship
Cause-probing research, 10, 12, 120, 127, 133
Cell
  crosstabs table and, 216
  risk indexes and, 218
Central (core) category, grounded theory, 267
Central tendency, 213–214. *See also* Mean
Certificate of Confidentiality, 66
Change score, 251–252
Charmaz, constructivist grounded theory, 169, 267–268
ChatGPT, 260
Checklist, observational research, 152
Chi-squared (χ^2) test, 227
Children, as a vulnerable group, 67
CINAHL database, 93
Clarke's situational analysis, 169
Clinical experience
  EBP and, 14
  as knowledge source, 5
Clinical fieldwork, 32
Clinical nursing research, 2
Clinical practice guideline, 297
Clinical query, PubMed, 92
Clinical questions, 13
Clinical relevance, 4. *See also* Evidence-based practice; Nursing research
Clinical significance, 4, 34
  benchmarks and, 252–253
  conceptual definitions of, 252
  group-level indicators, 251
  individual-level indicators, 251–253
  statistical significance *vs.*, 247, 251
Clinical trial, 30, 200. *See also* Experimental research
  pragmatic, 320–321
  randomized controlled trial (RCT), 15, 120–121 (*See also* Randomized controlled trial)
Closed-ended question, 148
Cluster randomized design, 321
Cochrane Collaboration, 290, 293–294, 296, 297
Cochrane Database of Systematic Reviews, 92, 290
Code of ethics, 60
Codes, in grounded theory
  Charmaz's method, 267–268
  Corbin and Strauss's method, 168, 267
  Glaser and Strauss's method, 265–267
Coding
  levels of, grounded theory and, 266
  literature reviews and, 98
  quantitative data and, 34
  scheme, qualitative data and, 258
Coefficient(s)
  correlation, 217
  intraclass correlation (ICC), 231
  product–moment correlation (Pearson's *r*), 217 (*See also* Pearson's *r*)
  reliability, 155, 231
Coefficient alpha (Cronbach's alpha), 231
Coercion, 62
Cohen's kappa, 231
Cohort design, 127
Colaizzi's phenomenological method, 264
Comparative effectiveness research, 124, 202
  defining characteristics of, 319–320

Comparator, PICO framework and, 16. *See also* PICO framework
Comparison
   constant, 168, 265–267
   multiple, in ANOVA, 226
   qualitative studies and, 163
   research design and, 118
Comparison group, 125
Complex hypothesis, 82–83
Complex intervention, 201
Componential analysis, ethnography, 263
Composite scale, 150, 157. *See also* Scale
Computer. *See also* Internet
   analysis of qualitative data and, 259–260
   analysis of quantitative data and, 224
   electronic literature searches and, 91–96
Computer-assisted qualitative data analysis software (CAQDAS), 259
Concealment, 63
Concept
   as component of theories, 106
   concept *vs.* construct, 24
   measurement of, 33, 154
   models of nursing and, 107
   operational definitions and, 26–27, 154
   theories and models, 106–107
Concept analysis, 107
Concept coding, qualitative data, 258–259
Conceptual definition, 26–27, 32, 107
Conceptual description, grounded theory, 168, 267
Conceptual framework, 107, 113. *See also* Conceptual model; Theory
Conceptual integration, 105
Conceptual map, 106, 111
Conceptual model, 106. *See also* Theory
   models of nursing and, 108
   nonnursing models, 109
Concurrent validity, 156
Conference, professional, presentation at, 43
Confidence interval (CI)
   clinical significance and, 251
   level of significance and, 222–223
   odds ratios and, 219
   precision and, 221, 246–247
   t-tests and, 224–225
Confidentiality, 66
Confirmability, trustworthiness and, 276
Confirming case, 179
Confounding variable, 52. *See also* Control, research
   analysis of covariance and, 133, 230
   controls for, 131–133
ConQual, confidence ratings, meta-aggregation, 303
Consecutive sampling, 144
Consensus panel, clinical significance, 252
Consent, 64–65. *See also* Ethics, research
Consent form, 65
CONSORT flowchart, 244
CONSORT guidelines, 244
Constancy of conditions, 131
Constant, 24
   holding confounders, 53, 131
Constant comparison, 168, 265–267, 266–267
Construct, 24. *See also* Concept
Construct validity, 133
   interpretation and, 241–242

interventions and, 136, 201
measurement and, 156, 232
Constructivist grounded theory, 169, 268
Constructivist methods, 8. *See also* Qualitative research
Constructivist paradigm, 6–8
Consumers of nursing research, 3
   assistance for, 17–18
Content analysis, 170, 261–262
Content validity, 156
Content validity index (CVI), 232
Contexts, applicability and, 319
Continuous quality improvement, 197
Continuous variable, 210
Control group, 120–121
   control group condition, 125
   nonequivalent, 125–126
Control, research, 52–53
   evaluation of methods for, 133
   experimental design and, 29–30, 120–121
   of external confounding factors, 131
   internal validity and, 134–135
   of intrinsic confounding factors, 131–133
   as purpose of research, 10
   qualitative research and, 163
   quasi-experiments and, 125–126, 134
   statistical, 133
Convenience sampling, 143–144, 178
Convergent design, mixed methods and, 194
Corbin and Strauss' grounded theory method, 267
Core category (variable), 30, 168, 266
   coding and, 267
Correlation, 217. *See also* Correlation coefficient; Relationship
   causation and, 127, 247
Correlation coefficient, 216–217
   intraclass (ICC), 231
   Pearson's product–moment (r), 217 (*See also* Pearson's r)
   Spearman's rho, 217
Correlation matrix, 217
Correlational research, 127
   advantages and disadvantages, 128
   internal validity and, 134
   interpretation and, 241–242
   surveys and, 203–204
Corroboration of results, 246
Cost (economic) analysis, 200
Costs, EBP and, 316
Counterfactual, 119–120, 124
Covariate, 230
Covert data collection, 63
COVID-19 pandemic, 221, 249, 265
   artificial intelligence (AI), 96
Credibility
   bias and, 245–246
   corroboration and, 246
   proxies and interpretation, 243–245
   quantitative results and, 242–246
   researcher, 282–283
   trustworthiness and, 51, 275–276 (*See also* Trustworthiness, qualitative research)
   validity and, 245
Criterion sampling, 179
Criterion validity, 156, 232

Critical appraisal of research, 46–47
 applicability, relevance, and generalizability, 324
 data analyses qualitative and, 269
 data analyses, quantitative and, 235–236
 data collection plan, qualitative and, 188
 data collection plan, quantitative and, 157
 discussion section and, 253–254
 ethical issues and, 68–69
 hypotheses and, 84–85
 interpretation of quantitative results and, 241–242
 literature reviews and, 100
 meta-analysis and, 303–304
 metasynthesis and, 304
 mixed methods research and, 204–205
 research challenges and, 50–54
 research design, qualitative and, 172–173
 research design, quantitative and, 136–137
 research problems and, 84–85
 sampling plan, qualitative and, 182
 sampling plan, quantitative and, 146–147
 systematic reviews and, 303–304
 theoretical framework and, 113
Critical Appraisal Skills Programme (CASP), 299
Critical ethnography, 171
Critical theory, 112, 171
Critique, 47. *See also* Critical appraisal of research
Cronbach's alpha, 231
Cross-sectional design, 129–130, 134
 qualitative research and, 164
Crossover design, 123, 132–133
Crosstabs table, 216
Crosstabulations, 216
Cultural theory, ethnography and, 110–111
Culture, 31, 164–166, 172, 180–181. *See also* Ethnography
Cumulative Index to Nursing and Allied Health Literature (CINAHL), 92–93

D

Data, 27–28. *See also* Qualitative data; Quantitative data
 analysis of (*See* Data analysis)
 assessment of quality (*See* Data quality)
 coding of, 258–259 (*See also* Coding)
 collection of (*See* Data collection)
 existing *vs.* original, 147
 extraction and encoding of for meta-analysis, 294
 narrative, 28
 qualitative, 28, 35 (*See also* Qualitative data)
 quantitative, 27, 33 (*See also* Quantitative data)
 raw, 45
 saturation of, 36, 180
Data analysis. *See also* Qualitative analysis; Quantitative analysis
 descriptive statistics, 211–219 (*See also* Descriptive statistics)
 inferential statistics, bivariate, 219–224 (*See also* Inferential statistics)
 meta-aggregation and, 301–302
 meta-analysis and, 294
 metasynthesis and, 298–300
 mixed methods and, 195
 multivariate statistics, 229–231
 qualitative, 36, 257–269 (*See also* Qualitative analysis)
 qualitative, secondary, 268

quantitative, 33, 209–236 (*See also* Quantitative analysis; Statistic[s])
Data collection. *See also* Measurement
 biophysiologic measures, 33, 148, 154
 goal of, 157
 measurement and, 33, 154 (*See also* Measurement)
 methods, overview, 147–148
 mixed methods research and, 195–196
 observational methods, 33, 151–152, 186–187 (*See also* Observation, data collection)
 plan for, 33, 147–157
 protocols, 152
 qualitative research and, 188
 quantitative research and, 147–157
 self-report methods, 33, 148–151, 183–185
 triangulation of methods, 51, 188, 279
Data quality
 critical appraisal of, quantitative, 157
 measurement and, 154–157 (*See also* Measurement)
 qualitative data and, 280 (*See also* Trustworthiness, qualitative research)
 quantitative data and, 151–153, 231–232 (*See also* Reliability; Validity)
Data saturation, 35, 180
Data set, 204
Data triangulation, 279
Database, bibliographic, 91–96
Debriefing
 peer, qualitative research and, 281–282
 study participant, ethics and, 66–67
Deception, 63
Decision trail, 279
Declaration of Helsinki, 60
Deductive reasoning, 24
 theory testing and, 106 (*See also* Hypothesis)
Definitions, variables and
 conceptual, 26–27, 32, 107
 operational, 27, 154
Degrees of freedom (*df*), 224–225, 228
Delayed treatment design, 121, 321
Delphi survey, 204
Dependability, trustworthiness and, 276
Dependent groups *t*-tests, 225, 232
Dependent variable, 26. *See also* Independent variable; Outcome (variable)
 control and, 52–53
 hypotheses and, 82
 keywords and, 91
 PICO framework and, 25–26
 relationships and, 27
 research questions and, 79
Descendancy approach, literature search, 91
Description
 clinical questions and, 12
 conceptual, grounded theory and, 168, 267
 interpretive, 170
 qualitative, 170–171
 as research purpose, 12, 81–82
 thick, 182, 276, 282
Descriptive coding, qualitative data, 258
Descriptive correlational study, 128
Descriptive notes, observation and, 187
Descriptive phenomenology, 166–167. *See also* Phenomenology
Descriptive qualitative study, 30, 170–171
Descriptive questions, 12, 30, 79

Descriptive research
    correlational, 127–128 (*See also* Correlational research)
    qualitative, 170–171
Descriptive statistics
    bivariate, 216–217
    central tendency and, 213–214
    frequency distribution and, 211–213
    risk indexes and, 218
    variability and, 214–215
Descriptive theory, 106
Design. *See* Research design; Sampling
Detailed approach, phenomenological analysis, 264
Determinism, 6, 119
Deviant case analysis, 281
Diagnostic accuracy, 232
Diagnostic/assessment questions, 11, 29
Diary
    data collection and, 184
    field, 187
    historical research and, 184
    reflexivity and, 278
Dichotomous question, 148
Dichotomous variable, 232
Diffusion of Innovations Model (Rogers), 313
Dilemma, ethical, 60–61
Directional hypothesis, 82
Disabled people, as a vulnerable group, 67
Disclosure, full, 63
Disconfirming case, 179, 281
Discussion section, research report, 45–46, 241–250
    interpretation of results and, 253–254
    systematic reviews and, 304
Disproof, hypothesis testing and, 222
Dissemination of research results. *See also* Research report
    journal article, 43–47
    professional conferences and, 43
    qualitative studies, 35
    quantitative studies, 34
Dissertations, 293, 299
Distribution
    central tendency and, 213–214
    frequency, 211–213 (*See also* Frequency distribution)
    normal (bell-shaped curve), 213 (*See also* Normal distribution)
    sampling, 219–220
    theoretical, 220, 223, 224
    unimodal *vs.* multimodal, 211
    variability of, 214–215
Documentation
    literature reviews and, 97–98
    trustworthiness and, 282
Domain, 263
Domain analysis, ethnographic, 263
Dominant status, mixed methods research, 194
Donabedian framework, 203
Double blind, 124
d statistic, 228, 295
Duquesne school of phenomenology, 264

E
EBP. *See* Evidence-based practice
Economic (cost) analysis, 200
Effect(s)
    average treatment, 318
    carryover, 121, 133
    causality and, 119
    heterogeneity of, 319
    interaction, 226, 322
    intervention, 118, 120–122
    magnitude of, 228, 247, 316 (*See also* Effect size)
    main, 226
    meta-analysis and, 290, 294–295
Effect size (ES), 316
    clinical significance and, 251, 316
    d statistic, 228, 295
    interpretation of, 228
    meta-analysis and, 290, 294–295
    metasynthesis and, 301
    odds ratio, 228, 295
    Pearson's *r*, 228, 295
    power analysis, 228
Effectiveness study, intervention research and, 200
Efficacy study, intervention research and, 200
Element, sampling and, 142
Eligibility criteria, 142, 178
    meta-analysis and, 292–293
Embase, 92
Embedded design, mixed methods, 195
Emergent design, 36, 162
Emergent fit, 266–267
Emic perspective, 165
Empirical evidence, 7, 9
Equal status, mixed methods research, 194
Error(s)
    and biases, quantitative studies, 245–246
    measurement, 154
    sampling, 145, 220
    standard, 220
    standard error of the mean (SEM), 220
    Type I and Type II, 222, 245–246, 321
Essence, 31, 166. *See also* Phenomenology
Estimation of parameters, 221
Ethical dilemma, 60–61
Ethics, research, 33, 59, 69–70
    animals and, 68
    code of ethics, 60
    confidentiality procedures, 65–66
    critical appraisal of, 68–69
    debriefings and referrals, 66–67
    ethical principles, 61–64
    experimental research and, 124
    external review and, 67–68
    federal regulations (U.S.) and, 60
    historical background of, 59–60
    informed consent, 63, 64–65, 67
    Institutional Review Board, 68
    Internet research and, 63
    qualitative research and, 36
    research design and, 123–124
    risk/benefit assessments, 64
    vulnerable groups, 67
Ethnography, 31. *See also* Qualitative research
    autoethnography, 165
    critical, 171
    data analysis and, 263
    data collection and, 165
    ethnursing research, 165, 263
    focused, 165
    institutional, 166

Ethnography (*continued*)
  interviews and, 183
  online, 166
  participant observation and, 165, 186–187 (*See also* Participant observation)
  photo elicitation and, 184
  purpose statement and, 78
  research questions and, 79–80
  sampling and, 180–181
  theoretical framework and, 110
Ethnonursing research, 165, 263
Etic perspective, 165
Etiology (causation)/harm questions, 11, 79
  research design and, 29, 119, 124, 127
Evaluation research, 200
Event sampling, 153
Evidence
  appraising, 315–317
  empirical, 7, 9
  finding and acquiring, 314
  integrating, 98, 290 (*See also* Systematic review)
  literature reviews and, 89–100 (*See also* Literature review)
  pre-appraised, 14, 311–312
  probabilistic, 6, 119, 248
  qualitative, 317
  quality of, 292, 299, 315–316
  quantity and consistency of, 316
  research design and, 119, 124, 128, 133, 135
  sources of, 4–5, 14–15, 312
Evidence-based practice (EBP), 2
  applicability and, 319
  asking well-worded questions, 16, 310
  basics of, 13–16, 310
  clinical practice guidelines, 311–312
  clinical significance and, 251
  costs and, 316
  definition of, 13
  external validity and, 318
  individual and organizational, 314
  Iowa model of, 313
  limitations, 317
  literature reviews and, 90
  models of, 313
  PICO framework for formulating questions, 16, 228, 315 (*See also* PICO framework)
  population models of evidence, 318
  practice-based evidence and, 317–324
  quality improvement and, 196
  research utilization and, 313
  risk indexes and, 217
  sources of evidence, 4–5, 312
  steps in, 314–317
  study purposes and, 12–13
  systematic reviews and, 290
  tips for nurses, 324
Evidence hierarchy, 15, 120, 124, 289–290, 315–316, 318
Exclusion criteria, sampling, 142
Exemplar, hermeneutic analysis, 265
Expectation bias, 118
Experience
  EBP and, 14
  phenomenology and, 31
  source of research problem and, 74–75
Experimental group, 120–121

Experimental intervention (treatment), 118, 120–123. *See also* Intervention
Experimental research, 29–30. *See also* Intervention research
  advantages and disadvantages of, 124
  causation and, 30, 120, 127
  characteristics of, 120–121
  clinical trial, 30, 200
  control and, 120
  control conditions and, 123–124
  designs for, 120–123, 320
  evaluation research and, 200
  evidence hierarchy and, 15, 124
  internal validity, 134–135
  quality improvement and, 200
  quasi-experiments and, 125–126 (*See also* Quasi-experiment)
  randomized controlled trials, 120–123
  Therapy/intervention questions and, 29–30, 119, 124
Experts, as knowledge source, 5
Explanation, as research purpose, 10
Explanatory sequential design, mixed methods, 195
Explanatory trial, 320, 321. *See also* Randomized controlled trial
Exploitation, protection from, 62
Exploration, as research purpose, 10
Exploratory sequential design, mixed methods, 195
External review, ethics and, 67–68
External validity, 135–136, 245, 276, 318. *See also* Generalizability
Extraneous variable, 52. *See also* Confounding variable
Extreme (deviant) case sampling, 179
Extreme response set bias, 151

F

Face-to-face (personal) interview, 148–149, 203. *See also* Interview
Face validity, 156
Fair treatment, right to, 63–64
Feasibility, pilot study and, 201, 228
Feminist research, 171–172
Field diary, 187
Field notes, 187
Fieldwork
  clinical, 31
  ethnography, 31, 164–165
Findings, 43. *See also* Interpretation of results; Results
  generalizability and transferability of, 54, 276, 282, 284
  statistical, 44–45, 233
Fit, grounded theory and, 266
5As, EBP and, 16, 314
5 Whys, root cause analysis, 198
Fixed effects model, 295
Flexible research design, qualitative research, 35
Flowchart, CONSORT, 244
Focus group interview, 184
Focused coding, Charmaz, 268
Focused ethnography, 165
Focused interview, 183
Follow-up study, 130
Forced-choice question, 148
Forest plot, 295
Framework, 31, 107, 110–112. *See also* Conceptual model; Theory

critical appraisal of, 113
F ratio, analysis of variance, 226
Frequency distribution. *See also* Distribution
   central tendency of, 213–214
   shapes of, 211
   variability of, 214–215
Frequency effect size, 301
Frequency polygon, 211
Full disclosure, 63
Functional relationship, 29

G

Gaining entrée, 36
   participant observation and, 186
Gatekeeper, 36
Generalizability, 319
   external validity and, 135–136, 319
   in literature themes, 98
   qualitative research and, 8, 276 (*See also* Transferability)
   quantitative research and, 7, 54
   quasi-experiments and, 125
   of results, 54, 245, 250
   sampling and, 243, 318
Giorgi's phenomenological method, 264
Glaser and Strauss's grounded theory method, 168, 265–267
Google Scholar, 92, 94–96
GRADE-CERQual, qualitative evidence syntheses, 303
GRADE, systematic reviews and, 297, 302, 316, 318
Grand theory, 106
Grand tour question, 183
Gray literature, 293, 301, 302
Grounded theory, 30. *See also* Qualitative research
   constructivist (Charmaz), 168, 268
   Clarke's situational analysis, 169
   Corbin and Strauss's method and, 168, 267
   data analysis and, 265–268
   Glaser and Strauss's method, 264–267
   interviews and, 182
   literature reviews and, 90
   purpose statements and, 78
   research questions and, 79–80
   sampling and, 179, 181–182
   substantive theory, 111–112
   symbolic interactionism and, 111, 168
   theory and, 111–112

H

Harm
   protection from, 61–62
   research questions about, 11
Health Belief Model (HBM), Becker, 109
Health Insurance Portability and Accountability Act (HIPAA), 64
Health Promotion Model (HPM), Pender, 108
Health services research, 202–203
Hermeneutic circle, 167, 265
Hermeneutics, 166–167. *See also* Phenomenology
   data analysis and, 265
Heterogeneity, 214
   statistical, 293, 295–296
   of treatment effects, 319
Heterogeneity of treatment effects (HTE), 318
HIPAA, 64
Historical research, 170

History threat, internal validity, 134
Holistic approach, phenomenological analysis, 264–265
Homogeneity, 214
   research design and, 133
Human rights, research and, 61–64. *See also* Ethics, research
Human subjects committee, 68
Humanbecoming Paradigm (Parse), 106
Hypothesis, 33
   characteristics of, 81
   corroboration and, 246
   critical appraisal of, 84–85
   directional *vs.* nondirectional, 82
   function of, 80–81
   generation of, in qualitative research, 193
   interpretation and, 241–242
   null, 84, 221–222
   research, 84, 221
   rival, 126
   simple *vs.* complex, 82–83
   testing of, 84, 221–224 (*See also* Hypothesis testing)
   theories and, 80
   wording of, 82
Hypothesis testing. *See also* Inferential statistics; Statistic(s)
   construct validity and, 156, 227
   disproof and, 222
   level of significance and, 223
   null hypothesis and, 84, 222–223
   overview of procedures for, 223–224
   parametric and nonparametric tests and, 224
   proof and, 84, 100–101, 248
   tests of statistical significance and, 223
   Type I and Type II errors and, 222, 245–246

I

ICMJE, 97
Ideational theory, 111
Identification (ID) number, 66
Identification, as research purpose, 10
Ideological perspectives, research with
   critical theory, 112, 171
   feminist research, 171–172
   participatory action research (PAR), 172
Implications of results, 251, 284
Implied consent, 65
Improvement science, 197
IMRAD format, 43
In-depth interview, 182, 185. *See also* Interview
In-person interview, 203. *See also* Interview
In Vitro measure, 154
In vivo codes, grounded theory, 266
In vivo measure, 154
Inclusion criteria, sampling and, 142
Incubation, qualitative interpretation and, 283
Independent groups *t*-test, 225, 232
Independent variable, 26. *See also* Dependent variable
   experimental research and, 30, 120
   hypotheses and, 82–83
   keywords and, 91
   nonexperimental research and, 127
   PICO framework and, 25–26
   quasi-experimental research and, 124, 135
   relationships and, 27
   research questions and, 79

Inductive reasoning, 24
   theory development and, 106
Inference, 50
   interpretation and, 242
   statistical, 84, 211, 221 (*See also* Inferential statistics)
   validity and, 51, 133–136
Inferential statistics. *See also* Statistic(s)
   analysis of variance, 225–226
   assumptions and, 219, 224
   bivariate, 224–229
   chi-squared test, 227
   confidence interval (CI), 221
   correlation coefficients, 227–228
   effect size indices, 228, 290, 294–295
   estimation of parameters, 221
   guide to tests, 228–229
   hypothesis testing and, 84 (*See also* Hypothesis testing)
   multivariate, 229–231
   probability and, 219, 224
   sampling distributions and, 219–220
   t-tests, 224–225
Informant, 24. *See also* Study participants; Subject(s)
   key, 165, 180–181, 187
Informed consent, 63, 64–65, 67
Initial coding, Charmaz, 268
Inquiry audit, 282
Insider research, 165
Institutional ethnography, 166
Institutional Review Board (IRB), 68
Institutionalized people, as a vulnerable group, 67
Instrument, 148–149, 152. *See also* Data collection; Measurement; Scale
   assessment of (*See* Data quality; Reliability; Validity)
   development, mixed methods research and, 193
   psychometric assessment, 155, 204, 231, 233, 252
   screening, 156
Integrative review, 89
Intensity effect size, 301
Interaction effect, 226, 322
Intercoder reliability, 277
Internal consistency, 157, 231
Internal validity, 134–135
   evidence hierarchies and, 318
   interpretation and, 241–242
   pragmatic clinical trials and, 321
   qualitative research and, 274–275
The International Committee of Medical Journal Editors (ICMJE), 97
International Council of Nurses (ICN), 60
Internet
   ethics and data collection, 63
   literature searches and, 91, 93–94
   open-access journals, 97
   questionnaires/interviews and, 149, 185
   surveys and, 203–204
Interobserver reliability, 157
Interpretation of results, 34. *See also* Results
   critical appraisal of, 253–254
   literature reviews and, 89 (*See also* Literature review)
   nonexperimental research and, 127–128, 246
   in qualitative research, 261, 265, 274–275
   in quantitative research, 242–246
   theory and, 106, 111–112

Interpretive description, 170
Interpretive phenomenology, 167, 264–265. *See also* Hermeneutics; Phenomenology
Interrater reliability, 157, 231, 280, 294
Interval estimation, 221
Interval measurement, 210
Intervention, 10–11, 118, 125–126. *See also* Intervention research
   complex, 201
   development of, 194, 201
   PICO framework and, 17, 119–121 (*See also* PICO framework)
   protocol for, 33, 123, 131
   theory-based, 106, 112, 201
Intervention fidelity, 131, 134
Intervention protocol, 33, 123, 131
Intervention research, 200–201. *See also* Intervention
   clinical trials and, 201
   comparative effectiveness research, 202, 319–320
   ethical constraints and, 127
   experimental research and, 120–123
   mixed methods research and, 194
   qualitative research and, 201
   quasi-experimental research and, 125–126
Intervention theory, 201
Interview. *See also* Self-report(s)
   face-to-face, 148–149, 203
   focus group, 184
   focused, 183
   in-depth, 182, 185
   personal (face-to-face), 148
   photo elicitation, 184
   questionnaire *vs.*, 149
   semi-structured, 185
   structured, 148–149
   telephone, 148–149, 203
   unstructured, 185
Interview schedule, 148
Intraclass correlation coefficient (ICC), 231
Introduction, research report, 43–44
Intuiting, 166–167
Inverse relationship, 217
Investigation, 24
Investigator, 24
Investigator triangulation, 280–281, 298
Iowa Model of Evidence-Based Practice, 313
IRB, 68
Item(s). *See also* Question(s); Scale
   content validity and, 156, 232
   internal consistency and, 157
   scales and, 149

J

Jargon, research, 7, 23, 46
Joanna Briggs Institute (JBI), 297, 301–302
Johns Hopkins Nursing Evidence-Based Practice Model, 313
Journal article, 42. *See also* Research report
   content of, 43–46
   critical appraisal of, 46–47
   style of, 46
   tips on reading, 46–47
Journal club, 3
Journal, reflexive, 166, 278
Justice, ethics and, 63

K

Kappa, Cohen's, 231
Key informant, 165, 180–181, 187
Keyword, 91–94
Knowledge-focused trigger, EBP and, 313
Knowledge, sources of, 4–5
Knowledge translation (KT), 311
Known-groups validity, 156, 232

L

Latent content, content analysis, 261
Lean approach, quality improvement, 198
Leininger's ethnonursing method, 165, 263
Level of evidence (LOE) scales, 15, 315
Level of measurement, 210–211
Level of significance, 44, 222
Levels of coding, grounded theory, 266
Likert scale, 150
Limitations
    constructivist approach and, 8, 9
    critical appraisals and, 253–254
    discussion section and, 46, 253–254
    EBP and, 4, 317
    scientific approach and, 7–9
Lincoln and Guba's trustworthiness framework, 275–276. *See also* Trustworthiness, qualitative research
Literature review, 32. *See also* Systematic review
    abstracting and recording notes for, 98
    appraising and analyzing evidence for, 98–99
    bibliographic databases, 91–96
    content of, 99
    critical appraisal of, 100
    documentation, 97–98
    electronic literature search, 91–92
    flow of tasks in, 90
    grounded theory and, 90
    locating sources for, 91–98
    meta-analysis (*See* Meta-analysis)
    metasynthesis (*See* Metasynthesis)
    preparing written review, 99–100
    problem statements and, 77
    purposes of, 89–90
    qualitative research and, 36
    research problem source, 74–75
    screening references for, 97
    search strategies for, 91–98
    steps and strategies for, 90–91
    style of, 99–100
    systematic review, 4, 289–304 (*See also* Systematic review)
    themes in, 98–99
    types of information to seek in, 90
Log, observational, 187
Logical reasoning, 24
Logistic regression, 231
Longitudinal design, 119, 130–131
    prospective *vs.*, 131
    qualitative studies and, 164

M

Macroethnography, 165
Macrotheory (grand theory), 106
Magnet Recognition Program, 2, 4
Main effect, ANOVA, 226
Manifest content, content analysis, 261

Manifest effect size, 301
Manipulation, experimental research and, 120. *See also* Experimental research
Manuscript, research report, 43, 47
Map, conceptual, 106, 111, 269
Mapping, electronic searches and, 92
Masking, 53
Matching, 132
Materialistic theory, 111
Matrix, correlation, 217
Maturation threat, 134–135
Maximum variation sampling, 179–181
Mean, 214
    confidence intervals and, 221
    standard error of, 221
    testing differences between groups, 224–225
Meaning, research purpose, 12, 78. *See also* Phenomenology
Meaning unit, content analysis, 261
Meaning/process questions, 12, 31, 79
Measure. *See also* Data collection; Instrument; Measurement; Scale
    biophysiologic (biomarkers), 148, 154
    observational, 155
    psychometric assessment of, 154, 204, 231, 233, 252
    self-report, 148–151
Measurement, 33. *See also* Data collection; Instrument; Measure
    change scores and, 251–252
    interval, 210
    levels of, 210–211
    nominal, 210
    operational definitions and, 27, 154
    ordinal, 210, 211
    problems of, 7
    ratio, 210–211
    reliability of instruments and, 155, 231 (*See also* Reliability)
    statistics for assessing, 231–232
    validity of instruments and, 156–157 (*See also* Validity)
Measurement error, 154
Measurement property, 154, 210, 231
Median, 213
Mediating variable, 52
Medical subject headings (MeSH), 94, 96, 299
MEDLINE database, 92–94, 96
Member check, 280
Memos, in qualitative research, 266
MeSH, 94, 96
Meta-aggregation, 15, 297, 301–302
Meta-analysis, 15. *See also* Systematic review
    advantages of, 290–291
    assessment of confidence- GRADE, 296–297, 316
    calculation of effects, 294–295
    criteria for undertaking, 291
    critical appraisal of, 303
    data analysis, 294
    data extraction and encoding, 294
    design of, 292–293
    metasynthesis *vs.*, 289–290
    power and, 291
    question formulation, 292
    sampling, 292–293
    search for evidence in, 293

Meta-analysis (*continued*)
  steps involved in, 292–297
  study quality in, 296
Meta-ethnography, 299–300
Meta-summary, 301
Metaphor, qualitative research and, 261
Metasynthesis, 15
  critical appraisal of, 304
  data analysis, 298–300
  definition, 298
  meta-analysis *vs.*, 289–290
  Noblit and Hare approach, 300
  problem formulation in, 298
  sampling in, 299
  Sandelowski and Barroso approach, 301
  search for evidence in, 299
  study quality in, 299
Method section, research reports, 44
Method triangulation, 279
Methodological study, 204
Methods, research, 6–9. *See also* Data collection; Measurement; Qualitative analysis; Quantitative analysis; Research design; Sampling
Middle-range theory, 106, 108–109
Minimal clinically important difference (MCID), 252
Minimal important change (MIC), 252
Minimal risk, 64
Mishel's Uncertainty in Illness Theory, 108
Mixed methods (MM) research, 9
  applications and purposes of, 193
  critical appraisal of, 204–205
  designs and strategies, 194–195
  notation for, 194
  rationale for, 193
  sampling and, 195–196
Mixed methods research synthesis, 290
Mixed research synthesis, 290
Mixed studies review, 15, 290
Mobile positioning, 187
Mode, 213
Model(s)
  conceptual, 107–110 (*See also* Conceptual model; Theory)
  of research utilization/EBP, 313
  schematic, 106
Moderator analysis, meta-analysis, 296
Moderator, focus group, 184
Mortality threat, 135
Multimodal distribution, 211
Multiple choice question, 148
Multiple comparison procedure, 226
Multiple positioning, 187
Multiple regression, 229–230
Multisite study, 24, 246
Multistage sampling, 145
Multivariate statistics, 229–231

N

Narrative analysis, 170
Narrative data, 27. *See also* Qualitative data
Narrative literature review. *See* Literature review
National Center for Nursing Research (NCNR), 3
National Institute of Nursing Research (NINR), 3, 63
National Institutes of Health (NIH), 3, 63
Naturalistic paradigm, 6. *See also* Constructivist paradigm

Naturalistic setting, 126, 164
Naysayers bias, 151
Negative case analysis, 281
Negative relationship, 217
Negative skew, 211
Nested sampling, mixed methods, 196
Netnography, 166
Network sampling, 178
Nightingale, Florence, 3, 210
NIH, 3, 63
NINR, 3, 63
NNT, 219, 251
Noblit and Hare meta-ethnographic approach, 299, 300
Nominal measurement, 210
Noncompliance bias, 246
Nondirectional hypothesis, 82
Nonequivalent control group design, 125–126
Nonexperimental research, 29–30
  advantages and disadvantages, 128–129
  correlational research, 127 (*See also* Correlational research)
  descriptive research, 127–128, 170–171
  qualitative research and, 163
Nonparametric test, 224
Nonprobability sampling, 143–144, 146. *See also* Sampling
Nonresponse bias, 147
Nonsignificant results, 223, 233, 235
  interpretation, 248–249
  systematic reviews and, 293
Normal distribution, 213
  sampling distributions and, 220
  standard deviations and, 214–215
Norms, 223
Notes, observational, 187
Null hypothesis, 84, 222, 223, 225–228, 233. *See also* Hypothesis testing
  interpretation and, 248
Number needed to treat (NNT), 219, 251
Nuremberg Code, 60
Nursing literature. *See* Literature review; Research report
Nursing practice
  conceptual models of, 108 (*See also* Conceptual model; Theoretical framework)
  evidence-based practice in, 2 (*See also* Evidence-based practice)
  as source of research problems, 74–75
Nursing research. *See also* Research
  clinical, 2
  conceptual models for, 107–110 (*See also* Conceptual model; Theory)
  consumers of, 17–18
  evidence-based practice and, 2, 4, 10–16 (*See also* Evidence-based practice)
  funding for, 4
  future directions for, 4
  history of, 45
  paradigms for, 6–9
  priorities for, 4
  purposes of, 153
  quantitative *vs.* qualitative, 6–8
  sources of evidence/knowledge and, 4–5
  utilization of, 3, 311, 313 (*See also* Research utilization)

Nursing sensitive outcome, 203
NVivo software, 259

O
Objective, research, 77
Objectivity
 blinding, 53, 131
 data collection and, 148
 hypothesis testing and, 221–222
 literature reviews and, 90, 99
 meta-analysis and, 290
 paradigms and, 6
 participant observation and, 187
 purpose statements and, 77
 qualitative research and, 276
 research reports and, 42, 46
Observation, data collection, 33
 bias and, 153
 categories and checklists, 152
 equipment for, 152
 ethical issues and, 63
 evaluation of method, 153
 participant, 165, 186–187 (*See also* Participant observation)
 persistent, 278
 qualitative research and, 186–187
 quantitative research and, 151–153
 sampling and, 154
Observational (nonexperimental) research, 30, 127–128. *See also* Nonexperimental research
Observational notes, 187
Observer, 152
 bias, 153
 interobserver reliability, 157
Odds, 230
Odds ratio (OR), 219, 228, 230
 meta-analysis and, 294
One-group pretest–posttest design, 126, 135
Online ethnography, 166
Open-access journal, 97
Open AI, 259
Open coding, 266–267
Open-ended question, 148
Operational definition, 27. *See also* Measurement
Operationalization, 27. *See also* Measurement
Ordinal measurement, 210, 211
Outcome (variable)
 dependent variable, 25–26 (*See also* Dependent variable)
 experimental research and, 120–122
 hypotheses and, 81
 nursing sensitive, 203
 PICO framework and, 17, 25–26 (*See also* PICO framework)
 research questions and, 79
Outcomes research, 202–203

P
Paired *t*-test, 225
Paradigm, 9
 constructivist, 6–8
 grounded theory and, 267
 mixed methods and, 193
 positivist, 6–8
 research methods and, 6–8
 research problem and, 74

Paradigm case, Benner and, 265
Parallel perspective, 275
Parameter, 211
 estimation of, 221
Parametric test, 224
PARIHS EBP model, 313
Parse's Humanbecoming Paradigm, 106
Participant. *See* Study participants
Participant observation, 165, 186–187
Participatory action research (PAR), 172, 184
Passive voice, research reports and, 46
Patient-centered outcomes research, 202
Patient centeredness, 4, 319
Patient preferences, EBP and, 14
Patient-reported outcome (PRO), 148, 320. *See also* Self-report(s)
Pattern of association, qualitative research, 29, 164
 ethnographic analysis and, 263
PCORI, Patient-Centered Outcomes Research Institute, 202
PDSA (Plan-Do-Study-Act), 198–199
Pearson's *r*, 217, 228. *See also* Correlation
 effect size index, 295
 effect size indices, 228
 measurement statistics and, 231–232
Peer debriefing, 281
Peer reviewer, 42–43, 47
Pender's Health Promotion Model (HPM), 108
Percentage, 211, 215, 227
Perfect relationship, 216
Persistent observation, 278
Person triangulation, 279
Personal (face-to-face) interview, 148–149, 203. *See also* Interview; Self-report(s)
Personalized health care, 319, 322–323
Phenomenology, 31, 166–167
 artistic expressions and, 167, 181, 264
 data analysis and, 264–265
 descriptive, 166–167
 Duquesne school, 264
 hermeneutics and, 167, 265
 interpretive, 167, 264
 literature reviews and, 90
 purpose statements and, 78
 research questions and, 78
 sampling and, 181
 theory and, 111
 Utrecht school, 264–265
Phenomenon, 6, 24
Photo elicitation, 184
Photographs, as data, 184, 187
Photovoice, 184
Physiologic measure, 153–154
PICO framework, 16, 315
 comparator and, 16
 dependent variable and, 25–26
 effect size indices and, 228
 experimental design and, 120
 hypotheses and, 81
 independent variable and, 26
 intervention and, 16, 119–121
 keywords for a search and, 315
 meta-analysis and, 292
 nonexperimental/observational design and, 127–128
 outcome variable and, 16, 26

PICO framework (*continued*)
   population and, 16, 142
   purpose statement and, 77
   quasi-experimental design and, 124
   research question and, 76, 84–85
Pilot study (test), 200–201, 228
Placebo, 53, 123
Plan-Do-Check-Act model, 198–199
Plan-Do-Study-Act (PDSA) model, 198–199
Point estimation, 221
Population, 33, 142, 145–147. *See also* Sampling
   estimation of values for, 221 (*See also* Inferential statistics)
   parameters and, 221
   PICO framework and, 16, 142 (*See also* PICO framework)
   target *vs.* accessible, 142
Positionality statement, 278
Positive relationship, 216
Positive skew, 211
Positivist paradigm, 6–7
Post hoc test, 226
Poster session, 43
Postpositivist paradigm, 6
Posttest data, 120–121
Posttest-only design, 121
Power
   meta-analysis and, 291
   statistical conclusion validity and, 133–134, 146, 245
   Type II errors and, 222, 228, 245, 321
Power analysis, 223
   sample size and, 146, 223
Practice-based evidence, 16, 310, 317, 319, 324
Practice guidelines, clinical, 311–312
Pragmatic clinical trial, 320–321
Pragmatism paradigm, 193
Pre-appraised evidence, EBP and, 14
PRECIS-2, 320
Precision
   confidence intervals and, 221 (*See also* Confidence interval)
   interpretation of results, 241–242
Precision health care, 319, 322–323
Predatory journals, 97
Prediction
   hypotheses and, 80–81
   multiple regression and, 229–230
   as research purpose, 10
   theory and, 25, 105–106
Predictive validity, 156
Predictor variable, 230
Pregnant women, as a vulnerable group, 67
Pretest
   baseline measure and, 121, 125
   trial run of an instrument, 149
Pretest–posttest design, 121, 125, 135
Primary qualitative validity, 276
Primary source, 90
Primary study, 14, 289, 292–295, 297–301
Priorities for nursing research, 4
Priority, mixed methods designs and, 194
PRISMA guidelines, 297
Privacy, study participants and, 64. *See also* Confidentiality
Probabilistic evidence, 6, 119, 248

Probability, 6, 11
   laws of, 219
Probability level. *See* Level of significance
Probability sampling, 144–145. *See also* Sampling
Probing, 278, 280
Problem-focused trigger, EBP and, 313
Problem statement, 76–77, 90. *See also* Hypothesis; Research problem
Process analysis, 200
Process consent, 65
Prochaska's Transtheoretical Model, 109
Producers of nursing research, 3
Product–moment correlation coefficient (r), 217. *See also* Correlation; Pearson's r
Professional conference, 43
Prognosis questions, 11, 79
   research design and, 29, 119, 126–127
Program of research, 7
Prolonged engagement, 278
Proof, hypothesis testing and, 84, 100–101, 248
Proportions
   chi-squared test and, 227
   risk indexes and, 218
Proposal, 34
Proprietary AI, 259
Prospective design, 127
   longitudinal design *vs.*, 130–131
PROSPERO, 293
Protocol
   intervention, 33, 123, 131
   systematic review, 293
Psychometric assessment, 154, 233
Psychometrics, 154
Psychosocial scale, 149. *See also* Scale
Publication bias, 293
PubMed, 93–97
Purpose, statement of, 77–78
Purposes of research, 153
Purposive (purposeful) sampling, 144, 179
P value, 45, 225, 228, 233. *See also* Statistical significance

Q

Q sort, 151
Qualitative analysis, 35, 257–258. *See also* Qualitative research
   analytic overview, 260–261
   analytic procedures, 260–269
   computers and, 259
   content analysis, 170, 261–262
   critical appraisal of, 269
   data management and organization, 258–260
   ethnographic analysis, 263
   grounded theory analysis, 265–268
   literature reviews and, 90, 97–98
   phenomenologic analysis, 264–265
   thematic analysis, 170, 261–262
   trustworthiness and, 37, 280–282
Qualitative content analysis, 170, 261–262
Qualitative data, 27. *See also* Qualitative analysis; Unstructured (qualitative) data collection
   analysis of (*See* Qualitative analysis)
   coding of, 258–259
   methods of data collection, 35, 182–188
   mixed methods research and, 197
   organization of, 259–260

quality enhancement and, 278–280 (*See also* Trustworthiness, qualitative research)
secondary analysis, 204
Qualitative descriptive research, 30, 170–171
Qualitative evidence syntheses (QES), 290, 298, 302
Qualitative research, 9. *See also* Qualitative analysis; Qualitative data
  activities in, 35–37
  analysis and, 257–269 (*See also* Qualitative analysis)
  case studies, 169
  causality in, 29, 164
  credibility of results, 282–283
  critical appraisal of, 172–173
  critical research and, 171
  data collection and, 35, 182–188 (*See also* Unstructured [qualitative] data collection)
  descriptive, 30, 170–171
  disciplinary traditions and, 30–31, 164–169
  ethical issues and, 70
  ethnography and, 31, 265–268 (*See also* Ethnography)
  frameworks for, 275–276
  grounded theory and, 30, 168–169, 265–268 (*See also* Grounded theory)
  historical research, 170
  hypotheses and, 193, 281
  ideological perspectives and, 171–172
  interpretation of findings, 283–284
  literature reviews and, 36, 89–90
  metasynthesis, 15
  mixed methods and, 192–196 (*See also* Mixed methods [MM] research)
  narrative analysis, 170
  paradigms and, 8
  phenomenology and, 31, 166–167 (*See also* Phenomenology)
  problem statement, 77
  purpose statement, 78
  quality and integrity in, 284–285 (*See also* Trustworthiness, qualitative research)
  research design and, 36, 162–173 (*See also* Research design, qualitative studies)
  research problems and, 36, 74
  research questions and, 79–80
  sampling and, 36, 177–182
  systematic reviews and, 297–303
  theory and, 24, 110–112 (*See also* Theory)
  triangulation in, 51, 163, 188, 279
  trustworthiness and, 51, 274–287
Quality Health Outcomes Model, 203
Quality improvement (QI), 4, 197
  approaches and models, 198–199
  features of, 197
  planning tools for, 197–198
Quality, in qualitative research, 274–275. *See also* Trustworthiness, qualitative research
Quantitative analysis, 32, 44. *See also* Hypothesis testing; Statistical test; Statistic(s)
  credibility of results, 242–246
  critical appraisal of, 235–236
  descriptive statistics, 211–219 (*See also* Descriptive statistics)
  inferential statistics, 219–224 (*See also* Inferential statistics)
  interpretation of results, 34, 241–242
  measurement levels and, 210–211
  measurement statistics and, 231–232
  multivariate statistics, 229–231
Quantitative data, 27. *See also* Measurement
  analysis of, 34 (*See also* Quantitative analysis; Statistic[s])
  assessment of data quality, 154–157
  measurement and, 154 (*See also* Measurement)
  methods of data collection, 34, 148–151
  secondary analysis, 204
Quantitative research. *See also* Quantitative analysis
  data collection and, 34, 148–151 (*See also* Structured data collection)
  experimental *vs.* nonexperimental, 29–30, 120–129
  hypotheses and, 33, 80–84 (*See also* Hypothesis)
  meta-analysis and, 15, 290–297
  mixed methods research and, 192–196 (*See also* Mixed methods [MM] research)
  paradigms and, 6–7
  research designs and, 36, 117–137 (*See also* Research design, quantitative studies)
  research problems and, 31, 74
  research questions and, 31, 79
  sampling in, 33, 142–147
  scientific method and, 6–7
  statement of purpose and, 77
  steps in, 31–35
  theory and, 24, 112 (*See also* Theory)
Quasi-experiment, 125–126
  advantages and disadvantages, 126
  evidence hierarchy and, 15, 120
  internal validity and, 135
  quality improvement and, 199
Question(s), 148. *See also* Item(s); Scale
  clinical, 16
  closed-ended *vs.* open-ended, 148–149
  grand tour, 183
  participant observers', 187
  PICO, 16 (*See also* PICO framework)
  research, 74, 78–80
  types of, structured, 148–149
  wording of, 148–149
Questionnaire, 148. *See also* Self-report(s)
  anonymity and, 149
  implied consent and, 65
  Internet, 149, 203–204
  interviews *vs.*, 149
  scales and, 149–151
  surveys and, 203–204
Quota sampling, 143–145

R

Random assignment/allocation, 5. *See also* Randomization
  random sampling *vs.*, 121, 144–145
Random effects model, 295
Random sampling (selection), 53, 145. *See also* Probability sampling
  random assignment *vs.*, 121, 144
Randomization, 120
  constraints on, 125, 128
  experimental designs and, 121–123
  internal validity and, 132
  quasi-experimental design and, 125–126
  research control and, 132

Randomized controlled trial (RCT), 120–122, 199,
        200, 202. *See also* Clinical trial; Experimental
        research; Intervention research
    evidence hierarchies and, 15, 118, 124
    flowchart for, 244
    meta-analysis and, 289, 297
    sampling problems and, 318
Randomness, 53
Range, 214
Rapid cycles, quality improvement, 198–199
Rapid review, 290
Rating question, 148
Rating scale, 152
Ratio measurement, 210–211
Raw data, 45
RCT. *See* Randomized controlled trial
Reactivity, 153
Readability, 34, 149
Realist evaluation, 201
Reasoning. *See* Logical reasoning
Recall bias, 246
Receiver operating characteristic (ROC) curve, 232
Records, as data sources, 148, 181
References
    in research report, 46, 90, 99
    screening and organizing for literature review, 99
Reflective notes, observations and, 187
Reflexive journal, 166, 278
Reflexivity, 54, 278
Registered Nurses' Association of Ontario (RNAO), 312
Relationship
    associative, 29
    causal (cause-and-effect), 28–29, 119 (*See also*
        Causal [cause-and-effect] relationship)
    correlation and, 127 (*See also* Correlation)
    hypotheses and, 33, 80–84
    independent variables and, 28
    interpreting, 246–250
    negative, 217
    outcome variables and, 28
    perfect, 216
    positive, 216
    qualitative analysis and, 260
    research questions and, 78
    statistical analysis of, 33, 221–222
    theories and models and, 106–107
Relative risk (RR), 219, 295
Relevance, patient centeredness and, 319
Reliability, 50–51, 54
    dependability and, qualitative research, 276, 279
    internal consistency, 155, 231
    interrater/interobserver, 155, 157, 231, 280
    test–retest, 155, 231
Reliability coefficient, 155
Repeated measures ANOVA, 226
Replication
    causal inferences and, 129
    credibility of results and, 242–246
    external validity and, 135
    reliability and, 155
Report. *See* Research report
Representative sample, 143
Representativeness, 143
Research
    cause-probing, 10, 12, 118, 126–127, 133
    challenges in, 50–54

clinical, 2
comparative effectiveness, 124, 202, 319–320
correlational, 127
critical appraisal of (*See* Critical appraisal of research)
critical theory and, 171
descriptive, 128, 170–171
evidence-based practice and, 2, 10–13
    (*See also* Evidence-based practice)
experimental, 29–30, 120–123
    (*See also* Experimental research)
health services, 202–203
historical, 170
intervention, 200–201 (*See also* Intervention
    research)
knowledge source and, 5
mixed methods (MM), 51, 192–196 (*See also* Mixed
    methods research)
new directions in, 319–323
nonexperimental, 29–30, 127–128
    (*See also* Nonexperimental research)
observational (nonexperimental), 29–30, 127–128
outcomes, 202–203
purposes of, 10–13
qualitative, 8–9, 162–173 (*See also* Qualitative
    research)
quantitative, 6–7, 10 (*See also* Quantitative research)
quasi-experimental, 125–126 (*See also*
    Quasi-experiment)
survey, 203–204
terminology, 23–29
theory and, 25, 105–110
Research critique. *See* Critical appraisal of research
Research design, 33, 117–137. *See also* Research
    design, qualitative studies; Research design,
    quantitative studies
Research design, mixed methods studies, 194–195. *See
    also* Mixed methods (MM) research
Research design, qualitative studies, 36, 173. *See also*
    Qualitative research
    causality and, 164
    characteristics of, 163
    critical appraisal of, 172–173
    disciplinary traditions and, 164–169
    ethnography, 164–166
    features of, 163–164
    grounded theory, 168–169
    ideological perspectives and, 171–172
    mixed methods and, 194–195
    phenomenology, 166–167
Research design, quantitative studies, 33
    causality and, 119–120
    characteristics of good design, 133
    construct validity and, 136
    controls for external confounding factors, 131
    controls for intrinsic confounding factors, 131–133
    critical appraisal of, 136–137
    ethics and, 123–124, 127
    evidence hierarchy and, 15, 120
    experimental design, 29–30, 120–123
    external validity and, 135–136
    internal validity and, 134–135
    key features, 118–119
    longitudinal *vs.* cross-sectional, 130–131
    mixed methods and, 194–195
    nonexperimental/observational research, 29–30,
        127–128

quasi-experimental design, 125–126, 135
statistical conclusion validity and, 133–134
Research Ethics Board, 68
Research findings, 43–46, 233. *See also* Interpretation of results; Results
Research Gate, 97
Research hypothesis, 80–84, 219, 221, 242, 248, 249. *See also* Hypothesis
Research methods, 6–9, 33. *See also* Data collection; Measurement; Qualitative analysis; Quantitative analysis; Research design; Sampling
Research, nursing. *See* Nursing research
Research problem
  communication of, 76
  critical appraisal of, 84–85
  development and refinement of, 75
  paradigms and, 74
  qualitative studies and, 36, 74
  quantitative studies and, 33, 74
  significance of, 84–85
  sources of, 74–75
  terms relating to, 74
Research program, 75
Research question, 33, 74, 78–80. *See also* Research problem
  research design and, 119–120
Research report. *See also* Dissemination of research results
  abstracts in, 43
  content of, 43–46
  critical appraisal of, 47 (*See also* Critical appraisal of research)
  discussion section in, 45–46, 254
  IMRAD format, 43
  introduction in, 43–44
  journal article, 43–47
  locating, 91–98
  method section in, 44
  qualitative studies and, 37
  quantitative studies and, 36
  references in, 46
  results section in, 44–45, 241
  style of, 46
  tips on reading, 46–47
  tips on reading statistical information, 233
  titles of, 43
  types of, 42–43
Research review. *See* Literature review; Systematic review
Research setting, 24, 135, 164. *See also* Setting, research
Research utilization, 311, 313. *See also* Evidence-based practice
Researcher, 25
Researcher credibility, 282–283
Respondent, 148–149. *See also* Study participants
Responder analysis, 253
Response bias, 147
Response option, 148
Response rate
  nonresponse bias and, 147
  questionnaires *vs.* interviews, 149
Response set bias, 151
Results
  credibility of, 242–246, 282

dissemination of, 35 (*See also* Dissemination of research results; Research report)
evidence-based practice and, 13 (*See also* Evidence-based practice)
generalizability of, 7, 54, 250 (*See also* Generalizability)
hypothesized, 246
interpretation of, 34, 241–254 (*See also* Interpretation of results)
nonsignificant, 223, 233, 235, 248–249
positive, 247
qualitative, 261, 264
statistical, 44–45, 241
transferability and, 54, 275, 284 (*See also* Transferability)
unhypothesized, 249–250
Results section, research report, 44–45, 241
Retrospective design, 127
Review. *See also* Critical appraisal of research
  blind, 43
  ethical issues and, 67–68
  integrative, 89
  literature, 32, 36, 89–100 (*See also* Literature review)
  narrative, 290–291
  peer, 42–43, 47, 281–282
  rapid, 290
  scoping, 292
  systematic, 4, 289–304 (*See also* Systematic review)
  umbrella, 290
Rho, Spearman's, 217
Rights, human subjects, 61–64. *See also* Ethics, research
Rigor
  qualitative research and, 274 (*See also* Trustworthiness, qualitative research)
  quantitative research and, 245 (*See also* Reliability; Validity)
Risk
  absolute (AR), 217–218
  indexes of, 218
  minimal, 64
  relative (RR), 219
Risk of bias assessment, Cochrane reviews, 293–294
Risk/benefit assessment, 64
Risk/benefit ratio, 64
Rival hypothesis, 126
RM-ANOVA, 226
ROC curve, 232
Rogers' Diffusion of Innovations Model, 313
Root cause analysis (RCA), 194–198
Roy's Adaptation Model, 108

S

Sample, 33. *See also* Sample size; Sampling
  representativeness of, 143
Sample size
  meta-analysis and, 294
  metasynthesis and, 299
  power analysis and, 146, 220
  qualitative studies, 180
  quantitative studies, 146
  standard errors and, 221
  statistical conclusion validity, 134–135, 146, 245
  statistical power and, 133–134
  Type II errors and, 228, 322

Sampling
    basic concepts, 142–143
    bias and, 143, 145
    consecutive, 144
    construct validity and, 245
    convenience, 143, 146, 178
    criterion, 179
    critical appraisal of, 146–147
    ethnography and, 180–181
    external validity and, 135–136, 245
    extreme/deviant case, 179
    grounded theory studies and, 181–182
    inference and, 242
    maximum variation, 179–181
    meta-analysis and, 292–293
    metasynthesis and, 299
    mixed methods research, 195–196
    multistage, 145
    nested, 196
    network, 178
    nonprobability, 143–144
    observational, 153
    phenomenological studies and, 181
    probability, 144–145
    purposive, 144, 179
    qualitative research and, 36, 177–182
    quantitative research and, 33, 142–147
    quota, 143–144
    random, 144–145
    RCTs and, 318
    sample size and, 146, 180 (*See also* Sample size)
    simple random, 145
    snowball, 178
    strata and, 143
    stratified random, 145
    systematic, 145
    theoretical, 179–180, 181
    typical case, 179
    volunteer, 178
Sampling bias, 143, 145
Sampling distribution, 219–220, 223
Sampling error, 145, 220
Sampling frame, 144–145
Sampling plan, 33, 143, 145, 146–147, 182. *See also* Sampling
    critical appraisal of, 146–147, 182
Sandelowski and Barroso metasynthesis approach, 301
Saturation, data, 35, 180
Scale. *See also* Psychometric assessment
    internal consistency and, 155, 231
    Likert, 150
    rating, observational, 153
    response set bias and, 151
    summated rating, 149–151
    visual analog, 151
Schematic model, 106
Scientific merit, 47
Scientific method, 6–7. *See also* Quantitative research
Scientific research. *See* Research
Scientist. *See* Researcher
Scoping review, 292
Scopus, 92
Score(s)
    change, 251–252
    scales and, 149–151
Screening instrument, 156

Search, electronic literature, 91–97
Search engine, Internet, 91
Secondary analysis, 204
Secondary qualitative analysis, 268
Secondary qualitative validity, 276
Secondary source, 90
Selection, random, 53, 144–145. *See also* Sampling
Selection threat (self-selection), 134
Selective approach, phenomenological analysis, 265
Selective coding, grounded theory, 266
Self-administered questionnaire, 149. *See also* Questionnaire
Self-determination, right to, 62
Self-efficacy theory, 108, 112
Self-report(s), 183–185. *See also* Interview; Questionnaire; Scale
    evaluation of method, 153
    interviews, 149, 183–184
    Q sorts, 151
    qualitative methods and, 183–184
    quantitative methods and, 148–151
    questionnaires *vs.* interviews, 149
    response set bias, 151
    scales, 149–151
    structured, 148–149
    survey research and, 203
    types of question, 148–149
    unstructured and semi-structured, 183
    vignettes, 151
Self-selection (selection threat), 128, 134
Semi-structured interview, 183
Sensitivity analysis, 296
Sensitivity, criterion validity and, 232
Sequential design, mixed methods, 194
Setting, research, 24
    qualitative research and, 164
    quantitative research and, 135
Sigma Theta Tau, 4
Significance, clinical, 4, 34, 251–253. *See also* Clinical significance
Significance of research problems, 84–85
Significance, statistical, 44–45
    clinical significance *vs.*, 250–253
    interpretation and, 241–242
    tests of, 223 (*See also* Statistical test)
Simple hypothesis, 82
Simple random sampling, 144
Single positioning, 187
Site, 24
6S hierarchy, evidence sources, 118
Skewed distribution, 211
Snowball sampling, 178
Social Cognitive Theory (Bandura), 109
Social desirability response set bias, 151
Space triangulation, 279
Spearman's rho, 217
Specificity, criterion validity and, 232
Spradley's ethnographic method, 263
Stages of change, 109
Stakeholder, 201, 311, 319
Standard deviation (SD), 214–215
    minimal important change and, 252–253
Standard error, 221
Standard error of the mean (SEM), 220
Standardized mean difference (SMD), 295
Statement of purpose, 74, 77–78

Statistic(s), 44, 211
    bivariate descriptive, 216–217
    critical appraisal of, 235–236
    descriptive, 211–219 (*See also* Descriptive statistics)
    inferential, 219–224 (*See also* Inferential statistics)
    measurement and, 231–232
    multivariate, 229–231
    parametric *vs.* nonparametric, 224
    tips on understanding, 233–235
Statistical analysis, 34, 44, 209–239. *See also*
        Quantitative analysis; Statistical test; Statistic(s)
Statistical conclusion validity, 133–134, 146, 245
Statistical control, 133
Statistical heterogeneity, meta-analysis, 293, 295–296
Statistical inference, 84, 221, 222, 233–235. *See also*
        Inferential statistics
Statistical power, 133–134. *See also* Power
Statistical significance, 44–45, 223
    clinical significance *vs.*, 250–253
    interpretation and, 241–242
    level of, 44–45, 222–223
    tests of (*See* Statistical test)
Statistical tables, 233–235
Statistical test, 44–45, 222, 223, 228–229. *See also*
        Inferential statistics; *specific tests*
    guide to bivariate tests, 228–229
    Type I and Type II errors, 222, 245–246, 321
Stepped wedge design, 321
Stetler model of research utilization, 313
Stipend, 62
Stories, narrative analysis and, 170
Strands, mixed methods research, 194
Strata, 143
Stratified health care, 322
Stratified random sampling, 145
Strauss and Corbin, grounded theory, 168
Structured (quantitative) data collection, 34. *See also*
        Data collection; Measurement
    biophysiologic measures (biomarkers), 148, 153–154
    observations and, 151–153 (*See also* Observation,
        data collection)
    self-reports, 148–151 (*See also* Self-report[s])
Study, 24. *See also* Research
Study participants, 24–25
    controlling intrinsic factors and, 131–133
    rights of, 61–64
Style. *See* Writing style
Subgroup analysis, 321–322
    meta-analysis and, 296
Subject(s), 24. *See also* Study participants
Subject heading, literature search, 92, 94
    MeSH, 94, 96, 299
Subject search, literature review, 92
Subjectivity, paradigms and, 8. *See also* Objectivity
Subscale, 150
Substantive codes, 266
Substantive theory, 111–112
Summated rating scale, 150–151
Survey research, 203–204. *See also* Self-report(s)
Symbolic interactionism, 111, 168
Symmetric distribution, 211
Systematic bias, 52
Systematic review, 4, 15
    aggregative *vs.* interpretive, 297
    clinical practice guidelines and, 312
    critical appraisal of, 303–304
    evidence-based practice and, 15
    meta-analyses, 15, 290–297 (*See also* Meta-analysis)
    meta-summary, 301
    meta-syntheses, 15
    metasyntheses, 290, 297–303 (*See also*
        Metasynthesis)
    mixed studies review, 15
    reports for, 303
Systematic sampling, 145

T
Table(s)
    crosstabs, 216, 227
    statistical, tips on reading, 233–235
Tacit knowledge, 165
Target population, 142, 147
Taxonomic analysis, 263
Taxonomy, 263
Telephone interview, 149, 203
Temporal ambiguity, internal validity and, 134
Terminally ill patients as a vulnerable group, 67
Test statistic, 223. *See also* Statistic(s)
Test–retest reliability, 155, 231
Textword search, 92
Thematic analysis, 170, 261–262
Theme, 36, 260
    analysis, ethnographic, 263
    cultural, 263
    in literature reviews, 98–99
    phenomenology and, 166, 265
    in qualitative analysis, 261
Theoretical code, grounded theory, 266
Theoretical distribution, 223–224
Theoretical framework, 32, 107. *See also* Conceptual
        model; Theory
Theoretical sampling, 179–180, 181
Theory, 113. *See also* Conceptual model; *specific theories*
    critical, 112, 171 (*See also* Critical theory)
    critical appraisal of, 113
    descriptive, 106
    ethnography and, 110
    grounded, 30, 111–112, 168–169 (*See also*
        Grounded theory)
    hypotheses and, 80–81, 105–107, 112–113
    interventions and, 108, 201
    middle-range, 106, 108–109
    nursing and, 108–109
    phenomenology and, 110
    qualitative research and, 24, 35, 110–112
    quantitative research and, 24, 32, 112
    research and, 108, 110–112
    as source of research problems, 74–75
    substantive, 111–112
    testing, 106, 107, 112
Theory of Planned Behavior (Ajzen), 110
Theory of Reasoned Action, 110
Theory triangulation, 279
Therapy/intervention questions, 10–11, 15, 79
    meta-analysis and, 289
    research design and, 29, 119, 124 (*See also*
        Experimental research)
Thick description, 182, 282, 284–285
    trustworthiness and, 276
Think-aloud method, 184
Threat to validity
    internal validity, 134–135

Time sampling, 153
Time-series design, 126, 134
  quality improvement and, 199
Time triangulation, 279
Title, research report, 43
Tool. *See* Instrument
Topic guide, 184
Topic, research, 73–74, 76. *See also* Research problem
Toyota Production System, quality improvement, 198
Tradition, knowledge source, 5
Traditions, disciplinary, qualitative research and, 30–31, 164–169
Transcriptions, interviews, 185, 279
Transferability, 54
  literature themes, 98
  qualitative findings and, 182, 284
  trustworthiness and, 276, 282
Translational science, 118
Transtheoretical Model (Prochaska), 109
Treatment, 10–11. *See also* Experimental research; Intervention
Trial and error, knowledge source, 5
Trials without randomization, 125
Triangulation, 52, 163
  corroborating evidence and, 246
  data, 279
  of data collection methods, 51, 188, 279
  investigator, 280–281, 298
  method, 279
  mixed methods research, 51, 197
Truncation symbol, 92
Trustworthiness, qualitative research, 37, 51, 275
  critical appraisal of, 284–285
  interpretation of findings, 283–284
  Lincoln and Guba's framework, 275–276
  strategies for enhancing, 276–283
t-Test, 224–225
Tuskegee syphilis study, 60
Type I error, 222, 248
  subgroup analysis and, 321
Type II error, 222, 228, 245, 248–249
  subgroup analysis and, 321
Typical case sampling, 179

U

Umbrella review, 290
Uncertainty in Illness Theory (Mishel), 108
Unhypothesized significant results, interpretation, 249–250
Unimodal distribution, 211
Univariate descriptive statistics, 216
Unstructured (qualitative) data collection, 35
  critical appraisal of, 188
  evaluation of, 185
  observation and, 186–187
  self-reports and, 183–185
  triangulation and, 163, 188, 279
Unstructured interview, 183

Unstructured observation, 186–187. *See also* Participant observation
Utilization. *See* Research utilization
Utrecht school of phenomenology, 264

V

Validity
  adulatory, 280
  concurrent, 156
  construct, 136, 156, 201, 232, 245
  content, 156, 232
  credibility and, 245–246
  criterion, 156, 232
  cross-cultural, 156–157
  external, 135–136, 200, 245, 276, 318
  face, 156
  inference and, 51, 135, 242
  internal, 134–135, 199, 245
  known groups, 156, 232
  measurement and, 156–157, 231–232
  mixed methods research and, 193
  predictive, 156
  qualitative research and, 274–275
  statistical conclusion, 133, 146, 245
Van Kaam's phenomenological method, 264
Van Manen's phenomenological method, 264
Variability, 214–216
  control over (*See* Control, research)
Variable(s), 24
  conceptual definition of, 27, 33
  confounding, 52, 118 (*See also* Confounding variable)
  continuous, 210
  core, 30, 168, 266
  dependent, 25–26 (*See also* Dependent variable)
  extraneous, 52
  independent, 25–26 (*See also* Independent variable)
  mediating, 52
  operational definitions of, 27
  outcome, 25–26 (*See also* Outcome [variable])
  predictor, 230
Variance, analysis of, 225–226
Vignette, 151
Visual analog scale, 151
Volunteer sample, 178
Vulnerable group, 67

W

Wait-listed control group design, 123
Web of Knowledge, 92
Web of Science, 92
Whittemore, quality criteria framework, 275
Writing style
  journal articles, 46
  literature reviews, 99–100

Y

Yea-sayer bias, 151